Cognitive Informatics in Biomedicine and Healthcare

Series Editor

Vimla L. Patel, Center for Cognitive Studies in Medicine and Public Health, New York Academy of Medicine, New York, NY, USA

Enormous advances in information technology have permeated essentially all facets of life. Although these technologies are transforming the workplace as well as leisure time, formidable challenges remain in fostering tools that enhance productivity, are sensitive to work practices, and are intuitive to learn and to use effectively. Informatics is a discipline concerned with applied and basic science of information, the practices involved in information processing, and the engineering of information systems.

Cognitive Informatics (CI), a term that has been adopted and applied particularly in the fields of biomedicine and health care, is the multidisciplinary study of cognition, information and computational sciences. It investigates all facets of computer applications in biomedicine and health care, including system design and computer-mediated intelligent action. The basic scientific discipline of CI is strongly grounded in methods and theories derived from cognitive science. The discipline provides a framework for the analysis and modeling of complex human performance in technology-mediated settings and contributes to the design and development of better information systems for biomedicine and health care.

Despite the significant growth of this discipline, there have been few systematic published volumes for reference or instruction intended for working professionals, scientists or graduate students in cognitive science and biomedical informatics, beyond those published in this series. Although information technologies are now in widespread use globally for promoting increased self-reliance in patients, there is often a disparity between the scientific and technological knowledge underlying healthcare practices and the lay beliefs, mental models, and cognitive representations of illness and disease. The topics covered in this book series address the key research gaps in biomedical informatics related to the applicability of theories, models, and evaluation frameworks of HCI and human factors as they apply to clinicians as well as to the lay public.

Andre W. Kushniruk • David R. Kaufman
Thomas G. Kannampallil • Vimla L. Patel
Editors

Human Computer Interaction in Healthcare

The Role of Cognition

Second Edition

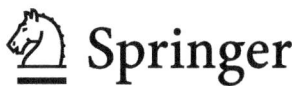

Editors
Andre W. Kushniruk
School of Health Information Science
University of Victoria
Victoria, BC, Canada

Thomas G. Kannampallil
Department of Anesthesiology
Washington University School of Medicine
St Louis, MO, USA

David R. Kaufman
Health Informatics Program, School of Health Professions
SUNY Downstate Health Sciences University
New York, NY, USA

Vimla L. Patel
Center for Cognitive Studies in Medicine and Public Health
New York Academy of Medicine
New York, NY, USA

ISSN 2662-7280 ISSN 2662-7299 (electronic)
Cognitive Informatics in Biomedicine and Healthcare
ISBN 978-3-031-69946-7 ISBN 978-3-031-69947-4 (eBook)
https://doi.org/10.1007/978-3-031-69947-4

© The Editor(s) (if applicable) and The Author(s), under exclusive license to Springer Nature Switzerland AG 2015, 2024

This work is subject to copyright. All rights are solely and exclusively licensed by the Publisher, whether the whole or part of the material is concerned, specifically the rights of translation, reprinting, reuse of illustrations, recitation, broadcasting, reproduction on microfilms or in any other physical way, and transmission or information storage and retrieval, electronic adaptation, computer software, or by similar or dissimilar methodology now known or hereafter developed.

The use of general descriptive names, registered names, trademarks, service marks, etc. in this publication does not imply, even in the absence of a specific statement, that such names are exempt from the relevant protective laws and regulations and therefore free for general use.

The publisher, the authors and the editors are safe to assume that the advice and information in this book are believed to be true and accurate at the date of publication. Neither the publisher nor the authors or the editors give a warranty, expressed or implied, with respect to the material contained herein or for any errors or omissions that may have been made. The publisher remains neutral with regard to jurisdictional claims in published maps and institutional affiliations.

This Springer imprint is published by the registered company Springer Nature Switzerland AG
The registered company address is: Gewerbestrasse 11, 6330 Cham, Switzerland

If disposing of this product, please recycle the paper.

William (Bill) J Clancey

His prescient use of cognitive models to enhance our understanding of human cognition and to develop better tools for student learning in medicine have greatly influenced our research on medical cognition.

James (Jim) J Cimino

His keen insight into the importance of the user experience, and his efforts to promote cognitive research in clinical practice, have affected the way clinical systems are perceived and used.

Foreword

When I was first introduced to computing (in university, not on my parents' laps the way it happens today), the notion of interface design was pretty much irrelevant. Initially (1966), I wrote my programs on paper and then translated them onto punch cards that were run through mainframe computers in batch mode. A direct human interface with the computer did not actually occur. Within a few years, I was able to type code into minicomputers using teletype machines—all uppercase, noisy, and certainly not mobile. The results of a program then came back as scrolling text on paper produced by the same teletype. And, a few years after that, we had moved on to the use of video display terminals although the screens still displayed only ASCII characters, and efforts to draw pictures were achieved solely by using keyboard characters aligned above or adjacent to others to suggest an image of some sort.

I moved in the early 1970s to what would soon become known as Silicon Valley, and there (as a Stanford medical student and computer science graduate student) I was exposed to remarkably inventive activities at Stanford Research Institute (now known simply as SRI International). Developed in their Artificial Intelligence Center, "Shakey the robot" was demonstrating whole new ways to interact with computing devices (this computer-on-wheels had "sensory" inputs, could solve problems, and then would perform their solution by moving in a room with a platform and pushing objects up or down ramps as required)[1]. A few years earlier, SRI scientist Doug Engelbart had developed a new way to interact with characters and activities on a display screen utilizing a manual device that rolled on a desktop and used a button to make selections—a creation that he wistfully called a "mouse" because of the wire "tail" that emerged from it to connect to the display device[2]. But most of us were still using keyboards for all our work, depending on paper printouts to review our programs and their results (initially produced on large line-printers, next on portable thermal-paper devices, and then on early laser printers).

---

[1] http://en.wikipedia.org/wiki/Shakey_the_robot. Accessed 30 Apr 2023.
[2] http://www.dougengelbart.org/firsts/mouse.html. Accessed 30 Apr 2023.

Nearby SRI was Xerox's Palo Alto Research Center, known simply as Xerox PARC, and we at Stanford had close interactions with many of the creative developers there. By 1973 we had been exposed to their work on the Xerox Alto, the first computer to use a desktop metaphor and incorporating a mouse pointing device of the sort that Engelbart had invented at SRI.[3] And, by the end of that decade, two other key innovations were unveiled: (1) the introduction of commercial microcomputers (notably the Apple II, first presented to the public in April 1977[4], and the first IBM PC, which did not appear until four years later[5]), and (2) the introduction of local area networking (LANs) in the form of Ethernet technology, developed by Bob Metcalfe at Xerox PARC and then spun off into a company called 3Com in 1979.[6]

But even at the end of that decade, most of us were still using character-based devices without graphical capabilities, and our access to networks was limited to the wide-area technology of the ARPANET[7]. I do not remember any discussions of interface design or human-computer interaction during most of the 1970s, although pertinent notions were beginning to develop, mostly at Xerox PARC in light of their Alto experience. Everything changed in the following decade. Xerox did introduce commercial products based on its Alto work (an office document-management system known as the Star[8], and a set of machines that were designed to support work coded in the Lisp programming language[9]), but their innovations had led to expensive special-purpose machines and failed to succeed in the marketplace [1]. The 1983 introduction of the Apple Lisa[10] (a personal computer with a graphical user interface, icons, and mouse pointing device), followed a year later by a less expensive and commercially successful successor, the Apple Macintosh[11], changed computing (and human-computer interaction) in key ways. Before long the notion of a computer "desktop" became standard, with icons, files, folders, and images. It was in this context that it became clear that programmers needed to understand their intended users and to design systems that would be intuitive, usable, and well matched with the user's needs and assumptions.

I have summarized this history here because I fear that we too often forget that our remarkable advances in computing and communications happened gradually, with key early insights and inventions that led incrementally to the interconnected world of ubiquitous computing that we expect and accept today. The same is true of our knowledge of human–computer interaction, which began as a subject of study

---

[3] http://en.wikipedia.org/wiki/Xerox_Alto. Accessed 30 Apr 2023.
[4] http://en.wikipedia.org/wiki/History_of_Apple_Inc.#Apple_II. Accessed 30 Apr 2023.
[5] http://www-03.ibm.com/ibm/history/exhibits/pc25/pc25_birth.html. Accessed 30 Apr 2023.
[6] https://history-computer.com/ethernet/. Accessed 30 Apr 2023.
[7] http://en.wikipedia.org/wiki/ARPANET. Accessed 30 Apr 2023.
[8] http://en.wikipedia.org/wiki/Xerox_Star. Accessed 30 Apr 2023.
[9] http://en.wikipedia.org/wiki/Lisp_machine. Accessed 30 Apr 2023.
[10] http://oldcomputers.net/lisa.html. Accessed 30 Apr 2023.
[11] http://apple-history.com/128k. Accessed 30 Apr 2023.

(as I have stressed) decades after we first began to work with early computing devices. Most of us began with highly intuitive notions of how a computer should interact with its users, and there were no courses or principled books to guide us. It was largely with the introduction of graphical user interfaces that notions of right and wrong ways to build interfaces began to emerge.

I was accordingly impressed, in 1980, when I encountered the first of Ben Shneiderman's books on psychological issues and human factors in the design of computer systems [2]. This initial volume focused more on programming styles, team organization, and personality factors, but I was intrigued and inspired by the psychological emphasis and the notion that cognition was a crucial consideration in the design and construction of computing systems. It was his landmark book on user interface design, which appeared in its first edition in 1986, that ultimately persuaded me that there was an important set of scientific issues to be explored and that building the interface to a computer system should be based on theory and established principles rather than intuition. Now in its sixth edition, that book continues to be a classic volume for those interested in how to achieve effective human-computer interaction through principled interface design [3]. Shneiderman has further built on this landmark volume with his recent important and influential book on human-centered artificial intelligence [4].

As a physician and computer scientist who has watched biomedical informatics evolve from an exploratory discipline to a more mature field that feeds into a vibrant health information technology industry, I can identify poor human engineering as a key barrier to the successful fielding of computer systems for health care and biomedicine. Physicians and other health professionals, who too often despise or reject the systems they are asked to use, will almost always focus on problems with the interface design and performance: "confusing," "inefficient," "slow," "difficult to learn," "annoying," "condescending," "unusable," and many more similar characterizations. With the introduction of electronic health records (EHRs) in recent decades—ones that have interfaces that too often generate similar outcries from physicians and other clinical users—we have seen common human-interface limitations emerge as complaints associated with the notion of clinician "burnout." I accordingly applaud efforts to focus on human-computer interaction and usability in the design and implementation of clinical systems and would like to see commercial developers embrace these concepts more aggressively in their design and introduction of systems for clinical use.

The best of intentions, and great cleverness in information and knowledge management, will come to naught if the systems that provide clinical functionalities are constructed without deep insight into the cognitive issues that affect the intended users. The growing field of cognitive informatics, with its focus on health and biomedicine as demonstrated in the current updated volume, is accordingly a crucial element in the evolution and success of the informatics field [5]. As this book makes clear, there are core principles and theories that need to be understood, and a set of methods for exploring the cognitive processes of both users and system developers, that will determine the utility and success of the systems that are built for use in healthcare settings, thereby demonstrating the importance of these cognitive principles. Their importance cannot be overstated, and it will be crucially important for students of biomedical informatics to learn these skills and insights and to bring them to bear in future work. I applaud the efforts of Drs. Kushniruk, Kaufman, Kannampallil, and Patel, and all the chapter authors, for compiling a second edition of their important and influential book on this topic. I commend this updated edition to all those who want to assure that the systems they build, and the interactive environments that they promote, will reflect the rigor and dedication to human-computer interaction principles, including cognitive informatics, that will ultimately enhance both the user's experience and the quality and safety of the care that we offer to patients.

References

1. Smith DK, Alexander RC. Fumbling the future: how Xerox invented, then ignored, the first personal computer. iUniverse; 1999. ISBN-13: 978-1583482667.
2. Shneiderman B. Software psychology: human factors in computer and information systems. Winthrop Publishers; 1980. ISBN-13: 978-0876268162.
3. Shneiderman B, Plaisant C, Cohen M, et al. Designing the user interface: strategies for effective human-computer interaction. London: Pearson; 2016. ISBN-13: 978-0134380384.
4. Shneiderman B. Human-centered AI. Oxford University Press; 2022. ISBN-13: 978-0192845290.
5. Shortliffe EH. Reflections on the role of cognitive science in biomedical informatics (Chapter 23). In: Patel VL, Kaufman D, Cohen T, editors. Cognitive informatics in health and biomedicine: case studies on critical care, complexity and errors. London: Springer; 2013. p. 467–75. ISBN-13: 978-1447154891.

Chair Emeritus and Adjunct Professor, Edward H. Shortliffe
Department of Biomedical Informatics
Columbia University,
New York, NY, USA
May 2023

Preface

One might ask why cognitive scientists have prepared a book that deals with a topic—human-computer interaction (HCI)—that has typically been the purview of computer scientists. Computer science is of course well represented in this volume, but the orientation of the discussion is distinctly cognitive. Some background may be helpful in explaining how this cognitive focus has emerged as we consider the realities of human-computer interaction within the context of medicine and health care.

As my team and I embarked on investigations into the nature of cognitive complexity and error in medicine, I became aware that the work would need to consider the pervasive roles of computers and other technology in high intensity settings such as emergency departments and intensive care units. However, given my major focus on the role of cognition, I did not fully anticipate the central role that technology would begin to play in our discussions and, in turn, in our studies. Our 6-year journey into these multi-site, team-based investigations quickly showed us that technology could either overwhelm or be taken for granted by clinical teams, occasionally exacerbating typical errors or leading to new ones. However, it also became clear that technology could play a major role in error mitigation if human cognition and its interaction with the socio-cultural environment were seriously considered in the context of system design and use. Furthermore, it was evident that advances in technology could support data collection and analyses, as well as the modeling of human behavior, to help us to make better predictions regarding the use and impact of patient oriented decision tools, and, in turn, the outcomes of care. In addition, new sensor-based methods allowed us to track healthcare providers in naturalistic practice settings, observing unobtrusively how they worked in the context of clinical workflow. We leveraged these methods to capture real-world data in a more precise way (at one- or two-second intervals), and then used visualization methods to display and support the analysis in our laboratory, studying the subjects' two-dimensional movement patterns within the clinical units.

During this time, we also saw a dramatic change in patient behavior, wherein patients increasingly came to the emergency room, or to see their personal physicians, bringing pieces of paper with information that they had gathered from the

Internet. Similarly, an increase in the use of social media to seek and share health information became apparent. We accordingly asked whether health information technology could help to mitigate errors by providing cognitive support to both healthcare providers and patients, in part by facilitating the delivery of information and computer-supported care without generating unintended negative consequences, even in the patients' homes. There were other questions about the effect of technology in shaping human behavior, especially in terms of how information is organized, retrieved, and used safely, which influenced our thoughts throughout the process.

Then, during the next few years, I became actively involved in teaching a course on *Human-Computer Interaction and Human Factors in Health Care*, offered to both biomedical informatics and computer science graduate students. We soon found that there were no books that covered this field in a coherent, systematic way, especially ones that offered a cognitive perspective that resonated with our view of the field. Most also offered no special insights or examples drawn from the healthcare environment. I co-taught the class with my colleague, David R. Kaufman, an educational and cognitive psychologist interested in both HCI and medical applications. We had no choice but to use papers from a diverse collection of journals and books, each of which generally covered HCI from a single perspective: biomedical informatics, psychology, computer science, engineering, or cognitive anthropology. I increasingly viewed HCI as having a major cognitive component, not solely as a technical topic. I accordingly reached out to my colleague, Thomas Kannampallil, who has a background in both computer science and cognition, as a logical person to work with me on a first edition of an HCI resource that would take a cognitive perspective while also elucidating the technical components of the field. We then extended our invitation to David R. Kaufman, who agreed to join us as a third co-editor. The resulting first edition has served as a useful resource for researchers seeking to understand the cognitive issues that arise when designing interfaces for medical and healthcare applications. It has also facilitated new types of courses developed to educate those who are designing or building systems that reflect cognitive considerations in the construction of medical applications.

Now, for the book's second edition, we have sought a pair of fresh eyes to evaluate the current field. I could not think of a more suitable person to lead this second edition than André W. Kushniruk. André, with a background in both psychology and computer science, has special expertise in HCI in healthcare and biomedicine. The next step was to review the topics covered in the first edition, identifying updates or additional issues that needed to be included in the new volume. Next, we invited the original chapter authors to update the current chapters and invited new authors to address the topics in additional chapters. Then, as we edited the revised chapters, we focused on cognitive themes and particularly asked how these technologies and methods influence and respond to the human mind and how they facilitate the effective completion of the tasks to be addressed by users.

We were delighted that the chapter authors enthusiastically agreed to participate in the book's second edition, seeing the need for such an updated volume. The resulting book highlights the current state of the art in HCI. It offers subject reviews, drawing from the current research in HCI and providing a graduate-level volume suitable for use in an introductory HCI course for biomedical informatics, cognitive science, computer science, or social science students. The volume is particularly pertinent for biomedical informatics students because most of the examples are drawn from medicine and health. Still, our classroom experience has shown us that medical examples can offer concrete motivation for students in computer science or other fields, even if they may not have a long-term professional interest to work in the healthcare arena.

This work would not have been possible without dedicated support and collegial brainstorming with my colleagues and co-editors, André, Thomas, and David. We spent many hours communicating and providing timely input to the authors. All chapters were reviewed by one of the editors and one additional reviewer. We are grateful for the input in the first edition of the book by our research center's advisory board members (Bill Clancey, Alan Lesgold, Randy Miller, Michael Shabot, and Ted Shortliffe), who shaped our thoughts regarding the developing volume while offering advice and guidance regarding the role of technology in mitigating errors as well as in providing cognitive support. I am indebted to John Bruer, former president of the James S. McDonnell Foundation, who influenced much of my thinking about cognition and education. His vision, commitment, and support of this field—especially with an emphasis on biomedicine and health care—provided the foundation that allowed us to create this book on HCI and cognition.

New York, NY, USA
June 2023

Vimla L. Patel

Contents

Part I Foundations

1 **A Multi-Disciplinary Science of Human Computer Interaction in Biomedical Informatics** 3
Vimla L. Patel, Thomas G. Kannampallil, and David R. Kaufman

2 **Cognition and Human Computer Interaction in Healthcare** 11
David R. Kaufman, Thomas G. Kannampallil, and Vimla L. Patel

3 **Theoretical Foundations for Health Communication Research and Practice**... 37
Daniel G. Morrow and Karen Dunn Lopez

4 **Applications and Challenges of Human Computer Interaction and AI Interfaces for Health Care**........................... 63
Meghan R. Hutch and Yuan Luo

Part II Approaches to Evaluation

5 **Evaluation of Health Information Technology: Methods, Frameworks and Challenges** 93
Thomas G. Kannampallil and Joanna Abraham

6 **Computational Ethnography: Automated and Unobtrusive Means for Collecting Data *In Situ* for Human–Computer Interaction Evaluation Studies** 121
Kai Zheng, David A. Hanauer, Nadir Weibel, and Zia Agha

7 **Analyzing Video-Based Human-Computer Interaction Data in Healthcare Using a Cognitive-Socio-Technical Framework**...... 151
Andre W. Kushniruk and Elizabeth M. Borycki

8 **A Cognitive Approach to Understanding and Mitigating a Pernicious Infodemic** 181
David R. Kaufman and Tonya N. Taylor

9   Visual Analytics: Leveraging Cognitive Principles to Accelerate Biomedical Discoveries 209
Suresh K. Bhavnani

Part III   Design

10   User-Centered Design and Evaluation of Health Information Systems: A Rapid Usability Engineering Approach 235
Andre W. Kushniruk, Helen Monkman, Elizabeth M. Borycki, and Joseph Kannry

11   Human Factors and Design for Supporting Healthcare Teams 263
Charlotte Tang, Yan Xiao, Yunan Chen, and Paul N. Gorman

12   Designing and Deploying Mobile Health Interventions 291
Meghan Reading Turchioe, Albert M. Lai, and Katie A. Siek

Part IV   Applications

13   Human-Computer Interaction in Medical Devices 319
Todd R. Johnson, Harold Thimbleby, Peter Killoran, and Franck Diaz-Garelli

14   Applying HCI Principles in Designing Usable Systems for Dentistry 345
Elsbeth Kalenderian and Muhammad F. Walji

15   The Unintended Consequences of the Technology in Clinical Settings 371
Amy Franklin and Jeritt Thayer

16   The Role of Human Computer Interaction in Consumer Health Applications: Current State, Challenges and Future 391
Holly B. Jimison and Misha Pavel

17   Intelligent Decision Support in Personal Health: Personalized Health Coaching in Type 2 Diabetes 413
Lena Mamykina, Elliot Mitchell, Pooja Desai, and David Albers

Part V   Future Directions

18   Looking Forward: The Role of Human Computer Interaction and Cognition in Healthcare 441
Andre W. Kushniruk, David R. Kaufman, Thomas G. Kannampallil, and Vimla L. Patel

Index 455

About the Editors

Andre W. Kushniruk, PhD, FACMI is the Director and Professor in the School of Health Information Science at the University of Victoria. He holds undergraduate degrees in Psychology and Biology, an MSc in Computer Science from McMaster University, and a PhD in Cognitive Psychology from McGill University. An elected member of the International Academy of Health Sciences Informatics, the Canadian Academy of Health Sciences, he is a Fellow of the American College of Medical Informatics. He conducts research in several areas, including evaluation of the effects of technology, human-computer interaction in health care, and usability engineering. Dr. Kushniruk's research focuses on developing new methods for evaluating information technology and conducting video analysis of computer users. He is currently extending this research to remote studies of e-health applications, virtual healthcare, and advanced information technologies, including electronic health record systems. He has been a key researcher on several national and international collaborative projects and has held academic positions at several Canadian universities. Besides his research with the publication of over 200 scholarly peer-reviewed articles and as a co-editor of several books in health informatics, Dr. Kushniruk has mentored numerous students and is actively involved with teaching, bridging academia to industry.

Thomas G. Kannampallil, PhD, FAMIA is an Associate Professor in the Washington University School of Medicine's (WUSM) Department of Anesthesiology and the Institute for Informatics. He also holds joint appointments in the Department of Computer Science and Engineering, and the Division of Biology and Biomedical Sciences. He is the Associate Chief Research Information Officer (CRIO) at WUSM. His research interests lie at the intersection of computer science, cognitive science, and clinical informatics, focusing on developing and evaluating intelligent computational tools for improving clinical decision-making and patient safety. More recently, Dr. Kannampallil's research has focused on developing artificial intelligence (AI)-based tools for improving postoperative and mental health outcomes. He is currently the *Associate Editor* for the *Journal of Biomedical Informatics* and serves on ONC and PCORI technical expert panels on health information technology. He was elected as a Fellow of the American Medical Informatics Association (FAMIA) in 2021. His research is supported by funding from the Agency for Healthcare Research and Quality (AHRQ), National Institute of Aging and National Library of Medicine.

David R. Kaufman, PhD, FACMI is an Associate Professor in Health Informatics at SUNY Downstate Health Sciences University. Previously, he was an Associate Professor of Biomedical informatics and the Director of the Graduate Training Program at Arizona State University (ASU). With an undergraduate degree in psychology, he received his masters and doctorate in educational psychology, both from McGill University. In 2017, he was elected a Fellow of the American College of Medical Informatics. Dr. Kaufman worked in human-computer interaction (HCI) and human factors for about 25 years. He has extensive experience conducting cognitive research concerning informatics initiatives and evaluating various health information technologies (HIT) developed for clinicians, patients, and health consumers. Since 1994, his involvement in HCI projects on the evaluation of electronic health records, computer-provider order entry systems, and a large-scale telemedicine system for patients with diabetes has transitioned to a recent NIH-funded telehealth clinical trial for stroke disparity patients. Dr. Kaufman was the principal investigator on a Mayo Clinic-ASU ROOT project, which characterized the EHR workflows during the transition to another EHR. He is currently leading an AHRQ-funded effort to characterize pandemic workflow at a Brooklyn safety-net hospital, with the objective to fashion technology-mediated solutions that will enhance data collection, aggregation, synthesis, and visualization to support decision-making.

Vimla L. Patel, PhD, DSc, FACMI is the Director and Senior Research Scientist at the Center for Cognitive Studies in Medicine and Public Health at the New York Academy of Medicine. She has adjunct professorial appointments at Columbia University, Arizona State University, and Weill Cornell Medical College in New York. Trained as a cognitive and educational psychologist at McGill University, Dr. Patel served as a Professor of Medicine and Psychology. She has expertise in using cognitive methods to capture and analyze data to model clinical decision-making and explore ways to augment human intelligence. Her recent research addresses the nature of complexity in the healthcare environment and the use of appropriate methods of investigation for health information technology intervention and patient safety. She is an elected fellow of the Royal Society of Canada (Academy of Social Sciences), the American College of Medical Informatics, and the New York Academy of Medicine. An elected founding member of the International Academy of Health Sciences Informatics, she is the past Associate Editor of the *Journal of Biomedical Informatics* and on the editorial board of the *Journal of Intelligence-Based Medicine and Healthcare*. She is an editor or co-editor of eight books and the series editor of the Springer book series in *Cognitive Informatics in Biomedicine and Healthcare*.

Part I
Foundations

Chapter 1
A Multi-Disciplinary Science of Human Computer Interaction in Biomedical Informatics

Vimla L. Patel, Thomas G. Kannampallil, and David R. Kaufman

Human Computer Interaction in Healthcare

Modern healthcare relies on a connected, integrated and sophisticated backbone of health information technology (HIT). Clinicians rely on HIT (e.g., electronic health records, EHRs) to deliver safe patient care. As has been extensively documented in recent research literature, HIT use is fraught with numerous challenges, some that compromise patient safety [1, 2]. Usability and more specifically, workflow, data integration and data presentation are among the principal pain points identified by clinicians in a HIMSS survey [3]. These issues are the subject of a growing body of applied research in human-computer interaction (HCI) and allied disciplines.

HCI is an interdisciplinary science at the intersection of social and behavioral sciences, and computer and information technology. Drawing from the fields of psychology, computer and social sciences, HCI is concerned with understanding how people interact with devices and systems, and how to make these interactions more useful and usable [4].

HCI research was originally spurred by the advent of personal computers in the early 1980s and developed as an applied science, drawing heavily on software psychology, to enhance the design and evaluation of human-computer interfaces

---

V. L. Patel (✉)
Cognitive Studies in Medicine and Public Health, The New York Academy of Medicine, New York, NY, USA
e-mail: vpatel@nyam.org

T. G. Kannampallil
Institute for Informatics, Data Science, and Biostatistics, Washington University School of Medicine, St Louis, MO, USA

D. R. Kaufman
Health Informatics Program, School of Health Professions, SUNY Downstate Health Sciences University, Brooklyn, NY, USA

© The Author(s), under exclusive license to Springer Nature Switzerland AG 2024
A. W. Kushniruk et al. (eds.), *Human Computer Interaction in Healthcare*, Cognitive Informatics in Biomedicine and Healthcare,
https://doi.org/10.1007/978-3-031-69947-4_1

[5]. With early work rooted in modeling human performance and efficiency of using interfaces [6], HCI has been transformed by developments in technology and software. HCI also became both a focal area of inquiry and application for cognitive science, and a fertile test bed for evaluating cognitive theories.

The role of human cognition in Biomedical Informatics, relates to the scientific discipline of Cognitive informatics (CI), which is grounded in methods and theories from cognitive science. As an applied discipline, it draws on methods and theories from human factors and HCI. In turn, the influence of human cognition on HCI has been significant, and will likely continue to shape the field. The cognitive foundations of HCI are coextensive with the sociotechnical approach that draws a wider circle around people, settings and cultures that influence technology-driven performance. These approaches emphasize how people think, reason, and interact with technology and this enables designers to create more usable, effective, and engaging systems that meet the needs of users.

With advances in computing and technology, HCI research has greatly expanded, spawning several research genres: computer supported cooperative work (CSCW), mobile and ubiquitous computing (UbiComp), and intelligent user interfaces (IUI). While early work on HCI drew heavily on theories and empirical research in cognitive psychology (e.g., research on memory, perception and motor skills), and human factors to explain and improve human interactions with machines, the advent of personal computers transformed the field. Grudin [7] provides a comprehensive history and development of HCI. The transformation and development of HCI as a field had a profound impact in healthcare as it did in other professional sectors. An extended history is beyond the scope of this chapter. However, we provide a brief synopsis as an entry-point to discuss HCI in the context of healthcare.

HCI research in healthcare has paralleled the theoretical and methodological developments in the field beginning with cognitive evaluations of electronic medical records in the mid-90s [8], extending to a focus on distributed health information systems [1, 9], analysis of unintended sociotechnical consequences of computerized provider order entry (CPOE) systems [2], and analysis of user interface challenges in using CPOE system in ICU [1]. HCI work in biomedical informatics extends across clinical and consumer health informatics, addressing a range of user populations including providers, biomedical scientists and patients. While the implications of HCI principles for the design of HIT are acknowledged, the adoption of the tools and techniques among clinicians, informatics researchers and developers of HIT are limited. There is a general consensus that HIT has not realized its potential as a tool that facilitates clinical decision-making, coordination of care, and improvement of patient safety [10].

Theories and methods in HCI continue to evolve to better meet the needs of evaluating systems. For example, classical cognitive or symbolic information processing theory viewed mental representations as mediating all activity [6]. Although methods and theories emerging from the classical cognitive approach continue to be useful and productive, they are limited in their characterization of interactivity or of team/group activities. In more contemporary theories of HCI, such as distributed cognition, cognition is viewed as the process of coordinating internal (mental states) and external representations. The scope has broadened to include external mediators of cognition including artifacts and is also seen as stretched across social agents (e.g., a clinical care team). The socio-technical approach has further expanded the focus of HCI research to include a range of social and organizational factors that influence the productive use and acceptance of technology. A recent paper describes how such frameworks and methods can be used in the evaluation of AI systems [11]. AI systems may extend the relationship between a computational agent (e.g., conventional decision support tools) or it may reinvent it, for example requiring a rethinking of how dialogues with such a system can restructure or even supplant reasoning. As such, new models and frameworks for evaluation are necessary.

The scope of HCI in biomedicine and healthcare is currently very broad encompassing thousands of journal articles across medical disciplines and consumer health domains. Although the 14 chapters in this volume cover considerable terrain, it would not be possible to cover the full range of research and application of HCI in biomedicine and healthcare. In general, there is a strong focus in this volume on issues in clinical informatics. Some notable exceptions are the chapters by Jimison and colleagues on consumer health informatics (Chap. 16), and Turchioe and colleagues (Chap. 12) on mobile health, in this volume.

Human factors and HCI are sister disciplines and share many of the same methods and foci. Although they remain distinct disciplines, the boundaries of research have become increasingly blurred, often using similar theories and methods [12]. In addition, patient safety and clinical workflow are focal topics in applied human factors in healthcare. However, we elected not to specifically cover human factors research because of its immense scope. The handbook edited by Carayon and colleagues [13] provides excellent coverage (in the 50+ chapters) of this important field. Pervasive computing in healthcare is a burgeoning cutting-edge field of growing importance [14], but is only briefly addressed in a couple of chapters. Similarly, HCI and global health informatics is an important emerging field of research [15, 16] but is not dealt with in this volume. Finally, our focus is predominantly on evaluation of HIT in the modern healthcare environment rather than the design (or design approaches) for HIT. Although the chapters in this volume embrace a range of theoretical perspectives, it should be noted that this is part of the Cognitive Informatics series and the frameworks are somewhat skewed toward the cognitive rather than the social perspectives.

Scope and Purpose of the Book

This volume is somewhat unique in its focus on the role of cognition in HCI, a flourishing cross-disciplinary field that cuts across several academic and professional sectors. The chapters in this volume focus on motivating examples drawn from the application of theories and methods from CI to challenges related to the development and use of safer, useful, and usable HIT. The objective of this second edition is to update the pedagogical description of HCI within the context of healthcare settings and HIT. Although there is a growing awareness of the importance of HCI in biomedical informatics, there is limited training at the graduate level in HCI for biomedical informatics (BMI) students. An informal review of the curriculum of graduate programs led us to the conclusion that fewer than 20% of the US-based BMI programs had any course in HCI or related topics, and this percentage is even less on topics related to the role of cognition. This can be partly attributed to a shift towards a more data science-oriented approach, where the human part of the equation is not a focal point. Also contributing to the paucity of courses, is the relative inaccessibility of advanced level graduate materials for students. Although there are considerable original materials in the form of journal and conference articles, these are idiosyncratic in their coverage of issues and demand greater understanding of cognitive and informatics-related issues. There are useful contemporary textbooks on human-computer interaction [17], but the coverage of health-related content or examples are limited. Our purpose with this book is to provide an aggregated source of a collection of HCI topics that are relevant to BMI students and researchers. The role of HCI in the biomedical informatics curriculum is reflected in the presence of HCI-related courses in some academic graduate programs and in the growing number of research programs. Most courses are taught with a combination of research papers, general HCI textbooks with minimal focus on HIT, and instructor prepared material. Within this scope, we have identified a set of topics—both from a classical HCI perspective and others from an applied HCI in BMI focus, specifically assessing the role of human cognition in such interactions. These revised chapters, and several new ones as we acknowledged above, do not provide comprehensive coverage of all HCI topics. However, the selected topics represent a mix of themes that coalesces the past with the future of HCI.

Organization of Chapters

The book is organized in the following manner: the early Chaps. 1, 2, 3, and 4 focus on the theoretical and methodological basis of HCI, including a recent consideration of HCI and AI. The major themes covered include cognition, communication, socio-technical considerations, and evaluation methods for research. Chapters 5, 6, 7, 8, and 9 describe various approaches to evaluation of HCI, including an evaluation framework, recent trends in visualization, including the topic of misinformation. The next three Chaps. 10, 11, and 12) focus on design, describing the user-centered design for providing team support and the use of HCI for mobile devices and theories to address several key issues including usability, team activities, and unintended consequences of technology use. The final chapters on applications (Chaps. 13, 14, 15, 16, and 17) that address the current state and future challenges in HCI in consumer health applications, human-centered AI to support everyday decisions in health, and the HCI issues in the domain of clinical dentistry.

The themes that are addressed in the various chapters have been selected with the purpose of addressing specific biomedical informatics challenges related to HIT evaluation. As a result, key topics that are often covered in HCI books, such as motor and visual/perceptual theories, have not been discussed. We have also followed a specific structure: each chapter includes a description of the key HCI problem and its relevance to biomedical informatics and cognition, detailed examples where applicable (in some chapters, explicit case studies), and additional follow up readings for interested readers. A brief overview of each of the chapters is provided below.

In Chap. 2, Kaufman, Kannampallil and Patel describe these cognitive foundations within the context of biomedicine and healthcare. Cognitive theories relevant to HCI including human information processing, interactive environments, mental models, role of external representation in HCI, and distributed cognition are described. In Chap. 3, Morrow and Dunn-Lopez describe the information processing and interactive approaches to communication, focusing on how these can be used to improve communication effectiveness, leading to more efficient work activities, collaboration and patient safety. Chapter 4 covers recent developments in applications and challenges of HCI for AI Interfaces. Hutch and Luo suggest that HCI tools and approaches can help overcome the complexity of developing and using AI systems in healthcare. They also advocate for making human-in-the-loop a standard feature in order to ensure that data conforms to societal norms and regulations.

In Chap. 5, Kannampallil and Abraham discuss the various methods for evaluating HIT. Methods of evaluation that encompass issues of HCI and those from a more contextual and situated perspective are described. The appropriateness of each method in various evaluation contexts is also described. In contrast to the traditional methods described in Chap. 5, Zheng and colleagues describe in Chap. 6 a new family of HCI methods called "computational ethnography." Computational ethnography relies on digital trace data available in healthcare environments to characterize human-computer interactions. Examples of such data include audit logs, motion capture, and Radio Frequency Identification (RFID). Examples from various clinical situations are used to illustrate how these methods have been applied in healthcare to study end users' interactions with technological interventions.

In Chap. 7, Kushniruk and colleagues describe the cognitive approaches to analyzing HCI data in improving the usability of clinical systems. A range of approaches including the use of laboratory style usability testing to the use of clinical simulations conducted in real-world clinical settings are described. The authors also introduce new approaches to low-cost rapid usability engineering methods that can be applied throughout the design and implementation cycle of clinical information systems. In Chap. 8, Kaufman and colleagues describe a cognitive approach to understanding and mitigating a rapid and far-reaching spread of both inaccurate information or misinformation. Believing in science is always challenging when scientific information is presented as evidence-based data and when powerful influencers offer counterarguments from inaccurate or misinformation, which are visually compellingly.

In Chap. 9, Bhavnani introduces a relatively new domain of biomedical visualization, specifically focusing on how visualization approaches can amplify our ability to analyze large and complex data. Using examples from network analysis, the significant power of visualization for data analysis and interpretation is demonstrated, from a scientific and translational perspective. Opportunities for visualization in biomedical informatics, available tools, and the challenges of biomedical visualization are also described.

User-centered design and evaluation of clinical Information systems from a usability engineering perspective is discussed by Kushniruk and colleague in Chap. 10. In Chap. 12, Turchioe and colleagues examine the use of mobile devices in healthcare both among consumers (e.g., patients) and clinicians, including design considerations, requirements and challenges of its deployment. Modern wearable devices, such as smart watches, and their potential applications within healthcare settings are also described. Johnson and colleagues in Chap. 13 provide an alternative perspective on the interaction challenges with medical devices—an almost ubiquitous component of clinical environments. They discuss the challenges of developing medical device interfaces as a function of the interplay between the complexities of the clinical environment, users of medical devices and the device constraints. The chapter weaves together a set of human factors issues pertaining to patient safety and HCI design considerations. Regulatory considerations and their impact on medical device HCI are also described.

In Chap. 14, Kalenderian and Walji provide an example of the application of HCI evaluation methods in the re-design of a dental EHR interface. In addition to showing how these principles can be applied for the design of dental EHRs, they describe the importance of the participatory design process for the design and development of HIT. The case study example provides further context for the methods described in Chap. 11. Tang and colleagues (Chap. 11) characterize the role of team activities and teamwork in modern healthcare practice. They discuss how team composition and interactions create significant challenges for maintaining seamless team activities in clinical settings. They draw on socio-technical systems theory to illustrate how team activities are situated within the context of HIT use. Case studies from the field are used to further exemplify the nuances of team activities and interactions in complex clinical settings.

In Chap. 15, Franklin provides an overview of the nature and types of unintended consequences of the use of HIT in clinical environments—both its positive serendipitous results, as well as negative, unintended, and potentially harmful consequences of technology in use. A review of different classification systems for studying the unanticipated effects of HIT, especially EHR and CPOE use, is described with several examples from the research literature.

In Chap. 16, Jimison and colleagues illustrate the challenges of designing healthcare solutions for consumers. They describe the issues of varying cultural backgrounds, levels of literacy and access that cause considerable challenges in design. The authors review these issues and describe the role of participatory user-centered design for developing safe and usable consumer health tools. Mamykina and her colleagues (Chap. 17) discusses the use of intelligent decision support in personal health, specifically personalized health coaching in type 2 diabetes. Personal informatics technologies facilitate self-management through reflection and increased self-knowledge. Machine learning can identify meaningful trends and patterns in self-monitoring data. Personal health coaching programs and digital health coaching are interventions for type 2 diabetes mellitus (T2DM) that have potential to provide patients with new tools for monitoring, understanding, and acting upon the state of their health. The final chapter by the editors, present a summary of the current status and some thoughts on the future of the field.

Future Directions for HCI in Healthcare: Role of Cognition

The range of users of HIT including clinicians, biomedical researchers, health consumers and patients continue to expand, as does the range of functions supported by HIT. The challenges of supporting these populations are well known. The advances in health technologies have not led to commensurate advances in usability or in cognitive support. HCI methods of evaluation and iterative design will play an increasingly pivotal role (Kushniruk et al., Chap. 10). The approaches encompass tried and tested methods that continue to yield valuable insight into system usability, and related matters such as learning, adoption and training. The approaches also include cutting-edge methodologies including computational ethnography (Zheng et al., Chap. 6), which continue to broaden the scope of applied HCI, and to ask questions about workflow and related matters that were not previously possible. Similarly, Hutch and Luo introduce the new challenges and opportunities presented by work at the intersection of AI and HCI. There is no doubt that these fields and that of mHealth (mobile Health) and pervasive computing will continue to push the envelope on creating new worlds in HIT. HCI methods will have to continue to advance to play a productive role and meet the new demands realized by these developments. More importantly, human-centered design with a focus and the mediating role of cognition, will continue to be a central concern.

We see future research to have a greater focus on the role of HIT and safe design of the healthcare workplace, including its involvement in patient safety. Although it has been shown that HIT has significant potential to improve safety, we have to acknowledge that it can also cause harm. One of our future challenges will be to ensure that we include both the private and public sectors in our efforts to understand the risks associated with HIT, including development of standards and criteria for safe design and implementation. The role of technology in healthcare is perpetually changing and advances in various areas are likely to be transformative.

References

1. Horsky J, Kuperman GJ, Patel VL. Comprehensive analysis of a medication dosing error related to CPOE. J Am Med Inform Assoc. 2005;12(4):377–82.
2. Koppel R, Metlay JP, Cohen A, et al. Role of computerized physician order entry systems in facilitating medication errors. JAMA. 2005;293(10):1197–203.

3. Ribitzky R, Sterling M, Bradley V. EHR usability pain points survey Q4 2009. Paper presented at: Oral presentation at the 2010 Annual HIMSS Conference & Exhibition. 2010.
4. Carroll JM. HCI models, theories, and frameworks: toward a multidisciplinary science. Elsevier; 2003.
5. Shneiderman B, Plaisant C, Cohen MS, Jacobs S, Elmqvist N, Diakopoulos N. Designing the user interface: strategies for effective human-computer interaction. Pearson; 2016.
6. Card S, Moran TP, Newell A. The psychology of human-computer interaction. Hillsdale, NJ: Lawrence Erlbaum Associates; 1983.
7. Grudin J. Introduction: a moving target: the evolution of human–computer interaction. In: Jacko JA, editor. The human–computer interaction handbook: fundamentals, evolving technologies, and emerging applications. Routledge; 2012. p. xxvii–lxi.
8. Kushniruk AW, Kaufman DR, Patel VL, Lévesque Y, Lottin P. Assessment of a computerized patient record system: a cognitive approach to evaluating medical technology. MD Comput. 1996;13(5):406–15.
9. Hazlehurst B, McMullen CK, Gorman PN. Distributed cognition in the heart room: how situation awareness arises from coordinated communications during cardiac surgery. J Biomed Inform. 2007;40(5):539–51.
10. Middleton B, Bloomrosen M, Dente MA, et al. Enhancing patient safety and quality of care by improving the usability of electronic health record systems: recommendations from AMIA. J Am Med Inform Assoc. 2013;20(e1):e2–8.
11. Shortliffe EH, Sepùlveda M-J, Patel VL. Framework for the evaluation of clinical AI systems. In: Cohen TA, Patel VL, Shortliffe EH, editors. Intelligent systems in medicine and health: the role of AI. Springer; 2022. p. 479–503.
12. Patel VL, Kannampallil TG. Human factors and health information technology: current challenges and future directions. Yearb Med Inform. 2014;23(01):58–66.
13. Carayon P, Wust K, Hose BZ, Salwei ME. Human factors and ergonomics in health care. In: Handbook of human factors and ergonomics. Wiley; 2021. p. 1417–37.
14. Orwat C, Graefe A, Faulwasser T. Towards pervasive computing in health care–a literature review. BMC Med Inform Decis Mak. 2008;8(1):1–18.
15. Chan CV, Kaufman DR. A technology selection framework for supporting delivery of patient-oriented health interventions in developing countries. J Biomed Inform. 2010;43(2):300–6.
16. Gulliksen J. Institutionalizing human-computer interaction for global health. Glob Health Action. 2017;10(sup3):1344003.
17. Preece J, Sharp H, Rogers Y. Interaction design: beyond human-computer interaction. Wiley; 2015.

Chapter 2
Cognition and Human Computer Interaction in Healthcare

David R. Kaufman, Thomas G. Kannampallil, and Vimla L. Patel

Introduction

Is a theory of cognition truly necessary? What benefits can be gained from having a cognitive theory or a collection of theories? How can cognitive theory contribute to our understanding of health information technology design and usage? Over the past three decades, a wealth of experiential and practical knowledge has accumulated regarding user experience, system design, and implementation, providing valuable insights to inform further advancements. This practical knowledge embodies the need for sensible and intuitive user interfaces, an understanding of workflow, and the ways in which systems impact individual and team performance [1]. Human-computer interaction (HCI) in health care and other domains are at least partly an empirical science where the growing knowledge base can be leveraged as needed. However, relying solely on practical or empirical knowledge, such as case studies, is insufficient for developing robust generalizations or establishing sound design and implementation principles.

We argue that there is a need for a theoretical foundation. Of course, theory is a core part of any basic or applied science and is necessary to advance knowledge, to test hypotheses and to discern robust generalizations from the increasingly idiosyncratic field of endeavor.

Cognitive theory has been a central part of HCI since its inception. However, HCI has expanded as a discipline focused on a small subset of interactive tasks such as text editing, information retrieval and software programming [2]. It is currently a flourishing area of inquiry that covers all manners of interactions with technology from smart phones to ticketing kiosks. In the field of healthcare, HCI research has encompassed a wide array of health information technologies, spanning from electronic health record (EHR) systems to consumer fitness devices like Fitbit, Apple Watch, and various devices designed for patients with chronic conditions or individuals seeking to improve their overall wellness. The scope of HCI research in healthcare has expanded to encompass an extensive range of technologies, aiming to enhance usability, effectiveness, and user experience across diverse healthcare settings and contexts. In addition, technology is no longer the realm of the solo agent; rather, it is increasingly a team game. This has led to the adaptation of cognitive theories to HCI that stress the importance of the social and/or distributed nature of computing [3, 4]. The rapid expansion of artificial intelligence (AI) is incontrovertible, and its integration into the health computing landscape is expected to accelerate. In order to establish a harmonious relationship between users and AI systems, it is essential to ensure a symmetrical dynamic where individuals can exert a certain level of control and understanding. Future AI systems in healthcare will need to incorporate explainable AI models, which enable users to comprehend and interpret the reasoning behind AI-generated recommendations or decisions [5]. By employing user-centered design principles, these systems can be tailored to prioritize the user's needs, preferences, and cognitive capabilities, fostering a more transparent and collaborative interaction between humans and AI technologies in the realm of health computing.

Rogers [3, 4] critiques the rapid pace of theory change. She argues "the paint has barely dried for one theory before a new coat is applied. It makes it difficult for anything to become established and widely used." Although we perceive this to be a legitimate criticism, we must acknowledge the extraordinary diversity in HCI subjects of inquiry. In addition, cognitive theories have endured, although they have evolved in response to new sets of circumstances such as the emphasis on real-world research in complex messy settings, on the role of artifacts as mediators of performance and on team cognition.

What role can theory play in HCI research and application? Bederson and Shneiderman [6] categorize five types of theories that can inform HCI practice:

- Descriptive—providing concepts, terminology, methods and focusing further inquiry;
- Explanatory—elucidating relationships and processes (e.g., explaining why user performance on a given system is suboptimal);
- Predictive—enabling predictions to be made about user performance or of a given system (e.g., predicting increased accuracy or efficiency as a result of a new design);

- Prescriptive—providing guidance for design from high level principles to specific design solutions;
- Generative—seeding novel ideas for design including prototype development and new paradigms of interaction.

Cognitive theories have played an instrumental role in all five categories, although predicting performance across a spectrum of users (e.g., from novice to expert) remains a significant challenge. In addition, generative theories have begun to play a more central role in HCI design. Although theoretical frameworks such as ethnomethodology, activity theory and ecological psychology, to name a few, have made substantive contributions to the field, this chapter is focused primarily on cognitive theories including classical human information processing, external cognition and distributed cognition.

The chapter takes a historical approach in documenting the evolution of cognitive theories beginning with the early application of information-processing theories and exploring external as well as distributed cognition. Each of these constitutes a family of theories or a framework that embraces core principles, but differs in important respects. A framework is a general pool of constructs for understanding a domain, but it is not sufficiently cohesive or fully realized to constitute a theory [7]. The field of HCI as applied to healthcare is remarkably broad in scope and the domain of medicine is characterized by immense complexity and diversity in both tasks and activities [8]. Specific HCI theories are often limited in scope especially as applied to a rich and complex knowledge domain. Patel and Groen [9] make an analogous argument for the use of cognitive theories as applied to medical education. Frameworks can provide a theoretical rationale for innovative design concepts and serve to motivate HCI experiments. They can become further differentiated into theories that cover or emphasize a particular facet of interaction (e.g., analyzing teamwork) in the context of a broader framework (e.g., distributed cognition).

We provide a survey of these different theories and illustrate their application with case studies and examples, focusing mostly on issues pertaining to health technology, but also drawing on other domains. The chapter is not intended to be comprehensive or a critical look at the state of the art on HCI in health and biomedicine. Rather, it is written for a diverse audience including those who are new to cognitive science and cognitive psychology. The scope of this chapter is limited with a primary focus on cognitive theories, as they have been applied in healthcare contexts.

A partial space of cognitive theories, as reflected in the chapter, is illustrated in Fig. 2.1. As described, it isn't intended to be exhaustive. It's illustrative of how to conceptualize the theoretical frameworks. It should also be noted that the boundaries between frameworks are somewhat permeable. For example, external and distribute cognition frameworks are co-extensive. However, it serves the purpose of emphasizing the evolution of cognitive theories and highlight specific facets such as the effect of representations on cognition or the social coordination of computer-mediated work. Although the theories within a framework may differ on key issues, the primary difference is in their points of emphasis. In other words, they privilege some aspect as it pertains to cognition and interaction.

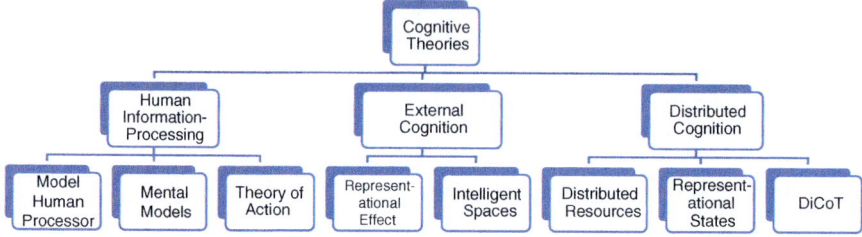

Fig. 2.1 Partial space of frameworks and cognitive theories

Human Information Processing

A computational theory of mind provides the fundamental underpinning for most contemporary cognitive theories. The basic premise is that much of human cognition can be characterized as a series of operations, computations on mental representations. Early theories and models of human performance were often described in terms of the perceptual and motor activities and assumptions by their structural components (e.g., limits of short-term memory). These were primarily derived from the stimulus-response paradigm, and considered the human as an "information processor." In other words, within this paradigm the human was an information controller, perceiving and responding to activities [10]. This approach led to the development of several commonly used models such as Fitts Law [11] and the theory of bimanual control [12]—that predict performance of human activities in a variety of tasks (e.g., task acquisition, flight controls, and air traffic control). Fitts Law, in particular has had an enduring impact with researchers exploring it's validity in reference to touchscreen computers [13], virtual-reality technology [14] and mobile devices for older adults [15]. Detailed descriptions of the use of these theories can be found in Chap. 5 of this volume.

With the advent of computers, and more recently significantly interactive environments, there was a need for more integrated information-processing models that accounted for the human-computer interaction (HCI). There were two important requirements: first, the models needed to account for the sequential and integrated actions that evolve during human-computer interactions; second, in addition to the layout and format of the interface, the models also needed to account for the content that was presented on the interfaces [16]. In its most general form, the human information processor consists of input, processing and output components (See Fig. 2.2). The input to the processor involves perception of stimuli from the external world; the input/stimuli would be processed by a processor and involves a series of processing stages. Typically, these stages include encoding of the perceived stimuli, comparing and matching it to known mental representations in memory, and selection and execution of an appropriate response. The response is realized through motor actions. For example, consider a clinician's interaction with an EHR interface, where he/she has to select a medication from a dropdown menu [17]. The input component would perceive the dropdown menu from the interface, which would be

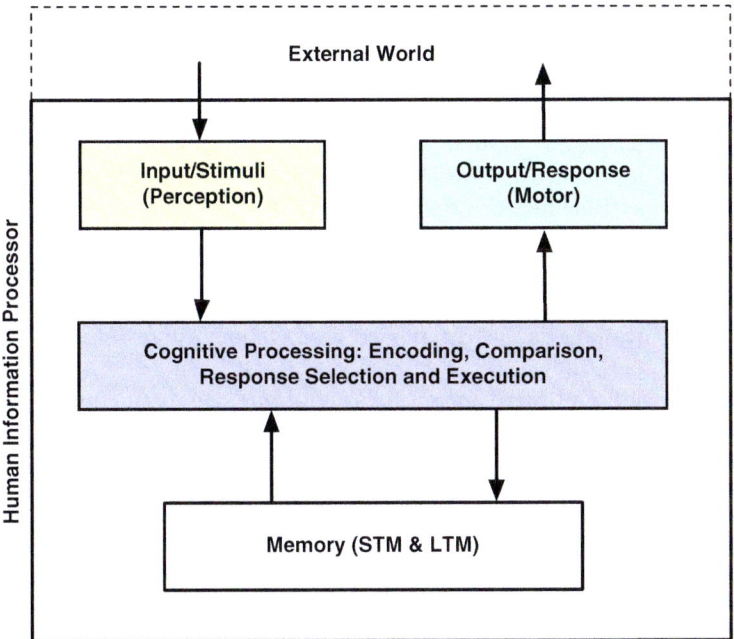

Fig. 2.2 Input-output model of human information processing. STM refers to short-term memory and LTM is an abbreviation for long-term memory

matched in memory and click action response would be triggered. This click action would be relayed as to the motor components (output), which executes the action by clicking the dropdown menu item. This cycle repeats till the entire task of selecting the medication is completed. In the next sections, we consider core constructs associated with this approach including the model human processor, Norman's theory of action, and mental models.

Model Human Processor

One of the earliest and most commonly described instantiations of a theoretical human information processing system is the Model Human Processor (MHP). The Model Human Processor (MHP) can be described as a set of processors, memories and their interactions that operate based on a set of principles [18]. As per MHP, the human mind consists of three interacting processors: perceptual, cognitive and motor. These processors can operate in serial (e.g., pressing a key) or in parallel (e.g., driving a car and listening to radio). Information processing of MHP occurs in cycles. First, the perceptual processor retrieves sensory (visual or audio) information from the external world and is transmitted to the working memory (WM). Once the information is in the WM, information is processed using a *recognize-act* cycle of cognitive processor. During each cycle, contents of WM are connected to actions that are linked to them (from long term memory). These actions, in turn, modify the contents of the WM resulting in a new cycle of actions. MHP can be used to develop an integrated description regarding the psychological effects of human computer interaction performance. While it is considered a significant oversimplification for general users, it provided a preliminary mechanism on which much of the human performance modeling research was developed. MHP is useful to predict and compare different interface designs, task performance and learnability of user interfaces. It can be used to develop guidelines for interface design such as spatial layout, response rates and recall. It also provides a significant advantage, as these human performance measures can be determined even without a functional prototype or actual users.

Although the use of MHP approach has not commonly been applied in healthcare contexts, there have been a few noteworthy studies. For example, Saitwal et al. [19] used the keystroke level model (KLM, an instantiation of the GOMS approach; See Chap. 5) to compute the time taken, and the number of steps required to complete a set of 14 EHR-based tasks. Using this approach, they characterized the challenges of the user interface and identified opportunities for improvement. Detailed description of this study and the use of the GOMS approach can be found in Chap. 5.

Norman's Theory of Action

In the mid 1980s, cognitive science was beginning to flourish as a discipline and HCI was viewed as both a test bed for these theories and as a domain of practice. The MHP work was indicative of those efforts. At the same time, microcomputers were becoming increasingly common in homes, work and school. As a result, computers were transitioning from being a tool that was used by experts (i.e., computer scientists and those with high degrees of technical expertise) exclusively to one that was used broadly by individuals in all walks of life. Systems at that point in time were particularly unwieldy and often, extremely difficult to learn. In a seminal paper on cognitive engineering [20], Norman sought to craft a theory "to understand the fundamental principles behind human action and performance that are relevant for the development of engineering principles of design" (p. 32). A second objective was to devise systems that are "pleasant to use."

A critical insight of the theory is the discrepancy between psychologically expressed goals and the physical controls and variables of a system. For example, a goal may be to scroll down towards the bottom of a document, and a scroll bar embodies the physical controls to realize such a goal. Shneiderman presented a similar analysis in his theory of direct manipulation [21]. The key question is how an individual's goals and intensions get expressed as a set of physical actions that transform a virtual system and result in the desired change of state (e.g., reaching the intended section of the document). The Norman model draws on many of the same basic cognitive concepts as the MHP model, but embodies it in a seven stage model of action.

The action cycle begins with a *goal*, for example, retrieving a patient's surgical history. The goal is a generic one independent of any system. In this context, let's presuppose that the clinician has access to paper record as well as those in an EHR. The second stage involves the formation of an *intention*, which in this case might be to retrieve the patient record in an EHR. The intention leads to the *specification of an action* sequence, which may include signing on to the system (which in itself may necessitate several actions), engaging a component system or simply a field that can be used to locate a patient in the database, and entering the patient's identifying information (e.g., last name or medical record number, if it is known). The specification results in *executing an action*, which may necessitate several actions. The system responds in some way or in the case of a failed attempt, may not respond at all. A change in system state may or may not provide a clear indication of the new state or a failure to provide feedback as to why the desired state has not appeared (e.g., system provides no indicators of a wait state or why no response is forthcoming). The perceived system response must then be *interpreted* and *evaluated* to determine whether the goal has been achieved. If the response provided by the system is "record not found," that could mean a number of things including that a name was mistyped or the number was incorrectly listed. On the basis of this determination, a next action will be chosen.

Any task of moderate complexity will involve substantial nesting of sub-goals, requiring a series of actions. To an experienced user, the action cycle may appear as a completely transparent and seamless process. However to a less experienced user, the process may breakdown at any of the seven stages. Norman [20] describes two primary means in which the action cycle can break down. The *gulf of execution* reflects the difference between the goals and intentions of the user and the kinds of actions enabled by the system. For example, a user may not know the appropriate action sequence or the interface may not provide discernible clues to make such sequences transparent. For instance, a transaction may appear to be complete, but further action is needed to execute the selection process (e.g., pressing enter to accept a transaction).

The *gulf of evaluation* reflects the degree to which the user can make sense of the state of a system and determine how well their expectations have been met. For example, it is sometimes difficult to interpret a state transition and to know whether one has arrived at the correct state or whether the user has chosen an incorrect path. Goals that necessitate multiple state or screen transitions are more likely to present difficulties for users, especially as they learn the system. Bridging gulfs involves both bringing about changes to the system design and training users to become better attuned to the affordances offered by a system resources. Gulfs can be partially explained by differences in the designer's models and the users' mental models, as discussed in the next section. The designer's model is the conceptual model to be built, based on analysis of the task, requirements, and an understanding of the users' capabilities [20]. The users' mental models of system behavior are developed through interacting with similar systems and gaining an understanding of how actions (e.g., selecting an item from a menu) will produce predictable and desired outcomes. Graphical user interfaces that involve direct manipulation of screen objects and widgets represent an attempt to reduce the distance between a designer's and user's model [21]. Obviously, the distance is likely to be more difficult to bridge in a system like an EHR that incorporates a wide range of functions and components that may provide different layouts and forms of interaction.

Norman's theory of action has given rise, or in some cases, reinforced the need for sound design principles. For example, the state of a system should be plainly visible to the user and feedback should be transparent. In illustration, dialog boxes or alert messages can trigger the intention of reminding users to what is possible or needed to complete the task. There is a need to provide good mappings between the actions (e.g., clicking on a tab) and the results of the action as reflected in the state of the system (e.g., providing access to the expected display).

Norman's theory of action informed a great deal of research and design across domains. The seven-stage action theory was used to good effect by Zhang and colleagues in their development of a taxonomy of errors [22]. The theory also draws on Reason's categorization of errors as either slips or mistakes [23]. Slips result from the incorrect execution of a correct action sequence and mistakes are the product of the correct completion of an incorrect action sequence. Slips and mistakes are further categorized into execution errors and evaluation errors. They are further categorized into each of the descriptors that correspond to the Norman's seven stages (e.g., goals, intentions, etc.). Zhang et al. [22] provide the following example of an intention slip: A" nurse intended to enter the rate of infusion using the up–down arrow keys, because this is the technique on the pump she most frequently uses; however, on this pump the arrow keys move the selection region instead of changing the selected number" (p. 98). An example of an evaluation/intention slips is that a nurse interprets a yellow flashing light on a device analogically (based on prior knowledge of yellow as a warning) and interprets it as noncritical when it is in fact signaling a critical event. Norman's seven-stage action theory proved to be a useful model for characterizing a wide range of medical error types. The model has broad applications, for example, in the design of assistive and rehabilitation system for disabled individuals [24].

Although theory of action has been very influential in the world of design and research, it also has shortcomings [25]. The theory proposes that stages are followed sequentially. However, users do not necessarily proceed in such a sequential manner, especially in a domain such as medicine, which is constituted by numerous and complex nonlinear tasks. Contemporary GUIs, for example, web-based or app-based systems provide users with greater flexibility in achieving the desired state or access the needed information. As discussed in subsequent sections, external representations (e.g., as expressed in text displays or visualizations) offer guidance to the user or even structure their interactions in such a way that a planned action sequence may not be necessary.

Mental Models

Mental models are an important construct in cognitive science and have been widely used in HCI research [26]. Mental models are a conceptual framework used to describe how individuals develop internal representations of systems, often relying on analogies and comparisons as building blocks. They are envisioned to answer questions such as "how does it work?" or "what will happen if I make the following move?" "Analog" suggests that the representation explicitly shares some aspect of the structure of the world it represents. For example, one can envision in the mind's eye a set of connected visual images of the succession of ATM screens one has to negotiate to get $200 out of one's checking account or buildings one passes on the way home from a local grocery store. This is in contrast to an abstraction-based form such as propositions or schemas in which the mental structure consists of either the gist, or a summary representation, for example, the procedures needed to complete an ATM transaction. Like other forms of mental representation, mental models are invariably incomplete, imperfect and subject to the processing limitations of the cognitive system [27]. Mental models can be derived from perception, language or from one's imagination [28]. Running of a model corresponds to a process of mental simulation to generate possible future states of a system from observed or hypothetical state.

The constructs discussed in the prior sections emphasize how the general limits of the human-information processing system (e.g., limits in perception, attention and retrieval from memory) influence performance on a given task in a particular context [20]. On the other hand, mental models emphasize mental content, namely, knowledge and beliefs. An individual's mental model provides predictive and explanatory capabilities regarding the functions of a particular system. The construct has been used to characterize differences in expertise in a range of knowledge domains such as physics [29]. Experts have richer and more robust models of a range of phenomena, whereas novices are more prone to imprecision and errors. Mental models has been used to characterize models that have a spatial and temporal context, as is the case in reasoning about the behavior of electrical circuits [29]. The model can be used to simulate a process (e.g., predict the effects of network interruptions on downloading a movie from www.amazon.com).

Mental models are a particularly useful explanatory device in understanding human-computer interaction. The premise is that by exploring what users can understand and how they reason about the systems, it is possible to design them in a way that support the acquisition of the appropriate mental model and to reduce errors while performing with them. It is also useful to distinguish between a designer's conceptual model of a given system and a user's mental model [30]. The wider the gap, the more difficulties individuals will experience in using the system. For example, Kaufman and colleagues [31] evaluated the usability of a home-based telemedicine system targeting older adults with diabetes. The study documented a substantial gulf between patients' mental models of the system and the designer's intent of how the system should be used. Although most of the participants had a shallow understanding of how such systems worked, there were some who possessed more elaborate mental models, and were better able to negotiate the system to perform a range of tasks including uploading blood glucose values and monitoring one's condition over time.

It is believed that novice users of a system can benefit from instructions that imparts a conceptual model or supports a mental simulation process (i.e., helping the users mentally step through problem states) [28]. Diagrammatic models of the device or system are often used to support such a learning process. For example, Halasz and Moran [32] found that such a model was particularly beneficial to students learning to use a programmable calculator. Kieras and Bovair [33] demonstrated a similar benefit for students learning to master a simple control panel device. They conducted a series of studies contrasting two groups learning to use a device. One group was trained to operate the device through learning the procedures by rote. The second group was trained using a model of how the device works. The model group learned the procedures faster, executed them more rapidly and improvised when necessary, e.g., replacing inefficient procedures with simple ones. The study provides an illustration of how having a more robust mental model of a system can impact performance. A more advanced model can enable a user to discover alternative ways to achieve the same goal and overcome obstacles.

For a time, the concept of mental models has declined in popularity as theories highlighting the importance of interaction and externalization of representations gained prominence and flourished. However, the construct has resurfaced in recent years as a means to characterize how individuals' conceptualizations differ from representations in systems. For example, Smith and Koppel [34] take the approach a step further in that they conceptualize three models: the patient's reality, that reality as represented in an EHR and as reflected in a clinician's understanding or mental model of the problem. Drawing on data from a wide range of sources (e.g., observations and log files) and findings, they constructed "scenarios of misalignment" or misrepresentation including categories such as "IT data too broadly focused" (i.e., lacking precise descriptions). For example, medical problem lists that do not permit sufficient qualification or classification illustrate an example of IT as being too broad or coarse. For instance, clinicians were not able to specify that a stroke resulted from a left-sided cerebrovascular accident. The typology provides a useful basis for IT designers to potentially reduce the gaps, better support users and diminish the potential for unintended consequences. The enduring value of the mental model constructs is that it is intuitive and has broad explanatory capabilities across a span of interface challenges [35, 36].

Shared mental models (SMM) represent an extension of the concept of mental models. The construct is rooted in research on teamwork in areas such as aviation [37]. Clinical care is recognized as a highly collaborative practice and there is a need to develop shared understanding about the processes involved in patient care as well as the evolving conditions of patients that are currently under their care. Breaks in communication among team members are known to be significant contributors to medical errors [38]. There are only a few studies to date that demonstrate a relationship between SMM and clinical performance [39]. Mamykina and colleagues [40] investigated the development of SMM in an intensive care unit. The data included observations, audio recorded transcripts of patient handoff (i.e., transfer of patient during shift change) and rounds. In a recent paper, the analysis focused on a single care team including an attending physician, residents, nurses, medical students and physician assistants. The results indicated that the team initially had rather divergent perspectives on how well patients were doing, and the relative success of the treatment. Rounds served as an important coordinating event and the team endeavored to construct shared mental models (i.e., achieving a shared understanding) through an iterative process of resolving discrepancies. There was substantial evidence of change in SMM and in the coordination of patient care over a three-day period. Whereas conversations on the first day focused on creating basic alignment and making immediate modifications to the care, discussions on the third day focused on understanding of underlying reasons for the situation, and developing a long-term plan more consistent with this collective causal understanding [40].

Mental models are not observable and can only be inferred indirectly. However, we believe that it has enduring value as an explanatory device for characterizing how individuals understand a system. The construct is too often used as a synonym for understanding, or for generic mental representation (i.e., with no commitment to the form of the representation). We favor the more specific instantiation of it as a model that can be used to simulate a process and project forward to predict events or outcomes or to explain why a particular outcome occurred. This enables us to develop theories or models for a given domain and then be able to predict and explain variation in performance. This should apply to a wide range of contexts whether the goal is to teach patients with diabetes to understand the basic physiology of their disease or clinicians to use a newly implemented EHR. There is also evidence to suggest that a model-centric approach to teaching, in which an effort is made to foster an understanding of how a system works, confers some advantages over rote learning approaches in which the goal is to acquire the procedures needed to complete a task [28, 41].

External Cognition

Internal representations reflect mental states that correspond to the external world. The term external representation refers to any object in the external world that has the potential to be internalized or to be used to augment cognitive processes (without internalizing). External representations such as images, graphs, icons, audible sounds, texts with symbols (e.g., letter and numbers), shapes and textures are vital sources of knowledge, means of communication and cultural transmission. The classical model of information-processing cognition viewed external representations as mere inputs to the mind that were processed and then internalized [42]. The landscape began to change in the early 1990s when new cognitive theories focused on interactivity rather than solely modeling what was assumed to happen inside the head. Rogers [4] cites Larkin and Simon's [43] classic paper on "why a diagram may be worth a thousand words" as seminal to researchers in HCI. It offered the first alternative empirical account that focused on how people interact with external representations. The core idea was that cognition can be viewed as the interplay between internal and external representations, rather than only about modeling what was assumed to happen inside the head. Similar ideas had been put forth by others [44], but Larkin and Simon provided an explicit computational account that inspired the HCI community [4]. Larkin and Simon [43] made an important distinction between two kinds of external representation: diagrammatic and sentential representations. Although they are informationally equivalent, they are considered to be computationally different. That is, they contain the same information about the problem but the amount of cognitive effort required to come to the solution differs. For example, effective displays facilitate problem solving by allowing users to substitute perceptual operations (i.e., recognition) for effortful cognitive operations (e.g., memory retrieval and computationally-intensive reasoning) and effective displays can reduce the amount of time spent searching for critical information [45]. On the other hand, cluttered or poorly organized displays may increase the burden.

In the next two sections, we consider two extensions of external cognition, namely, the representational effect and the theory of intelligent spaces.

Representational Effect

The representational effect can be construed as a generalization of Larkin and Simon's [43] conceptualization of the cognitive impact of external representations [46]. It is well-known that different representations of a common abstract structure can have a significant impact on cognition [46, 47]. For example, different forms of displaying patients' medications can be more or less efficient for tasks [48]. A display may be oriented to support a quick readout of discrete values or alternatively, one that allows clinician to discern trends over a period of time. A simple illustration of the effect is that Arabic numerals are more efficient for arithmetic calculations (e.g., 26 x 92) than Roman numerals (XXVI x XCII) even though the representations are identical in meaning. Similarly, a digital clock provides a quick readout for precisely determining the time at a glance [49]. On the other hand, an analog clock enables one to more easily determine time intervals (e.g., elapsed or remaining time) without recourse to mental calculations. Norman [49] proposed that external representations play a critical role in enhancing cognition and intelligent behavior. These durable representations (at least those that are visible) persist in the external world and are continuously available to augment memory, reasoning, and computation. Imagine the cognitive burden of having to do multi-digit multiplication without the use of external aids. Even a pencil and paper will allow you to hold partial results (interim calculations) externally. Calculations can be extremely computationally intensive without recourse to external representations (or memory aids).

Zhang and colleagues [42, 50, 51] summarized the following properties of external representations:

- Provide memory aids so that cognitive load can be reduced.
- Provide information that can be directly perceived and used such that minimal processing is needed to explicitly interpret the information.
- Support perception so that one can recognize features easily and make inferences directly.
- Structure cognitive behavior without cognitive awareness
- Change the nature of a task by generating more efficient action sequences.

Several researchers have described the mediating role of information technology on clinical reasoning. For example, Kushniruk et al. [52] studied how clinicians learned to use an EHR over multiple sessions. They found that as users familiarized themselves with the system, their sequential information-gathering and reasoning strategies were driven by the organization of information on the user interface. In other words, the users followed a "screen-driven" strategy when taking a medical history from a patient. This had both positive consequences in that it promoted a more thorough consideration of the patient history, as well as negative consequences in that the clinician failed to search for findings not available on the display or inconsistent with their operative diagnostic hypothesis. In general, a screen-driven strategy can enhance performance by reducing the cognitive load imposed by information-gathering goals and enable the physician to allocate more cognitive resources toward patient evaluation [45]. On the other hand, this strategy can induce a certain sense of complacency or excessive reliance on the display to guide the process.

Similar results were found by Patel et al. [53] in a study contrasting the use of EHRs with paper records in a diabetic clinic setting. For example, physicians entered significantly more information about the patient's chief complaint using the EHR similarly following a screen-driven strategy. Likewise, the structure of the paper records document was such that physicians represented more information about the history of present illness and review of systems using paper-based records. The introduction of an EHR changed information-gathering and documentation strategies, thereby changing the information representation and meaning. The effects of the EHR persisted even after the re-introduction of paper records.

External representations can mediate cognition in a number of ways with both positive and negative impact. The following real-world example was drawn from a study related to a comprehensive causal analysis of a medication dosing error, in which an overdose of Potassium Chloride (KCl) was administered through a commercial computer order entry system (CPOE) in an ICU [54]. The authors' detailed analysis included the use of inspection of system logs, interviews with clinicians and a cognitive evaluation of the order-entry system involved. For the purpose of this paper, we highlight one element of the error to illustrate the interplay between technology and user interaction for clinical decision-making. In this case, the system provided screen order entry forms for medication with intravenous drip and IV bolus orders that were superficially similar, yet required different calculations to estimate the dose. In this case, orders for IV bolus were specified by dose. In contrast, orders for other intravenous drip administration were indicated by duration, rather than by volume of administered fluid as suggested by the order-entry field "Total Volume." The latter referred to the size of the IV bag rather than the total amount of fluid to be delivered, which may exceed the volume indicated. In addition, intravenous fluid orders were not displayed on the medication review screen, further complicating the task of calculating an appropriate KCl bolus for a patient receiving intravenous medications. Calculating the correct infusion dosage was a vitally important task. However, not only did the interface not provide tools to facilitate this process, but also proved to be an obstacle.

It is well documented that IV medication errors commonly result in potentially harmful events [52, 53]. The configuration of external resources or representations, for example on a visual display, can have a significant impact on how the system facilitates (or alternatively, hinders) cognition. Critical care settings are immensely complex environments and medical error can be the product of a host of factors including workflow and communication [55–57]. As discussed in subsequent sections, the organization of displays are just one of several facets that mediate interaction.

Intelligent Use of Space

Theories of external cognition tend to emphasize the computational offloading that eases the cognitive burden of a user. However, external representations can also be manipulated by individuals in a variety of ways to facilitate creative thinking as well [4, 46, 58]. According to Kirsh, "cognitive processes flow to wherever it is cheaper to perform them. The human 'cognitive operating system' extends to states, structures, and processes outside the mind and body" [59] (p. 172). For example, one may choose to create a diagram to help interpret a complex sentence and that will alleviate some of the cognitive burden of sense-making. Kirsch draws on a range of examples, in illustration, how people follow a cooking recipe by arranging and rearranging items (e.g., utensils and ingredients) to coordinate their activities. The central premise is that people interact and create external structure (or representations) because through these interactions, it is easier to process more efficiently and more effectively than by working inside the head alone. In essence, individuals are able to improve their thinking and comprehension by creating and using external representations [59].

Kirsh [60] studied how individuals restructured their environments when performing a range of tasks. He found that they constantly rearrange items to track the task state, support memory, predict effects of actions, and so forth. Restructuring often can reduce the cost of visual search, make it easier to notice, identify and remember items, and simplify task representation [61]. The theory of intelligent spaces is an extension of this idea. Kirsh classified intelligent uses of space into three categories: (1) arrangements that simplify choice, (2) arrangements that simplify perception (e.g., calling attention to a group of items), and (3) spatial dynamics that simplify mental computation. The theory of intelligent spaces suggests that the idiosyncratic arrangements of individuals including clinicians may serve to simplify inferences or computations. The theory is potentially extensible across a range of domains including health information technology (HIT).

Although EHRs are very elaborate complex systems that support a wide range of functions, they often fail to support the varied needs of healthcare practitioners. Systems often fail to take into consideration the significant variability of medical information needs, which differ according to setting, specialty, role, individual patient and institution [62]. In addition, they are not responsive to the highly collaborative nature of the work. In response to these challenges, Senathirajah and colleagues [61, 62] developed a new model for health information systems, embodied in MedWISE, a widget-based highly configurable EHR platform. MedWISE supports drag/drop user configurations and the sharing of user-created elements such as custom laboratory result panels and user-created interface tabs. It was hypothesized that such a system could afford the clinician greater flexibility and better fit to the tasks they were required to perform. The intelligent spaces theoretical framework informed the design of MedWISE.

In an experiment conducted by Senathirajah et al. [62], 13 clinicians used the MedWISE system to review four patient cases. The data included video recordings of clinicians' interactions with the system and the screen layouts they created via the drag/drop capabilities. The focus here was on the creation of spatial layouts. The study documented three strategies which were labeled "opportunistic selection" (rapidly gathering items on the screen and reviewing), structured (organizing the layout categorically) and "dynamic stage" approach. The latter approach involved the user interacting with small groups of widgets at a time, using the space as a staging area to examine a specific concern and then shift to the next. An example of dynamic stage approach was that the clinician kept the index note (initial note) open at the bottom of column 2 (middle column) and stacked the unexamined labs and reports, closed, in column 1 (leftmost column), opened them in column 2 to compare them with the index note, and closed and moved them to column 3. This interaction pattern could reflect examination of specific diagnostic concerns (e.g., ruling out a diagnostic hypothesis). An example of the structured approach is indicated in Fig. 2.3. The clinician has stated that he is keeping the right side as a free space for thinking space, for studies, and for to-do items. A to-do list is at upper right (in the yellow sticky note), while orienting items including the primary provider clinic note is at left, with lab data down the middle. This reflects a common pattern found of going from left to right with orienting material, data, and then action items. The clinician has grouped labs according to related diagnostic facets, for example, the HbA1c and micro albumin (diabetes-related) are together, and then thyroid-related results (TSH, T3 and T4) are grouped at the bottom of the center column.

The clinicians employed spatial arrangement in ways consistent with theory and research on workplace spatial arrangement [62]. This includes assignment of screen regions for particular purposes, juxtaposition of elements to facilitate calculation (e.g., ratios), and grouping elements with common meanings or relevance to the diagnostic facets of the case (e.g., thyroid findings). Clinicians also made deliberate

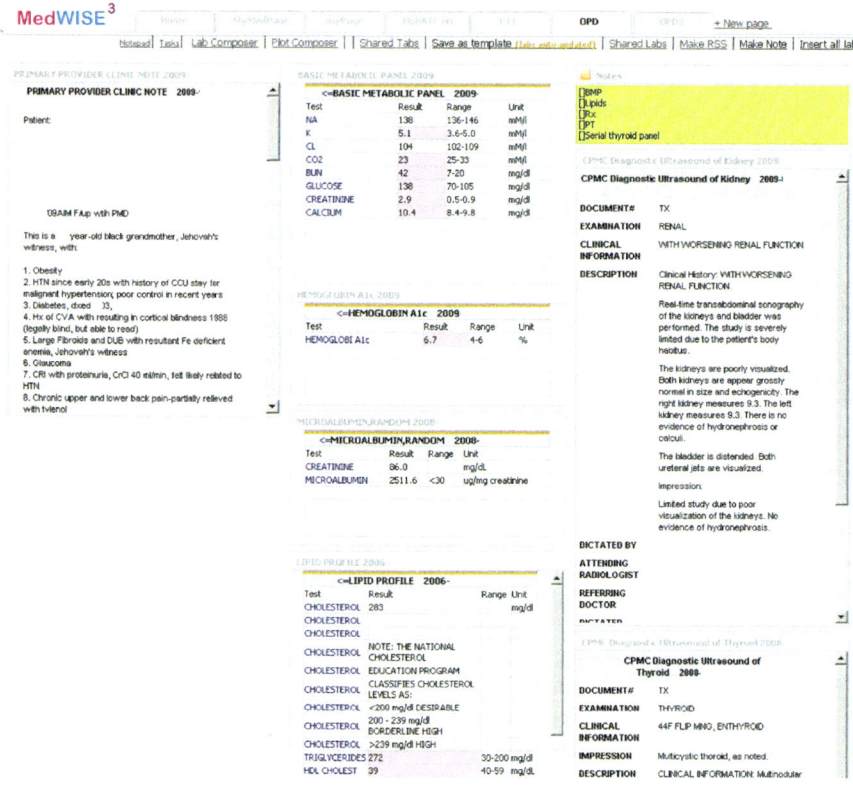

Fig. 2.3 An illustration of a physician using a structured approach in MedWISE. Reproduced with permissions from MedWISE

use of the space following a common pattern of left-to-right progression of orienting materials, data, and action items or reflection space. Widget selection was based on an assessment of what information was useful or relevant immediately or likely to be in the near future (as more information is gathered). The study demonstrated how a user-composable EHR in which users have substantial control over how a display is populated and arranged can embody the advantages predicted by the intelligent use of space theory.

The external cognition framework has introduced a set of concepts that has enabled researchers and designers to characterize designs in ways not previously accessible to them [4]. As evidenced in the work on MedWISE, it provided a language that framed how people manipulate representations, interact with objects, and organize their space. This provides a basis for designing tools that facilitate different kinds of interaction. It also suggests that there are more and less optimal ways to configure a display for particular tasks and that the impact of such configurations are measurable.

Distributed Cognition

The external cognition framework seeded important design concepts. It also provides a means to engage in a more rigorous approach to evaluation. The distributed cognition (DCog) approach takes the argument further beyond the internal-external representation divide [4]. DCog re-conceptualizes cognitive phenomena in terms of individuals, artifacts, and internal and external representations and their interactions [4]. It provides a more extensive account than external cognition. The fundamental approach involves describing a "cognitive system," which encompasses the dynamic interactions among individuals, the artifacts they utilize, and the environment in which they are situated. Hutchins and colleagues proposed a new paradigm for fundamentally rethinking our assumptions about cognition [63].

DCog represents a shift in the study of cognition from an exclusive focus on the mind of the individual to being "stretched" across groups, material artifacts and cultures [63, 64]. This paradigm has gained substantial currency in HCI research. In the distributed approach, cognition is viewed as a process of coordinating distributed internal (i.e., what's in the mind) and external representations (e.g., visual displays, post-it notes, paper records). Distributed cognition has two focal points of inquiry, one that emphasizes the inherently social and collaborative nature of cognition (e.g., attending physicians, residents, nurses and respiratory therapists in cardiothoracic intensive care unit jointly contributing to a decision process), and one that characterizes the mediating effects of technology (e.g., EHRs, mobile devices apps) or other artifacts on cognition.

Hollan et al. [65] emphasize that distributed cognition is more than the social distribution of cognitive processes; rather it is a broader conceptualization that includes emergent phenomena in social interactions as well as interactions between people and the structure of their environment. According to Hollan et al., the perspective "highlights three fundamental questions about social interactions: (1) how are the cognitive processes we normally associate with an individual mind implemented in a group of individuals, (2) how do the cognitive properties of groups differ from the cognitive properties of the people who act in those groups, and (3) how are the cognitive properties of individual minds affected by participation in group activities?" [65] (p. 177).

DCog is concerned with representational states and the informational flows around the media carrying these representations [66]. The framework enables researchers to consider all factors relevant to a task, coalescing individuals, the problem and the tools into a single unit of analysis. This makes it a productive means to develop an understanding of how representations act as intermediaries in the dynamically changing and coordinated processes of work activities [63].

Hutchins' [63] seminal analysis of ship navigation of a U.S. navy vessel provided a compelling account of how crews took the ships bearing and how this information was interpreted processed, and transformed across representational states (embodied in media and technology such as ship navigation instruments like the ship's compass and communication among interdependent actors that constitute the ship's crew). The succession of states resulted in the determination of a ship's location, progress and how they could be aligned with intended trajectories. The entities operating within the functional system are not viewed from the perspective of the individual, but as a collective [66]. Both people and artifacts are considered as representational components of the system. As should be clear at this point, external representations are not mere inputs or stimuli to the mind but play a more instrumental role in cognition.

In the next sections, we review two extensions of DCog including the distributed resource model and the propagation of representational states.

Distributed Resources Model

One of the strengths of the DCog, as applied to HCI, is that it can be used to understand how properties of objects on the screen (e.g., links, menus) can serve as external representations and reduce cognitive load. Wright et al. [67] proposed a distributed resources model to address the question of the information needed to carry out a task and where it should be located: as an interface object or as knowledge that a user brings to the task. The relative difference in the distribution of representations is pivotal in determining the efficacy of a system designed to support a complex task such as computer provider entry [68]. The distributed resources model includes two primary components. The first is a characterization of information structures (i.e., resource types), pertaining to the control of action and the second is a process-oriented description of how these information structures can be used for action (interaction strategies) to complete a task. The information structures can be embodied in any artifact (e.g., paper charts or an EHR). Wright et al. enumerated several of these information structures including plans, goals, history and state. Plans include possible sequence of actions, events, and anticipated states. Goals refer to the desired states the user wants to accomplish. They may be generated internally or emerge from the interaction with the system. History refers to the part of a plan that has already been accomplished. The history of past actions may be maintained in a web browser, for example, as a list of previously visited pages that can be accessed via a drop-down list. State is the current configuration of resources, for example, as represented in the display screen at a given point in time. These are all considered to be resources for action rather than static structures. They can be externalized, manipulated and subjected to evaluation [64].

Horsky et al. [68] employed the distributed resource model to investigate the usability of a CPOE system. The goal was to analyze order-entry tasks and to identify areas of complexity that may impede performance. The research consisted of two component analyses: a cognitive walkthrough evaluation that was modified based on the distributed resource model and an experiment involving a simulated clinical ordering task performed by seven physicians who were experienced users of the CPOE. The walkthrough analysis revealed that the configuration of resources (e.g., very long menus and complexly configured screens) placed an unnecessarily heavy cognitive load on the user. In addition, successful interaction was too often dependent on the recall of system-related knowledge. The resources model was also used to explain patterns of errors produced by clinicians including, selecting an inappropriate order set, omissions and redundant entries. The authors concluded that the reconfiguration of resources may yield guiding principles and design solutions in the development of complex interactive systems [65]. In addition, system design that better reflects the constraints of the task (e.g., hospital admission) and domain (e.g., internal medicine) may minimize the need for more robust mental models or extensive system knowledge.

Propagation of Representational States

Horsky et al. conducted a DCog analysis that emphasized the technology-mediating effects of a CPOE interface on clinical performance. Hazlehurst and colleagues [69] emphasize both the socially-distributed nature and mediating impact of artifacts on communication during cardiac surgery. Towards that end, they employed a cognitive ethnography method to understand how system resources are configured and used for cardiac surgery and to prevent adverse events. DCog focuses on the activity system as the unit of analysis and seeks to understand how properties of this system determine performance [63, 66, 69].

Following Hutchins [63], Hazlehurt views the 'propagation of representational states' through activity systems as explanatory of cognitive behavior and sought to investigate the organizing features of this propagation as an explanation of system and human performance [69]. Accordingly, "a representational state is a particular configuration of an information-bearing structure, such as a monitor display, a verbal utterance, or a printed label, that plays some functional role in a process within the system [69] (p. 540)". They identified six patterns of communication between surgeon and perfusionist that relate to the functional properties of the activity system. For example, *direction* is a pattern that seeks to transition the activity system to a new state (e.g., administering medications that affect blood coagulation). *Goal sharing* involves creating an expectation of a desired future, but not specifically the action sequence necessary to achieve the target state. These patterns of communication serve to enhance situation awareness, for example, by making the current situation clear and mutually understood.

The distributed cognition approach has been widely used in HCI to examine existing practices and workflow [4]. It has also been used to inform the iterative design process by characterizing how the quality and configuration of resources and representations might be transformed and how this change may impact work practices. It is an approach that is inherently well suited to a complex, media-rich and collaborative domain such as medicine. However, a distributed cognitive analysis can be extremely difficult to conduct (requiring substantial specialized knowledge of the analytic approach as well as the knowledge domain), rather complex and very time consuming. In the next section, we describe an approach which endeavors to make the DCog approach more tractable and bring it closer to the design process [70].

Distributed Cognition of Teamwork (DiCoT)

DCog's has developed a rather comprehensive and penetrating approach to understanding the different dimensions of human-computer interaction. However, there is no 'off-the-shelf' methodology for using it in research or as a practitioner [68]. According to Rogers, the application of DCog theory and methods are complicated by the fact that there are no set of features to attend to and no checklist or prescribed method to follow [4]. In addition, the analysis and abstraction requires a very high level of skill. However, there have been various structured approaches to gathering and analyzing data including the Distributed Resources (DR) Model [67] described in a previous section. DiCoT (Distributed Cognition for Teamwork) was developed to provide a structured approach to analyze work systems and teamwork [68, 69] The approach is informed by theoretical principles from the DCog literature.

The DiCoT framework focuses on developing five interdependent models with different foci: artifacts, physical, information flow, social and evolutionary [71]. Each of the models is informed by a set of principles. For example, the artifacts model includes the premise that mediating artifacts are brought into coordination (e.g., paper and electronic health records) in the completion of a task. A second principle is reflected in the fact that we use our environment continuously by "creating scaffolding" to simplify cognitive tasks [65]. The physical model refers to the physical organization of work. It is guided by principles such as space and cognition, which states how humans manipulate space towards the facilitation of decision making or problem solving (e.g., grouping objects into categories). This is similar to the intelligent uses of space [60]. Information transformation is one of the principles of information flow. It suggests that transformation occurs when the representation of information changes. As described previously, more effective representations provide better support for reasoning.

DiCoT has been used to analyze complex systems in a range of healthcare contexts including ambulance control room dispatch [72] and infusion pump use in intensive care [73]. Emergency medical dispatch (EMD) is constituted by a team that coordinates the delivery of services (e.g., dispatching an ambulance) to respond to a call for medical assistance. Furniss and Blandford [72] conducted a study of an EMD team using the DiCoT approach. The focus was on describing the work system, identifying sources of weakness and projecting the likely consequences of a redesign (e.g., what is likely to happen when a centrally available shared display is visible or accessible to each member of the team). On the basis of characterizing systemic weaknesses, they suggested changes to the physical layout that could enhance "cross-boundary working". Their observations revealed a discontinuity between the central ambulance control and the crews in the field. In response, Furniss and Blandford [72] proposed the use of more flexible communication channels so the crew could be contacted whether they are at a station or are mobile. The multifaceted model enables the researchers to envision a set of consequences to the redesign scheme along a range of dimensions (e.g., information flow). Clinical practitioners and other stakeholders review and comment on the concrete redesign solutions. Drawing on a similar approach, Rajkomar and Blandford [73] used the DiCot model to study the use of infusion pumps by nurses in an Intensive Care Unit. The investigators constructed representational models using the with a specific focus on information flows, physical layouts, social structures, and artifacts. The findings reveal a significant distribution of cognition within the ICU setting, socially among nurses, as well as physically through the environment and technological artifacts present.

The DCog framework, which incorporates a number of interrelated theories, offers the most comprehensive and in our view, the most compelling theoretical approach to explain the technology-mediated and social/collaborative nature of clinical work. Each theory with this framework privileges different aspects of interactions. The methods identified areas of improvements that could increase patient safety and workflow efficiency.

Conclusions

It is reasonable to conclude that we need a theory (or theories) of cognition in the context of HCI and health care. Although we have learned much from empirical studies and applied work, a theoretical framework is needed to account for the broad scope of the field and the complexity that is inherent in the domain of medicine. Without a sound theoretical framework, generalizations would be limited, and principled approaches to design would be largely illusory. In this chapter, we traced the evolution of cognitive theory from the classical information-processing approach to external cognition through distributed cognition. The information-processing approach drew extensively on concepts from cognitive psychology and embraced a computational approach to the study of interaction. The MHP theory [18] provides insight into cognitive processes and provides a predictive model of behavior, albeit one that is limited in scope. Norman's theory of action [20] offers an explanatory account of the challenges involved in using systems. It also offers general prescriptions, for example, emphasizing the importance of quality feedback to the user. The theory of mental models as applied to HCI builds on the idea of gulfs to further explicate the kinds of knowledge needed to productively use a system. It also broadly prescribes how to narrow the divide between designer models and users' mental models. Although these theories are inherently incomplete in their focus on the solitary individual, they continue to be productive as explanatory theories of HCI.

Theories of external cognition expanded the scope of analysis to include a focus on external representations. Several studies have demonstrated how representations mediate cognition and how differential mediation (as reflected in display configurations) can contribute to medical errors. The theory of intelligent spaces [60] is a generative theory, which seeded concepts that were realized in the design of the MedWISE system. DCog theories are the most encompassing in their focus on both technology-mediated and socially distributed cognition. The theories offer rich descriptive and explanatory accounts of technology use in the medical workplace. Distributed resource theory [67] works both as a descriptive theory characterizing the state of affairs and a prescriptive theory that can be used to reconfigure interfaces to alleviate some of the cognitive burden on users. Significant challenges remain in the domain of health information technology. The increasing presence of AI in healthcare, the ubiquity of mobile phones and the expanded use of medical devices greatly advance the capability of users and present opportunities for theory-driven user-centered design to further enhance their experience. While cognitive theory may not offer all-encompassing solutions, it remains a potent tool for advancing knowledge and propelling scientific inquiry and its associated practical applications.

Discussion Questions
1. What role can cognitive theory play in HCI research and application? Describe the different kinds of theories that can inform HCI in practice situations.
2. Explain the gulfs of execution and evaluation and how they can be used to inform HCI design.
3. Mental models are an analog-based construct for describing how individuals form internal models of systems. Explain what is meant by analog. How can mental models inform our understanding of the user experience?
4. Describe the meaning and significance of the representational effect. How can it influence the design of visual displays to represent lab results?
5. What implications can one draw from the theory of intelligent spaces? How can it be used to seed design concepts in health care?
6. What are the essential differences between theories of external representation and theories of distributed cognition?

References

1. Patel V, Kaufman D. Cognitive science, and biomedical informatics. In: Shortliffe EHC, Cimino JJ, Chiang M, editors. Biomedical informatics. 4th ed. Basel: Springer; 2021. p. 122–53.
2. Grudin J. A moving target: the evolution of human-computer interaction. In: The human-computer interaction handbook–fundamentals, evolving technologies, and emerging applications. Mahwah, NJ: Erlbaum Associates; 2008. p. 1–24.
3. Rogers Y. New theoretical approaches for human-computer interaction. Annu Rev Inf Sci Technol. 2004;38(1):87–143.
4. Rogers Y. HCI theory: classical, modern, and contemporary. Synth Lect Hum-Centered Inform. 2012;5(2):1–129.
5. Lee S. AI as an explanation agent and user-centered explanation interfaces for trust in AI-based systems. In: Nam CS, Jung JY, Lee S, editors. Human-centered artificial intelligence. Academic Press; 2022. p. 91–102. https://doi.org/10.1016/B978-0-323-85648-5.00014-1.

6. Bederson BB, Shneiderman B. The craft of information visualization: readings and reflections. Morgan Kaufmann; 2003.
7. Anderson JR. The architecture of cognition. Cambridge, MA: Cambridge University Press; 1983.
8. Kannampallil TG, et al. Considering complexity in healthcare systems. J Biomed Inform. 2011;44(6):943–7.
9. Patel VL, Groen GJ. Cognitive framework for clinical reasoning: application for training and practice. In: Evans DA, Patel VL, editors. Advanced models of cognition for medical training and practice. Heidelberg: Springer-Verlag GmbH; 1992. p. 193–212.
10. Anderson JR. Cognitive psychology and its implications. Macmillan; 2005.
11. Mackenzie IS. Fitts' law as a research and design tool in human-computer interaction. Hum-Comput Interact. 1992;7(1):91–139.
12. Mackenzie IS. Motor behavior models for human-computer interaction. In: Carroll JM, editor. HCI models, theories, and frameworks: toward a multidisciplinary science. San Francisco, CA: Morgan Kaufmann; 2003.
13. Chakraborty P, Yadav S. Applicability of Fitts' law to interaction with touchscreen: review of experimental results. Theor Issues Ergon Sci. 2023;24(5):532–46.
14. Clark LD, Bhagat AB, Riggs SL. Extending Fitts' law in three-dimensional virtual environments with current low-cost virtual reality technology. Int J Hum-Comput Stud. 2020;139:102413.
15. Lin CJ, Ho S-H. Prediction of the use of mobile device interfaces in the progressive aging process with the model of Fitts' law. J Biomed Inform. 2020;107:103457.
16. John BE. Information processing and skilled behavior. In: Carroll JM, editor. HCI models, theories and frameworks: towards a multidisciplinary science. San Francisco, CA: Morgan Kaufmann; 2003. p. 55–102.
17. Duncan BJ, Kaufman DR, Zheng L, et al. A microanalytic approach to understanding EHR navigation paths. J Biomed Inform. 2020;110:103566.
18. Card SK, Newell A, Moran TP. The psychology of human-computer interaction. New York: L. Erlbaum Associates; 1983.
19. Saitwal H, Feng X, Walji M, Patel V, Zhang J. Assessing performance of an electronic health record (EHR) using cognitive task analysis. Int J Med Inform. 2010;79(7):501–6.
20. Norman DA. Cognitive engineering. In: Norman DA, Draper SW, editors. User centered system design. Hillsdale, NJ: Erlbaum Associates; 1986. p. 31–61.
21. Shneiderman B. The future of interactive systems and the emergence of direct manipulation. Behav Inform Technol. 1982;1(3):237–56.
22. Zhang J, Patel VL, Johnson TR, Shortliffe EH. A cognitive taxonomy of medical error. J Biomed Inform. 2004;37(3):193–204.
23. Reason J. Human error. Cambridge, UK: Cambridge University Press; 1992.
24. Guffroy M, Nadine V, Kolski C, Vella F, Teutsch P. From human-centered design to disabled user & ecosystem centered design in case of assistive interactive systems. Int J Sociotechnol Knowl Dev (IJSKD). 2017;9(4):28–42.
25. Sharp H, Rogers Y, Preece J. Interaction design: beyond human-computer interaction. New York: Wiley; 2007.
26. Van der Veer GC, Melguizo P. Mental models. In: Sears A, Jacko JA, editors. The human-computer interaction handbook: fundamentals, evolving technologies, and emerging applications. Mahwah, NJ: Erlbaum Associates; 2003. p. 58–80.
27. Norman DA. Some observations on mental models. In: Gentner D, Stevens AL, editors. Mental models. Hillsdale, NJ: Erlbaum Associates; 1983. p. 7–14.
28. Payne SJ. Users' mental models: the very ideas. In: Carroll JM, editor. HCI models, theories, and frameworks: toward a multidisciplinary science. San Francisco, CA: Morgan Kaufmann; 2003. p. 135–56.
29. White BY, Frederiksen JR. Causal model progressions as a foundation for intelligent learning environments. Artif Intell. 1990;42(1):99–157.

30. Staggers N, Norcio AF. Mental models: concepts for human-computer interaction research. Int J Man-Mach Stud. 1993;38(4):587–605.
31. Kaufman DR, Patel VL, Hilliman C, et al. Usability in the real world: assessing medical information technologies in patients' homes. J Biomed Inform. 2003;36(1):45–60.
32. Halasz FG, Moran TP. Mental models and problem solving in using a calculator. Paper presented at: Proceedings of the SIGCHI Conference on Human Factors in Computing Systems. ACM; 1983.
33. Kieras DE, Bovair S. The role of a mental model in learning to operate a device. Cogn Sci. 1984;8(3):255–73.
34. Smith SW, Koppel R. Healthcare information technology's relativity problems: a typology of how patients' physical reality, clinicians' mental models, and healthcare information technology differ. J Am Med Inform Assoc. 2014;21(1):117–31.
35. Cho J. Mental models and home virtual assistants (HVAs). Paper presented at: Extended Abstracts of the 2018 CHI Conference on Human Factors in Computing Systems. 2018.
36. Zhou J, Chourasia A, Vanderheiden G. Interface adaptation to novice older adults' mental models through concrete metaphors. Int J Hum–Comput Interact. 2017;33(7):592–606.
37. Orasanu JM. Shared mental models and crew decision making (CSL tech. rep. no. 46). Princeton, NJ: Princeton University, Cognitive Sciences Laboratory; 1990.
38. Coiera E. When conversation is better than computation. J Am Med Inform Assoc. 2000;7(3):277–86.
39. Custer JW, et al. A qualitative study of expert and team cognition on complex patients in the pediatric intensive care unit. Pediatr Crit Care Med. 2012;13(3):278–84.
40. Mamykina L, Hum RS, Kaufman DR. Investigating shared mental models in critical care. In: Patel VL, Kaufman DR, Cohen T, editors. Cognitive informatics in health and biomedicine. New York: Springer; 2014. p. 291–315.
41. Gott SP, Lesgold AM. Competence in the workplace: how cognitive performance models and situated instruction can accelerate skill acquisition. In: Glaser R, editor. Advances in instructional psychology: educational design and cognitive science. Mahwah, NJ: Erlbaum Associates; 2000. p. 239–327.
42. Zhang J. The nature of external representations in problem solving. Cogn Sci. 1997;21(2):179–217.
43. Larkin JH, Simon HA. Why a diagram is (sometimes) worth ten thousand words. Cogn Sci. 1987;11(1):65–100.
44. Hutchins EL, Hollan JD, Norman DA. Direct manipulation interfaces. Hum–Comput Interact. 1985;1(4):311–38.
45. Patel VL, Kaufman DR. Cognitive science and biomedical informatics. In: Shortliffe EH, Cimino JJ, editors. Biomedical informatics: computer applications in health care and biomedicine. New York: Springer; 2014. p. 133–85.
46. Zhang J, Norman DA. Representations in distributed cognitive tasks. Cogn Sci. 1994;18(1):87–122.
47. Kahneman D. Thinking, fast and slow. New York: McMillan Farrar, Straus and Giroux; 2011.
48. Duncan BJ, Zheng L, Furniss SK, et al. Perioperative medication management: reconciling differences across clinical sites. Paper presented at: Proceedings of the International Symposium on Human Factors and Ergonomics in Health Care. New Delhi: Sage India. 2018
49. Norman DA. Cognition in the head and in the world: an introduction to the special issue on situated action. Cogn Sci. 1993;17(1):1–6.
50. Zhang J, Johnson KA, Malin JT, Smith JW. Human-centered information visualization. Paper presented at: International Workshop on Dynamic Visualizations and Learning, Tubingen, Germany.
51. Zhang J, Patel VL. Distributed cognition, representation, and affordance. Pragmat Cogn. 2006;14(2):333–41.

52. Kushniruk AW, Kaufman DR, Patel VL, Lévesque Y, Lottin P. Assessment of a computerized patient record system: a cognitive approach to evaluating medical technology. MD Comput. 1996;13(5):406–15.
53. Patel VL, Kushniruk AW, Yang S, Yale JF. Impact of a computer-based patient record system on data collection, knowledge organization, and reasoning. J Am Med Inform Assoc. 2000;7(6):569–85.
54. Horsky J, Kuperman GJ, Patel VL. Comprehensive analysis of a medication dosing error related to CPOE. J Am Med Inform Assoc. 2005;12(4):377–82.
55. Taxis K, Barber N. Causes of intravenous medication errors: an ethnographic study. Qual Saf Health Care. 2003;12(5):343–7.
56. Husch M, Sullivan C, Rooney D, et al. Insights from the sharp end of intravenous medication errors: implications for infusion pump technology. Qual Saf Health Care. 2005;14(2):80–6.
57. Patel VL, Kaufman DR, Cohen T, editors. Cognitive informatics in health and biomedicine: case studies on critical care, complexity and errors. London: Springer; 2014.
58. Kirsh D. Metacognition, distributed cognition and visual design. In: Gardenfors P, Johansson P, editors. Cognition, education, and communication technology. London: Routledge; 2005. p. 147–80.
59. Kirsh D. Thinking with external representations. AI Soc. 2010;25:441–54.
60. Kirsh D. The intelligent use of space. Artif Intell. 1995;73(1):31–68.
61. Senathirajah Y, Bakken S, Kaufman D. The clinician in the Driver's Seat: part 1–a drag/drop user-composable electronic health record platform. J Biomed Inform. 2014;52:165–76.
62. Senathirajah Y, Kaufman D, Bakken S. The clinician in the Driver's Seat: part 2–intelligent uses of space in a drag/drop user-composable electronic health record. J Biomed Inform. 2014;52:177–88.
63. Hutchins E. Cognition in the wild. Cambridge, MA: MIT press; 1995.
64. Suchman L. Plans and situated actions: the problem of human machine interaction. Cambridge, MA: Cambridge University; 1986.
65. Hollan J, Hutchins E, Kirsh D. Distributed cognition: toward a new foundation for human-computer interaction research. ACM Trans Comput-Hum Interact (TOCHI). 2000;7(2):174–96.
66. Perry M. Distributed cognition. In: Carroll JM, editor. HCI, models, theories, and frameworks: toward a multidisciplinary science. San Francisco, CA: Morgan Kaufmann; 2003. p. 193–223.
67. Wright PC, Fields RE, Harrison MD. Analyzing human-computer interaction as distributed cognition: the resources model. Hum-Comput Interact. 2000;15(1):1–41.
68. Horsky J, Kaufman DR, Oppenheim MI, Patel VL. A framework for analyzing the cognitive complexity of computer-assisted clinical ordering. J Biomed Inform. 2003;36(1–2):4–22.
69. Hazlehurst B, McMullen CK, Gorman PN. Distributed cognition in the heart room: how situation awareness arises from coordinated communications during cardiac surgery. J Biomed Inform. 2007;40(5):539–51.
70. Blandford D, Furniss D. DiCoT: a methodology for applying distributed cognition to the design of teamworking systems. In: Gilroy SW, Harrison MD, editors. Interactive systems: design, specification, and verification. Berlin: Springer; 2006. p. 26–38.
71. Furniss D, Masci P, Curzon P, Mayer A, Blandford A. Exploring medical device design and use through layers of distributed cognition: how a glucometer is coupled with its context. J Biomed Inform. 2015;53:330–41.
72. Furniss D, Blandford A. Understanding emergency medical dispatch in terms of distributed cognition: a case study. Ergonomics. 2006;49(12–13):1174–203.
73. Rajkomar A, Blandford A. Understanding infusion administration in the ICU through distributed Cognition. J Biomed Inform. 2012;45(3):580–90.

Further Reading

Carroll JM. HCI models, theories, and frameworks: toward a multidisciplinary science. San Francisco, CA: Morgan Kaufmann; 2003.

Patel VL, Kaufman DR. Cognitive science and biomedical informatics. In: Shortliffe EH, Cimino JJ, editors. Biomedical informatics: computer applications in health care and biomedicine. New York: Springer; 2014. p. 133–85.

Patel VL, Kaufman DR. Cognitive science and biomedical informatics. In: Shortliffe EH, Cimino JJ, Chiang M, editors. Biomedical informatics: computer applications in health care and biomedicine. 5th ed. New York: Springer-Verlag; 2021. p. 121–52.

Rogers Y. HCI theory: classical, modern, and contemporary. Synth Lect Hum-Centered Inform. 2012;5(2):1–129.

Chapter 3
Theoretical Foundations for Health Communication Research and Practice

Daniel G. Morrow and Karen Dunn Lopez

Introduction

At first glance, communication among clinicians may seem to be the least complicated component of the health care domain, which involves providing care for a wide variety of illnesses, disease intensity, age groups using an array of low and high technology diagnostics and treatment, and a continually mounting base of clinical evidence. Yet, there is growing evidence that points to serious problems in communication within health care. Annually, at least 98,000 deaths are attributed to errors in health care [1, 2], with an estimated 60% attributed to avoidable communication failures [3]. Other research using root cause analysis revealed that approximately 70% of sentinel events (serious negative consequences involving the unexpected occurrence or risk of death or serious injury) are caused by poor communication [4] and that poor information sharing and coordination is linked to patient mortality in multiple settings [5–8]. These findings should not be surprising given the evidence that miscommunication is an important contributor to errors in other complex and high stakes domains such as aviation [9].

These failures are brought about by multiple challenges of communicating in the high stakes health care domain. A key challenge is the high cognitive demands associated with managing biological complexity in health care. This task requires interpreting and sharing uncertain and dynamic patient information, including frequent

---

D. G. Morrow (✉)
Department of Educational Psychology, University of Illinois at Urbana-Champaign, Champaign, IL, USA
e-mail: dgm@illinois.edu

K. D. Lopez
University of Iowa, College of Nursing, Iowa City, IA, USA
e-mail: karen-dunn-lopez@uiowa.edu

© The Author(s), under exclusive license to Springer Nature Switzerland AG 2024
A. W. Kushniruk et al. (eds.), *Human Computer Interaction in Healthcare*, Cognitive Informatics in Biomedicine and Healthcare, https://doi.org/10.1007/978-3-031-69947-4_3

unplanned and interruptive communication among clinicians from different disciplines who must collaborate despite discipline-specific terminologies and taxonomies. These challenges are exacerbated by rapid diffusion of health information and communication technologies that can increase communication complexity. In addition, the round-the-clock nature of health care requires frequent complete transfer of responsibility for patients within disciplines, or handoffs that increase the number of clinicians from different disciplines who take care of a single patient. The consequences of interdisciplinary communication problems are dire, with poor interdisciplinary communication leading to diagnostic errors up to over 40 per 1000 for patients that experience adverse events [10].

Compounding the aforementioned challenges is the unsustainably high cost of health care, which leads to multiple federal regulations that directly impact how care is delivered [11, 12]. For all these reasons, communication challenges may be even greater in health care than in other domains that involve managing complex engineered systems. For example, in aviation, pilots' interaction with aircraft usually yield predictable consequences with swift feedback, while in health care the effects of clinicians' decisions are much less predictable, with more variable and sometimes delayed feedback [13].

Given the vast differences between patient-provider communication, provider-informal caregiver communication, communication about health in the media, communication within health care organizations between clinicians and non-clinicians, communication between clinicians, and communication across disciplines, we focus our discussion on the communication between clinicians across many disciplines who are involved in direct patient care. Despite the volume of research related to inter-and intra-disciplinary communication in patient care, this work is often not theoretically-based. For example, a systematic review of hand-off communication research found that only 34% of studies were guided by theoretical frameworks ([14]; also see Patterson and Wears [15]). Therefore, we will focus on existing theoretical foundations that can inform research to address these key challenges in health care that hold strong potential for improving the quality and safety of patient care. In the next section, we describe information processing and interactive theories of communication. We then summarize some important challenges related to communication in health care contexts and argue for the importance of communication theory for addressing these challenges. We will suggest several ways that the theories discussed in this chapter can be leveraged to improve clinical work.

Theories of Communication Relevant to Health Care

Several theoretical approaches help identify processes involved in health communication as well as factors that influence these processes and thus the success of communication. In this section, we review approaches that tend to view communication as information processing or communication as interaction, which have influenced research about performance in complex domains such as aviation, and increasingly in health care (Fig. 3.1).

Communication as Information Processing

A longstanding and fruitful approach assumes that communication can be explained in part in terms of mental processes involved in information exchange by producing and understanding messages. This approach has its origins in information theory, developed by Shannon and Weaver [17]. They distinguished the following types of communication:

- Technical communication (how accurately information is encoded, transmitted by sending them through a communication medium or channel, and decoded by interpreting the coded message);
- Semantic communication (how well these codes convey meaning); and
- Communication effectiveness (how well the message has the intended effect).

Information theory most directly addressed the technical level. The approach has been successful in many ways, for example by guiding development of communication technology (e.g., speech synthesis and recognition systems) and explaining some aspects of communication success such as reducing the impact of channel capacity, noise, and related factors on speech comprehension. A good example is provided by radio-based communication in the Air Traffic Control system [18]. Health care as well as other domains have greatly benefited from these improvements because of its reliance on many forms of voice communication (e.g., Interactive Voice Response systems, mobile phones, and dictation systems).

The information processing approach was elaborated during the cognitive revolution in which the mind was understood metaphorically in terms of the computer, and drawing upon linguistic theories of mental structures [19]. Communication was explained in terms of the cognitive processes required to produce and understand linguistic messages, as well as the cognitive abilities and resources that are required by and constrain these processes.

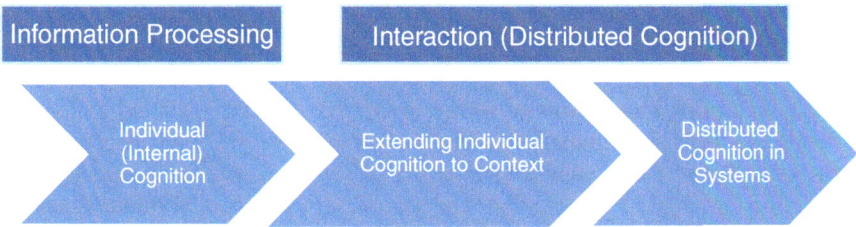

Fig. 3.1 Communication theories relevant to health care (adapted from Morrow [16])

Speakers (or writers) generate ideas by activating concepts in long-term memory and assembling these concepts (and associated words) into ideas (represented as propositions) that are mapped onto syntactic structures to convey the ideas through speech [20]. Word access and propositional encoding processes involved in speech planning are shaped by our cognitive architecture, such as the capacity of working memory, which constrains how much conceptual context can be active at one time, and thus the size of the planning unit, as revealed in patterns of pausing when talking [20]. To understand these messages, listeners (readers) recognize spoken (printed) words, activate the corresponding lexical codes and concepts in long-term memory, and integrate these concepts into propositions or idea units. Understanding extended discourse involves identifying relationships among these ideas, often driven by identifying referents of co-referring expressions and drawing on knowledge to identify temporal, causal, and other relationships among the ideas [21]. Comprehension requires more than assembling concepts into propositions: The network of propositions (the textbase) must be interpreted in terms of what we know about the concepts in order to develop a situation model, or representation of the described events and scenes ([21]; for application to issues of comprehension and knowledge representation in the medical domain, see Patel et al. [22]). Situation models may be concrete, reflecting our perceptual experience of the described situation [23], or more abstract, capturing the essential 'gist' of the message [24]. Understanding as well as producing messages is constrained by limited cognitive resources. For example, readers tend to pause at the end of clauses and sentences, presumably to 'wrap up' conceptual integration, so that the pattern of pausing when reading mirrors the pauses when producing the message [25].

Individual differences in cognitive resources such as working memory capacity help explain differences in successful communication. For example, age differences in understanding complex messages (e.g., conceptually dense text) often reflect age-related differences in cognitive resources [25]. Knowledge, on the other hand, can facilitate comprehension, reducing need for effortful conceptual integration and inference processes [21]. Age differences in comprehension are often reduced for texts that are organized to match knowledge organization [25].

While the information processing approach has been successful both theoretically (supporting a large body of empirical research on language understanding and production processes and how they are shaped by cognitive resources) and practically (e.g., spurring development of communication technology), it is incomplete as an account of communication in complex domains. It is based on and guided by a conduit metaphor of communication, which assumes communication depends on how precisely linguistic codes match speaker ideas and how accurately listeners decode these ideas, or how well they 'take away' the message [26]. Thus, the focus is more on participants' processes and resources than on communication medium, context, and purpose. Although this approach recognizes the importance of pragmatic as well as semantic views of language (e.g., explaining message effectiveness is an important goal of information theory), much of the work within this framework has focused on how people represent message meaning, more than on the actions performed by speakers when using language; e.g., semantic rather than pragmatic effects of discourse [27].

Other theories within this tradition focus on affective as well as cognitive processes in communication, how these processes interact to influence addressees, and how speakers design messages to influence addressee beliefs and actions. For example, the elaboration-likelihood model argues that persuasive effects of messages depend on both a direct route (addressee's deliberative processing of message meaning) and on peripheral routes (addressee's responses to indirect, secondary aspects of the message context) [28]. This research addressed social-psychological problems related to attitude change, but the mechanisms presumed to underlie persuasive effects of messages were similar to information processing models of text processing. Similarly, cognitive models of risk communication focus both on how addressees represent message meaning and how these representations interact with beliefs and domain knowledge in order to influence behavior. For example, mental model theory focuses on how to design messages to target addressees' conceptions of risk in order to improve decision making [29]. The fuzzy trace memory theory argues that addressees can understand risk at both verbatim and gist-based levels, which have different effects on decision making and action [24]. A large body of research that builds on such theories investigates how to leverage technology to deliver health-related messages tailored to specific addressee characteristics [30].

Communication as Interaction (Distributed Cognition)

Interactive theories analyze how meaning emerges from coordination of communication partners' actions ("sense-making in the moment"), and how this activity is influenced by constraints imposed by communication media and context as well as by speakers' and addressees' cognitive resources. An important idea is that communicative success depends on the interaction of participants' cognitive resources in context, with joint attention as a key resource. Therefore, interactive theories can be interpreted within the framework of distributed cognition, which analyzes human performance, including communication, as emerging from cognitive resources and representations distributed across social contexts such as conversational partners, and external contexts such as tools ([31]; a detailed description can be found in Chap. 2 in this volume). In the following sections, we first describe distributed cognition theories that tend to focus on individual cognition interacting with a dyad partner, technology, or other local context, and then describe distributed cognition theories that focus on a more systems-level of analysis that includes broader context.

Distributed Cognition: Individual Cognition in Context

Common Ground

Conversational partners communicate by coordinating cognitive effort in order to construct meaning [32]. To do this, they 'ground' information, or agree that the information is mutually understood and accepted (as accurate and relevant to joint goals). Grounding rests on and contributes to shared situation models [33]. In this view, speakers not only ensure that they are understood, but collaborate with their addressees to create meaning. For example, speakers may implicitly invite their addressees to co-construct their message by presenting an intentionally 'underdeveloped' contribution, encouraging their addressees to help specify the content. For example, a resident might say "I checked that patient", prompting a nurse to complete the contribution: "The one with edema?" "Right. It's down". Speakers may also present a message they think is clear, but the addressee's request for clarification reveals that it is not [32, 34]. Thus, ongoing feedback is essential to communication. For example, stories are more understandable when speakers receive immediate feedback from their addressees [35].

Communication depends on joint or collaborative effort, as well as the individual effort involved in producing and understanding messages [32]. Developing common ground itself requires effort. Pre-emptive grounding involves devoting effort ahead of time to develop shared knowledge about the message domain, communication strategies, and other aspects of communication [34]. The upfront work involved in pre-emptive grounding facilitates communication as it occurs (e.g., little cost to grounding during communication). For example, aviation communication depends heavily on shared knowledge about aviation concepts, terminology, and communication procedures that is acquired by Air Traffic Controllers and pilots as part of their professional training and experience. This shared knowledge often enables rapid and efficient communication during flight operations [33]. Similarly, in health care, two providers may discuss patients before a formal hand-off, "the process of passing information, responsibility and control from one caregiver to the next during care transitions", in order to expedite the official hand-off [36]. Just-in-time grounding, on the other hand, involves devoting effort during, rather than before, communication. In this case, partners may share less knowledge about the domain and/or the conventions of communication, and so must devote more effort 'on the fly' during communication [34]. For example, communication between domain experts and novices or between experts from different subdomains (e.g., physicians and nurses) often requires partners to be more explicit, devoting more effort to ground contributions.

Common ground theory helps to refine the view of how cognitive resources constrain communication:

- Speakers *initiate* contributions by getting their addressee's attention using verbal or nonverbal (e.g., gestures) cues.

- They then *present* messages that are designed to be understood based on common ground (shared knowledge of the language, cultural context, as well as more specific concepts that are relevant based on the prior discourse and context of communication). Listeners not only understand the message (which involves activating and integrating concepts, as described above), but also signal to the speaker that they do or do not understand. In the latter case, they may implicitly (e.g., puzzled expression) or explicitly request clarification.
- The speaker and addressee *accept* the message as mutually understood and relevant, so that the contribution enters common ground.

These phases typically overlap: speakers often initiate contributions by presenting messages, and listeners often signal acceptance by responding to the message with a relevant contribution [32].

Collaborative Effort and Communication Success

Interactive approaches emphasize that communication depends on partners' collaborative or joint effort. For example, Air Traffic Controllers communicate by radio with many aircraft in the same air space in order to manage the flow of traffic. They may try to reduce their own effort by presenting one long, rapidly delivered message to a pilot rather than breaking this message into several shorter messages that require more radio time and complicates the task of talking to multiple pilots on a single radio line. However, this strategy may increase the addressed pilot's effort involved in understanding and accepting the long message (by 'reading back' or repeating key concepts from the message in order to demonstrate understanding and to help establish common ground). It also increases the likelihood that the pilot misunderstands and requests clarification, or that the pilot does not explicitly accept the message at all (responding with minimal or no acknowledgement). The controller in turn must then spend more radio time in order to 'close the communication loop' by clarifying their message and seeking confirmation that the pilot understood. The upshot is increased collaborative effort [37].

In health care, outgoing ICU nurses who hand off patients to incoming nurses may overestimate common ground when the incoming nurses are already familiar with the patients, so that they present overly abbreviated reports. This strategy can minimize their own effort involved in hand-offs, but at the expense of the incoming nurse, who is likely to misunderstand and to request clarification, resulting in increased collaborative effort ([38]; also see Abraham et al. [39]). In short, successful communication depends on how well partners coordinate contributions through shared attention and collaborative effort. Such communication problems in turn contribute to adverse events that reduce patient safety [40–42].

Common Ground and Technology in Health Care

Common ground theory (and distributed cognition theories more generally) is important for identifying factors that influence communication in health care settings, which depends heavily on technology and is often distributed over space (synchronous remote) and time (asynchronous remote), as well as occurring face-to-face. Next, we consider how collaborative effort and communication success depend on resources related to communication media, participants (e.g., cognition), and health care tasks. We also consider the role of technology as an external resource that shapes communication.

Communication Media Media differ in terms of the opportunities they afford for, and constraints they impose on, establishing common ground [43, 44]. In face-to-face communication, the most basic communication situation, partners are co-present and typically see and hear each other as well as the referent situation. They can use nonverbal (gesture and facial expression) as well as verbal resources in order to coordinate attention on linguistic information as well as the nonlinguistic context when presenting and accepting messages. Communication can be efficient, with less need for elaborate verbal description compared to other media [45, 46]. Turn-taking is rapid, with messages received almost as they are produced (contemporality), the possibility of signaling that a message is understood as it is presented (simultaneity), and the order of contributions easily determined (sequentiality) [43]. Face-to-face communication is especially suited for accomplishing complex joint tasks such as performing surgery. In these situations, nonverbal cues such as joint gaze and body posture help coordinate attention to task-critical information, which can predict success in clinical tasks such as handoffs [47]. These cues, as well as nonverbal cues such as tempo, voice fluctuation and tone are also important for expressing emotion, which can be critical for communication among clinicians. For example, in a peri-operative context, a two-challenge rule (CUS protocol, I am Concerned, I am Uncomfortable, Stop!) can be used to escalate the assertiveness and tone of a member of the surgical team who believes that an error is imminent (e.g., wrong leg draped; [48]).

Face-to-face communication also has drawbacks. Communication at work is often complex, with partners having to keep track of interacting topics or conversational threads. This complexity requires partners to frequently access concepts from prior discourse (reviewability) and revise contributions in light of the evolving discourse (revisability) [43]. The transient nature of speech challenges comprehension of complex messages because of listeners' working memory limits. More generally, the time pressure of face-to-face communication may preclude the deliberation needed to craft complex messages, as well as to understand them.

Other media may impose more constraints on communication, providing fewer resources for grounding. Synchronous communication between partners at different locations (e.g., telephone), like face-to-face communication, allows rapid turn-taking, contemporality, and simultaneity that support grounding (e.g., immediately indicating and repairing comprehension problems). On the other hand, it eliminates visual cues (unless using videophone), which can increase collaborative effort involved in accepting contributions [43]. Synchronous remote communication has become pervasive with mobile phone technology, and is frequently used in hospitals and other complex health environments because it allows clinicians to communicate while performing other tasks at geo-physically different locations [49]. However, when partners are not visually co-present, this medium may increase overall workload because speakers cannot modulate their communication as required by listener context. A good example comes from driver distraction research. Driver-passenger conversation is less likely to disrupt driving (e.g., lane control; likelihood of seeing highway exit) compared to cell phone conversation, in part because driver and passenger are co-present and the passenger can modulate their talk as required by the situation [51]. Texting, like online chat, is similar to synchronous remote communication because proficient texters use compressed language that allows rapid turn-taking, although this medium does not allow contemporality. Texting also eliminates auditory (e.g., speech prosody) cues for grounding and for affective messages, which may be remediated in part by innovative use of punctuation, emojis, or other symbols that convey affect. Texting also provides a record of the message, which supports reviewability.

Grounding can be even more challenging for asynchronous remote communication such as email, which lacks contemporality, simultaneity, and sometimes sequentiality. More effort is needed to produce messages (typing vs speaking), which influences individual and collaborative effort involved in grounding. Asynchronous voice communication (such as exchanging pre-recorded messages) is often less effective than synchronous communication (telephone conversation). For example, introducing an EHR system in an Emergency Department may increase the use of EHR-based emails between nurses and physicians about patient treatment plans, which reduces the face-to-face communication that can help clarify and elaborate shared treatment plans. On the other hand, email supports message reviewability and revisability and affords time for deliberation, which may result in more comprehensive and understandable messages [50].

The effects of media-related constraints on communication also depend on the tasks that people communicate about [52]. For example, remote communication may be more appropriate for tasks that hinge on message reviewability and revisability, such as integrating multiple sources of complex information in order to diagnose an illness or troubleshoot a problem. Face-to-face or synchronous remote media may be more effective for tasks requiring frequent interaction to accomplish goals or to resolve conflicting goals (negotiation, persuasion). For example, an unstable ICU patient receiving provisional treatment that requires close monitoring would be better served by a face-to-face nurse handoff rather than an asynchronous handoff based on a phone message from the outgoing nurse.

Participant Resources While information processing theories focus on the cognitive resources (e.g., attention, working memory) needed to produce (speakers) and understand (listeners) messages, interactive theories emphasize that resources are also essential for grounding contributions to build a shared situation model, so that communication success depends on collaborative effort. For example, speakers with fewer cognitive resources, either because of long-term effects such as aging or short-term effects such as fatigue or distraction, may take more short-cuts when producing messages (resulting in more elliptical or vague messages) potentially complicating message comprehension and grounding. Conversely, listeners with fewer resources may be less likely to explicitly acknowledge contributions, providing less evidence for comprehension and undermining grounding. Older adults with fewer cognitive resources may be less adept at tailoring message presentation to listeners based on common ground [53]. On the other hand, shared knowledge about language, the discourse topic, and other aspects of communication can reduce effort and support grounding. This knowledge arises from partner familiarity and membership in a variety of linguistic/cultural communities and includes social norms and conversational conventions [32]. Partners who share knowledge about the discourse topic more quickly establish co-reference [54] and more effectively perform joint tasks by coordinating attention to key information [55], suggesting that knowledge reduces collaborative effort. The benefits of shared knowledge for communication partly reflect enhanced retrieval of previously mentioned information [56]. These advantages may explain why experts sometimes benefit more than novices from collaboration (compared to working alone) when recalling and acting on domain-relevant information [57].

Technology and Communication Technology shapes communication in many ways, especially by expanding the repertoire of media options that create new communication opportunities and constraints. In complex environments such as hospitals, where work is typically done by multiple distributed and interacting teams, technology provides options for remote communication, both synchronous (chat, texting, videophone, electronic status boards) and asynchronous (voicemail, email, clinical messaging in EHRs).

Technology, broadly considered as "cognitive artifacts," includes paper-based tools such as notes or whiteboards in addition to electronic-based tools [31, 58]. Distributed cognition theories analyze how artifacts, a pervasive part of work environments, reduce the need for mental computation, memory search, and other effortful cognitive processes involved in producing and understanding messages. They can support grounding by providing easily shared external referents that reduce need for explicit description [44]. They also support reviewability in face-to-face communication [46] and visibility in synchronous remote communication such as teleconferencing because speakers can gesture to guide attention to information on the tool [44]. They may especially benefit older adults by reducing demands of speech production and comprehension on cognitive resources [59].

However, it is important to note that the benefits of technology-based tools can be overestimated. For example, using video-conferencing or other technology to distribute information to remote team members does not in itself ensure that people will work together to effectively ground and act on this information. Electronic white boards can lead to ineffective grounding because they may not be updated as frequently as the comparatively lower-tech physical dry erase board. Such displays can also be cluttered, leading to inaccurate interpretation of information and have been found to be less effective in providing information related to care coordination in some circumstances [60, 61]. More generally, such technology may tempt us to distribute large amounts of information to as many people as possible. This strategy may undermine communication and reduce safety if information distribution is not guided by strategies to manage joint attention to the information that is most relevant within an evolving mental model organized around shared goals. In addition, the use of technology-based tools often contributes to work interruptions that increase clinicians' cognitive workload [62].

Distributed Cognition: Systems-Level Analysis

Technology has transformed health care communication, and work processes more broadly, in many ways. Therefore, there is great interest in designing health information technology that flexibly supports a range of communication and task goals in different workflow situations. An important challenge for communication theory and research is to understand and predict strengths and limitations of different communication technologies in complex environments such as the ICU or primary care clinics, where communication interacts with many social-organizational processes. This requires integrating more individual-level theories that identify how participant-related and media-related resources influence work, with macro-level, systems-based analysis of work processes in organizations. Systems theories such as the Systems Engineering Initiative for Patient Safety (SEIPS) model [63] investigate how system outcomes such as safety and efficiency emerge from the interaction of multiple system levels, e.g., individuals interacting with devices in the context of tasks, environments, teams, management, organizational policies and practices. Such an approach would analyze communication in organizations, with technology-related factors at different system levels interacting to influence communication between dyads, teams, etc. [64]. Therefore, communication is analyzed both as an input to and outcome of work processes.

Hazlehurst et al. [65] developed a systems theory that is directly rooted in the distributed cognition approach. The unit of analysis is the activity system, composed of agents, tools, and environment, organized around shared goals. Like interactive approaches that focus on individuals in context, behavior is viewed as emerging in part from an internal/mental organization that responds to external demands. However, rather than driven primarily by individuals' mental processes, behavior depends on distribution of information representations through physical media (e.g., digital tools) across the activity system, as influenced by physical and social structures [65]. This view broadens investigation from how individuals extend their own internal resources to task or collaborative contexts, to a system of interacting agents and external resources in which collaborative action is coordinated through external representations over time, in response to constraints from tools, environment, tasks, and multiple goals at multiple system levels (e.g., accomplishing patient care, managing errors, training novices). The activity system approach has provided a valuable lens for analyzing how medication orders are accomplished in ICUs [65], how clinicians coordinate during surgery [66], and other aspects of clinical work.

Related to this approach, the Interactive Team Cognition theory analyzes team cognition (including patterns of communication needed to accomplish team goals) as emergent team-level activity, rather than cognition (e.g., mental models) that is shared by individual team members [67]. Team performance is evaluated by dynamic measures of team processes such as coordination (often based on communication patterns) rather than by static performance measures such as conceptual overlap in team member mental models. This theory has been influential in developing and evaluating approaches to team training for a variety of collaborative tasks (e.g., Unmanned Aerial Vehicle control; [67]).

System-based interactive communication theories highlight many communication issues that have emerged as clinicians increasingly rely on technology to get their work done. For example, because clinicians routinely collaborate with technology itself as well as using technology to collaborate with each other, common ground must be established between clinicians and this technology. In general, people tend to take a 'social stance' toward technology and treat it as they would a human partner [68]. Technology in turn must be able to reciprocate by building up and acting on common ground with their human partners, which requires technology to update and reason from a model of the user's context during communication [34]. Because collaborative success turns on trust, a critical issue is the extent to which humans trust their automated partners. People are more likely to trust robots and other technology to the extent this technology behaves like a human, such as responding in a conversational style [69]. Teams composed of human and automated members are also likely to be more successful to the extent team interaction is predictable over time, including how well humans and automated agents recover from automation failure, so that partners can calibrate their trust to support coordination [70].

Systems-based theories also highlight the importance of organizational factors for communication efficiency and patient safety. For instance, the HITECH (Health Information Technology for Economic and Clinical Health) Act in 2009 required EHRs to have specific functions (e.g., electronic medication prescribing), with the goal of improving the safety, quality and efficiency of care. This regulation dramatically transformed how computers are used by clinicians during routine clinical workflow, which tended to increase provider workload [71].

Key Challenges for Health Care Communication

The High Cognitive Demands Associated with Biological Complexity

Health care is an information-intensive domain that includes knowledge of normal and abnormal physiology, pharmacology, multiple treatment options and health specialties, health system and organizational infrastructure, a high volume of new clinical evidence, and longitudinal information about patients, families and their communities. Delivering care to patients and communicating about care is therefore a highly complex endeavor characterized by both uncertain responses to treatment interventions and changing patient conditions [72]. For acutely ill patients, each change in their condition requires the clinicians to reorganize and reinterpret multiple sources of data (e.g., lab values, physical exam, vital signs and patient's subjective responses) to inform their next decision [73], which further increases cognitive demands. Thus the potential for information overload and its associated safety implications is very high [74–76].

The cognitive complexity of health care both reflects, and in turn contributes to, the need to perform multiple, interleaved tasks, often for multiple patients, which result in pervasive interruptions [77]. Interruptions increase clinicians' cognitive load because of the need to recall the interrupted tasks, introducing risk for hazards [78] such as reduced diagnostic accuracy [79] and forgetting critical tasks [80]. Interruptions also increase the complexity of communication, making it more vulnerable to error during hand-offs [81], when caring for patients in ICUs [82], and in many other clinical tasks. Cognitive load can be exacerbated by poorly designed information displays and electronic interfaces that fragment, rather than integrate, information needed to perform multiple tasks, which can increase the frequency and consequences of interruption. A multi-site study of EHRs found that health care workers waste much time sifting through multiple sources of the information to get a true picture of a patient's situation, which is needed for effective communication [83]. Similarly, a study of intensive care nurses found that information needed to perform many of the common nursing tasks was inaccessible, difficult to see, and/or located in multiple displays [84]. In sum, problems associated with cognitive demands in health care have important implications for communication and lead to ineffective decision making, important tasks left undone and high potential for error.

Interactive theories of communication are essential for explaining how cognitive and communication complexity reduces work efficiency and safety, which in turn provides a foundation for improving communication. For example, the need to switch topics when discussing patient care, or to interleave communication with other clinical tasks, complicates processes involved in grounding information and developing a shared mental model of the task. In face-to-face communication, speakers may truncate contributions or listeners may fail to acknowledge these contributions in an attempt to manage their own workload, which ends up increasing the collaborative workload involved in effective communication, or increasing the chance of inaccurate or incomplete communication that undermines patient care. The impact of interruption on these grounding processes may be greater for remote (e.g., telephone) communication because speakers and listeners do not share a visual context, and therefore cannot modulate communication to accommodate each other's workload.

Given the high cognitive demands in health care and its relationship to quality and safety in health care, the application of information processing and interactive theories can aid in the design of tools to help clinicians manage the demands of communication during complex work. For example, large electronic status boards in ICUs or other environments in which multiple clinicians must coordinate care can support the ability to jointly attend to critical information, a pre-requisite for grounding information to develop a shared mental model that supports team performance. Tools that allow communication partners to electronically share and update care plans can also support grounding during asynchronous remote communication. For example, electronic checklists that saliently indicate the currently performed subtask can remind clinicians where they left off in a task when they are interrupted. However, it is important for procedures that support explicit grounding to be integrated into these tools in order to guard against a tendency to assume that information shared through technology is automatically understood by all team members. The potential benefits of such guidelines are especially important when communication is analyzed as emerging from, as well as contributing to, clinical workflow, as suggested by system-based theories of communication interaction [63, 64]. As a final example, interface designers often leverage cognitive load theory in order to minimize extraneous cognitive load, in part by limiting the number of data elements per screen in order to avoid overloading clinicians' working memory [85].

The Pervasive Nature of Interdisciplinary Work

The promotion of health and treatment of illness often involves multiple members of a health care team. Ambulatory patient care is most often led by a "team" of clinicians from the medical or nursing discipline. All hospitalized patients also require the care of medical, nursing, and pharmacy practitioners and many need the additional support from physical therapy, occupational therapy, social work, and other health disciplines. In both ambulatory and hospitalized patients, the complexity and acuity of the patient's condition is often reflected by the number of additional disciplines involved in their care, which may also require one or more medical subspecialties (e.g., cardiology, endocrinology, hematology) as well as a combination of care from other disciplines such as physical, occupational, and or respiratory therapy, dietary counseling, pharmacy, and social service. This means that the most complex patients are more likely to have complex interdisciplinary teams that must communicate effectively in order to coordinate care by performing interdependent tasks. Moreover, although members of the "team" have different roles, there is increasingly blurred boundaries between some disciplines that have overlapping expertise [86]. Finally, because many patients have multiple chronic illnesses, this type of interdisciplinary work is pervasive in our health care system.

Unfortunately, the term "team" in health care often does not mean that the group involved in care effectively communicates, collaborates, and coordinates care together based on shared mental models and goals [87]. Despite calls for teamwork [1, 88] and significant research to improve teamwork in healthcare [89–91], there are multiple barriers to effective teamwork [92, 93]. In practice, team members often partake in silo-ed work on the patient's behalf, sharing information passively through the health record or reactively interrupting a "team" member's work when there is an urgent need [94, 95]. When "team" members have the opportunity to communicate, many clinicians favor face-to-face communication, perhaps because this medium affords rapid turn-taking and a wealth of nonverbal as well as verbal cues that support interpretation and grounding of information [8]. However, this practice is challenging because the "team" members often work in geo-physically separate places and may work only temporarily together on a single patient during hospitalization or during the course of an illness. In addition, the composition of hospital teams are subject to frequent, sometimes daily, changes due to limitations in duty hours, changing schedules, and personnel rotations.

For ambulatory patients with chronic conditions, the "team" may be formed over longer periods of time, but may be assembled by the patient, such that the same team members, including different disciplines and subspecialists, may only have one patient in common. Another challenge of patient-assembled teams is that team members may work in different organizations with different medical record systems that do not readily share information across settings. Finally, ambulatory schedules are generally clinician-driven with little to no time for synchronous collaborative discussions.

Inadequate communication between health care team members can harm patients. For example, a study of incident reports found limited transfer of information and lack of shared understanding between physicians and nurses. Of the communication failures, approximately 40% caused delays in needed care and 20% resulted in physical harm [96]. Inadequate interdisciplinary communication has also been found to be the root cause of diagnostic error (41 errors per 1000 patients; [10]).

Although more research on interdisciplinary teamwork is needed, there are some examples of positive outcomes related to teamwork training or interventions. A number of formal teamwork trainings exist (e.g., TeamSTEPPS) as well as simulation based training that have a positive impact. A recent meta-analysis of 1390 teams found that teamwork in healthcare is positively correlated with performance [97]. Interventions to promote shared goals have been shown to reduce postoperative complication rates [98]. Improved delivery of care may reflect the use of tools (e.g., checklists) and explicit communication procedures that help team members from different disciplines coordinate their attention on critical information, reducing the collaborative effort required to update a shared mental model of the task at hand. However, effective use of checklists can sometimes itself require coordination that adds complexity to joint work [99]. Specialized teams in hospitals with shared goals, training and tools, and that work together over time (e.g., rapid response teams) have been shown to improve some teamwork processes [100]. In addition to training and specialization, well-designed technologies can also have a positive impact on clinical teamwork [101].

Discipline-Specific Terminologies and Taxonomies

Given that interdisciplinary work is pervasive in health care, it is somewhat surprising that each discipline uses specific and different terminologies and taxonomies, which contributes to the challenge of effectively communicating and coordinating across disciplines [102]. Some of these differences relate to discipline-specific knowledge, traditions, and education and training practices. Clinicians from different disciplines may interpret the same information differently or make different assumptions about which information is most relevant, reflecting these differences [103]. There is also limited history of interaction as well as varying education among team members that can create barriers to developing shared mental models because of limited shared experience related to communication conventions and knowledge. In other words, there is less opportunity for pre-emptive grounding that would reduce effort during communication [34]. Furthermore, each discipline focuses on interrelated but different information and aspects of patient care. This has been demonstrated through natural language processing analysis of nursing and physician discharge notes that revealed minimal overlap in terms mapped to similar or related concepts between nurses and physicians caring for the same patients [104]. Therefore, given that knowledge guides attention to and decisions about relevant information in complex situations, these knowledge and linguistic differences between disciplines can undermine grounding processes, making communication challenging unless it is very explicit, which may be too inefficient when health care work is demanding and urgent. Discipline-based differences among team members [105] may also challenge the ability to develop predictable communication patterns over time, which may disrupt the coordination needed to successfully accomplish collaborative tasks [67].

Rapid Diffusion of Health Information Technologies

Communication technologies are important for addressing some of these challenges, particularly the need for frequent interdisciplinary communication. These technologies allow rapid exchange of, and negotiation about, information among team members that address the challenges of both interdependence and uncertainty. While many clinicians favor face-to-face communication [8], this is often not possible in health care where individual work is highly mobile [106]. Physicians in hospitals often divide their time among several units, or in different buildings for their ambulatory versus hospitalized patients, resulting in limited direct contact with individual nurses throughout the day [105]. In addition, to promote patient privacy, interaction with patients is most often in individual rooms such that clinician team members may be geo-physically close to each other, but unaware of their proximity, which would offer opportunity for care coordination discussions. As mentioned above, technologies such as EHR systems may reinforce discipline-based practices rather than bridge discipline-based differences in order to support coordinated care [95].

Pagers and telephones remain ubiquitous for nurse and physician communication [107, 108]. More recently, communication platforms have been developed to improve team communication and address some of the deficits of pagers and telephones [107], including wearable devices (e.g., vocera https://www.vocera.com/), shared task lists (e.g., CareAlign https://carealign.ai/clinicians/), and EHR-based instant messaging (e.g., Sticky notes https://enigmaforensics.com/blog/epic-software/). While these technologies are promising, they have not been subject to independent peer-reviewed research and may have unidentified limitations.

Although there is evidence for benefits of communication technologies, there are also unintended consequences that promote errors and inefficiency ([109–111]; a detailed description regarding the role of unintended consequences in health care environments can be found in Chap. 11). Communication technologies have rapidly diffused into health care from other domains. There is need for theoretically-based and empirically-derived guidelines to determine which technologies are most effective in different clinical situations. Traditionally, synchronous communication modes such as face-to-face or telephone that occur in real-time have been relied on by clinicians [94] and are perceived by many to offer more complete information transfer [8]. While these modes offer many resources for grounding information, which supports collaboration (e.g., nonverbal as well as verbal cues, rapid turn-taking), synchronous communication in the fast-paced, multi-task health care domain can also be interruptive, inefficient, and distracting, which can increase cognitive workload, miscommunication, and risk for error [94, 112–114]. Synchronous communication may also contribute to burnout among clinicians, in part because of increased workload [115]. More recently, asynchronous modes (transmit messages to be received at a later time) are increasingly used. These include email and texting, and are less interruptive and more appropriate for non-urgent clinical matters ([94]; also refer to Chaps. 10 and 13 in this volume). However, these asynchronous modes may also pose threats to patient safety, including uncertain delivery, missed messages, and delays in transmission [116, 117]. They also narrow the range of information that can be easily communicated (e.g., affective as well as cognitive meaning). Tasks that require negotiation, such as consults to interpret complex and uncertain patient information in order to come to a diagnosis, may be especially vulnerable to asynchronous communication. For example, technology-enabled remote synchronous communication, such as video telehealth appointments, may reduce patient-provider interaction compared to face-to-face appointments [118], and this challenge may be even more likely in asynchronous communication. Nonetheless, to the extent that technologies such as texting preserve aspects of face-to-face communication such as rapid turn-taking, they may combine flexibility of this communication while avoiding some drawbacks, such as limited message reviewability and revisability. Systems-based theories of interactive communication will be especially important for designing communication technology that meshes with the constraints and opportunities of workflows in health care organizations.

Frequent Complete Transfer of Responsibility Within Disciplines

The round-the-clock nature of health care makes it unsafe for individual clinicians to provide care every hour of every day. For this reason, patient care in acute settings is regularly and frequently (2–3 times per day for hospitalized patients) transferred between clinicians. This is commonly referred to as a "handoff", indicating that the responsibility and authority for care is transferred to another individual of the same discipline. These transitions are conducted between two people or in groups using a variety of communication media, including face-to-face, telephone, audio recording or electronic tools. They present a vulnerable time period for patient care [119, 120] for a variety of reasons, including the fact that they often occur in noisy environments with frequent interruptions [121]. Communication problems during handoffs, including omission of key information, occur frequently and lead to redundant work, missed care, delays in diagnosis and treatment, and medical errors such as near misses and sentinel events [40, 122].

Clinicians often prefer face-to-face handoffs, in part because of the rich nonverbal as well as verbal resources for grounding information. However, handoffs require communicating large amounts of patient information, which can hamper face-to-face communication because transient speech limits the ability to revise and review this complex information. Multiple efforts to improve the quality of handoffs, in part by reducing demands on memory, include low-tech memory aids such as mnemonics, checklists, or paper templates [123]. More recently, electronic handoff tools have emerged in practice [124–126]. These tools, when integrated into the electronic health record, may decrease clinical workload if information needed for handoff is incorporated in an automated manner into a handoff template.

Theories that articulate the impact of communication media and participant resource constraints guide analysis of how these support tools can improve or impair handoff communication. For example, electronic tools may impair communication accuracy, decrease situation awareness, and reduce the ability of incoming clinicians to assume responsibility for patient care to the extent they reduce the interactive synchronous communication needed to successfully ground information and negotiate shared goals. Moreover, some important functions of handoffs, such as discovering patient care errors when incoming clinicians review information, may be eliminated to the extent electronic tools reduce interaction during handoffs [127, 128]. Other design challenges include the importance of not adding to collaborative workload for outgoing and incoming clinicians during hand-offs, and ensuring the messages are received when using asynchronous communication technologies (closed loop communication). That being said, there are many opportunities to improve current communication with theory-based technology design, such as by automatically integrating key information that should be shared during handoffs and verifying that the information is grounded at the time of the hand-off.

Conclusion

The importance of communication in healthcare is reflected in the evidence that miscommunication often contributes to care errors, patient harm, and inefficiency. In response, there is growing attention to health care communication and communication technologies as a means to minimize inefficient and unsafe care related to poor communication processes. For example, it is hoped that the use of technology to increase the speed of information transfer and access to real-time information among team members will reduce delays in care and shorten hospital stays, potentially saving substantial costs. However, because there are drawbacks as well as benefits to any technology, research is needed to evaluate the effects of clinical communication technologies.

With the crisis in health care costs in the United States, attention to the field of health care communication extends beyond academics to regulators [129]. The Joint Commission has required implementation of a standardized handoff method since 2006, giving rise to the design and testing of tools for handoff communication [130]. To meet this requirement, many hospitals implemented measures that were not theoretically based [123]. In addition, The Center for Medicare and Medicaid Services introduced significant financial incentives to implement electronic health records, with some of the emphasis on clinical communication and communication with patients [131]. Again, the design, implementation, and evaluation of these tools are not often guided by communication theories.

In this chapter, we pointed out the need for, and value of, leveraging theories to guide research on communication in complex health care settings. These theories identify important characteristics of communication situations (e.g., media, participants, context) likely to impact the success of communication, as well as the processes underlying communication, which help explain why communication fails in particular situations. Such analyses in turn can guide development of design, training, and workflow approaches to improve communication in clinical environments. These theories are often overlooked, yet are valuable tools for explaining effects of technology on communication and delivery of patient care, and for anticipating potential effects of new technologies before they are implemented. Theories and models that have been effectively applied to the health domain often derive from analysis of conversation (typically between two people; [32]; see [44] for extensions to health care technology) and are used to analyze processes underlying exchange of information between patients and providers [132], incoming and outgoing clinicians during handoffs [133, 134], and for interdisciplinary communication [135]. An important challenge is to integrate such theories with more macro-level system theories in order to analyze processes and representations involved in communication among networks of people and technologies that coordinate to accomplish complex patient care tasks.

Acknowledgements Preparation of this chapter was supported by the National Institute of Aging (Grant R01 AG31718) and the National Institute of Nursing Research (Grant R01 NR011300). Any opinions, findings, and conclusions or recommendations expressed in this publication are those of the authors and do not necessarily reflect the views of the NIH.

Discussion Questions
1. What are the key challenges to clinical communication?
2. What are the concepts and theories that can be applied to communication research in healthcare?
3. What are ways that theory can be applied in communication technology design?

References

1. Kohn LT, Corrigan JM, Donaldson MS. To err is human: building a safer health system committee on quality of health care in America. Washington D.C.: Institute of Medicine; 2000.
2. Makary MA, Daniel M. Medical error—the third leading cause of death in the US. BMJ. 2016;353:i2139.
3. The Joint Commission on Accreditation of Healthcare Organizations. Root causes of medication errors (1995–2004). 2005 [cited 2005 Nov 2].
4. Cordero C. Advancing effective communication, cultural competence, and patient-and family-centered care: a roadmap for hospitals. 2011. Available from National Association of Public Hospitals and Health Systems: http://www.naph.org/Different-Formats/PowerPoint-Only/2711-Joint-Commission-Standards-Webinar.aspx
5. Kim M, Barnato A, Angus D, Fleisher L, Kahn J. The effect of multidisciplinary care teams on intensive care unit mortality. Arch Intern Med. 2010;170(4):369–76.
6. Knaus WA, Draper EA, Wagner DP, Zimmerman JE. An evaluation of outcome from intensive care in major medical centers. Ann Intern Med. 1986;104(3):410–8.
7. Shortell SM, Zimmerman JE, Gillies RR, et al. Continuously improving patient care: practical lessons and an assessment tool from the National ICU Study. Qual Rev Bull. 1992;18(5):150–5.
8. Williams R, Silverman R, Schwind C, et al. Surgeon information transfer and communication: factors affecting quality and efficiency of inpatient care. Ann Surg. 2007;245(2):159–69.
9. Barshi I, Farris C. Misunderstandings in ATC communication: language, cognition, and experimental methodology. Routledge; 2016.
10. Khan A, Spector ND, Baird JD, et al. Patient safety after implementation of a coproduced family centered communication programme: multicenter before and after intervention study. BMJ. 2018;363:k4764. https://doi.org/10.1136/bmj.k4764.
11. Congress.Gov. H.R.34 - 21st Century Cures Act. 2016. https://www.congress.gov/bill/114th-congress/house-bill/34
12. US Department of Health and Human Services. HITECH act enforcement interim final rule. 2009. https://www.hhs.gov/hipaa/for-professionals/special-topics/hitech-act-enforcement-interim-final-rule/index.html
13. Durso FT, Drews FA. Health care, aviation, and ecosystems a socio-natural systems perspective. Curr Dir Psychol Sci. 2010;19(2):71–5.

14. Abraham J, Kannampallil T, Patel VL. A systematic review of the literature on the evaluation of handoff tools: implications for research and practice. J Am Med Inform Assoc. 2014;21(1):154–62.
15. Patterson ES, Wears RL. Patient handoffs: standardized and reliable measurement tools remain elusive. Jt Comm J Qual Patient Saf. 2010;36(2):52–61.
16. Morrow DG. Cognitive ergonomics: application of cognitive theories to patient work. In: Holden R, Valdez R, editors. The patient factor: a handbook on patient ergonomics, vol. 1. CRC Press; 2021. p. 21–36.
17. Shannon CE, Weaver N. The mathematical theory of communication. Urbana: University of Illinois Press. 1949.
18. Wickens C, Hollands J. Engineering psychology and human performance. Psychology Press; 2000.
19. Miller GA. The cognitive revolution: a historical perspective. Trends Cogn Sci. 2003;7(3):141–4.
20. Levelt WJ. Speaking: from intention to articulation. ACL: MIT Press series in natural-language processing. Cambridge, MA: MIT Press; 1989.
21. Kintsch W. Comprehension: a paradigm for cognition. Cambridge University Press; 1998.
22. Patel VL, Kaufman DR, Arocha JF. Emerging paradigms of cognition in medical decision-making. J Biomed Inform. 2002;35(1):52–75.
23. Zwaan RA, Taylor LJ. Seeing, acting, understanding: motor resonance in language comprehension. J Exp Psychol Gen. 2006;135(1):1–11.
24. Reyna VF. A theory of medical decision making and health: fuzzy trace theory. Med Decis Mak. 2008;28(6):850–65.
25. Stine-Morrow EAL, Radvansky GA. Discourse processing and development through the adult lifespan. In: Schober MF, Rapp DN, Britt MA, editors. The Routledge handbook of discourse processes. Routledge/Taylor & Francis Group; 2018. p. 247–68. https://doi.org/10.4324/9781315687384-14.
26. Reddy M. The conduit metaphor: a case of frame conflict in our language about language. In: Metaphor and thought. Cambridge University Press; 1979. p. 164–201.
27. Austin JL. How to do things with words. Harvard university press. 1975.
28. Petty R, Cacioppo J. The elaboration likelihood model of persuasion. Springer; 1986.
29. Morgan KM, DeKay ML, Fischbeck PS, Morgan MG, Fischhoff B, Florig HK. A deliberative method for ranking risks (II): evaluation of validity and agreement among risk managers. Risk Anal. 2001;21(5):923–37.
30. Kreuter MW, Wray RJ. Tailored and targeted health communication: strategies for enhancing information relevance. Am J Health Behav. 2003;27(Suppl 3):S227–32.
31. Hutchins E. Cognition in the wild, vol. 262082314. Cambridge, MA: MIT press; 1995.
32. Clark H. Using language. Cambridge University Press; 1996.
33. Morrow DG, Fischer UM. Communication in socio-technical systems. In: The Oxford handbook of cognitive engineering. Oxford University Press; 2013. p. 178–99.
34. Coiera E. When conversation is better than computation. J Am Med Inform Assoc. 2000;7(3):277–86.
35. Bavelas JB, Coates L, Johnson T. Listeners as co-narrators. J Pers Soc Psychol. 2000;79(6):941–52.
36. O'Rourke J, Abraham J, Riesenberg LA, Matson J, Lopez KD. A Delphi study to identify the core components of nurse to nurse handoff. J Adv Nurs. 2018;74(7):1659–71.
37. Morrow D, Rodvold M, Lee A. Nonroutine transactions in controller-pilot communication. Discourse Process. 1994;17(2):235–58.
38. Carroll JS, Williams M, Gallivan TM. The ins and outs of change of shift handoffs between nurses: a communication challenge. BMJ Qual Saf. 2012;21(7):586–93.
39. Abraham J, Kannampallil T, Brenner C, et al. Characterizing the structure and content of nurse handoffs: a sequential conversational analysis approach. J Biomed Inform. 2016;59:76–88.

40. Desmedt M, Ulenaers D, Grosemans J, Hellings J, Bergs J. Clinical handover and hand-off in healthcare: a systematic review of systematic reviews. Int J Qual Health Care. 2021;33(1):mzaa170.
41. Galatzan BJ, Carrington JM. Exploring the state of the science of the nursing hand-off communication. Comput Inform Nurs. 2018;36(10):484–93.
42. The Joint Commission. Inadequate hand-off communication. Sentinel Event Alert. 2017;58(1):6.
43. Clark H, Brennan S. Grounding in communication. In: Resnick LB, Levine JM, Teasley SD, editors. Perspectives on socially shared cognition. Washington: APA Books; 1991. p. 127–49.
44. Monk A. Common ground in electronically mediated conversation. Synth Lect Human-centered Inform. 2008;1(1):1–50.
45. Convertino G, Mentis HM, Rosson MB, Carroll JM, Slavkovic A, Ganoe CH. Articulating common ground in cooperative work: content and process. Paper presented at: Proceedings of the SIGCHI Conference on Human Factors in Computing Systems. 2008.
46. Gergle D, Kraut RE, Fussell SR. Language efficiency and visual technology minimizing collaborative effort with visual information. J Lang Soc Psychol. 2004;23(4):491–517.
47. Frankel RM, Flanagan M, Ebright P, et al. Context, culture and (non-verbal) communication affect handover quality. BMJ Qual Saf. 2012;21(Suppl 1):i121–8.
48. Guttman OT, Lazzara EH, Keebler JR, Webster KL, Gisick LM, Baker AL. Dissecting communication barriers in healthcare: a path to enhancing communication resiliency, reliability, and patient safety. J Patient Saf. 2021;17(8):e1465–71.
49. Aziz S, Barber J, Singh A, Alayari A, Rassbach CE. Resident and nurse perspectives on the use of secure text messaging systems. J Hosp Med. 2022;17(11):880–7.
50. Olson GM, Olson JS. Computer-support cooperative work. In Handbook of applied cognition. Chichester, England: Wiley; 2007. pp. 497–526.
51. Drews FA, Pasupathi M, Strayer DL. Passenger and cell phone conversations in simulated driving. J Exp Psychol Appl. 2008;14(4):392.
52. Zigurs I, Buckland B. A theory of task/technology fit and group support systems effectiveness. MIS Q. 1998;22:313–34.
53. Horton W, Spieler D. Age-related differences in communication and audience design. Psychol Aging. 2007;22(2):281.
54. Isaacs EA, Clark HH. References in conversation between experts and novices. J Exp Psychol Gen. 1987;116(1):26.
55. Richardson D, Dale R, Kirkham N. The art of conversation is coordination common ground and the coupling of eye movements during dialogue. Psychol Sci. 2007;18(5):407–13.
56. Ericsson KA, Kintsch W. Long-term working memory. Psychol Rev. 1995;102(2):211–45.
57. Nokes-Malach TJ, Meade ML, Morrow DG. The effect of expertise on collaborative problem solving. Thinking & Reasoning. 2012;18(1):32–58.
58. Nemeth CP, Cook RI, O'Connor M, Klock PA. Using cognitive artifacts to understand distributed cognition. IEEE Trans Syst Man Cybern Part A Syst Hum. 2004;34(6):726–35.
59. Graumlich J, Wang H, Madison A, et al. Effects of a patient-provider collaborative education tool: a randomized, controlled trial. J Diabetes Res. 2016;2016:2129838.
60. Rasmussen R, Hertzum M. Details that matter: a study of the reading distance and revision time of electronic over dry-erase whiteboards. Paper presented at: Proceedings of the 10th Asia Pacific Conference on Computer-Human Interaction. New York: ACM; 2012. p. 663–4.
61. Wears RL, Perry SJ, Shapiro M, Beach C, Croskerry P, Behara R. A comparison of manual and electronic status boards in the emergency department: what's gained and what's lost? Proc Hum Factors Ergon Soc Annu Meet. 2003;47(12):1415–9. https://doi.org/10.1177/154193120304701208.
62. Danesh V, Sasangohar F, Kallberg AS, Kean EB, Brixey JJ, Johnson KD. Systematic review of interruptions in the emergency department work environment. Int Emerg Nurs. 2022;63:101175.

63. Holden RJ, Carayon P. SEIPS 101 and seven simple SEIPS tools. BMJ Qual Saf. 2021;30(11):901–10.
64. Kaufman DR, Mamykina L, Abraham J. Communication and complexity: negotiating transitions in critical care. In: Patel VL, Kaufman D, Cohen T, editors. Cognitive informatics in health and biomedicine: case studies on critical care, complexity and errors. London: Springer; 2014.
65. Hazlehurst B, McMullen C, Gorman P, Sittig D. How the ICU follows orders: care delivery as a complex activity system. AMIA Annu Symp Proc. 2003;2003:284–8.
66. Hazlehurst B, McMullen CK, Gorman PN. Distributed cognition in the heart room: how situation awareness arises from coordinated communications during cardiac surgery. J Biomed Inform. 2007;40(5):539–51.
67. Cooke NJ, Gorman JC, Myers CW, Duran JL. Interactive team cognition. Cogn Sci. 2013;37(2):255–85.
68. Reeves B, Nass C. How people treat computers, television, and new media like real people and places. CSLI Publications and Cambridge University Press; 1996.
69. Morrow DG, Lane HC, Rogers WA. A framework for design of conversational agents to support health self-care for older adults. Hum Factors. 2021;63(3):369–78.
70. Demir M, McNeese NJ, Gorman JC, Cooke NJ, Myers CW, Grimm DA. Exploration of teammate trust and interaction dynamics in human-autonomy teaming. IEEE Trans Human-machine Syst. 2021;51(6):696–705.
71. Lopez KD, Chin CL, Azevedo RFL, et al. Electronic health record usability and workload changes over time for provider and nursing staff following transition to new EHR. Appl Ergon. 2021;93:103359.
72. Glouberman S, Mintzberg H. Managing the care of health and the cure of disease: part 1. Health Care Manag Rev. 2001;23(1):56–69.
73. Yee A. Clinical decision-making in the intensive care unit: a concept analysis. Intensive Crit Care Nurs. 2023;77:103430.
74. Beasley JW, Wetterneck TB, Temte J, et al. Information chaos in primary care: implications for physician performance and patient safety. J Am Board Fam Med. 2011;24(6):745–51.
75. Ehrmann DE, Gallant SN, Nagaraj S, et al. Evaluating and reducing cognitive load should be a priority for machine learning in healthcare. Nat Med. 2022;28(7):1331–3.
76. Pollack AH, Pratt W. Association of health record visualizations with physicians' cognitive load when prioritizing hospitalized patients. JAMA Netw Open. 2020;3(1):e1919301.
77. Walter SR, Raban MZ, Westbrook JI. Visualising clinical work in the emergency department: understanding interleaved patient management. Appl Ergon. 2019;79:45–53.
78. Drews FA, Markewitz BA, Stoddard GJ, Samore MH. Interruptions and delivery of care in the intensive care unit. Hum Factors. 2019;61(4):564–76.
79. Balint BJ, Steenburg SD, Lin H, Shen C, Steele JL, Gunderman RB. Do telephone call interruptions have an impact on radiology resident diagnostic accuracy?. Acad Radiol. 2014;21(12):1623–8.
80. Froehle CM, White DL. Interruption and forgetting in knowledge-intensive service environments. Prod Oper Manag. 2014;23(4):704–22.
81. Behara R, Wears RL, Perry SJ, Eisenberg E, Murphy L, Vanderhoef M. et al. Advances in Patient Safety: From Research to Implementation. 2, AHRQ Publication Nos. 050021 (1-4). Rockville, MD: Agency for Healthcare Research and Quality; 2005.
82. Grundgeiger T, Sanderson P. Interruptions in healthcare: theoretical views. Int J Med Inform. 2009;78(5):293–307.
83. Stead W, Lin H, editors. Computational technology for effective health care: immediate steps and strategic directions. Washington D.C.: National Academies Press; 2009.
84. Koch SH, Weir C, Haar M, et al. Intensive care unit nurses' information needs and recommendations for integrated displays to improve nurses' situation awareness. J Am Med Inform Assoc. 2012;19(4):583–90.

85. Harry EM, Shin GH, Neville BA, et al. Using cognitive load theory to improve posthospitalization follow-up visits. Appl Clin Inform. 2019;10(04):610–4.
86. Liberati EG, Gorli M, Scaratti G. Invisible walls within multidisciplinary teams: disciplinary boundaries and their effects on integrated care. Soc Sci Med. 2016;150:31–9.
87. Schoen C, Osborn R, Squires D, Doty M, Pierson R, Applebaum S. New 2011 survey of patients with complex care needs in eleven countries finds that care is often poorly coordinated. Health Aff. 2011;30(12):2437–48.
88. Corrigan JM. Crossing the quality chasm. In: Building a better delivery system: a new engineering/health care partnership. Washington (DC): National Academies Press (US); 2005.
89. Hughes AM, Gregory ME, Joseph DL, et al. Saving lives: a meta-analysis of team training in healthcare. J Appl Psychol. 2016;101(9):1266.
90. Hysong SJ, Amspoker AB, Hughes AM, et al. Improving team coordination in primary-care settings via multifaceted team-based feedback: a non-randomised controlled trial study. BJGP Open. 2021;5(2):BJGPO.2020.0185.
91. Stevens EL, Hulme A, Salmon PM. The impact of power on health care team performance and patient safety: a review of the literature. Ergonomics. 2021;64(8):1072–90.
92. Etherington C, Burns JK, Kitto S, et al. Barriers and enablers to effective interprofessional teamwork in the operating room: a qualitative study using the theoretical domains framework. PLoS One. 2021;16(4):e0249576.
93. Sherman JM, Chang TP, Ziv N, Nager AL. Barriers to effective teamwork relating to pediatric resuscitations: perceptions of pediatric emergency medicine staff. Pediatr Emerg Care. 2020;36(3):e146–50.
94. Coiera E, Tombs V. Communication behaviours in a hospital setting: an observational study. Bmj. 1998;316(7132):673–6.
95. Stoller J. Electronic siloing: an unintended consequence of the electronic health record. Cleve Clin J Med. 2013;80(7):406–9.
96. Umberfield E, Ghaferi AA, Krein SL, Manojlovich M. Using incident reports to assess communication failures and patient outcomes. Jt Comm J Qual Patient Saf. 2019;45(6):406–13.
97. Buljac-Samardzic M, Doekhie KD, van Wijngaarden JD. Interventions to improve team effectiveness within health care: a systematic review of the past decade. Hum Resour Health. 2020;18(1):1–42.
98. Sun R, Marshall DC, Sykes MC, Maruthappu M, Shalhoub J. The impact of improving teamwork on patient outcomes in surgery: a systematic review. Int J Surg. 2018;53:171–7.
99. Drews F. Human factors in critical care medical environments. Rev Hum Factors Ergon. 2013;8:103–48.
100. Mackintosh N, Rainey H, Sandall J. Understanding how rapid response systems may improve safety for the acutely ill patient: learning from the frontline. BMJ Qual Saf. 2012;21(2):135–44.
101. Tang T, Heidebrecht C, Coburn A, et al. Using an electronic tool to improve teamwork and interprofessional communication to meet the needs of complex hospitalized patients: a mixed methods study. Int J Med Inform. 2019;127:35–42.
102. Boyd AD, Lopez KD, Lugaresi C, et al. Physician nurse care: a new use of UMLS to measure professional contribution: are we talking about the same patient a new graph matching algorithm? Int J Med Inform. 2018;113:63–71.
103. Vatani H, Sharma H, Azhar K, Kochendorfer KM, Valenta AL, Dunn Lopez K. Required data elements for interprofessional rounds through the lens of multiple professions. J Interprof Care. 2024;38(3):453–9.
104. DiEugenio B, Lugaresi C, Keenan G, et al. Integrating physician discharge notes with coded nursing care data to generate patient-centric summaries. Paper presented at: the American Medical Informatics Association, Washington DC. 2013.
105. Manojlovich M, Harrod M, Hofer T, Lafferty M, McBratnie M, Krein SL. Factors influencing physician responsiveness to nurse-initiated communication: a qualitative study. BMJ Qual Saf. 2021;30(9):747–54.

106. Welton J, Decker M, Adam J, Zone-Smith L. How far do nurses walk? Medsurg Nurs. 2006;15(4):213–6.
107. Lafferty M, Harrod M, Krein S, Manojlovich M. It's like sending a message in a bottle: a qualitative study of the consequences of one-way communication technologies in hospitals. J Am Med Inform Assoc. 2021;28(12):2601–7.
108. Manojlovich M, Harrod M, Hofer TP, Lafferty M, McBratnie M, Krein SL. Using qualitative methods to explore communication practices in the context of patient care rounds on general care units. J Gen Intern Med. 2020;35:839–45.
109. Ash J, Sittig D, Dyskstra R, Campbell E, Guappone K. The unintended consequences of computer provider order entry: findings from a mixed methods exploration. Int J Med Inform. 2009;78(Suppl 1):S69–76.
110. Ash J, Sittig D, Dyskstra R, Guappone K, Carpenter J, Seshadri. Categorizing the unintended sociotechnical consequences of computerized provider order entry. Int J Med Inform. 2007;76(Suppl 1):S1–S27.
111. Melby L, Hellesø R. Introducing electronic messaging in Norwegian healthcare: unintended consequences for interprofessional collaboration. Int J Med Inform. 2014;83(5):343–53.
112. Coiera E. Communication systems in healthcare. Clin Biochem Rev. 2006;27:89–98.
113. Karsh B, Holden R, Alper S, Or C. A human factors engineering paradigm for patient safety: designing to support the performance of the healthcare professional. Qual Saf Health Care. 2006;15(Suppl):i59–65.
114. Tucker A, Spear S. Operational failures and interruptions in hospital nursing. Health Serv Res. 2006;41(3):643–62.
115. Gardner RL, Cooper E, Haskell J, et al. Physician stress and burnout: the impact of health information technology. J Am Med Inform Assoc. 2019;26(2):106–14.
116. Colicchio TK, Cimino JJ, Del Fiol G. Unintended consequences of nationwide electronic health record adoption: challenges and opportunities in the post-meaningful use era. J Med Internet Res. 2019;21(6):e13313.
117. O'Malley A, Grossman J, Cohen G, Kemper N, Pham H. Are electronic medical records helpful for care coordination? Experiences of physician practices. J Gen Intern Med. 2010;25:177–85.
118. Gordon HS, Solanki P, Bokhour BG, Gopal RK. "I'm not feeling like I'm part of the conversation" patients' perspectives on communicating in clinical video telehealth visits. J Gen Intern Med. 2020;35:1751–8.
119. Arora V, Johnson J, Meltzer D, Humphrey H. A theoretical framework and competency-based approach to improving handoffs. Qual Saf Health Care. 2008;17(1):11–4.
120. Santhosh L, Lyons PG, Rojas JC, et al. Characterising ICU–ward handoffs at three academic medical centres: process and perceptions. BMJ Qual Saf. 2019;28(8):627–34.
121. Kitch BT, Cooper JB, Zapol WM, et al. Handoffs causing patient harm: a survey of medical and surgical house staff. Jt Comm J Qual Patient Saf. 2008;34(10):563–570D.
122. Turner JS, Courtney RD, Sarmiento E, Ellender TJ. Frequency of safety net errors in the emergency department: effect of patient handoffs. Am J Emerg Med. 2021;42:188–91.
123. Riesenberg LA, Leitzsch J, Little BW. Systematic review of handoff mnemonics literature. Am J Med Qual. 2019;34(5):446–54.
124. Benton SE, Hueckel RM, Taicher B, Muckler VC. Usability assessment of an electronic handoff tool to facilitate and improve postoperative communication between anesthesia and intensive care unit staff. Comput Inform Nurs. 2020;38(10):500–7.
125. Motulsky A, Wong J, Cordeau JP, Pomalaza J, Barkun J, Tamblyn R. Using mobile devices for inpatient rounding and handoffs: an innovative application developed and rapidly adopted by clinicians in a pediatric hospital. J Am Med Inform Assoc. 2017;24(e1):e69–78.
126. Shah AC, Oh DC, Xue AH, Lang JD, Nair BG. An electronic handoff tool to facilitate transfer of care from anesthesia to nursing in intensive care units. Health Informatics J. 2019;25(1):3–16.

127. Clark JR, Stanton NA, Revell KM. Identified handover tools and techniques in high-risk domains: using distributed situation awareness theory to inform current practices. Saf Sci. 2019;118:915–24.
128. Staggers N, Blaz JW. Research on nursing handoffs for medical and surgical settings: an integrative review. J Adv Nurs. 2013;69(2):247–62.
129. Holman HR. The relation of the chronic disease epidemic to the health care crisis. ACR Open Rheumatol. 2020;2(3):167–73.
130. Agency for Healthcare Quality and Research. Handoffs and signouts. Patient safety: primer. 2012 Oct [2014 May 19]. Available from: http://psnet.ahrq.gov/primer.aspx?primerID=9
131. Turner K, Hong YR, Yadav S, Huo J, Mainous AG III. Patient portal utilization: before and after stage 2 electronic health record meaningful use. J Am Med Inform Assoc. 2019;26(10):960–7.
132. Cuffy C, Hagiwara N, Vrana S, McInnes BT. Measuring the quality of patient–physician communication. J Biomed Inform. 2020;112:103589.
133. Galatzan BJ, Carrington JM. Communicating data, information, and knowledge in the nursing handoff. Comput Inform Nurs. 2022;40(1):21–7.
134. Kannampallil T, Abraham J. Listening and question-asking behaviors in resident and nurse handoff conversations: a prospective observational study. JAMIA Open. 2020;3(1):87–93.
135. Forbes TH III, Larson K, Scott ES, Garrison HG. Getting work done: a grounded theory study of resident physician value of nursing communication. J Interprof Care. 2020;34(2):225–32.

Further Reading

Coiera E. Communication systems in healthcare. Clin Biochem Rev. 2006;27(2):89–98.
Lafferty M, Harrod M, Krein S, Manojlovich M. It's like sending a message in a bottle: a qualitative study of the consequences of one-way communication technologies in hospitals. J Am Med Inform Assoc. 2021;28(12):2601–7.
Rouleau G, Gagnon MP, Côté J, Payne-Gagnon J, Hudson E, Dubois CA. Impact of information and communication technologies on nursing care: results of an overview of systematic reviews. J Med Internet Res. 2017;19(4):e122. https://doi.org/10.2196/jmir.6686.
Weigl M, Catchpole K, Wehler M, Schneider A. Workflow disruptions and provider situation awareness in acute care: an observational study with emergency department physicians and nurses. Appl Ergon. 2020;88:103155.

Chapter 4
Applications and Challenges of Human Computer Interaction and AI Interfaces for Health Care

Meghan R. Hutch and Yuan Luo

Introduction

Medical doctors and scientists increasingly find themselves trying to stay abreast of a ceaseless flood of health-related data. The influx of such data is due in large part to improved data capture methods, including implementation of electronic health record systems in the hospital setting, advances in genomic and proteomic sequencing of biologic samples, and the popularity of smartwatches for monitoring daily activity. Additionally, massive expansions in technology including computing power and memory have powered advancements in both the fields of human computer interaction (HCI) and artificial intelligence (AI). Accordingly, the medical and research community have surged to leverage the availability of these large health-related datasets and computational developments in order to solve a myriad of complex biomedical problems such as:

- Which patients are at risk for life-threatening diseases like sepsis?
- Can we predict the emergence and trajectory of viral infections?
- What can spatial gene expression tell us about the interactions between cells in cancerous tissues?

The unification of HCI and AI (HCI-AI) is a promising means for answering these and other important health care related questions. This chapter will review the emergence, evolution, and unification of HCI-AI systems in the health care domain. Additionally, we will present current applications of HCI-AI systems designed to support clinical, public health, and biomedical research settings. We will also

---

M. R. Hutch · Y. Luo (✉)
Department of Preventive Medicine, Feinberg School of Medicine, Northwestern University, Chicago, IL, USA
e-mail: meghan.hutch@northwestern.edu; yuan.luo@northwestern.edu

© The Author(s), under exclusive license to Springer Nature Switzerland AG 2024
A. W. Kushniruk et al. (eds.), *Human Computer Interaction in Healthcare*, Cognitive Informatics in Biomedicine and Healthcare, https://doi.org/10.1007/978-3-031-69947-4_4

discuss historical and current challenges of designing and implementing HCI-AI systems that are clinically useful.

First, Section "Emergence and Evolution of Artificial Intelligence and Human Computer Interaction" will lead with a historical review of the mid-to-late twentieth century, which began to see HCI and AI advancements booming, albeit independently. This subsection will first focus on early tensions between these two fields as a byproduct of opposing objectives and philosophies. We will also introduce the ideas and frameworks proposed by scientists that advocated for HCI-AI unification.

Next, Section "Twentieth Century: Early Intelligent Systems for Health Care" will focus on twentieth century efforts to apply HCI-AI for the development of intelligent clinical decision support systems for health care. These early intelligent systems intended to improve clinical decision making by transforming a physician's decision making process into a simplified mathematical problem. This section will also discuss the efforts and challenges of incorporating HCI principles in order to improve these systems and ensure their clinical utility.

Section "Twenty-First Century: Advances in AI and Applications for Health Care" will introduce AI in the twenty-first century, which has massively expanded owing to advances in present-day computing and memory. This section aims to provide a brief primer on the types of AI frequently used today and to describe the ways in which they can assist health care research.

Next, Sections "HCI-AI in the Clinical Setting", "HCI-AI for Public Health", and "HCI-AI for Biological Research", will discuss current efforts to develop and unify HCI-AI systems to solve and to support present-day health care challenges. First, Section "HCI-AI in the Clinical Setting" will present recent HCI-AI systems that can support the diagnosis of complex medical conditions, optimize treatment strategies, and alert physicians to patients at risk for a poor disease course. Of special importance, we will demonstrate that unification of HCI and AI has resulted in systems that are easy to use, understandable, and time and cost effective. Section "HCI-AI for Public Health" will then proceed with a discussion on the deployment of HCI-AI systems to improve public health, with a special focus on disease surveillance and improved efforts to facilitate data collection and dissemination of health information. Finally, Section "HCI-AI for Biological Research" will conclude with an overview of HCI-AI applications to support biomedical research, with an emphasis on the growing number of online tools to help analyze large 'omics' datasets.

In Section "Challenges and Barriers to HCI-AI Implementation" we will discuss the remaining technical, social, and ethical challenges with regard to the deployment and use of HCI-AI systems in health care. We will also highlight important policy designs for navigating and mitigating these challenges.

Lastly, Section "Conclusions: Future Directions & Recommendations" will conclude with a discussion on future efforts and recommendations for successful and ethical implementation of HCI-AI systems for health care applications.

While a comprehensive background on AI and its varied methods is regrettably out of the scope of this chapter, we will introduce key terms and main concepts of AI as needed. We encourage readers to study formative textbooks including Russel and Norvig's introduction to AI [1] and Goodfellow, Bengio, and Courville's textbook on Deep Learning [2].

Emergence and Evolution of Artificial Intelligence and Human Computer Interaction

First coined in 1955 by John McCarthy [3], 'Artificial Intelligence' (AI), described the "conjecture that every aspect of learning or any other feature of intelligence can in principle be so precisely described that a machine can be made to simulate it". McCarthy, considered one of the founding fathers of AI, subsequently called for an assembly of scientists to convene for a discussion on the challenges and solutions to the emerging field of AI and to study 'how to make machines use language, form abstractions and concepts, solve kinds of problems now reserved for humans, and improve themselves [3]." In other words, AI was conceptualized as a means of developing machines (i.e. computers) to solve problems with human, or above human, intelligence [4–6]. The algorithms underlying these machines were envisioned to solve problems too complicated or time consuming for humans to discern. Notably, these algorithms were predicted to become powerful and complex enough to improve themselves, subsequently enhancing their problem solving capabilities.

Excitement about AI flourished over the course of the 1950s due in part to the pioneering efforts of its founding fathers: Alan Turing [4], John McCarthy [7], Herbert Simon [5, 8], Marvin Minksy [9], and Allen Newell [8]. These scientists demonstrated foundational support for AI's ability to develop intelligent systems that would aid or surpass human decision making. Indeed, Alan Turing described his 'imitation game' as an example that machines would one day 'think', or in other words, perform in such a way in which a human could not distinguish whether he was interacting with another human or a machine [4]. Even in its early days, the implications of such technology was predicted to benefit a myriad of fields including business, government, science, and health care [10–12].

During this time, Human Computer Interaction (HCI) was also a burgeoning field. However, despite their rapid and emerging developments, both disciplines often remained separate and even competed against one another [13]. Jonathan Grudin, a prolific historian on the evolution of HCI and AI, explains that these two fields experienced alternating winters and summers throughout the latter half of the twentieth century [13, 14]. In other words, when developments flourished in one field (summer), the other field correspondingly fell victim to a period of withering advancements (winter) [13]. AI summers saw heightened interest, excitement and research funding distributed to scientists and AI focused laboratories. During AI winters, interest and funding of AI declined due in large part to the realization that computational power and memory capabilities were not yet advanced enough to support such systems [13, 15]. However, AI winters often spurred rejuvenated support and efforts aimed at advancing HCI.

Seasons of growing or withering interest in AI and HCI cycled consistently throughout the twentieth century, at approximately 10-year intervals. Alternating periods of success and failure between these similar, but competing fields may be surprising, however, each was rooted with contrasting philosophies and goals [13]. Moreover, each field was pillared by different definitions of 'intelligence' and perspectives as to where humans stood in relation to machines.

For example, HCI derived heavily from the study of human psychology and behavior in order to understand how humans could most effectively interact with machines. In his perspective detailing the difference between HCI and AI, Winograd [16] explained that HCI advocated for a 'design' approach for modeling the interactions between humans and machines: "In design, we often work in areas of human interpretations and behaviors for which we do not have predictive models. The question of 'Does it work?' is not approached as a calculation before construction, but as an iterative process of prototype testing and refinement [13, 16]." Hence, HCI emphasized the need for repeated testing and revised systems to ensure they were compatible with the needs of its users. Within HCI, human input and cognition was fundamental for successful development of 'intelligent' machine programs.

In contrast, early AI pioneers were largely mathematicians, engineers, and logicians [13]. AI originated with a 'rationalistic' approach [16], which envisioned the construction of intelligent machines that could model human thought processes. Human intelligence, it was believed, could be delineated into symbolic processes that a machine could understand in order to perform human tasks with ease [8, 13, 16]. Thus, to the AI researcher, intelligence was defined as the ability to break down and solve the underlying mathematical problems of these tasks [14].

Despite an emphasis on logic and mathematics, AI founding fathers Simon and Newell [17] proposed leveraging concepts from human psychology to improve AI's ability to solve ill-structured and qualitative problems: "There are many important situations in everyday life where the objective function, the goal, is vague and non-quantitative. How, for example, do we evaluate the quality of an educational system or the effectiveness of a public relations department?" [17] Simon and Newell recommended applying human-like heuristic problem solving in order to aid in the development of intelligent machines which would one day replace the human's need for solving ill-structured qualitative problems.

Rather than replace the human in his role to solve complex and elusive problems, other scientists anticipated that AI would augment a human's decision making, rather than replace it. In 1960, Licklider described a vision for the coupling of humans and intelligent machines, where humans would direct the machine to perform the redundant and clerical tasks which often impede the human's time to think [15]. Similarly, in 1962 Engelbart described a framework for augmenting human intelligence with computers [18]. His proposal discussed the potential of computers to solve complex problems, expedite human decision making, and provide humans with more space and time for creative thinking. These frameworks were among the earliest proposals advocating for HCI-AI unification to augment human decision making.

It was not long before scientists recognized the utility of AI and its coupling with HCI for solving health care problems. Technology bolstered by HCI-AI can more adequately expedite diagnostics, optimize treatment strategies, and alert health care professionals to patients who are at risk for a poor disease course. Further, intelligent systems that can alleviate the burden of tedious and time consuming tasks, can provide the physician with more time to spend on the deep thinking required to develop testable hypotheses and experiments, and to forge meaningful relationships with patients. As the following section will detail, clinical decision support (CDS) systems emerged soon after the inception of AI during the mid-to-late half of the twentieth century.

Twentieth Century: Early Intelligent Systems for Health Care

In his landmark essay *Man-Computer Symbiosis*, Licklider advocated for the need for improved intelligent machines which could help military commanders make time-sensitive and critical decisions [15]. Analogous to the military commander, medical physicians also must make timely diagnostic and treatment decisions for patients, especially those in intensive care units who are critically ill and at risk for further clinical deterioration. AI systems that seamlessly integrate into a physician's clinical workflow can expedite the time to diagnosis, treatment, and provide alerts as to which patients may be at risk for poor health outcomes.

The utility of CDS to enhance medical decision making was recognized as early as the 1950s [19]. Aligned with the founding hypothesis of AI which stated that human intelligence could be modeled through a set of symbolic processes [8], in 1959 Ledley and Lusted demonstrated that the complex medical decision making processes by physicians could be transformed into logical symbols and probabilities [20]. In other words, they advocated that machines, or computers, could help distill a physician's complex diagnostic and treatment decisions into simplified mathematical problems. With what seems like incredible foresight as to present-day hospital and doctor's offices, Ledley and Lusted wrote frequently on the potential applications of electronic computers in the health care setting [20–22].

Early CDS systems were simple computer programs that aimed to transform medical decision making into mathematical models. Such CDS systems were envisioned to record patient diagnoses, compute diagnostic probabilities, and inform optimal treatment strategies to aid in the timeliness of medical decision making [20, 21, 23, 24]. In their review of the evolution of CDS, Wright and Sittig describe these early models as 'Stand-alone systems' [19]. Early CDS systems were often individual programs that required a physician or other health care professional to manually record information about a patient. Thus, unlike present-day CDS systems which we will discuss later on in this chapter, these systems did not integrate within the electronic health record or other hospital-wide systems.

By the early 1960s, the earliest CDS systems were evaluated in health care settings. Although these early systems did not have the technology to incorporate the type of AI that exists today, the challenges in their usability and clinical utility underscore the need for HCI-AI unification. For instance, Warner and colleagues proposed a CDS system that could assist physicians in diagnosing patients with congenital heart disease based on the incidence of heart-related diseases and the presence of associated symptoms [24]. Warner's system relied on incidence rates to be recorded on punch cards that were read by a computer. After seeing a new patient, a physician added the patient's symptoms to a new card in order to update the information contained in the system. Similarly, Collen proposed an electronic, automated multiphasic screening and diagnostic system that computed likely diagnoses based on a patient's symptoms as determined by self-reports and physical measurements of vital signs and laboratory tests [25]. The system was designed to determine the likelihood of a diagnosis based on the pre-specified probability that a symptom is associated with a specific diagnosis. Like Warner's system [24], the multiphase screening and diagnosis system also operated with a set of punch cards which required the patient to answer survey questions related to their symptoms. A box containing a section for 'yes' responses and a separate section for 'no' responses collected the punch cards. While both proposed systems were promising proof-of-concepts, record keeping on cards was time consuming for both physicians and patients, requiring answering hundreds of questions across hundreds of punch cards.

As early intelligent systems continued to emerge, developers focused their efforts on HCI principles to improve system usability. For example, Bleich described the development and use of an intelligent rule-based system that could evaluate possible acid-base disorders and generate evaluation notes that detailed a patient's differential diagnosis (i.e. all of the possible diagnoses a doctor will consider based on a patient's demographics, clinical history, and presenting symptoms), suggested laboratory tests to remeasure, and recommended therapeutics [26]. The study describes essential HCI components that were integrated into the system, including an easy-to-use interface and prompts that alerted physicians to missing or inconsistent information. Rather than replace the physician's need to think critically about acid-base disorders, the program was also employed as an educational tool to augment the physician's ability to think more critically about the pathophysiology of acid-base disorders and promote more careful data entry.

The importance of integrating HCI principles into intelligent systems can be further observed through the development of INTERNIST [27]. Similar to the aforementioned early CDS systems, INTERNIST was a system designed to diagnose patients seeking internal medicine care, which covers an extensive list of possible conditions. In fact, INTERNIST's knowledge-base contained the relationships of 400 diagnoses and >2000 symptoms/physical measurements [28]. While the system was able to indicate the most likely diagnoses, it became apparent that the system was neither time-efficient nor as effective as a physician at solving complex cases, especially for patients who had concurrent diagnoses. For these reasons, future iterations of INTERNIST focused on modifying the system to behave as a physician would when evaluating a patient's differential diagnosis [28]. This prompted refining the system's underlying heuristics and problem solving strategies to focus on multi-problem solving and the probability of each symptom being related to a specific disease. The revised system, INTERNIST-II, provided users with suspected diagnoses within 20 s–2 min, compared to the 3–7 min required by the initial system.

Like INTERNIST, additional systems focused on the incorporation of HCI in order to enhance the user's experience. For example, EMERGE was another rules-based system that performed repeated studies to evaluate its usability and improve its functioning [29, 30]. EMERGE was designed to support the decision making process of health care professionals who were examining patients with chest pain [29]. For an individual patient, users could change the system's display mode to capture a patient's clinical presentation either through answering a series of yes/no questions or by entering free text. The entered information prompted the system to traverse the EMERGE knowledge-base and provide a risk assessment as to whether the patient should be admitted to the hospital, and/or which treatments should be considered [29]. In subsequent studies, it became clear that the user interface of EMERGE influenced the ease of the tool's use and the understanding of its decisions [30]. Indeed, users found that answering individual yes/no questions made the system's decisions more intuitive and logical. In contrast, interacting with the free text mode engendered the perception that users were merely searching for and directing the system's eventual choice of treatment plan.

Additionally, the Medical Emergency Decisions Assistance System (MEDAS) was an intelligent pattern-based system designed to aid in the diagnosis of 53 different diagnoses [31]. MEDAS was structured with a knowledge-base of almost 600 symptoms of clinical findings that were used to identify the most likely diagnosis. MEDAS supported an easy-to-use interface that even non-technically savvy physicians could operate. Moreover, while MEDAS could make diagnostic and treatment recommendations, the user could override the system. The override functionality supported the perception that MEDAS was designed to augment a physician's decision making process. Impressively, MEDAS also allowed the user to retrieve the information within its knowledge-base in order to aid in the physician's understanding of the system's decision making process. This retrieval of information from the knowledge-base is an early example of explainable intelligent systems which continues to be an area of consideration in light of today's AI black-box algorithms that often obfuscate the salient patterns used for decision making.

The Need for a More Unified Model of HCI-AI in Health Care

Although these initial intelligent systems could not yet leverage the powerful and complex AI that exists today, they emerged as early evidence that humans could develop intelligent machines to support clinical decision making. However, transforming a physician's differential diagnosis and optimal treatment strategies into equations was not an easy task even for a computer.

Furthermore, while the aforementioned studies frequently noted that the integration of HCI could enhance intelligent systems, the actual implementation of intelligent support systems into the clinical health care setting was infrequent. Heather Heathfield advocated for more robust cooperation between AI scientists and physicians in order to implement clinically useful CDS systems [32]. Indeed, Heathfield proposed a cooperative model that was designed to exploit the strengths of both computers and pathologists for diagnosing breast cancer [33, 34]. For example, due to information storage capabilities, computers can alleviate the need for pathologists to remember and recall every possible diagnosis, especially for conditions that are rarely seen. On the other hand, similar to the challenges noted during the development of INTERNIST [27, 28], Heathfield's study observed that diagnostic support tools often took much longer than a pathologist to evaluate all of a patient's possible differential diagnoses [33]. Heathfield's proposed system allowed a pathologist to first enter their suspected differential diagnoses. The system then used the initial differential to identify additional diagnoses that a pathologist may want to add to their differential. Once again, such a system aims to foster cooperation and augmentation between humans and machines.

Similarly, Miller stressed the importance of developing clinically useful systems that were synergized by both humans and AI [35]. Miller advocated for continuous evaluation of HCI-AI systems in order to ensure their utility in enabling health care providers to solve clinically important problems. The proposed evaluation framework called for continued assessment of a system's intended clinical use case, users, beneficiaries, and potential limitations, in order to ensure that systems were operating as designed and continued to support clinical decision making. Moreover, this framework paved the way to Charles Friedman's fundamental theorem of biomedical informatics: "A person working in partnership with an information resource is 'better' than that same person unassisted" [36]. Such sentiments continue to remain foundational and essential for the robust design and implementation of clinically useful HCI-AI systems.

Twenty-First Century: Advances in AI and Applications for Health Care

Current advances in computing power and memory have moved us closer to the types of AI-based systems envisioned decades ago. While the aforementioned systems were deemed 'intelligent' in that they could aid in the decision making process of health care providers, these systems often relied on rule-based systems, Bayesian statistics, and large matrices of pre-defined incidence rates and correlations between symptoms and diseases.

In contrast, today we commonly refer to intelligent systems as those composed of more complex AI algorithms. In fact, we frequently interact with AI on a daily-basis when using our smartphones, activity trackers, computers, and cars. In brief, 'AI' in current everyday language, typically refers to algorithms (i.e. mathematical functions) that are trained on copious amounts of data in order to learn the underlying relationships of the data as they relate to an outcome, objective, or to the dataset as a whole. By 'training,' we refer to the process of iteratively passing data through an algorithm in order that it learns these relationships (Fig. 4.1). Through this training process, the algorithm iteratively makes predictions on the data it receives and updates its

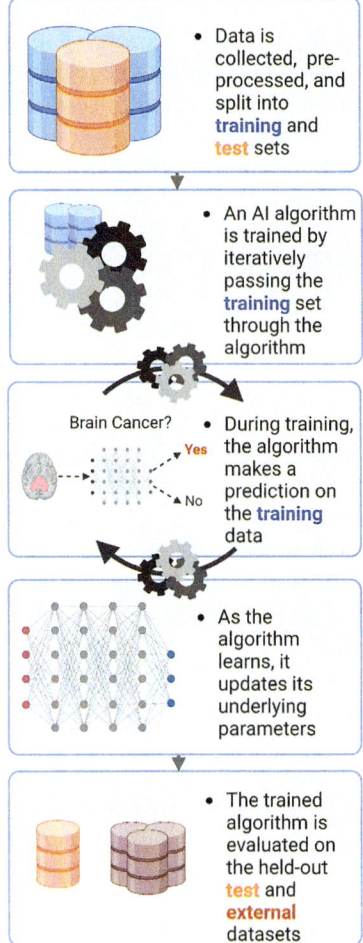

Fig. 4.1 Process of training an Artificial Intelligence (AI) algorithm. While there are numerous approaches for training an AI algorithm, this figure depicts a high-level overview of a general training process. First, data is collected, pre-processed, and split into training and test sets. Subsequently, the training set is iteratively passed through an AI algorithm. In this example, the algorithm is trained to predict whether a patient has brain cancer from an image of their brain. With each image the algorithm receives, it makes a prediction as to whether the image belongs to a patient with or without cancer. The algorithm subsequently compares each of its predictions to a ground-truth label (e.g. clinical documentation of a patient's cancer status). As the algorithm evaluates its correct and incorrect predictions, it updates its underlying parameters to more accurately reflect the complex relationships between images with and without cancer. Once the algorithm begins to make fewer mistakes during the training (as measured by metrics including accuracy, area under the receiver operating curve, sensitivity, specificity, etc.) the algorithm's final performance is evaluated on the held-out test set and, ideally, an external dataset (if available) that it has not seen before. Created with BioRender.com

underlying parameters as it begins to learn which parts of the data are associated with each outcome. As the algorithm learns, the accuracy of its predictions increase.

Although the previous paragraph is a gross simplification of how AI algorithms are trained, it is important to recognize that these algorithms are complex. Commonly referred to as 'black boxes,' AI algorithms get their nickname due to the frequent difficulty in understanding how they made their predictions. AI algorithms can contain hundreds to even millions of parameters that are updated and tuned during training. Trying to untangle these parameters can be an enormously difficult to impossible task. While the complexity of such algorithms can help us derive powerful insights from equally complex health care data, it is important to recognize the challenges and consequences that can derive from models whose predictions are difficult to explain. In later sections, we will discuss efforts aimed at leveraging HCI-AI systems to aid in increasing AI explainability.

Despite a trade-off with explainability, AI algorithms are powerful tools in that their large network of parameters aid in their ability to learn non-linear relationships. This particular benefit of AI is especially attractive for the field of health care. Historically, there have been many linear-based models which have been developed to evaluate a patient's probable health outcome (e.g. death, survival, optimal treatments, etc.) [37, 38]. However, linear-based models are not able to delineate complex relationships between variables. This is especially problematic in the context of health where even the same disease may have varying etiologies derived from a myriad of molecular pathways and genetic factors which do not often share a linear relationship with a single diagnosis. As such, patients with the same diagnosis often present with diverse symptoms and clinical phenotypes (i.e. manifestations of the disease). AI algorithms or systems that can traverse the various molecular and clinical data to identify disease subtypes, or patients who are at risk for poor health outcomes, are a promising means of achieving personalized medicine [39].

As AI continues to expand into the next quarter of the twenty-first century, it is critical to continue discussions and evaluations focused on human interaction with this technology. Conventional means of interacting with AI can be broadly stratified into three categories (Fig. 4.2). First, as demonstrated in the previous section, rule-based systems were the foundation of many early intelligent systems and continue to be employed in today's health care systems. As the name suggests, rule-based systems operate with a set of predefined rules that determine the relationship between a system's inputs and outputs. Importantly, humans are essential for determining these rules by transforming domain expertise into logical and mathematical relationships. Moreover, such systems can be thought of as decision trees, where a set of inputs trigger a cascade of if-else statements that further define the relationship of an input to its associated output. Due to the inherent explainability within rule-based systems, this approach has the added benefit of helping humans understand the way in which a system has arrived at a certain output or decision.

Second, humans also interact with AI through the training and use of machine and deep learning algorithms. These algorithms are often referred to as 'black boxes,' in that their complex architecture typically obfuscates the way in which the algorithm determined its prediction. Humans typically guide the training of machine

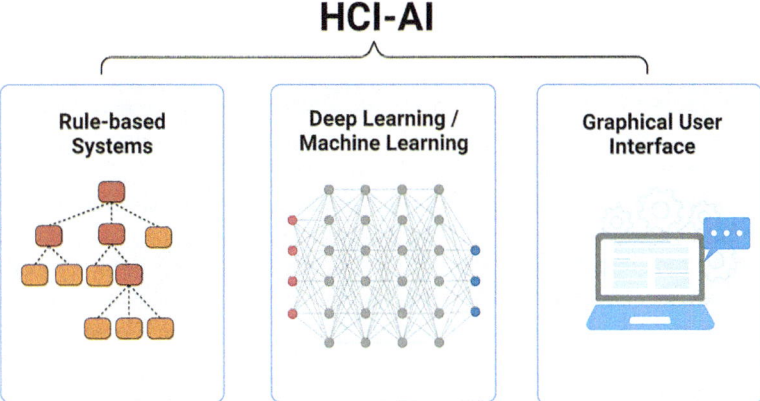

Fig. 4.2 Human interaction with artificial intelligence (AI). Here we present three common approaches for facilitating human interaction with intelligent systems. First, humans can interact with intelligent rule-based systems that are constructed through a series of predefined rules that relate a user's inputs to an associated outcome. Human guidance is critical for determining these rules through the transformation of domain expertise into logical and mathematical relationships. Rule-based systems help facilitate explainability of a system's outputs and decisions, through the decision tree-like cascade of if-else statements that rule-based systems often employ. Second, complex machine and deep learning algorithms are trained by humans to evaluate the relationship between inputs and outputs. Often referred to as black boxes, these algorithms make it more difficult to understand how a system arrived as its final output or decision. Moreover, machine and deep learning algorithms are often trained locally, outside of the clinical setting, before they are implemented into a clinical program or system. For example, the trained algorithms can be integrated within the hospital's electronic health record, where they work behind the scenes evaluating inputs in real time and making predictions. The clinical system or program can subsequently display these AI-derived predictions to support clinical decision making. Third, graphical user interfaces (GUIs) can allow humans to more directly and intuitively interact with AI. For example, GUIs have been designed to allow physicians to interact with AI chat bots, which can mimic human-to-human interactions. Created with BioRender.com

and deep learning models locally before implementing them into a clinical program or system, such as a patient's electronic health record [19]. Once implemented in the clinical setting, these algorithms often work behind the scenes where they evaluate input entered directly by the physician, or input automatically captured by medical devices such as blood pressure cuffs. The AI-derived outputs and predictions are displayed within the clinical system or program to inform a physician's decision making process.

Lastly, graphical user interfaces (GUIs), a conventional HCI component, can allow humans to more intuitively interact and control AI. For example, ChatGPT is an online GUI which allows humans to directly interact with a large language model (LLM), a type of algorithm trained on large amounts of text data [40, 41]. The GUI consists of a text box and an output box that allows humans to type questions or prompts and receive outputs generated by the algorithm. This design allows humans to interact with AI in an approach that mimics human-to-human interaction. As AI technology continues to advance and expand into the clinical health care setting, the use of such GUIs housing LLMs could mitigate the need to develop many different clinical systems. Instead, health care providers could interact with a single system and direct it to perform different clinical tasks.

As mentioned in the introduction of this chapter, a deep dive into distinct types of AI algorithms is outside the scope of this text. However, it is important to recognize that there are a myriad of AI algorithms that have been developed for varied data types and applications. Each algorithm is composed of a constellation of different parameters and relies on different training strategies and objectives. Subsequently, these algorithms can be further sub-categorized under several different, but often overlapping domains including machine learning, deep learning, and natural language processing. As we introduce recent examples of HCI-AI applications for health care, we will explain relevant terms and concepts as needed. However, readers are also encouraged to review the papers cited throughout the chapter and the foundational texts listed in the introduction.

HCI-AI in the Clinical Setting

Continued unification of HCI-AI with today's computing technology promises expansive utility in the clinical health care setting. Section "HCI-AI in the Clinical Setting" will review recent demonstrations of HCI-AI systems that were developed to support physicians in their efforts to diagnose, prognosticate, and administer appropriate interventions and therapies for their patients. Moreover, with the development of more complex AI methods, HCI-AI unification has the potential to improve model explainability and to peek inside the notorious black box of AI algorithms. This section will review several HCI-AI systems intended for the clinical health care setting, which have been designed to be clinically useful, easy to use, resource preserving, and explainable.

Diagnostic and Prognostic Support

In today's clinical setting, the importance of HCI-AI unification is increasingly recognized to enhance diagnostic support. In particular, HCI-AI systems have shown promise for specialties that require imaging to diagnose patients. Tschandl and colleagues reported that an HCI-AI system improved the accuracy of skin cancer diagnosis by 13.3% when paired with an interactive website displaying the neural network derived probabilities associated with each skin cancer type [42]. The study also reported that early stage physicians were much more likely to benefit from the aid of the HCI-AI system and to leverage its estimated probabilities in order to increase the accuracy of their diagnosis. In a separate study, Hekler and colleagues presented an HCI-AI system for classifying skin images as cancerous vs noncancerous [43]. The proposed system demonstrated that fusion of separate classifications performed by both a dermatologist and a convolutional neural network (CNN), a type of deep learning algorithm that is especially apt at handling imaging data, was more sensitive at correctly classifying cancerous skin images (89%) compared to the CNN (86%) or dermatologist (66%) alone. Although the use of a CNN alone was found to be fairly sensitive, its diagnostic ability was significantly enhanced when supplemented with human input. Thus, systems that require both humans and AI to work together may achieve better results than either one alone.

Indeed, Patel reported superior performance of an HCI-AI system that was augmented with physician feedback [44]. Specifically, the study used a deep learning model to evaluate chest x-rays and evaluate the probability that a patient had pneumonia. Images deemed to have low-confidence predictions from the deep learning model, were sent for further evaluation by physicians using the Swarm platform [45]. Swarm, an online platform designed to leverage the wisdom of a crowd, allowed physicians to work together when reviewing the low-confidence x-rays. Through Swarm's GUI, physicians could visualize the estimated probabilities entered by their colleagues. The human augmented system was found to significantly increase diagnostic sensitivity (88%, 95% Confidence Intervals (CI): 78–96%) compared to physician diagnosis alone (70%, 95% CI: 58–82%), and significantly increased diagnostic specificity (93%, 95% CI: 88–98%) compared to the deep learning model alone (0.77%, 95% CI: 67–86%).

HCI-AI systems which improve diagnostics, subsequently also optimize resource utilization. Raja and colleagues demonstrated the utility of a rule-based HCI system designed to help physicians decide whether to order a CT pulmonary angiography for patients with suspected pulmonary embolism [46]. The three rule-based system supported a simple user interface where the first rule prompted physicians to indicate whether a patient's D-dimer levels were elevated and their level of clinical suspicion for pulmonary embolism. Based on these selections, the second and third rules were triggered to provide decision support to users in the form of brief explanations as to whether or not the patient's D-dimer should be tested or whether a CT pulmonary angiography should be ordered. The system also provided functionality for users to submit an imaging order or cancel the initial intended order based on the system's feedback. The authors demonstrated that the integration of their three-rule system decreased unnecessary image ordering by 20% and increased the number of images positive for a pulmonary embolism by 69%. Notably, the authors attributed their success to the design of their system which focused on a single clinical diagnostic objective. The simple design of the system not only enforced its clinical utility, but also helped improve education and outreach among multiple stakeholders within the hospital who were able to successfully use the system and recognize its value.

Such simple rule-based systems are often desirable to physicians who can more easily understand how a system came to its decision. This is especially important when physicians need to explain how a system may have informed their decision making process to other health care providers or to their patients. Explainable systems can be especially difficult in the setting of complex HCI-AI systems that leverage machine and deep learning. Despite these challenges, recent efforts have demonstrated successful techniques to improve explainability of such systems. For example, Pantanowitz and colleagues demonstrated the performance of an explainable HCI-AI system that was deployed into the pathology lab to improve the diagnosis of prostate cancer [47]. The deployed system was referred to as a 'second read system', meaning that it alerted pathologists when there was a discrepancy between their diagnosis and that of the deep learning algorithm. Upon the trigger of a discrepancy alert, a second review of the image provided pathologists with a AI-derived heatmap that overlaid the pathology slides to highlight the discrepant areas. This technique was able to visually guide the pathologists to re-examine specific areas the algorithm detected as cancerous. Incredibly, the system's ability to steer the pathologist to potentially cancerous regions of the image only added about 1% extra time to the pathologist's workflow.

Developing explainable AI predictions was also a crucial objective of the CAD-DL system for diagnosis of coronary artery disease (CAD) [48]. CAD-DL was trained to diagnose CAD from myocardial perfusion images. The system was implemented into standard clinical software with a user interface designed to aid in explainability of deep learning predictions. Specifically, CAD-DL overlays heatmaps onto the image to help physicians understand the areas the neural network paid the most attention to when making its predictions. CAD-DL was found to be significantly superior to cardiology experts alone (Area under the receiver operating curve (AUROC): 0.80 vs 0.65). Additionally, CAD-DL supported diagnostic efficiency; it computed predictions in <12 s and automatically abstracted demographic data from the image's metadata, hence minimizing the physician's need to manually enter information.

Recent CDS systems have also shown applications to support prognostication. For example, Farzaneh developed a machine learning HCI-AI system to predict functional outcome in patients six months following a traumatic brain injury [49]. Importantly, model development was augmented by human clinical domain experts to identify the salient clinical variables during the course of the algorithm's training process. The resulting machine learning model was found to have an AUC of 0.81 and to be 75% accurate when predicting a patient's functional outcome. Importantly, the model also utilized SHAP [50] values as an explainability technique to help physicians identify the salient variables that the AI model relied on for its prognosis prediction. Remarkably, SHAP values can be visualized collectively across all variables or within a single patient. Explainability techniques such as SHAP can help physicians better understand the system they are working with.

Interventions and Therapeutics

HCI-AI systems are increasingly designed to support decisions involving clinical interventions and therapeutics. For example, advanced heart failure requires timely therapeutic interventions in order to optimize patient health outcomes. Cheema and colleagues developed and implemented an HCI-AI system within the electronic health record that could identify patients with chronic or advanced heart failure [51]. The system's alert triggered a cascade of coordinated clinical care workflows which consisted of: (1) chart review by the nurse and subsequent documentation of recommended next steps for the patient, (2) triage of the most at-risk patients for expedited evaluation by the heart failure team, and (3) electronic health record mediated inquiry to the patient's primary care doctor or cardiologist to approve the patient's visit to a heart failure clinic. Importantly, the described system required human guidance throughout the system's life cycle. For example, the AI model was trained with validated heart failure risk factors and salient variables chosen by the clinical experts in the study team. Moreover, at-risk patients who triggered the alert were carefully evaluated by clinical experts who prescribed the appropriate level of follow-up care (e.g. expedited evaluation, evaluation at three months, follow-up in a general cardiology clinic, or no follow-up needed).

As another example, a randomized control trial reported that the use of an HCI-AI system, Asthma-Guidance and Prediction System (A-GPS), significantly decreased the time needed for physicians to review a patient's electronic health record (3.5 vs 11.3 min) [52]. For patients enrolled in the intervention arm, A-GPS provided physicians with a customized report containing a summary of the patient's historical and current care plan, risk factors, a machine-learning derived risk score, a visual timeline of the patient's clinical course, and asthma management plans. Notably, the study did not find a significant difference between the occurrence of asthma exacerbation between the control and intervention groups. However, there was a significant decrease in the occurrence of asthma exacerbation in both the control and intervention groups compared to the baseline rates prior to A-GPS implementation. Due to the nature of the single-blind study, where the physicians must be aware of which patients were in the intervention group, it is suspected that the benefits of the A-GPS summary reports may have trickled down to the control group. This finding may suggest that HCI-AI systems that involved coordination of care teams can have far reaching benefits, even to patients who may not directly be assessed by them. Moreover, as with previous studies, the implementation of the HCI-AI system relied on clinical experts who engaged in focus groups and surveys to identify which data to use and prioritize during system development.

HCI-AI for Public Health

In the public health setting, HCI-AI systems are used to facilitate data collection, analysis, and health information dissemination. Additionally, HCI-AI systems have increased surveillance efforts for a number of diseases including viral infections, cancer, and mental health. This next section will review HCI-AI systems that aim to support and strengthen public health responses.

Surveillance Systems

Lee and colleagues developed an interactive web application to demonstrate the utility of their HCI-AI system for enabling prostate cancer surveillance [53]. The system leverages AI to more effectively learn a patient's suspected clinical trajectory. The interactive website allowed physicians to visualize the machine learning derived trajectories, which encouraged increased understanding of the model predictions. With such a system, physicians could more easily monitor patients, while simultaneously understanding the clinical factors and trajectories that implicate a high-risk patient.

The utility of interactive websites for disseminating complex results derived by AI, can be further seen in efforts by Marvel who released an interactive dashboard to allow users to evaluate machine learning derived COVID-19 Pandemic Vulnerability Index scores across counties in the United States [54]. The index for each county is computed from a myriad of data to inform a county's vulnerability to COVID-19. These include a county's infection rates, demographics, health and environmental factors. The dashboard is meant to serve as a dynamic visualization tool to help monitor a county's vulnerability risk for COVID-19. By providing users with simple and easy to understand visualizations, the dashboard can help users identify potential risk attributes contributing to a country's vulnerability level. Importantly, the authors describe the use of their dashboard as a tool to aid in public health dissemination to inform community and local public health responses.

Similarly, Villavicencio developed a COVID-19 machine learning prediction model and associated web application to help identify patients with COVID-19 from user-reported symptoms [55]. The web application was designed to be visually appealing and intuitive for users. After submitting symptoms, the application provided a user with the model predicted COVID-19 positive or negative status, in addition to links to direct the user to the World Health Organization (WHO) COVID-19 guidelines. Importantly, the study underscored the careful consideration of the application's useability, including from the back-end development perspective, and the front-end user perspective. Technical details of the web application's development and implementation were heavily detailed, which could serve as a helpful framework for researchers developing new HCI-AI systems.

The Semantic Platform for Adverse Childhood Experiences Surveillance (SPACES) system also leveraged interactive web applications to facilitate explainable mental health surveillance [56]. SPACES supported a virtual chat bot, which mapped user input to a custom ontology of concepts related to adverse childhood experiences such as risk factors, social determinants of health, chronic diseases, and stress. A rule-based system was developed to contextualize the relationships of these concepts to one another. Additionally, the system contained a knowledge-base of geographic information that allowed it to recommend resources such as schools, health clinics, or housing options to its users. The system also constructed a personalized knowledge graph which allowed users to visually understand how the information they entered was connected to the system's recommended resources.

Additionally, the system was designed to store a user's interactions within the system and to tabulate the types of concepts most commonly mapped. The system's data collection capabilities aim to aid policymakers in disseminating information, designing interventions, and allocating resources.

In contrast to the aforementioned interactive web-based systems, Low piloted a study to explore the utility of passive smartwatch and mobile phone data collection for estimating symptom burden during chemotherapy [57]. The study team leveraged the AWARE framework [58], which was designed to passively collect information from mobile phone use including statistics about communications, mobility, activity and location. AWARE also enabled participants to rate their symptoms each day which was used to compute daily symptom burden. A machine learning model achieved 88% accuracy in predicting symptom burden based on passively collected smartwatch and mobile phone data. This study provides an example of supporting public health goals by passively engaging humans in HCI-AI systems that learn from popular forms of technology already frequently used throughout their day. Such systems may be preferable monitoring tools due to the minimal effort needed by users.

HCI-AI for Biological Research

Recently, there has been a surge of development focused on the curation of databases and interactive web-based applications that help users access and interrogate high dimensional biomolecular data. The successful use of such tools rely on core HCI components to ensure their utility, usability, and explainability. In the next section, we will introduce several interactive web-based databases that allow users to access molecular data and results from offline AI experiments. By offline, we mean that scientists first deployed AI algorithms on biological data and have subsequently constructed databases for users to explore, download, and further analyze these results through the use of interactive modules. Additionally, we will introduce examples of HCI-AI systems designed to foster explainability of biological data.

Databases and Interactive Web-Based Applications

Spatial transcriptomics is an exploding area of biological research which makes it possible to capture gene expression at specific locations within cells of a tissue sample [59]. The high dimensionality of such data can greatly benefit from the use of AI and interactive tools that can help researchers unveil and understand its latent biological insights [60]. Indeed, Li and colleagues, developed SOAR: a spatial transcriptomics analysis resource to model spatial variability and cell type interactions [61]. SOAR is an interactive application which currently houses the results of >2700 spatial transcriptomics samples. The use of different bioinformatics AI methods were used to evaluate the spatial variability and cell-cell interaction of these samples. The web application was developed to be a comprehensive, one-stop resource housing the vast majority of publicly available spatial transcriptomics datasets. SOAR is interactive, user-friendly, and enables researchers to analyze their own genes and samples of interest to support their research needs.

Similarly, there have been databases developed to store AI derived protein structure predictions. For example, AlphaFold is an AI algorithm designed to predict protein structure [62]. The accompanying AlphaFold Protein Structure Database allows users to search >200 million protein structures predicted by AlphaFold, visualize the structures with interactive modules, and evaluate the algorithm's confidence and errors [63]. Even more recently, the EMS Metagenomic Atlas is a database containing >615 million metagenomic protein structures predicted through the use of a large language model [64]. The interactive atlas allows users to search and download sequences of interest to support their own research needs.

The St. Jude Cloud Ecosystem is a recent cloud-based interactive application which allows users to access, analyze, and visualize genomic data curated from >10,000 pediatric cancer patients [65]. Notably, the application was designed to be easy to use by researchers with limited to extensive computational abilities. The application allows users to upload their own data and to subsequently analyze and visualize it with a machine-learning tool that identifies differentially expressed genes and allows for cancer subtyping.

There has also been increasing interest in developing applications that allow users to directly interact and modify the performance of AI to aid in biomedical research. For example, PEAX is an interactive web-based application that leverages deep learning and a human-in-the-loop framework to support pattern detection in sequential data, such as genomic data [66]. The development of PEAX was motivated by the authors' recognition that while there are many similarity measurements like Euclidean distance which identify objectively similar sequences, the definition of 'similar' may be perceived differently from person-to-person. For this reason, PEAX employs an active learning sampling strategy which allows users to manually label salient patterns throughout the sequence, which in turn informs the algorithm's identification of other potential patterns. Through an evaluation study with computational biologists, PEAX was concluded to be easy to use and biologically useful; a classifier trained with the computational biologists' labels resulted in an increased AUC (0.93 vs 0.80) and average precision (0.56 vs 0.41) for the classifiers' ability to detect patterns compared to the performance when training on the ground-truth labels alone.

Furthermore, DrugExplorer was designed as an explainable AI system for drug repurposing [67]. To facilitate explainable AI, the authors leveraged a scaffolding-design approach by sequentially considering the following attributes: (1) the user and target domain, (2) the format and granularity of data abstraction that will best help the target domain understand the explanations, and choice of (3) visualization, and (4) algorithm. This approach, which underscores the necessity of usable and explainable HCI-AI systems, is the reverse workflow of many examples reviewed previously, which typically try to add explanations after model development. The study evaluated the usability of the system with medical professionals who had limited machine learning knowledge. Medical professionals were found to have more accurate, confident, and faster understanding of AI predictions when results were presented as path-based visualizations (e.g. Drug A is predicted to target Gene/Protein B which is associated with Disease C), as compared to more complicated graph-based visualizations or simple numeric confidence scores.

Open source tools for deploying visually appealing dashboards locally have also gained traction. For example, Lanchantin and colleagues constructed the Deep Motif Dashboard (DeMo) for visualizing deep learning results on classifiers trained to predict transcription factor binding sites [68]. This tool can be downloaded to a researcher's local system and makes available several visualization methods for identifying salient motifs that are predictive of transcription factor binding sites. These visualizations include (1) saliency maps for identifying the nucleotides most important for driving the network's prediction, (2) temporal outputs which take into account the sequential order of the genetic information, and (3) class optimization that identifies the most predictive sequence. The authors concluded that DeMo's visualizations can help humans better understand how neural networks make their predictions.

Challenges and Barriers to HCI-AI Implementation

Even now as AI becomes more commonplace in society, its role in medicine remains uncertain. Currently, development and implementation of HCI-AI systems is challenging for a number of reasons. First, successful development and implementation of HCI-AI systems is dependent on ensuring that proposed systems are clinically useful and practical for the designed application. Additionally, rapid acceleration of HCI-AI systems and their underlying technology has far outpaced the implementation of rigorous policies and guidelines to ensure their safe and ethical use. Consideration of timely policies and guidelines is needed to ensure these systems remain safe and fair for patients, health care providers, researchers, and all additional stakeholders. This section will discuss the important technical, social, and policy considerations that are crucial for ensuring that implementable HCI-AI systems are (1) clinically useful, (2) generalizable, and (3) safe.

Technical Challenges

When it comes to successful implementation of HCI-AI systems, there are a number of necessary technical considerations to ensure that systems are clinically useful. First, HCI-AI systems need to be designed to ensure that they are understandable to users with limited computational backgrounds and technical training. This is especially important when considering integrating AI-derived results into systems that are designed to guide and inform patient care. Accordingly, there have been discussions regarding the redesign of medical school curriculums in order to ensure that medical students have exposure to AI and proper evaluation of HCI-AI based systems. For example, Ötleş and colleagues advocated for the need to integrate AI education longitudinally throughout medical education and training [69]. In particular they suggested that medical education adopt an analytics hierarchy where initial exposure to descriptive analytics can set a foundation for more complex analytic methods including predictive and prescriptive analytics. Similarly, after evaluating a five week introductory AI workshop for medical students, Hu suggested 'literacy over proficiency' and identified heterogenous academic backgrounds as one of the primary challenges for introducing complex AI concepts [70]. As a result of often absent or informal AI education, it's important to recognize that many physicians and care providers have limited understanding as to how AI works. Incomplete education related to AI has likely driven mixed findings as to the perception and acceptance of AI within health care.

For instance, Henry and colleagues reported that emergency department physicians from a single health care center maintained positive sentiments towards an HCI-AI system for sepsis prediction, despite having a very limited understanding of AI [71]. Importantly, physicians did report appreciation that the system augmented their clinical judgment, rather than try and replace it. The study noted that the educational sessions and meetings with the CDS implementation team may have bolstered trust in the system, by providing opportunities for physicians to ask clarifying questions about the system or offer their advice on system implementation. This suggests that physicians and other health care providers have a significant role to play in guiding the implementation of HCI-AI systems across the entire training and implementation pipeline.

In contrast, while health care providers reported clinical care coordination and patient self-management improved after the implementation of an HCI-AI system for diabetic glycemic control, providers indicated low satisfaction with the system. Indeed, only 14% of survey participants indicated that they would recommend the system's adoption in other clinics [72]. Dissatisfaction of the system was largely attributed to inadequate patient recommendations. Although participants reported disenchantment over the prospect of AI and its clinical implications, participants did indicate the strength of the system in prompting discussions among the rest of a patient's care team. The contradictory nature of the findings reinforces the need to consider HCI-AI systems as augmenting the provider's role in treating the patient, rather than replacing. Moreover, the authors hypothesized that providers were more likely able to contextualize the patient's needs by considering social factors that were not able to be evaluated by the system, providing additional support for the need for humans and machines to work in tandem to support patient care.

Similarly, a study led by Liu demonstrated that ChatGPT can generate understandable and relevant CDS alerts, albeit such alerts may not always be useful without modifications [73]. Similar to Liu and colleagues, we propose that HCI-AI systems leveraging large language models (LLM) like ChatGPT, could be designed to function as iterative dialogue systems with the physician. In this framework, a

LLM could be integrated within the hospital's electronic health record to support real-time interaction with a physician as they document a patient's clinical status. As patient information is recorded, the LLM could simultaneously supplement a physician's initial treatment plans with additional recommendations or alert physicians to patients who are at risk for adverse health events. Importantly, this proposed system would enable the physician to steer the output of the system to remain more in line with his or her clinical suspicion. For example, the physician could modify recommendations as needed and instruct the LLM when its suggestions may be erroneous. Over time, through the physician's interactions with the electronic health record based LLM, the model will more robustly learn associations between a patient's clinical status and optimal treatment course. Through the generation of more clinically relevant alerts and recommendations, interactions with this type of HCI-AI system may be more tolerable, reducing commonly cited alert fatigue, while allowing the physician to remain in the loop and in the captain's seat when making critical clinical decisions. Moreover, as the system continues to learn, it ideally will facilitate the physician's clinical decision making abilities by adding intelligent AI-informed perspectives [73].

For widespread implementation, HCI-AI systems also must be generalizable. Thus, it is critical for systems to be tested on external datasets to validate their effectiveness, and thus, ability to treat patients across other health care systems safely and effectively. For example, an HCI-AI CDS sepsis prediction system deployed by Epic [74], a leading electronic health record platform, was found to have low generalizability, with poor discrimination and calibration, at an external hospital [75]. Indeed, an external evaluation of the model's performance reported that the system failed to identify 67% of patients with sepsis. Moreover, while the system alerted physicians to 18% of patients with suspected sepsis, only 7% of them were found to have sepsis. Unsurprisingly, the poor performance of the model was concluded to have caused high alert fatigue and raises serious concerns regarding patient safety due to a non-generalizable system.

Social Challenges

Overcoming technical challenges are also imperative for mitigating the influence of biases, especially those that could negatively impact patients of minority or other vulnerable populations. For example, in training the LLM underlying ChatGPT, Ouyang and colleagues discuss their efforts to reduce the potential of bias in the algorithm and to ensure its alignment with the intent of its users [40]. Accordingly, the training process of ChatGPT maintained a human-in-the-loop approach. Human labelers were recruited to aid in writing and rating prompts to fine-tune the performance of the LLM. The labelers were explicitly instructed to ensure that prompts were 'helpful, honest, and harmless'. [76] This study design was enacted to ensure that the resulting algorithm was unbiased and unharmful, especially towards different demographic or underrepresented groups. In Ouyan's discussion of the study, he discussed the challenge of ensuring that HCI-AI systems are aligned with ethical and moral human values. Focused efforts are still needed to ensure that LLMs are safe to all potential stakeholders.

Other efforts have strived to ensure that humans remain an essential focus amidst the expansion of AI technology. In fact, Chancellor sought to determine *Who is the 'Human' in Human-Centered Machine Learning* [77]. Indeed, Chancellor conducted a systematic review of studies that applied machine learning to predict the likelihood of mental illness of users who posted on social media. The authors categorized the studies by how each of them referred to the humans in the study. Commonly, humans were referred to by clinical terms such as 'patient' or grouped by mental illness (e.g. 'the Anxiety group' or 'the Depression group'). Alternatively, some studies deduced the human to analytical terms (e.g. 'data', 'sample', 'datapoint') or as social media terms (e.g. 'user', 'tweeter', 'post'). The authors warned that inconsistency with terminology to describe humans in AI studies, may lead to confusion by readers and downstream challenges in regard to scientific reproducibility. Moreover, the way in which humans are represented in studies that pertain to mental health is especially important in order to reduce the use of stigmatizing language and harmful perceptions of mental illness. The authors provided guidelines for how to report information about humans in machine learning studies, recommending: (1) clarity and consistency in how human data is represented and used, (2) collaborations with domain experts to identify an appropriate vocabulary, (3) to be mindful of harmful practices and stigmatization of language, and (4) maintaining the 'human' in human-centered machine learning in order to provide "insight into the context lost through mathematical translations."

Policy and Guidelines

Currently, AI is booming at a rate outpacing our abilities to define proper policies, guidelines, and regulations [78, 79]. As HCI-AI systems continue to emerge into the health care setting, the careful consideration of guidelines and policies to ensure safe systems is critical. To this end, large consortia have met to devise reporting guidelines for researchers implementing HCI-AI systems into the clinical setting. Recommended reporting guidelines aim to facilitate transparent systems that encourage clinical utility, patient safety, and physician confidence in AI-based methods and predictions. For example, CONSORT-AI leveraged Delphi consensus from a diverse group of stakeholders to develop guidelines for reporting clinical trials focused on evaluating HCI-AI interventions [80]. To aid in usability, the guidelines ask authors to explicitly explain if and how human-AI interaction was used in preparing data and the level of expertise expected of users. Moreover, the guidelines call for the specification of the AI intervention's output, how the output should be used to inform clinical decision making, whether human-AI interaction is needed for the outputs, and the expected experience of the user who may interpret the outputs and use them to guide clinical decision making. These guidelines exist to ensure usability of AI systems and to guide the development of transparent, reproducible, and generalizable systems. Cooperation with these guidelines overall seek to reduce patient harm from erroneously used systems and the development of systems that can inform clinical decision making.

Conclusions: Future Directions and Recommendations

As discussed in the beginning of this chapter, the present-day landscape of humans interacting with AI was envisioned decades ago. Even during its early days, AI was more fact than science-fiction. Kurt Vonnegut's 1952 debut novel *Player Piano*, explored the consequences of a society where most jobs have been taken over by machines [81]. *Player Piano*'s main character Paul Proteus laments that machines have replaced important aspects of what it means to be human: "The main business of humanity is to do a good job of being human beings," said Paul, "not to serve as appendages to machines, institutions, and systems." Later Vonnegut was quoted "I learned from the reviewers that I was a science-fiction writer. I didn't know that. I supposed that I was writing a novel about life." [82] Similarly, Donald A. Norman delineated the present and future challenges involving the development of human interaction with autonomous agents [83]. Norman's foreboding of the privacy and safety concerns regarding autonomous agents who can understand human language to the extent capable of offering suggestions and even writing computer programs, speaks to our present reality as AI becomes more embedded into society.

Today's students and researchers are witnessing a flourishing of activity in HCI-AI with the advent of large language models like OpenAI's ChatGPT, which debuted at the end of 2022 [40]. Within months of its release, its easy to use graphical user interface and powerful language modeling capabilities, is a realization of the future of HCI-AI unification that earlier scientists foreshadowed. Licklider lamented in his own assessment of his research time that: "About 85 per cent of my 'thinking' time was spent getting into a position to think, to make a decision, to learn something I needed to know. Much more time went into finding or obtaining information than into digesting it. Hours went into the plotting of graphs, and other hours into instructing an assistant how to plot" [15]. ChatGPT can summarize user requested information and write and help debug complex code, hence becoming an assistive tool to reduce the time burden of less important tasks that are critical to the research and scientific process.

Nevertheless, there remains an urgent need to devise policies to ensure ethical clinical and biomedical use of AI, especially in light of the rapid deployment of large language models. In a study by Gao and colleagues, ChatGPT was used to generate 50 scientific abstracts, 38% of which were believed to be real by a team of biomedical researchers [84]. While we commend the user friendly and intuitive interface of ChatGPT, it's critical to recognize that humans have a gap in their abilities to distinguish human vs AI. We echo the recommendations of other researchers and academic publishers who stress the importance of transparency when large language models are used in order to ensure accountability and ethical use of HCI-AI systems, especially as they continue to improve [85–87].

As underscored throughout many of the clinical, public health, and biological HCI-AI systems demonstrated throughout the chapter, continued unification of HCI-AI systems to support health care requires frequent and extensive communication with doctors, patients, and other stakeholders. Such conversations are necessary to not only identify clinically important problems and construct systems that address real-world needs, but to improve these systems overtime [32, 42, 88]. For more robust clinical utility, Luo recommends a transition from reactive HCI-AI systems to proactive HCI-AI systems [89]. Conventionally, many HCI-AI systems are designed and implemented using a reactive approach. By reactive, we refer to a training and implementation approach where human domain experts are heavily involved in each step of the AI workflow (e.g. beginning from initial stages of data collection and preparation to the latest stages of model evaluation and deployment). In contrast, proactive systems are designed with two levels which leverage human domain experts to facilitate improved automation and augmentation of a system throughout its life cycle. Level 1 refers to the role of human experts in automating feature engineering and model training and tuning. In level 2, continued model evaluation by human domain experts can facilitate targeted data collection and augment the data preparation process. This level ensures the continuous evaluation of the system once it has been implemented in the clinical setting. Proactive AI effectively completes the data-model-deployment-data feedback loop with humans organically embedded. Future developers of HCI-AI systems should consider more effective HCI design for proactive development in order to ensure that such systems can integrate successfully into our dynamic health landscape. Continuous evaluation and monitoring of HCI-AI systems is vital to ensuring that systems remain clinically useful and safe in their abilities to support accurate and precise clinical decision making.

References

1. Russell SJ, Norvig P, Davis E. Artificial intelligence: a modern approach. 3rd ed. Upper Saddle River: Prentice Hall; 2010. 1132 p. (Prentice Hall series in artificial intelligence).
2. Goodfellow I, Bengio Y, Courville A. Deep learning. MIT Press; 2016.
3. McCarthy J, Minsky ML, Rochester N, Shannon CE. A Proposal for the Dartmouth Summer Research Project on Artificial Intelligence AI Magazine. 2006;27(4):12. https://doi.org/10.1609/aimag.v27i4.1904
4. Turing AM. I.—Computing machinery and intelligence. Mind. 1950;LIX(236):433–60.
5. Herbert SA. The new science of management decision. Harper & Brothers; 1960. 50 p.
6. Good IJ. Speculations concerning the first ultraintelligent machine. In: Advances in computers [Internet]. Elsevier; 1966 [cited 2023 May 31]. p. 31–88. Available from: https://linkinghub.elsevier.com/retrieve/pii/S0065245808604180
7. McCarthy J. Programs with common sense. National Physical Laboratory. Mechanisation of thought processes: Proceedings of a symposium held at the National Physical Laboratory on 24th, 25th, 26th and 27th November 1958. H. M. Stationery Off. 1959. p. 1–15.

8. Newell A, Simon H. The logic theory machine--a complex information processing system. IEEE Trans Inform Theory. 1956;2(3):61–79.
9. Minsky ML. Computation: finite and infinite machines. Prentice-Hall; 1967. (Prentice-Hall series in automatic computation).
10. Bush V. As we may think. Interactions. 1996;3(2):35–46.
11. Simon HA. Organizational design: man-machine systems for decision making. In: The new science of management decision [Internet]. New York: Harper & Brothers; 1960 [cited 2023 Jun 11]. p. 35–50. Available from: http://content.apa.org/books/13978-005
12. Simon HA. The executive as decision maker. In: The new science of management decision [Internet]. New York: Harper & Brothers; 1960 [cited 2023 Jun 11]. p. 1–8. Available from: http://content.apa.org/books/13978-001
13. Grudin J. AI and HCI: two fields divided by a common focus. AI Mag. 2009;30(4):48.
14. Grudin J. Turing maturing: the separation of artificial intelligence and human-computer interaction. Interactions. 2006;13(5):54–7.
15. Licklider JCR. Man-computer symbiosis. IRE Trans Hum Factors Electron. 1960;HFE-1(1):4–11.
16. Winograd T. Shifting viewpoints: artificial intelligence and human–computer interaction. Artif Intell. 2006;170(18):1256–8.
17. Simon HA, Newell A. Heuristic problem solving: the next advance in operations research. Oper Res. 1958;6(1):1–10.
18. Engelbart DC. Augmenting human intellect: a conceptual framework. SRI summary report AFOSR-3223; 1962.
19. Wright A, Sittig DF. A four-phase model of the evolution of clinical decision support architectures. Int J Med Inform. 2008;77(10):641–9.
20. Ledley RS, Lusted LB. Reasoning foundations of medical diagnosis. Science, New Series. 1959;130(3366):9–21.
21. Ledley R, Lusted L. The use of electronic computers to aid in medical diagnosis. Proc IRE. 1959;47(11):1970–7.
22. Ledley RS, Lusted LB. The use of electronic computers in medical data processing: aids in diagnosis, current information retrieval, and medical record keeping. IRE Trans Med Electron. 1960;ME-7(1):31–47.
23. Crumb CB, Rupe CE. The automatic digital computer as an aid in medical diagnosis. Papers presented at the December 1–3, 1959, Eastern Joint IRE-AIEE-ACM Computer Conference on - IRE-AIEE-ACM '59 (Eastern) [Internet]. Boston, MA: ACM Press; 1959 [cited 2023 May 10]. p. 174–180. Available from: http://portal.acm.org/citation.cfm?doid=1460299.1460319
24. Warner HR, Toronto AF, Veasey LG, Stephenson R. A mathematical approach to medical diagnosis: application to congenital heart disease. JAMA. 1961;177(3):177–83.
25. Collen MF, Rubin L, Neyman J, Dantzig GB, Baer RM, Siegelaub AB. Automated multiphasic screening and diagnosis. Am J Public Health Nations Health. 1964;54(5):741–50.
26. Bleich HL. Computer evaluation of acid-base disorders. J Clin Invest. 1969;48:1689–96.
27. Pople HE, Myers JD, Miller RA. Dialog: a model of diagnostic logic for internal medicine. Paper presented at: IJCAI'75: Proceedings of the 4th International Joint Conference on Artificial Intelligence, vol. 1. 1975. p. 848–62.
28. Pople HE. The formation of composite hypotheses in diagnostic problem solving: an exercise in synthetic reasoning. Paper presented at: IJCAI'77: Proceedings of the 5th International Joint Conference on Artificial Intelligence, vol. 2. 1977. p. 1030–7.
29. Hudson DL, Estrin T. EMERGE-a data-driven medical decision making aid. IEEE Trans Pattern Anal Mach Intell. 1984;PAMI-6(1):87–91.
30. Hudson DL, Cohen ME. Human-computer interaction in a medical decision support system. Paper presented at: [1989] Proceedings of the Twenty-Second Annual Hawaii International Conference on System Sciences Volume II: Software Track [Internet]. Kailua-Kona, HI, USA. 1989 [cited 2023 Apr 28]. p. 429–35. Available from: http://ieeexplore.ieee.org/document/48023/

31. Ben-Bassat M, Carlson RW, Puri VK, et al. Pattern-based interactive diagnosis of multiple disorders: the MEDAS system. IEEE Trans Pattern Anal Mach Intell. 1980;PAMI-2(2):148–60.
32. Heathfield H. The rise and "fall" of expert systems in medicine. Expert Syst. 1999;16(3):183–8.
33. Heathfield HA, Winstanley G, Kirkham N. Decision support system for the differential diagnosis of breast disease. J Biomed Eng. 1991;13(1):51–7.
34. Heathfield H, Kirkham N. A cooperative approach to decision support in the differential diagnosis of breast disease. Med Inf. 1992;17(1):21–33.
35. Miller RA. Evaluating evaluations of medical diagnostic systems. J Am Med Inform Assoc. 1996;3(6):429–31.
36. Friedman CP. A "fundamental theorem" of biomedical informatics. J Am Med Inform Assoc. 2009;16(2):169–70.
37. Charlson ME, Pompei P, Ales KL, MacKenzie CR. A new method of classifying prognostic comorbidity in longitudinal studies: development and validation. J Chronic Dis. 1987;40(5):373–83.
38. Gage BF, Waterman AD, Shannon W, Boechler M, Rich MW, Radford MJ. Validation of clinical classification schemes for predicting stroke: results from the national registry of atrial fibrillation. ACC Curr J Rev. 2001;10(6):20–1.
39. Toward precision medicine: building a knowledge network for biomedical research and a new taxonomy of disease [Internet]. Washington, D.C.: National Academies Press; 2011 [cited 2023 May 9]. Available from: http://www.nap.edu/catalog/13284
40. Ouyang L, Wu J, Jiang X, et al. Training language models to follow instructions with human feedback [Internet]. arXiv. 2022 [cited 2023 Feb 14]. Available from: http://arxiv.org/abs/2203.02155
41. ChatGPT [Internet]. [cited 2023 Jun 24]. Available from: https://chat.openai.com
42. Tschandl P, Rinner C, Apalla Z, et al. Human–computer collaboration for skin cancer recognition. Nat Med. 2020;26(8):1229–34.
43. Hekler A, Utikal JS, Enk AH, et al. Superior skin cancer classification by the combination of human and artificial intelligence. Eur J Cancer. 2019;120:114–21.
44. Patel BN, Rosenberg L, Willcox G, et al. Human–machine partnership with artificial intelligence for chest radiograph diagnosis. NPJ Digit Med. 2019;2(1):111.
45. Rosenberg L. Artificial swarm intelligence, a human-in-the-loop approach to A.I. AAAI [Internet]. 2016 Mar 5 [cited 2023 Jun 1];30(1). Available from: https://ojs.aaai.org/index.php/AAAI/article/view/9833
46. Raja AS, Ip IK, Prevedello LM, et al. Effect of computerized clinical decision support on the use and yield of CT pulmonary angiography in the emergency department. Radiology. 2012;262(2):468–74.
47. Pantanowitz L, Quiroga-Garza GM, Bien L, et al. An artificial intelligence algorithm for prostate cancer diagnosis in whole slide images of core needle biopsies: a blinded clinical validation and deployment study. Lancet Digit Health. 2020;2(8):e407–16.
48. Otaki Y, Singh A, Kavanagh P, et al. Clinical deployment of explainable artificial intelligence of SPECT for diagnosis of coronary artery disease. JACC Cardiovasc Imaging. 2022;15(6):1091–102.
49. Farzaneh N, Williamson CA, Gryak J, Najarian K. A hierarchical expert-guided machine learning framework for clinical decision support systems: an application to traumatic brain injury prognostication. NPJ Digit Med. 2021;4(1):78.
50. Lundberg S, Lee SI. A unified approach to interpreting model predictions [Internet]. arXiv. 2017 [cited 2023 Jun 24]. Available from: http://arxiv.org/abs/1705.07874
51. Cheema B, Mutharasan RK, Sharma A, et al. Augmented intelligence to identify patients with advanced heart failure in an integrated health system. JACC Adv. 2022;1(4):100123.
52. Seol HY, Shrestha P, Muth JF, et al. Artificial intelligence-assisted clinical decision support for childhood asthma management: a randomized clinical trial. PLoS One. 2021;16(8):e0255261.

53. Lee C, Light A, Saveliev ES, van der Schaar M, Gnanapragasam VJ. Developing machine learning algorithms for dynamic estimation of progression during active surveillance for prostate cancer. NPJ Digit Med. 2022;5(1):110.
54. Marvel SW, House JS, Wheeler M, et al. The COVID-19 pandemic vulnerability index (PVI) dashboard: monitoring county-level vulnerability using visualization, statistical modeling, and machine learning. Environ Health Perspect. 2021;129(1):017701.
55. Villavicencio CN, Macrohon JJ, Inbaraj XA, Jeng JH, Hsieh JG. Development of a machine learning based web application for early diagnosis of COVID-19 based on symptoms. Diagnostics. 2022;12(4):821.
56. Ammar N, Shaban-Nejad A. Explainable artificial intelligence recommendation system by leveraging the semantics of adverse childhood experiences: proof-of-concept prototype development. JMIR Med Inform. 2020;8(11):e18752.
57. Low CA, Dey AK, Ferreira D, et al. Estimation of symptom severity during chemotherapy from passively sensed data: exploratory study. J Med Internet Res. 2017;19(12):e420.
58. Ferreira D, Kostakos V, Dey AK. AWARE: mobile context instrumentation framework. Front ICT [Internet]. 2015 Apr 20 [cited 2023 Jun 20];2. Available from: http://journal.frontiersin.org/article/10.3389/fict.2015.00006/abstract
59. Ståhl PL, Salmén F, Vickovic S, et al. Visualization and analysis of gene expression in tissue sections by spatial transcriptomics. Science. 2016;353(6294):78–82.
60. Zeng Z, Li Y, Li Y, Luo Y. Statistical and machine learning methods for spatially resolved transcriptomics data analysis. Genome Biol. 2022;23(1):83.
61. Li Y, Dennis S, Hutch MR, et al. SOAR elucidates disease mechanisms and empowers drug discovery through spatial transcriptomics. bioRxiv. 2023; https://doi.org/10.1101/2022.04.17.488596.
62. Jumper J, Evans R, Pritzel A, et al. Highly accurate protein structure prediction with AlphaFold. Nature. 2021;596(7873):583–9.
63. Varadi M, Anyango S, Deshpande M, et al. AlphaFold protein structure database: massively expanding the structural coverage of protein-sequence space with high-accuracy models. Nucleic Acids Res. 2022;50(D1):D439–44.
64. Lin Z, Akin H, Rao R, et al. Evolutionary-scale prediction of atomic-level protein structure with a language model. Science. 2023;379(6637):1123–30.
65. McLeod C, Gout AM, Zhou X, et al. St. Jude Cloud: a pediatric cancer genomic data-sharing ecosystem. Cancer Discov. 2021;11(5):1082–99.
66. Lekschas F, Peterson B, Haehn D, Ma E, Gehlenborg N, Pfister H. Peax: interactive visual pattern search in sequential data using unsupervised deep representation learning. Comput Graph Forum. 2020;39(3):167–79.
67. Wang Q, Huang K, Chandak P, Zitnik M, Gehlenborg N. Extending the nested model for user-centric XAI: a design study on GNN-based drug repurposing. IEEE Trans Vis Comput Graph. 2023;29(1):1266–76.
68. Lanchantin J, Singh R, Wang B, Qi Y. Deep Motif dashboard: visualizing and understanding genomic sequences using deep neural networks. Pac Symp Biocomput. 2017;22:254–65.
69. Ötleş E, James CA, Lomis KD, Woolliscroft JO. Teaching artificial intelligence as a fundamental toolset of medicine. Cell Rep Med. 2022;3(12):100824.
70. Hu R, Fan KY, Pandey P, et al. Insights from teaching artificial intelligence to medical students in Canada. Commun Med. 2022;2(1):63.
71. Henry KE, Kornfield R, Sridharan A, et al. Human–machine teaming is key to AI adoption: clinicians' experiences with a deployed machine learning system. NPJ Digit Med. 2022;5(1):97.
72. Romero-Brufau S, Wyatt KD, Boyum P, Mickelson M, Moore M, Cognetta-Rieke C. A lesson in implementation: a pre-post study of providers' experience with artificial intelligence-based clinical decision support. Int J Med Inform. 2020;137:104072.
73. Liu S, Wright AP, Patterson BL, et al. Using AI-generated suggestions from ChatGPT to optimize clinical decision support. J Am Med Inform Assoc. 2023;30:1237–45.

74. Epic. With the patient at the heart [Internet]. [cited 2023 Jun 25]. Available from: https://www.epic.com/
75. Wong A, Otles E, Donnelly JP, et al. External validation of a widely implemented proprietary sepsis prediction model in hospitalized patients. JAMA Intern Med. 2021;181(8):1065–70.
76. Askell A, Bai Y, Chen A, et al. A general language assistant as a laboratory for alignment [Internet]. arXiv. 2021 [cited 2023 Jun 25]. Available from: http://arxiv.org/abs/2112.00861
77. Chancellor S, Baumer EPS, De Choudhury M. Who is the "human" in human-centered machine learning: the case of predicting mental health from social media. Proc ACM Hum-Comput Interact. 2019;3(CSCW):1–32.
78. Klein E. The surprising thing A.I. engineers will tell you if you let them. The New York Times. 2023 Apr 16.
79. Li FF. How to make A.I. that's good for people. The New York Times. 2018 Mar 7.
80. Liu X, Cruz Rivera S, Moher D, et al. Reporting guidelines for clinical trial reports for interventions involving artificial intelligence: the CONSORT-AI extension. Nat Med. 2020;26(9):1364–74.
81. Vonnegut K. Player piano. New York: Random House Publishing Group; 2009.
82. Vonnegut K. Wampeters, foma & granfalloons (opinions). Dial Press trade paperback ed. New York: Dial Press; 2006. 288 p.
83. Norman DA. How might people interact with agents. Commun ACM. 1994;37(7):68–71.
84. Gao CA, Howard FM, Markov NS, et al. Comparing scientific abstracts generated by ChatGPT to real abstracts with detectors and blinded human reviewers. NPJ Digit Med. 2023;6(1):75.
85. Flanagin A, Bibbins-Domingo K, Berkwits M, Christiansen SL. Nonhuman "authors" and implications for the integrity of scientific publication and medical knowledge. JAMA. 2023;329(8):637.
86. Tools such as ChatGPT threaten transparent science; here are our ground rules for their use. Nature. 2023;613(7945):612.
87. Liebrenz M, Schleifer R, Buadze A, Bhugra D, Smith A. Generating scholarly content with ChatGPT: ethical challenges for medical publishing. Lancet Digit Health. 2023;5(3):e105–6.
88. Cai CJ, Reif E, Hegde N, et al. Human-centered tools for coping with imperfect algorithms during medical decision-making. Paper presented at: Proceedings of the 2019 CHI Conference on Human Factors in Computing Systems [Internet]. Glasgow: ACM; 2019 [cited 2023 May 5]. p. 1–14. Available from: https://dl.acm.org/doi/10.1145/3290605.3300234
89. Luo Y, Wunderink RG, Lloyd-Jones D. Proactive vs reactive machine learning in health care: lessons from the COVID-19 pandemic. JAMA. 2022;327(7):623.

Part II
Approaches to Evaluation

Chapter 5
Evaluation of Health Information Technology: Methods, Frameworks and Challenges

Thomas G. Kannampallil and Joanna Abraham

Introduction

The adoption and use of health information technology (HIT), especially Electronic Health Records (EHR), has increased over the last decade [1]. This increase, at least in part, has been spurred by recent federal mandates as part of the American Reinvestment and Recovery Act (ARRA). These mandates have incentivized the use of HIT with the goal of improving the quality and safety of healthcare. Though there are several positive reports of significant benefits in cost savings, quality and safety, persuasive evidence of the substantial impact of HIT is currently lacking. Most often, HIT implementation is characterized by inconsistent and mixed results regarding their utility and value [2]. A large body of research investigates the unintended and unanticipated consequences associated with the use of HIT that results in increased time spent on documentation, workarounds, communication failures, duplication and redundancy of information, and effort to maintain continuity of information and care (e.g., [3–5]; also see Chap. 11, on unanticipated consequences of HIT use). Furthermore, evaluation studies have also questioned the safety implications of EHR use (e.g., errors and adverse events) [6].

A recent Institute of Medicine (IOM) report (e.g., [7]) has highlighted the lack of effective integration of appropriate evaluation methods during the design and development phases of HIT. The IOM committee has also called for a systematic evaluation of not only the HIT systems, but also the context of clinical environments in

---

T. G. Kannampallil (✉) · J. Abraham
Department of Anesthesiology, Washington University School of Medicine, St Louis, MO, USA

Institute for Informatics, Data Science, and Biostatistics, Washington University School of Medicine, St Louis, MO, USA
e-mail: thomas.k@wustl.edu

© The Author(s), under exclusive license to Springer Nature Switzerland AG 2024
A. W. Kushniruk et al. (eds.), *Human Computer Interaction in Healthcare*, Cognitive Informatics in Biomedicine and Healthcare, https://doi.org/10.1007/978-3-031-69947-4_5

which these systems would be used. Nevertheless, the challenge that is faced by developers and researchers alike is to *identify, select* and *use* appropriate methods of HIT evaluation. In this chapter, our aims are two-fold: *first*, to provide an overview of the various methods that can be used for evaluating HIT systems. We have categorized evaluation methods under two general headings: (a) evaluation of systems, focusing on usability and other parameters related to human computer interaction (HCI)—these methods are analytic, and most often laboratory-based; (b) a more generic usability and situated testing of systems, focusing on a comprehensive perspective of the use of HIT systems within the context of clinical environments (e.g., the role of HIT on clinical workflow or its role in causing unintended consequences)—these methods are more open-ended, in-situ and field-based. It is important to note that these categorizations are not mutually exclusive—evaluation of systems often involve the use of one or more methods from both categories. *Second*, we discuss the challenges of conducting comprehensive evaluation studies in the clinical environment, and approaches to potentially overcome these challenges. In addition, we provide examples of the use of the specific methods, and cross-references to other chapters in this volume that have utilized the same methods in a clinical context.

Methods of Evaluation in Clinical Environments

A healthcare system is often considered a complex, socio-technical system consisting of many components—clinicians, patients, and HIT, to name a few [8, 9]. Among these, HIT is a key component that is necessary to ensure the smooth and effective functioning of the modern healthcare system. HIT incorporation into a clinical environment often transforms the structure, processes or outcomes—hence appropriate evaluation is often necessary to determine its viability or effectiveness [10]. The pertinent question is *how do we study the effects of HIT on structure, processes or outcomes—both directly, and indirectly*? HIT evaluation is often built on components assessing the: (1) system functionality, (2) impact of the user interface on the work activities, and (3) discovering specific interface and system issues that affect the contextual work activities of user [11].

In general, an evaluation would involve the following questions of what, why, when and how: (a) *what* to evaluate (e.g., an interface); (b) *why* should it be evaluated—it should be noted that given the breadth of biomedical informatics research, the purpose of the evaluation can include the following: as a promotional activity (e.g., reassuring patients or clinicians that resources are safe), part of scholarly work (e.g., a research project), a pragmatic activity (e.g., to evaluate whether a device is cost effective to purchase), ethical activity (e.g., to evaluate whether a medical device is functional and can be used as an alternative to an existing device), or medico-legal (e.g., to reduce legal liability) [12]; (c) *when* to evaluate (e.g., at what stage of the design or implementation process); and (d) *how* to evaluate (i.e., the methods and tools that should be used for evaluation).

In terms of "when to evaluate" a system, evaluation studies can be generally classified into two categories: formative or summative. *Formative evaluation* is defined as "*a rigorous assessment process designed to identify potential and actual influences on the progress and effectiveness of implementation efforts*" [13]. These evaluation studies are performed during the early stages of system design, and continue throughout the system development lifecycle. These evaluations are conducted to receive early feedback from potential users, and are mostly conducted with prototypes (using low-fidelity paper prototypes or hi-fidelity actual test interfaces). The purpose of these evaluations is to study the complexity of design and update the system before implementation through user feedback. In contrast, *summative evaluation* is performed at the completion of the design and development efforts. These are often considered comprehensive as it is expected to demonstrate the efficacy of a system in its environment of use.

In this chapter, we focus specifically on the "how to evaluate" aspect. We have classified evaluation methods into two categories: general analytic evaluation approaches and usability testing. This categorization was informally based on the type of participant in the evaluation. Analytic evaluation studies are, most often, using experts as participants—usability experts, domain experts, software designers—or in some cases, without participants. These techniques include task-analytic, inspection-based or model-based approaches and are most often conducted in laboratory-based (or controlled) settings.

In contrast, usability testing employs users and stakeholders in the evaluation process. Usability testing can be conducted in the field or in a controlled laboratory setting. For example, one can evaluate the use of a hand-held device in an Emergency Room (ER) using observational techniques. In contrast, EHR interfaces or other user interfaces can be tested in a laboratory environment where users are asked to complete specific simulated task scenarios. While certain methods of usability testing can be more effectively conducted in a laboratory setting, the settings are sometimes a matter of convenience (e.g., it is easier for a participant to complete a task with verbal think-aloud without interruptions in a laboratory setting than in a clinical setting). We have categorized usability testing into field-based studies (including general observational and other studies) that capture situated and contextual aspects of HIT use, and a general category of methods (e.g., interviews, focus groups, surveys) that solicit user opinions and can be administered in different modes (e.g., face-to-face or online). A brief categorization of the evaluation approaches can be found in Fig. 5.1. In the following sections, we provide a detailed description of each of the evaluation approaches along with research examples of its use.

Analytical Approaches

Analytical approaches rely on analysts' judgments and analytic techniques to perform evaluations on user interfaces, and often do not directly involve the participation of end users. These approaches utilize experts—usability, human factors, or

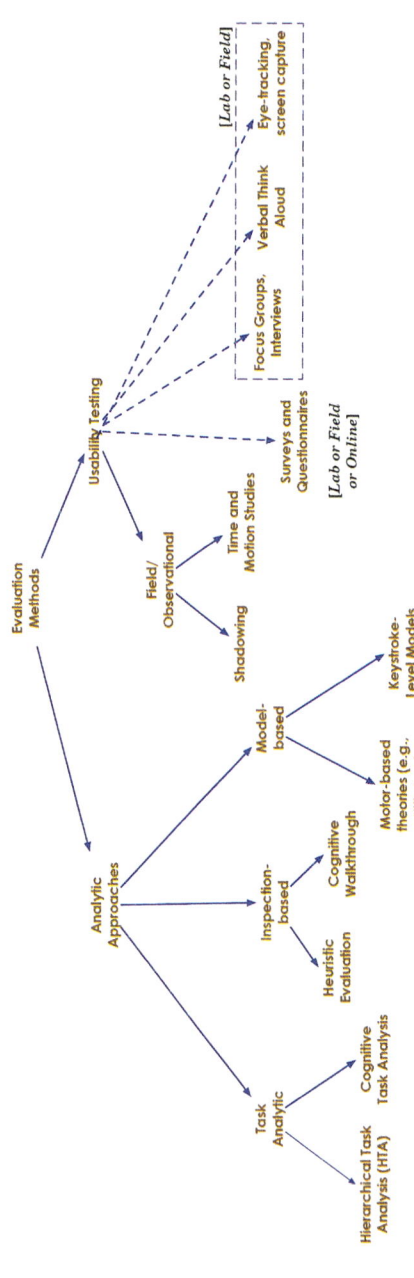

Fig. 5.1 Classification of evaluation methods

software—to conduct the evaluation studies. In general, analytical evaluation techniques involve *task-analytic* approaches (e.g., hierarchical and cognitive task analysis), *inspection-based* methods (e.g., heuristic evaluations and walkthroughs), and predictive *model-based* methods (e.g., keystroke models, Fitts Law). As will be described in the respective sections, the model-based techniques do not use any participants and relies on parameterized approaches for describing expert behavior. We describe each of these techniques, their applications, appropriate contexts of their use and examples from recent research literature.

Task Analysis[1]

Task analysis is one of most commonly used techniques to evaluate "existing practices" in order to understand the rationale behind people's goals of performing a task, the motivations behind their goals, and how they perform these tasks [14]. As described by Vicente [15], task analysis is an evaluation of the "trajectories of behavior." There are several variants of task analysis—hierarchical task analysis (HTA) and cognitive task analysis (CTA) being the most commonly used in biomedical informatics research.

Hierarchical Task Analysis

HTA is the simplest task analytic approach and involves the breaking down of a task into sub-tasks and smaller constituted parts (e.g., sub-sub-tasks). The tasks are organized according to specific goals. This method, originally designed to identify specific training needs, has been used extensively in the design and evaluation of interactive interfaces [16]. The application of HTA can be explained with an example: consider the goal of printing a Microsoft Word document that is on your desktop. The sub-tasks for this goal would involve finding (or identifying) the document on your desktop, and then printing it by selecting the appropriate printer. The HTA for this task can be organized as follows:

0. Print document on the desktop
1. Go to the desktop
2. Find the document

    2.1. Use "Search" function
    2.2. Enter the name of the document
    2.3. Identify the document

3. Open the document

---

[1] While GOMS is considered a task-analytic approach, we have categorized it as a model-based approach for predictions of task completion times. It is based on a task analytic decomposition of tasks.

4. Select the "File" menu and then "Print"
   4.1. Select relevant printer
   4.2. Click "Print" button
        Plan 0: do 1–3–4; if file cannot be located by a visual search, do 2–3–4
        Plan 2: do 2.1–2.2–2.3

In the above-mentioned task analysis, the task can be decomposed into the following: moving to your desktop, searching for the document (either visually or by using the search function and typing in the search criteria), selecting the document, opening and printing it using the appropriate printer. The order in which these tasks are performed may change based on certain situations. For example, if the document is not immediately visible on the desktop (or if the desktop has several documents making it impossible to identify the document visually), then a search function is necessary. Similarly, if there are multiple printer choices, then a relevant printer must be selected. The plans include a set of tasks that a user must undertake to achieve the goal (i.e., print the document). In this case, there are two plans: plan 0 and plan 2 (all plans are conditional on tasks having pertinent sub-tasks associated with it). For example, if the user cannot find a document on the desktop, plan 2 is instantiated, where a search function is used to identify the document (steps 2.1, 2.2 and 2.3). Figure 5.2 depicts the visual form of the HTA for this particular example.

HTA has been used significantly in evaluating interfaces and medical devices. For example, Chung et al. [17] used HTA to compare the differences between six infusion pumps. Using HTA, they identified potential sources for the generation of human errors during various tasks. While exploratory, their use of HTA provided insights into how the HTA can be used for evaluating human performance and for predicting potential sources of errors. Alternatively, HTA has been used to model information and clinical workflow in ambulatory clinics [18]. Unertl et al. [18] used direct observations and semi-structured interviews to create a HTA of the

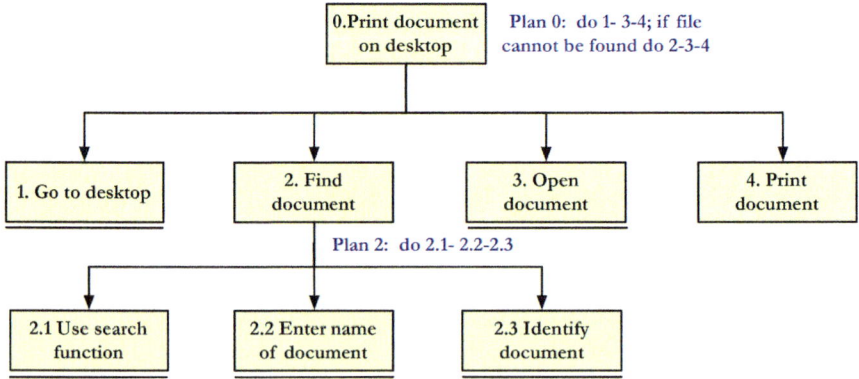

Fig. 5.2 Graphical representation of task analysis of printing a document: the tasks are represented in the boxes; the line underneath certain boxes represents the fact that there are no sub-tasks for these tasks

workflows. The HTA was then used to identify the gaps in existing HIT functionality for supporting clinical workflows, and the needs of chronic disease care providers.

Cognitive Task Analysis

CTA is an extension of the general task analysis technique to develop a more comprehensive understanding regarding the knowledge, cognitive/thought processes and goals that underlie observable task activities [19]. While the focus is on knowledge and cognitive components of the task activities and performance, CTA relies on observable human activities to draw insights on the knowledge based constraints and challenges that impair effective task performance.

CTA techniques are broadly classified into three groups based on how data is captured: (a) interviews and observations, (b) process tracing and (c) conceptual techniques [20]. CTA supported by interviews and observations involve developing a comprehensive understanding of the tasks through discussions with, and task observations of experts. For example, a researcher observes an expert physician performing the task of medication order entry into a CPOE (Computerized Physician Order Entry) system and asks follow up questions regarding the specific aspects of the task. In a study on understanding providers' management of abnormal test results, Hysong et al. [21] conducted interviews with 28 primary care physicians on how and when they manage alerts, and how they use the various features on the EHR system to filter and sort their alerts. The authors used the CTA approach supported by a combination of interviews and demonstrations. Participants were asked how they performed their alert management tasks and were asked to demonstrate these to the researcher. Based on the evaluation, they found that understanding of alert management differed (between 4 and 75%) between providers and most did not use these features.

CTA supported by process-tracing approaches relies on capturing task activities through direct (e.g., verbal think aloud) or indirect (e.g., unobtrusive screen recording) data capture methods. Whereas the process-tracing approach is generally used to capture expert behaviors, it has also been used to evaluate general users. In a study on experts' information seeking behavior in critical care, Kannampallil et al. [22] used the process-tracing approach to identify the nature of information-seeking activities including the information sources, cognitive strategies and shortcuts used by critical care physicians in decision making tasks. The CTA approach relied on the verbalizations of physicians, their access of various sources, and the time spent on accessing these sources to identify the strategies of information seeking. In a related study, the process-tracing approach was used to characterize the differences of information seeking practices of two groups of clinicians [23].

Finally, CTA supported by conceptual techniques rely on the development of representations of a domain (and their related concepts) and the potential relationships between them. This approach is often used with experts and different methods are used for knowledge elicitation including concept elicitation, structured interviews, ranking approaches, card sorting, structural approaches such as multi-dimensional scaling, and graphical associations [20]. While extensively used in general HCI studies, the use of conceptual techniques based CTA is much less prominent in biomedical informatics research literature. A detailed review of these approaches and their use can be found in Cooke [20].

Inspection-Based Evaluation

Inspection methods involve one or more experts appraising a system, playing the role of a user in order to identify potential usability and interaction problems with a system [24]. Inspection methods are most often conducted on fully developed systems or interfaces, but may also be used on prototypes or beta systems. These techniques provide a cost-effective mechanism for evaluation to identify the shortcomings of a system. Inspection methods rely on a usability expert, i.e., a person with significant training and experience in evaluating interfaces, to go through a system and identify whether the user interface elements conform to a pre-determined set of usability guidelines and design requirements (or principles). This method has been used as an alternative to recruiting potential users to test the usability of a system. The most commonly used inspection methods are heuristic evaluations (HE) and walkthroughs.

Heuristic Evaluation

HE techniques utilize a small set of experts to evaluate a user interface (or a set of interfaces in a system) based on their understanding of a set of heuristic principles regarding interface design [25]. This technique was developed by Jakob Nielsen and colleagues [24, 26], and has been used extensively in the evaluation of user interfaces. The original set of heuristics was developed by Nielsen [24] based on an abstraction of 249 usability problems. In general, the following ten heuristic principles (or a subset of these) are most often considered for HE studies: system status visibility; match between system and real world; user control and freedom; consistency and standards; error prevention; recognition rather than recall; flexibility and efficiency of use; aesthetic and minimalist design; help users recognize, diagnose and recover from errors; and help and documentation (retrieved from: http://www.nngroup.com/articles/ten-usability-heuristics/, on September 24, 2014; additional details can be found at this link). Conducting a HE involves a usability expert going through an interface to identify potential violations to a set of usability principles (referred to as the "heuristics"). These perceived violations could involve a variety of interface elements such as windows, menu items, links, navigation, and interaction.

Evaluators typically select a relevant subset of heuristics for evaluation (or add more based on the specific needs and context). The selection of heuristics is based on the type of system and interface being evaluated. For example, the relevant heuristics for evaluating an EHR interface would be different from that of a medical device. After selecting a set of applicable heuristics, one or more usability experts evaluate the user interface against the identified heuristics. After evaluating the heuristics, the potential violations are rated according to a severity score (1–5, where 1 indicates a cosmetic problem and 5 indicates a catastrophic problem). This process is iterative and continues till the expert feels that a majority (if not all) of the violations are identified. It is also generally recommended that a set of 4–5 usability experts are required to identify 95% of the perceived violations or problems with a user interface. It should be acknowledged that HE approach may not lead to the identification of all problems and the identified problems may be localized (i.e., specific to a particular interface in a system). An example of an HE evaluation form is shown in Fig. 5.3.

In the healthcare domain, HE has been used in the evaluation of medical devices and HIT interfaces. For example, Zhang et al. [27] used a modified set of 14 heuristics to compare the patient safety characteristics of two 1-channel volumetric infusion pumps. Four independent usability experts evaluated both infusion pumps using the list of heuristics and identified 89 usability problems categorized as 192 heuristic violations for pump 1, and 52 usability problems categorized as 121 heuristic violations for pump 2. The heuristic violations were also classified based on

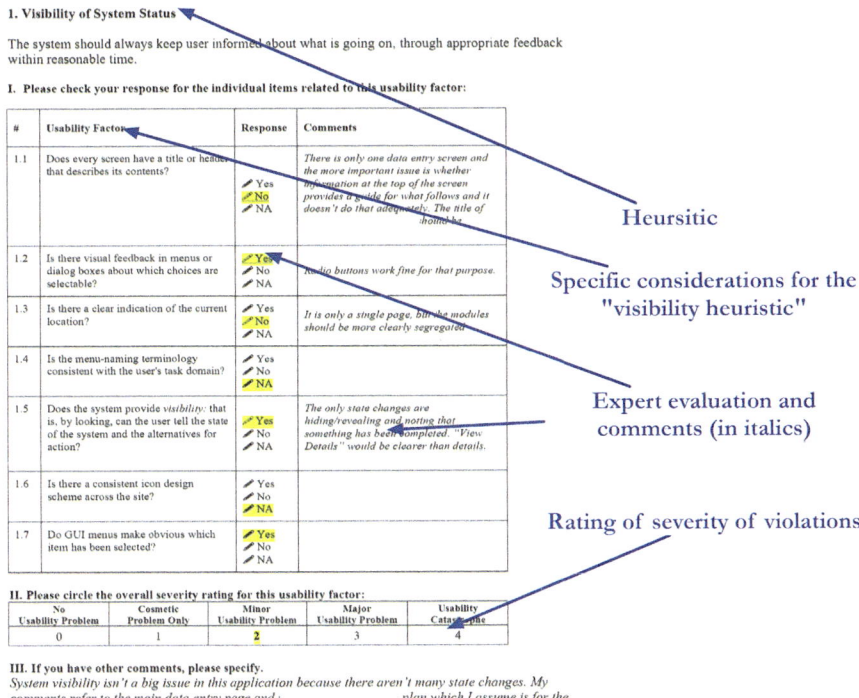

Fig. 5.3 Example of a HE form (for visibility) (Figure courtesy, David Kaufman, Personal communication)

their severity. In another study, Allen et al. [28] developed a simplified list of heuristics to evaluate web-based healthcare interfaces (printouts of each interface). Multiple usability experts assigned severity ratings for each of the identified violations and the severity ratings were used to re-design the interface. HE has also been used for evaluating consumer-based pages (e.g., see the use of HE by Choi et al. [29] on the evaluation of a web-based education portal for low-literate parents of infants). Variants of HE approaches have been widely used in the evaluation of HIT interfaces primarily because of its easy applicability. However, the ease of its application in a variety of usability evaluation scenarios often gives rise to inappropriate use. For example, there are several instances where only one or two usability experts (instead of the suggested 4–5 experts) are used for the HE. Other instances have used subject matter experts rather than usability experts for such evaluation studies.

Walkthroughs

Walkthroughs are another inspection-based approach that relies on experts to evaluate the cognitive processes of users performing a task. It involves employing a set of potential stakeholders (designers, usability experts) to characterize a sequence of actions and goals for completing a task. Most commonly used walkthrough, referred to as cognitive walkthrough (CW), involves observing, recording and analyzing the actions and behaviors of users as they complete a scenario of use. CW is focused on identifying the usability and comprehensibility of a system [30]. The aim of CW is to investigate and determine whether the user's knowledge and skills and the interface cues are sufficient to produce an appropriate goal-action sequence that is required to perform a given task [31]. CW is derived from the cognitive theory of how users work on computer-based tasks, using the exploratory learning approach, where system users continually appraise their goals and evaluate their progress against these goals [32].

While performing CW, the focus is on simulating the human-system interaction, and evaluating the fit between the system features and the user's goals. Conducting CW studies involves multiple steps. Potential participants (e.g., users, designers, usability experts) are provided a set of task sequences or scenarios for working with an interface or system. For example, for an interface for entering demographic and patient history details, participants (e.g., physicians) are asked to enter the age, gender, race and clinical history information. As the participants perform their assigned task, their task sequences, errors and other behavioral aspects are recorded. Often, follow up interviews or think aloud (described in a later section) are used to identify participants' interpretation of the tasks, how they make progress, and potential points of mismatches in the system. Detailed observations and recordings of these mismatches are documented for further analysis. While in most situations CWs are performed by individuals, sometimes groups of stakeholders perform the walkthrough together. For example, usability experts, designers and potential users could go through systems together to identify the potential issues and drawbacks. Such group walkthroughs are often referred to as pluralistic walkthroughs.

In biomedical informatics, it must be noted that CW has been used extensively in evaluating situations other than human computer interaction. For example, CW method (and its variants) has been used to evaluate diagnostic reasoning, decision-making processes and clinical activities. For example, Kushniruk et al. [33] used the CW method to perform an early evaluation on the mediating role of HIT in clinical practice. The CW was not only used to identify usability problems, but was instrumental in the development of a coding scheme for subsequent usability testing. Hewing et al. [34] used CW to evaluate an expert ophthalmologist's reasoning regarding the plus disease among infants. Using images, clinical experts were independently asked to rate the presence and severity of the plus condition and provide an explanation of how they arrived at their diagnostic decisions. Similar approaches were used by Kaufman et al. [31] to evaluate the usability of a home-based, telehealth system.

While extremely useful in identifying the key usability issues, CW methods involve significant investments in cost and time for data capture and analysis (for example, as compared to HE). However, it is a powerful approach for HIT evaluation.

Model-Based Evaluation

Model-based evaluation approaches use predictive modeling approaches to characterize the efficiency of user interfaces. Model-based approaches are often used for evaluating routine, expert task performance. For example, how can the keys of a medical device interface be optimally organized such that the users can complete their tasks quickly (and accurately)? Similarly, predictive modeling can be used to compare the data entry efficiency between interfaces with different layouts and organization. We describe two commonly used predictive modeling techniques in the evaluation of interfaces.

GOMS

Card, Moran and Newell [35, 36] proposed the GOMS (Goals, Operators, Methods and Selection Rules) analytical framework for predicting human performance with interactive systems. Specifically, GOMS models predict the time taken to complete a task by a skilled/expert user based on "the composite of actions of retrieving plans from long-term memory, choosing among alternative available methods depending on features of the task at hand, keeping track of what has been done and what needs to be done, and executing the motor movements necessary for the keyboard and mouse" [37]. In other words, GOMS assumes that the execution of tasks can be represented as a serial sequence of cognitive operations and motor actions.

GOMS is used to describe an aggregate of the task and the user's knowledge regarding how to perform the task. This is expressed in terms of the *G*oals, *O*perators, *M*ethods and *S*election rules. *Goals* are the expected outcomes that a user wants to achieve. For example, a goal for a physician could be documenting the details of a patient interaction on an EHR interface. *Operators* are the specific actions that can be performed on the user interface. For example, clicking on a text box or selecting a patient from a list in a dropdown menu. *Methods* are sequential combinations of operators and sub-goals that need to be achieved. For example, in the case of selecting a patient from a dropdown list, the user has to move the mouse over to the dropdown menu, click on the arrow using the appropriate mouse key to retrieve the list of patients. Finally, *selection* rules are used to ascertain which methods to choose when several choices are available. For example, using the arrow keys on the keyboard to scroll down a list versus using the mouse to select.

One of the simplest and most commonly used GOMS approaches is the Keystroke-Level Model (KLM), which was first described in Card, Moran and Newell [36]. As opposed to the general GOMS model, the KLM makes several assumptions regarding the task. In KLM, methods are limited to keystroke level operations and task duration is predicted based on these estimates. For the KLM, there are six types of operators: K for pressing a key; P for pointing the mouse to a target; H for moving hands to the keyboard or pointing device; D for drawing a line segment; M for mental preparation for an action; and R for system response. Based on experimental data or other predictive models (e.g., Fitts Law), each of these operators is assigned a value or a parameterized estimate of execution time. We describe an example from Saitwal et al. [38] on the use of the KLM approach.

In a study investigating the usability of EHR interfaces, Saitwal et al. [38] used the KLM approach to evaluate the time taken, and the number of steps required to complete a set of 14 EHR-based tasks. The purpose of the study was to characterize the issues with the user interface and also to identify potential areas for improvement. The evaluation was performed on the AHLTA (Armed Forces Health Longitudinal Technology Application) user interface. A set of 14 prototypical tasks was first identified. Sample tasks included entering patient's current illness, history of present illness, social history and family history. KLM analysis was performed on each of the tasks: this involved breaking each of the tasks into its component goals, operators, methods and selection rules. The operators were also categorized as physical (e.g., move mouse to a button) or mental (e.g., locate an item from a dropdown menu). For example, the selection of a patient name involved eight steps (M—mental operation; P—physical operation): (1) think of location on the menu [M, 1.2s], (2) move hand to the mouse [P, 0.4s], (3) move the mouse to "Go" in the menu [P, 0.4s], (4) extend the mouse to "Patient" [P, 0.4s], (5) retrieve the name of the patient [M, 1.2s], (6) locate patient name on the list [M, 1.2s], (7) move mouse to the identified patient [P, 0.4s] and (8) click on the identified patient [P, 0.4s]. In this case, there were a total of eight steps that would take 5.2s to complete. In a similar manner, the number of steps and the time taken for each of the 14 considered AHLTA tasks were computed.

In addition, GOMS and its family of methods can be effectively used to make comparisons regarding the efficiency of performing tasks interfaces. However, such approaches are approximations and have several disadvantages. While GOMS provides a flexible and often reliable mechanism for predicting human performance in a variety of computer-based tasks, there are several potential limitations. A brief summary is provided here, and interested readers can find further details in Card et al. [35]. GOMS models can be applied only to the *error-free*, *routine* tasks of *skilled* users. Thus, it is not possible to make time predictions for non-skilled users, who are likely to take considerable time to learn to use a new system. For example, the use of the GOMS approach to predict the potential time spent by physicians in using a new EHR would be inaccurate—owing to relative lack of knowledge of the physicians regarding the use of the various interfaces, and the learning curve required to be up-to-speed with the new system. The complexity of clinical work processes and tasks, and the variability of the user population create significant challenges for the effective use of GOMS in measuring the effectiveness of clinical tasks.

Fitts Law

Fitts Law is used to predict human motor behavior; it is used to predict the time taken to acquire a target [39]. On computer-based interfaces, it has been used to develop a predictive model of time it takes to acquire a target using a mouse (or another pointing device). The time taken to acquire a target depends on the distance between the pointer and target (referred to as amplitude, A) and the width of the target (W). The movement time (MT) is mathematically represented as follows:

$$\text{MT} = k . \log_2 \left(\frac{A}{W} + 1 \right)$$

where k is a constant, A—amplitude, W—width of target

In summary, based on Fitts law, one can say that the larger objects are easier to acquire while smaller, closely aligned objects are much more difficult to acquire with a pointing device. While the direct application of Fitts law is not often found in the evaluation studies of HIT or health interfaces in general, it has a profound influence in the design of interfaces. For example, the placement of menu items and buttons, such that a user can easily click on them for selection, are based on Fitts law parameters. Similarly, in the design of number keypads for medical devices, the size of the buttons and their location can be effectively predicted by Fitts law parameters.

In addition to the above-mentioned predictive models, there are several other less common models. While a detailed description of each of them or their use is beyond the scope of this chapter, we provide a brief introduction to another predictive approach: Hick-Hyman choice reaction time [40, 41]. Choice reaction time, RT, can be predicted based on the number of available stimuli (or choices), n:

$$\text{RT} = a + b . \log_2(n);$$

where a and b are constants.

Hick-Hyman law is particularly useful in predicting text entry rates for different keyboards [42], and time required to select from different menus (e.g., a linear vs. a hierarchical menu). In particular, the method is useful to make decisions regarding the design and evaluation of menus. For example, consider two menu design choices: 9 items deep/3 items wide and 3 items deep/9 items wide. The RT for each of these can be calculated as follows: $(3 * (a + b. \log_2(n)) < 9 * (a + b. \log_2(n))$. This shows that the access to menus is more efficient when it is designed breadth-wise rather than depth-wise.

Usability Testing/User-Based Evaluation

In this section, we have grouped a range of approaches that are generally used for evaluating the usability of HIT systems. In general, we have classified them into field/observational studies and general approaches for usability evaluation that can be utilized in both field and laboratory settings. While formal usability testing is often conducted in laboratory settings where user performance (and other selected variables) are evaluated based on pre-selected tasks, we have loosely classified the evaluation techniques that utilize users in the evaluation process into general approaches (those that can be used in both field and laboratory based studies) and field studies.

General Usability Testing Approaches

Interviews

Interviews are commonly used to elicit information about opinions and perspectives of participants and their work practices [43]. Within the context of HIT design and evaluation, interviews have been used to obtain clinicians' perspectives and their experiences within the context of the clinical workflow and its respective challenges and opportunities for design improvement. A study on physicians' use of EHR with particular emphasis on its barriers and solutions is a classic example of an interview study that investigates the impact of HIT on physician workflow. For example, Miller et al. [44] conducted over 90 interviews with physician champions and EHR managers. Through these interview sessions, they identified participant perceptions regarding barriers to EHR use including high initial set-up costs, slow and uncertain financial payoffs, high initial physician time costs related to challenges with the technology, attitudes and incentives to use the new system. Interview participants, when asked, suggested potential solutions such as performance incentives for achieving quality improvement, technical support for the system and incorporation of a community-wide data exchange.

Interviews are viewed as an approach to elicit additional information and are often used in concert with other field study methods (e.g., observation or shadowing). For example, Unertl et al. [45] investigated the use of health information exchange (HIE) technology, and its impact on care delivery at an e-health organization. Multi-faceted data collection methods including observations, informal and formal interviews, were used to examine workflow and information flow among team members and patients. While the interview findings illustrated the benefits of HIE technologies for communication and care continuity, their adoption in practice was limited. The integrated analysis highlighted the importance of moving away from a data and information "ownership" model to a "continuity and context-aware" model for the design and implementation of HIE technology.

Often, the data obtained from interviews are used to analyze the contextual language and meaning as quoted by participants. For example, in a qualitative study on patient transfers, Abraham et al. [46, 47] observed breakdowns in information flow between clinical units, despite the effective use of a care coordination system. Using follow-up interviews, the authors captured participants' perspectives on the underlying cause for the information breakdowns. For example, in one of the interviews, an emergency department charge nurse was asked to describe the information sharing issues that affected the coordination of patient transfers from her unit. Her response was: "*A lot of times the attending residents don't know to put in medication or change orders, additional labs and if we are busy with other patients, we don't have time to go to the computer and even though these screens help, they still don't alleviate the problem.*" She further added that: "*I think basically they don't understand how the emergency department works, how difficult it is to hold patients, I don't think they understand the concept like I said we don't have the ancillary staff and so they have this expectation of what the patient is going to be like when they come up, you know they are disheveled or haven't had a bath or like you know they think that's horrible* [47]."

Individual interviews can be classified into three major categories based on the format and level of standardization of the interview questions—structured, semi-structured and narrative (or unstructured). During *structured interviews*, all interviewees are asked the same questions in the same order. This allows for comparisons between responses across interviewees, which can be analyzed using qualitative and quantitative methods. *Semi-structured interviews*, unlike the structured interviews, are flexible and allow for probing of participants (i.e., with follow up questions) to discuss relevant issues.

In contrast to the structured methods of interviewing, narrative, open-ended, unstructured interviewing does not use any question-response structure. Instead, it adopts a storytelling and listening framework for obtaining participant perspectives. Narrative interviewing is typically comprised of four steps: (a) initiation (introduction of the topic for narration), (b) the main storytelling or narration, (c) questioning and clarification, and (d) concluding remarks [48, 49]. This particular type of interviewing allows participants to describe their story in their own spontaneous language. For instance, short HCI scenarios can be used to elicit participants' responses on how they react to a real-world situation. An example scenario can focus on the emergency medical service (EMS) personnel use of patient EHR to support handoff communication to an ER physician during a trauma patient drop-off. Some of the potential questions that follow the scenario could uncover the details of how the

EMS and ED team respond to the trauma situation, and the EHR functions and features that can support such emergent communication during trauma resuscitation.

Most interviews are audio-recorded for a variety of reasons: (a) the data can be transcribed verbatim, with limited chances of missing key points made by participants, (b) provides the ability for the researcher to listen to the audio files and (c) features such as voice tone and frequency may be of interest for researchers. It is recommended that interviews be conducted at locations selected by the participants to ensure that they feel comfortable to freely talk, without being concerned about other colleagues overhearing their conversations.

Focus Groups

Focus group is a type of interactive interviewing method that involves an in-depth discussion of a particular topic of interest with a small group of participants. Focus group method has been described as "a carefully planned discussion designed to obtain perceptions on a defined area of interest in a permissive, non-threatening environment" [50]. The central elements of focus groups as highlighted by Vaughn et al. [51] include: (a) the group is an informal assembly of target participants to discuss a topic; (b) the group is small, between 6 to 12 members and is relatively homogeneous; (c) the group conversation is facilitated by a trained moderator with prepared questions and probes; and (d) given that the primary goal of a focus group is to elicit the perceptions, feelings, attitudes, and ideas of participants about a selected topic, it can be used to generate hypotheses for further research [50].

Unlike individual interviews, focus group discussions allow the researcher to probe responses to a particular research topic while capturing the underlying group dynamics of the participants. According to Kitzinger [52], interaction is the crucial feature of focus groups because the interaction between participants views the group as a single unit and also captures their view of the world, the language they use about an issue and their values and beliefs about a situation [53]. For instance, a focus group involving usability experts, system designers and care providers can allow participants to share their varying perspectives on HIT system design based on their work role. This will enable them to voice the key issues on the fit or (lack thereof) between the functionalities of the system and the clinical workflow.

Many researchers have argued that focus group interviewing depends on the active discussion and engagement among participants, and therefore have strongly advocated for homogenous groups (similar participants) (e.g., [50]). Although the interaction between participants is considered a strength of the method, group participants and the setting can sometimes inhibit the group interaction [54], especially during instances when sensitive personal issues are discussed. A decision regarding the composition should be based on the specific research (or design) question at hand. For example, a qualitative study supported by a series of seven focus group interviews with emergency medical services (EMS) and emergency room (ER) teams were conducted to investigate their coordination practices in a crisis response situation. The focus group participants were presented with a mass casualty incident situation, and were asked to respond to a series of events that unfolded. The questions were related to the decision making process during a large-scale emergency situation, with particular emphasis on (a) their information and communication needs, (b) their information and communication technology use, and (c) their roles and responsibilities during the crisis. During the focus group sessions, two researchers moderated the discussion, and took detailed notes. Barriers perceived to impact coordination activities between EMS and ED teams included ineffective information and communication technologies, lack of common ground, and breakdowns in information flow. Furthermore, the focus group interview participants also jointly identified several key socio-technical requirements for inter-team coordination systems such as situation awareness, context, and workflow [55, 56].

Another important factor that plays a vital role in focus group sessions is the presence of a skilled moderator (or facilitator) [57] who manages the conversations and interactions between participants. Moreover, scheduling a convenient time and location for administering focus group interviews can be very difficult, given the number of participants that are involved.

Verbal Think Aloud

Verbal think aloud (or simply "think aloud") is often used to capture rich verbal data on the thought processes that underlie human actions. Analysis of these verbal reports can be used to characterize the underlying information and knowledge structures. Think aloud evaluations are generally characterized into two types: (1) concurrent and (2) retrospective [58]. A concurrent think aloud requires uninterrupted and direct verbalizations of participants as they perform a task, and is considered to be complete and consistent with their thought sequence. In contrast, a retrospective think aloud requires the researcher to ask and prompt subjects to recall their thought sequence while performing a task (or after completing a task). Ericsson and Simon [59], the original proponents of the verbal think aloud method, suggested the value of think aloud data is based on the following assumptions: (1) the verbalizations capture only a subset of the cognitive processes underlying behavior; (2) human mind is an information processor; and (3) the verbalizations capture contents of working memory (i.e., information recently acquired is accessed).

Think aloud studies are typically conducted to identify and characterize cognitive processes such as reasoning, problem solving, and decision-making processes. For example, Patel and colleagues [60–63] have conducted several studies using verbal think aloud that investigated the nature of reasoning using electronic tools, its effects of expertise and decision-making. Most of these studies relied on verbalizations by a participant (e.g., a physician), and in-depth linguistic analysis of the verbalizations to identify inherent strategies in their reasoning and decision-making. Similarly, Fonteyn and Grobe [64] utilized a think aloud study to understand the reasoning and decision-making behaviors of critical care nurses regarding unstable patients. Insights on the reasoning process of expert nurses informed the design of an expert system. Other examples of similar key studies can be found here [65–69].

One of the concerns that have been raised in evaluation studies using verbal think aloud method is the issue of sample size. While many researchers have used a small sample size of five participants to focus on in-depth analysis of the cognitive processes, others have critiqued the sample size (e.g., [70]). Lundgrén-Laine et al. [71] have suggested that the characteristics of the study participants in terms of their verbalization skills and the appropriate application of the think aloud is more important than the sample size [72–74]. Measures of information and participant saturation are often used to determine study completion. A detailed description of the think aloud method and approaches for its analysis can be found here [59].

Surveys and Questionnaires

Surveys and questionnaires are widely used in evaluation studies. Their widespread use is related to ease of administration (through multiple modes: online, face-to-face) and limited time required to complete (especially those that use Likert scale measures). In terms of usability evaluation, there are several surveys that are commonly used. A list of the commonly used usability surveys are provided below:

(a) *QUIS* (Questionnaire for User Interface Satisfaction: http://lap.umd.edu/quis/): measure user interface interaction and subjective satisfaction;
(b) *SUMI* (Software Usability Measurement Inventory: http://sumi.ucc.ie/): assess usability of software;
(c) *PSSUQ* (Post-Study System Usability Questionnaire), and *ASQ* (After Scenario Questionnaire: http://hcibib.org/perlman/question.cgi?form=ASQ) [75]: address global usability of a system along with specific scenarios of use;
(d) *SUS* (System Usability Scale: http://www.usability.gov/how-to-and-tools/methods/system-usability-scale.html) [76]: a general survey of system usability;
(e) *Subjective workload assessment* (NASA-TLX Workload Instrument: http://humansystems.arc.nasa.gov/groups/tlx/paperpencil.html) [77]: a multi-item scale to determine the physical, temporal, mental, effort, frustration and performance while working with interfaces.

Although most of the above-mentioned surveys are validated for their reliability, researchers often use a variety of self-created surveys and questionnaires. Questionnaires, as opposed to the surveys that use a specific scale (e.g., a scale of 1–7), often use open-ended questions to elicit responses from participants regarding system use (e.g., "Describe some of the challenges that you faced while using the system?").

Surveys are often used along with other data collection methods and are considered a complementary data collection method in HIT evaluation. For example, Karahoca and colleagues [78] used a generic survey along with system usage logs to characterize the usability of two mobile device prototypes. Similar open-ended questionnaires along with additional observational data was used by Holzinger and colleagues [79] to characterize patient interactions with a mobile interface. Dalai and colleagues [80] used the SUS scale and the NASA-TLX scales for comparing the effectiveness of two interfaces for comprehending psychiatric clinical narratives. These survey scales were used in concert with an analysis of verbal reports to evaluate the effectiveness of presented interfaces.

Field/Observational Approaches

In contrast to the analytic evaluation techniques that often yield objective data, there are several qualitative approaches that focus on the subjective and contextual assessments of system design and user interactions within the *context* of a real work environment [11]. These qualitative approaches are generally categorized as ethnographic-based methods and require an "immersion" in the field in order to understand the experiences and practices of the informants [81]. Ethnography is a widely accepted method for data collection in the field of anthropology [82]. An ethnographer obtains a firsthand experience by immersing herself in the research setting for an extended period of time. This helps in gaining an understanding of the particular social and cultural practices of the setting. Ethnographic methods are used in a variety of domains to gain meaningful insights on the nuances and complexities of work practices [83, 84].

Field studies using ethnographic methods allow for a situated, in-depth and in-situ evaluation of the clinical environments—providing insights on the use and interaction of care providers with the computer technologies and tools, situated within their organizational structures. Furthermore, field studies allow us to gain deeper insights on *not only* the interdependencies between the usability (ease of use, learnability and access) and the available functionality afforded by the technology, *but also*, the hidden tensions in the healthcare work practices arising from the contextual and environmental constraints that can potentially disrupt the user interaction with the technology. In other words, these methods provide an understanding of the effects of the user-system interaction on the end user *workflow* in actual practice. For instance, these methods can answer questions such as "how did the system change user behavior?"; "what are the reasons for poor task performance?"; "what are the unintended consequences or opportunities related to the system implementation in the work context?"; "what are the motivations behind the use of the system?" In contrast to the analytical approaches that are applicable only at an individual level, these empirical methods support the investigation of collaborative practices of work and the effect of technologies on coordination of work in these practices (e.g., [85, 86]).

Field studies have been extensively used in studying the unique characteristics and nuances of clinical environments (e.g., [47, 87], clinical and non-clinical activities and tasks surrounding clinical workflows such as information seeking practices of clinicians, coordination of patient transfer activities, decision making activities (e.g., [22, 23, 88, 89]), and HIT use in clinical environments (e.g., [90–92]). Several of the chapters in this volume have used one or more of these methods. In the following sections, we describe two commonly used forms of structured field study approaches—shadowing, and time and motion studies.

Shadowing

Shadowing techniques involve a researcher closely following a participant over an extended period of time. In contrast to general observations of the entire unit and patient care team, shadowing techniques focus on collecting data about a single participant. The data obtained through shadowing are mainly related to the steps (e.g., process, activities or tasks) performed by the selected participant during the observational period. Specific to the use of HIT in clinical environments, shadowing can be used to gather data on the activities of different clinicians (attending physicians, residents, nurses) as they carry out their patient-care tasks, and their use of health IT. For example, in a study evaluating the use of EHR systems in an emergency care setting, Abraham et al. [91, 93] shadowed attending physicians over multiple sessions. In addition to identifying the key activities around EHR use, they found that the use of the EHR led to additional "peripheral" activities that increased their work activities, consequently creating a fragmentation in the care process (e.g., the need to use multiple care artifacts, move across multiple locations and interact with several care providers). A similar shadowing study was conducted by Patterson et al. [94] to investigate the barriers to effective use of clinical reminders supported by clinical decision support systems at multiple study sites. Using detailed shadowing notes and interview data, the authors identified six barriers: (a) workload during patient visits, (b) time to document when a clinical reminder was not clinically relevant, (c) inapplicability of the clinical reminder due to context-specific reasons, (d) limited training on how to use the clinical reminder software for rotating staff and permanent staff, (e) perceived reduction of quality of provider–patient interaction, and (f) the decision to use paper forms to enable review of resident physician orders prior to order entry.

Time and Motion Studies

Time and Motion study is a specific shadowing approach that helps in developing a deeper understanding of the impact of clinical work activities; for example, the changes on clinical efficiency, team coordination, rounds communication due to the implementation of a new health technology such as the computerized physician order entry system or an EHR system [95]. In routine time and motion studies, a researcher shadows the participant, capturing the sequence of a particular process/activity/task, in conjunction with the time spent by participant (on the process/activity/task). Time and motion studies help in examining the nature of emerging practices around care provider's adoption and use of the HIT system (e.g., [96]). For instance, this method helps in understanding the role and the use of the EMR system for care activities such as developing an assessment and plan (in terms of distribution of time spent on clinical notes interface vs. patient labs interface). In addition to time, it is possible collect data on the locations traversed by the participant during the session. This provides an additional level of data on use and interaction of the HIT system within the context of its use, which can inform better design of health

IT that are integrated within the clinical workflow. This method was used in a study that evaluated the impact of complexity on physician activities in an emergency care setting [93]. Based on the study, the authors characterized the nature of physician activities, the time allocated for these activities, how these activities were distributed across the unit and the susceptibility of these activities for interruptions, and found that approximately one-fourth (~25%) of the physician activities (e.g., direct patient care) were localized at specific locations in the unit, while the rest of the activities (e.g., communication) were distributed across the unit and were less predictable. These non-localized activities also had a higher likelihood of interruptions. Based on the time and motion study, the authors highlight implications for mitigating the physician workload, and the design of technologies for monitoring such complex settings [93].

Similar to shadowing, time and motion studies often require the use of a pre-defined taxonomy to record and document the observational data. The accuracy of the taxonomy, and its fit for the particular work environment is critical to the evaluation. Time and motion studies are very useful for assessing efficiency and effectiveness of HIT systems and also, human-centered characteristics of such technologies. An example of a validated taxonomy used by researchers in the medical informatics field was developed by Overhage [97], and later refined by Pizziferri [98]. This taxonomy was recommended by the Agency for Healthcare Research and Quality (AHRQ) for collecting time-motion data in clinical workflow studies. This taxonomy has successfully been used to document the electronic documentation and note-writing practices of residents in a general medicine unit at a large teaching hospital [99]. Using this taxonomy, they conducted a time and motion study on 11 resident physicians that provided insights on: (a) When and in what circumstances did residents use the EHR to write a note? (b) What were the general steps of EHR note composition? (c) Were there common patterns of transitions between these steps among residents? (d) How did the EHR documentation system facilitate or inhibit their clinical tasks such as developing a patient assessment and plan of care? The authors identified that seven of the ten most common transitions between activities during note composition were between documenting, and gathering and reviewing patient data, and updating the plan of care. Through the fine-granular data collection on temporal properties of resident use of EHR system, the authors were able to find that clinical documentation on an EHR system was a *synthesis* activity, which was in contrast to the fundamental design of EHR systems that conceptualized clinical documentation as an uninterrupted composition. As highlighted in the above examples, time and motion studies solely depend on the observer to accurately document and record the participant time devoted to each task.

Shadowing and time and motion studies are labor-intensive and time-consuming, as they require continuous observation for extended periods of time by the researcher. Also, given that this method is a labor-intensive process, the sample size may be limited and may lead to questions regarding the generalizability of results. As with most observational studies, the presence of an observer can potentially impact the normal behavior of the participant due to awareness that he or she is being observed.

Considerations for Conducting HIT Evaluation Studies

In this chapter, we provided an overview of the range of methods that are available for conducting evaluation studies on HIT systems. The evaluation methods were classified into two general groups—analytical and user-based testing. While the methods are not truly mutually exclusive across these two groups, the classification provides a useful framework for selecting the appropriate method(s) for the evaluation of HIT systems. Additionally, given the complexities of the clinical environment, we have also adapted a more integrative perspective in terms of the applicable methods for HIT evaluation—acknowledging the importance of evaluation methods that capture the nuances of the work environment in which these systems are deployed. We highlight the role of field studies that capture the situated and contextual perspective of HIT including the effects of HIT implementations on clinical workflow, tasks and decision-making. Other chapters in this volume also provide extensions of these methods, both in terms of their use for evaluation and also for design. In Chap. 7, Kushniruk et al. (this volume) introduces and explains user-centered design (UCD), a design approach that relies on some of the above-mentioned methods for the usability evaluation and design of HIT systems. Similarly, in Chap. 9, Kalenderian et al. (this volume) describes the evaluation and re-design of a dental EHR interface.

In the rest of this section, we highlight some of the considerations for conducting HIT evaluation studies, directions of future evaluation studies and potential challenges for conducting these studies. One of the preliminary considerations for evaluations is to determine the environment in which the evaluation study will be conducted. As previously described, analytical evaluations are invariably conducted in a laboratory setting with experts. However, analytical evaluation studies would fail to capture the nuances and implications of the use of HIT within a clinical setting. For example, laboratory-based evaluations can identify most of the interface issues with a Computerized Physician Order Entry (CPOE) system, but long-term observational studies are possibly required for identifying the unintended effects of its use in clinical settings (as highlighted by [4, 92]). Similarly, remote usability evaluation studies are now routinely conducted using web-conference and screen sharing software (see for example, [100]; also see Chap. 7, this volume, for low-cost simulation and tele-evaluation studies).

Another important consideration is the use of a framework to guide the evaluation process. These frameworks provide a theoretical and methodological scaffold for conducting an evaluation for improving the design of a system. While there are several such design and evaluation frameworks in general HCI (e.g., Scenario-based Design [101]), they are far less prominent in the healthcare research literature. One recent framework is TURF: Task, User, Representation, and Function [102]. In addition to being a theoretical framework for describing and predicting usability differences between HIT systems, it also provides a framework for selecting appropriate evaluation methods, measuring the usability using these methods, and making design improvements based on the evaluation. Similar frameworks are likely to evolve with the widespread adoption of HIT and with the need for rapid evaluation protocols. Additionally, federally mandated programs such as the meaningful use (MU) of EHRs have furthered the adoption and use of HIT systems. However, with persistent concerns regarding EHRs (and HIT in general), further evaluation is very likely to continue. For example, EHR interfaces are still considered to have usability issues that require a redesign process. More research and development efforts, both from academia and healthcare industry partners, are likely to be forthcoming in this area.

Two other fast-growing fields within biomedical informatics are the use of mobile technology and consumer health informatics tools. The proliferation of mobile devices (phones, tablets) has provided a new approach for accessing and sharing health information between patients and their healthcare providers. Similarly, consumer health information tools have also been extensively used—for example, web-based social support tools, aggregated medical information tools and patient portals. These tools (both mobile and web-based) are still evolving and are likely an area of significant future design and evaluation (see Chaps. 12 and 13 in this volume for a detailed discussion of consumer informatics and mobile tools respectively).

Finally, it is also important to consider the challenges for conducting HIT evaluation studies. These require considerable investments in time, effort and planning, thoughtful considerations in selecting appropriate methods, and often require significant buy-ins from hospital administration and clinicians.

Conclusions

In this chapter, we described the traditional methods from usability engineering and HCI, and their applicability for HIT evaluation. The applicability of each of these methods for evaluation requires careful consideration. We have provided brief descriptions of these methods within the context of biomedical and healthcare applications. A detailed review is beyond the scope of this chapter (interested readers are encouraged to review the additional readings provided at the end of this chapter). Recently, more innovative techniques have been utilized for usability testing and evaluation. These have varied from general techniques such as eye-tracking, simulations and screen-capture tools to unobtrusive techniques that have used motion sensing (for a detailed review, see Chap. 6 in this volume by Zheng and colleagues). The scope of evaluation methods continues to expand in response to developing technologies, evolving health information tasks and changing circumstances (e.g., role of the health consumer).

Discussion Questions
1. Why is usability of systems a relevant topic for investigation? Why is evaluation of HIT a challenge to healthcare researchers?

2. When designing a new HIT system for a clinical vs. non-clinical setting, what are some of the considerations that must be made?
3. What are some of the considerations for evaluating a prototype vs. an actual, fully-developed system?
4. What methods will you use to evaluate a vendor-developed EHR?
5. How do usability issues manifest across professions? What can be done to mitigate them?

References

1. Blumenthal D. Stimulating the adoption of health information technology. N Engl J Med. 2009;360(15):1477–9.
2. Linder JA, Ma J, Bates DW, Middleton B, Stafford RS. Electronic health record use and the quality of ambulatory care in the United States. Arch Intern Med. 2007;167(13):1400–5.
3. Ash JS, Stavri PZ, Kuperman GJ. A consensus statement on considerations for a successful CPOE implementation. J Am Med Inform Assoc. 2003;10(3):229–34.
4. Koppel R, Metlay JP, Cohen A, et al. Role of computerized physician order entry systems in facilitating medication errors. JAMA. 2005;293(10):1197–203.
5. McDonald CJ, Callaghan FM, Weissman A, Goodwin RM, Mundkur M, Kuhn T. Use of internist's free time by ambulatory care electronic medical record systems. JAMA Intern Med. 2014;174(11):1860–3.
6. Sittig DF, Classen DC. Safe electronic health record use requires a comprehensive monitoring and evaluation framework. JAMA. 2010;303(5):450–1.
7. IOM. Health IT and patient safety: building safer systems for better care. Washington, DC: Institute of Medicine; 2011.
8. Kannampallil TG, Schauer GF, Cohen T, Patel VL. Considering complexity in healthcare systems. J Biomed Inform. 2011;44(6):943–7.
9. Patel VL, Kaufman DR, Cohen T. Cognitive informatics in health and biomedicine. London: Springer; 2014.
10. Donabedian A. Evaluating the quality of medical care. Milbank Meml Fund Q. 1966;44(3):166–206.
11. Assila A, de Oliveira KM, Ezzedine H. Towards qualitative and quantitative data integration approach for enhancing HCI quality evaluation. In: Human-computer interaction. Theories, methods, and tools. Springer; 2014. p. 469–80.
12. Friedman CP, Wyatt JC. Evaluation methods in biomedical informatics. Springer; 2006.
13. Stetler CB, Legro MW, Wallace CM, et al. The role of formative evaluation in implementation research and the QUERI experience. J Gen Intern Med. 2006;21(S2):S1–8.
14. Preece J, Rogers Y, Sharp H, Benyon D, Holland S, Carey T. Human-computer interaction. Addison-Wesley Longman Ltd.; 1994.
15. Vicente KJ. Cognitive work analysis. Mahwah, NJ: Lawrence Erlbaum Associates; 1999.
16. Annett J, Duncan KD. Task analysis and training design. Occup Psychol. 1967;41:211–21.
17. Chung P, Zhang J, Johnson T, et al. An extended hierarchical task analysis for error prediction in medical devices. AMIA Annu Symp Proc. 2003;2003:165–9.
18. Unertl KM, Weinger MB, Johnson KB, Lorenzi N. Describing and modeling workflow and information flow in chronic disease care. J Am Med Inform Assoc. 2009;16(6):826–36.
19. Chipman SF, Schraagen JM, Shalin VL. Introduction to cognitive task analysis. In: Schraagen JM, Chipman SF, Shute VJ, editors. Cognitive task analysis. Mahwah, NJ: Lawrence Erlbaum Associates; 2000. p. 3–23.

20. Cooke NJ. Varieties of knowledge elicitation techniques. Int J Hum-Comput Stud. 1994;41:801–49.
21. Hysong SJ, Sawhney MK, Wilson L, et al. Provider management strategies of abnormal test result alerts: a cognitive task analysis. J Am Med Inform Assoc. 2010;17(1):71–7.
22. Kannampallil TG, Franklin A, Mishra R, Cohen T, Almoosa KF, Patel VL. Understanding the nature of information seeking behavior in critical care: implications for the design of health information technology. Artif Intell Med. 2013;57(1):21–9.
23. Kannampallil TG, Jones LK, Patel VL, Buchman TG, Franklin A. Comparing the information seeking strategies of residents, nurse practitioners, and physician assistants in critical care settings. J Am Med Inform Assoc. 2014;21:e249–56.
24. Nielsen J. Usability inspection methods. Paper presented at: Conference Companion on Human Factors in Computing Systems. Boston, MA: ACM; 1994. p. 413–4.
25. Johnson CM, Johnson TR, Zhang J. A user-centered framework for redesigning health care interfaces. J Biomed Inform. 2005;38:75–87.
26. Nielsen J, Molich R. Heuristic evaluation of user interfaces. Paper presented at: Proceedings of the SIGCHI Conference on Human Factors in Computing Systems. Seattle, WA: ACM; 1990. p. 249–56.
27. Zhang J, Johnson TR, Patel VL, Paige DL, Kubose T. Using usability heuristics to evaluate patient safety of medical devices. J Biomed Inform. 2003;36(1):23–30.
28. Allen M, Currie LM, Bakken S, Patel VL, Cimino JJ. Heuristic evaluation of paper-based web pages: a simplified inspection usability methodology. J Biomed Inform. 2006;39(4):412–23.
29. Choi J, Bakken S. Web-based education for low-literate parents in Neonatal Intensive Care Unit: development of a website and heuristic evaluation and usability testing. Int J Med Inform. 2010;79(8):565–75.
30. Polson PG, Lewis C, Rieman J, Wharton C. Cognitive walkthroughs: a method for theory-based evaluation of user interfaces. Int J Man-Mach Stud. 1992;36(5):741–73.
31. Kaufman DR, Patel VL, Hillman C, et al. Usability in the real world: assessing medical information technologies in patients' homes. J Biomed Inform. 2003;36(1):45–60.
32. Kahn MJ, Prail A. Formal usability inspections. In: Usability inspection methods. Wiley; 1994. p. 141–71.
33. Kushniruk AW, Kaufman DR, Patel VL, Levesque Y, Lottin P. Assessment of a computerized patient record system: a cognitive approach to evaluating medical technology. MD Comput. 1996;13:406–15.
34. Hewing NJ, Kaufman DR, Chan RP, Chiang MF. Plus disease in retinopathy of prematurity: qualitative analysis of diagnostic process by experts. JAMA Ophthalmol. 2013;131(8):1026–32.
35. Card SK, Moran TP, Newell A. The keystroke-level model for user performance time with interactive systems. Commun ACM. 1980;23(7):396–410.
36. Card SK, Newell A, Moran TP. The psychology of human-computer Interaction. L. Erlbaum Associates Inc.; 1983. p. 469.
37. Olson GM, Olson JS. Human-computer interaction: psychological aspects of the human use of computing. Annu Rev Psychol. 2003;54(1):491–516.
38. Saitwal H, Feng X, Walji M, et al. Assessing performance of an electronic health record (EHR) using cognitive task analysis. Int J Med Inform. 2010;79(7):501–6.
39. Fitts PM. The information capacity of the human motor system in controlling the amplitude of movement. J Exp Psychol. 1954;47:381–91.
40. Hick WE. A simple stimulus generator. Q J Exp Psychol. 1951;3:94–5.
41. Hyman R. Stimulus information as a determinant of reaction time. J Exp Psychol. 1953;45:188–96.
42. MacKenzie IS, Zhang SX, Soukoreff RW. Text entry using soft keyboards. Behav Inf Technol. 1999;18:235–44.
43. Mason J. Qualitative researching. London: Sage Publications; 2002.

44. Miller RH, Sim I. Physicians' use of electronic medical records: barriers and solutions. Health Aff (Millwood). 2004;23(2):116–26.
45. Unertl K, Johnson K, Gadd C, Lorenzi N. Bridging organizational divides in health care: an ecological view of health information exchange. JMIR Med Inform. 2013;1(2):e3.
46. Abraham J. Meta-coordination activities: exploring articulation work in hospitals. In: Information sciences and technology (IST) [doctoral dissertation]. The Pennsylvania State University; 2010.
47. Abraham J, Reddy MC. Moving patients around: a field study of coordination between clinical and non-clinical staff in hospitals. Paper presented at: ACM Conference on Computer Supported Cooperative Work (CSCW). ACM; 2008.
48. Farr RM. Interviewing: the social psychology of the interview. In: Fransella F, editor. Psychology for occupational therapists. London: Macmillan; 1982. p. 151–70.
49. Hermanns H. Narratives interview. In: Flick U, van Kardorff E, Keupp H, von Rosenstiel L, Wolff S, editors. Handbuch qualitative socialforschung. Muenchen: Psychologie Verlags Union; 1991. p. 182–5.
50. Krueger RA. Focus groups: a practical guide for applied research. Sage; 2009.
51. Vaughn S, Schumm JS, Sinagub J. Focus group interviews in education and psychology. Thousand Oaks, CA: Sage; 1996.
52. Kitzinger J. Introducing focus groups. Br Med J. 1995;311:299–302.
53. Gibbs A. Focus groups. Soc Res Update. 1997;19:1–7.
54. Lewis A. Group child interviews as a research tool. Br Educ Res J. 1992;18:413–21.
55. Paul SA, Reddy M, Abraham J, DeFlitch C. The usefulness of information and communication technologies in crisis response. AMIA Annu Symp Proc. 2008;2008:561–5.
56. Reddy MC, Paul SA, Abraham J, McNeese M, DeFlitch C, Yen J. Challenges to effective crisis management: using information and communication technologies to coordinate emergency medical services and emergency department teams. Int J Med Inform. 2009;78(4):259–69.
57. Burrows D, Kendall S. Focus groups: what are they and how can they be used in nursing and health care research? Soc Sci Health. 1997;3:244–53.
58. Ericsson KA, Simon H. Verbal reports as data. Psychol Rev. 1980;87(3):215–50.
59. Ericsson KA, Simon H. Protocol analysis: verbal reports as data. Cambridge: MIT Press; 1984.
60. Patel VL, Arocha JF, Kaufman DR. Diagnostic reasoning and medical expertise. In: Douglas LM, editor. Psychology of learning and motivation. Academic Press; 1994. p. 187–252.
61. Patel VL, Arocha JF, Kaufman DR. A primer on aspects of cognition for medical informatics. J Am Med Inform Assoc. 2001;8(4):324–43.
62. Patel VL, Groen GJ. The general and specific nature of medical expertise: a critical look. In: Smith KAEJ, editor. Toward a general theory of expertise: prospects and limits. New York: Cambridge University Press; 1991. p. 93–125.
63. Patel VL, Groen GJ. Developmental accounts of the transition from medical student to doctor: some problems and suggestions. Med Educ. 1991;25(6):527–35.
64. Fonteyn ME, Grobe SJ. Expert system development in nursing: implications for critical care nursing practice. Heart Lung. 1994;23(1):80–7.
65. Fisher A, Fonteyn ME. An exploration of an innovative methodological approach for examining nurses' heuristic use in clinical practice. Sch Inq Nurs Pract. 1995;9(3):263–76.
66. Fowler LP. Clinical reasoning strategies used during care planning. Clin Nurs Res. 1997;6(4):349–61.
67. Funkesson KH, Anbäcken E-M, Ek A-C. Nurses' reasoning process during care planning taking pressure ulcer prevention as an example. A think-aloud study. Int J Nurs Stud. 2007;44:1109–19.
68. Grobe SJ, Drew JA, Fonteyn ME. A descriptive analysis of experienced nurses' clinical reasoning during a planning task. Res Nurs Health. 1991;14(4):305–14.
69. Simmons B, Lanuza D, Fonteyn M, Hicks F, Holm K. Clinical reasoning in experienced nurses. West J Nurs Res. 2003;25:720–4.

70. Lewis JR. Sample sizes for usability studies: additional considerations. Hum Factors. 1994;36:369–78.
71. Lundgrén-Laine H, Salanterä S. Think-aloud technique and protocol analysis in clinical decision-making research. Qual Health Res. 2010;20(4):565–75.
72. Caulton DA. Relaxing the homogeneity assumption in usability testing. Behav Inform Technol. 2001;20:1–7.
73. Fonteyn M, Kuipers B, Grobe S. A description of think aloud method and protocol analysis. Qual Health Res. 1993;3:430–41.
74. Hall M, De Jong M, Steehouder M. Cultural differences and usability evaluation: individualistic and collectivistic participants compared. Tech Commun. 2004;51(4):489–503.
75. Lewis JR. Psychometric evaluation of an after-scenario questionnaire for computer usability studies: the ASQ. ACM SIGCHI Bull. 1991;23(1):78–81.
76. Brooke J. SUS: a 'quick and dirty' usabiliy scale. In: Jordan PW, Thomas B, McClell IL, editors. Usability evaluation in industry. London: Taylor & Francis; 1996. p. 189–95.
77. Hart S, Staveland L. Development of NASA TLX (task load index): results of empirical and theoretical research. In: Hancock P, Meshkati N, editors. Human mental workload. Amsterdam: North Holland Press; 1988.
78. Karahoca A, Bayraktar E, Tatoglu E, Karahoca D. Information system design for a hospital emergency department: a usability analysis of software prototypes. J Biomed Inform. 2010;43(2):224–32.
79. Holzinger A, Kosec P, Schwantzer G, Debevc M, Hofmann-Wellenhof R, Frühauf J. Design and development of a mobile computer application to reengineer workflows in the hospital and the methodology to evaluate its effectiveness. J Biomed Inform. 2011;44(6):968–77.
80. Dalai VV, Khalid S, Gottipati D, et al. Evaluating the effects of cognitive support on psychiatric clinical comprehension. Aritif Intell Med. 2014;62(2):91–104.
81. Schatzberg M. Seeing the invisible, hearing silence, thinking the unthinkable: the advantages of ethnographic immersion. Paper presented at: APSA 2008 Annual Meeting. Hynes Convention Center, MA; 2008.
82. Fetterman DM, editor. Ethnography: step by step. 2nd ed. Thousand Oaks, CA: Sage; 1998.
83. Forsythe DE. "It's just a matter of common sense": ethnography as invisible work. Comput Support Coop Work. 1999;8(1–2):127–45.
84. Brixey JJ, Robinson DJ, Tang Z, Johnson TR, Zhang J, Turley JP. Interruptions in workflow for RNs in a level one trauma center. AMIA Ann Symp Proc. 2005;2005:86–90.
85. Aarts J, Ash J, Berg M. Extending the understanding of computerized physician order entry: implications for professional collaboration, workflow and quality of care. Int J Med Inform. 2007;76(Suppl 1):S4–S13.
86. Horsky J, Gutnik L, Patel VL. Technology for emergency care: cognitive and workflow considerations. Paper presented at: American Medical Informatics Association Symposium Proceedings, Washington, DC; 2006.
87. Malhotra S, Jordan D, Shortliffe E, Patel VL. Workflow modeling in critical care: piecing together your own puzzle. J Biomed Inform. 2007;40(2):81–92.
88. Patel VL, Kannampallil TG. Cognitive approaches to clinical data management for decision support: is it old wine in new bottle? In: Holzinger A, Simonic K-M, editors. Information quality in e-Health. Berlin Heidelberg: Springer; 2011. p. 1–13.
89. Patel VL, Kaufman DR, Kannampallil T. Diagnostic reasoning and decision making in the context of health information technology. Rev Hum Factors Ergon. 2013;8:149–90.
90. Abraham J, Kannampallil T, Patel B, Almoosa K, Patel VL. Ensuring patient safety in care transitions: an empirical evaluation of a handoff intervention tool. AMIA Annu Symp Proc. 2012;2012:17–26.
91. Abraham J, Kannampallil TG, Reddy M. Peripheral activities during EMR use in emergency care: a case study. AMIA Annu Symp Proc. 2009;2009:1–5.

92. Ash JS, Berg M, Coiera E. Some unintended consequences of information technology in health care: the nature of patient care information system-related errors. J Am Med Inform Assoc. 2004;11(2):104–12.
93. Abraham J, Kannampallil TG. Quantifying physician activities in emergency care: an exploratory study. Proc Hum Factors Ergon Soc Annu Meet. 2014;58(1):798–802.
94. Patterson ES, Nguyen AD, Halloran JP, Asch SM. Human factors barriers to the effective use of ten HIV clinical reminders. J Am Med Inform Assoc. 2004;11(1):50–9.
95. Zheng K, Guo MH, Hanauer DA. Using the time and motion method to study clinical work processes and workflow: methodological inconsistencies and a call for standardized research. J Am Med Inform Assoc. 2011;18(5):704–10.
96. Zheng K, Haftel HM, Hirschl RB, O'Reilly M, Hanauer DA. Quantifying the impact of health IT implementations on clinical workflow: a new methodological perspective. J Am Med Inform Assoc. 2010;17(4):454–61.
97. Overhage J, Perkins S, Tierney W, McDonald C. Controlled trial of direct physician order entry: effects on physicians' time utilization in ambulatory primary care internal medicine practices. J Am Med Inform Assoc. 2001;8(4):361–71.
98. Pizziferri L, Kittler A, Volk L, et al. Primary care physician time utilization before and after implementation of an electronic health record: a time-motion study. J Biomed Inform. 2005;38(3):176–88.
99. Mamykina L, Vawdrey D, Stetson P, Zheng K, Hripcsak G. Clinical documentation: composition or synthesis? J Am Med Inform Assoc. 2012;19(6):1025–103.
100. Kushniruk AW, Borycki EM, Kuwata S, Watanabe H. Using a low-cost simulation for assessing the impact of a medication administration system on workflow. Stud Health Technol Inform. 2008;136:567–72.
101. Rosson MB, Carroll JM. Usability engineering: scenario-based development of human-computer interaction. Elsevier; 2009.
102. Zhang J, Walji MF. TURF: toward a unified framework of EHR usability. J Biomed Inform. 2011;44(6):1056–67.

Further Reading

Johnson CM, Johnston D, Crowle PK. EHR usability toolkit: a background report on usability and electronic health records. Rockville, MD: Agency for Healthcare Research and Quality; 2011.
Kushniruk AW, Patel VL. Cognitive and usability engineering methods for the evaluation of clinical information systems. J Biomed Inform. 2004;37(1):56–76.
Preece J, Rogers Y, Sharp H, Benyon D, Holland S, Carey T. Human-computer interaction. Addison-Wesley Longman Ltd.; 1994.
Shortliffe EH, Patel VL. Generation and formulation of knowledge: human-intensive techniques. In: Greenes RA, editor. Clinical decision support: the road ahead. Academic Press; 2011.

Chapter 6
Computational Ethnography: Automated and Unobtrusive Means for Collecting Data *In Situ* for Human–Computer Interaction Evaluation Studies

Kai Zheng, David A. Hanauer, Nadir Weibel, and Zia Agha

Introduction

Health information technology (IT) holds great promise to cross the quality chasm of the US healthcare system and to bend the curve of ever-rising costs. However, many successfully deployed health IT systems have failed to generate anticipated benefits [1]; some are even associated with unintended adverse consequences [2]. It has been extensively documented that the lack of usability is one of the key factors accounting for the suboptimal outcomes of implementing the current generation of health IT systems [1]. Human–computer interaction (HCI) evaluation studies, which help designers and researchers assess the effectiveness of competing designs and identify potential usability pitfalls, are therefore of vital importance. HCI evaluation

---

K. Zheng (✉)
Department of Informatics, Donald Bren School of Information and Computer Science, University of California, Irvine, CA, USA
e-mail: kai.zheng@uci.edu

D. A. Hanauer
Department of Learning Health Sciences, University of Michigan Medical School, Ann Arbor, MI, USA
e-mail: hanauer@umich.edu

N. Weibel
Department of Computer Science and Engineering, Jacobs School of Engineering, University of California, San Diego, La Jolla, CA, USA
e-mail: weibel@ucsd.edu

Z. Agha
West Health Institute, La Jolla, CA, USA

Department of Medicine, School of Medicine, University of California, San Diego, La Jolla, CA, USA
e-mail: zagha@westhealth.org

studies in healthcare have been traditionally conducted in the following four forms: (1) expert inspection (e.g., heuristic evaluation), (2) usability experiments carried out in laboratory settings, (3) field studies (e.g., ethnographical observation and contextual inquiries), and (4) perception solicitation through questionnaire surveys, interviews, or focus groups.

In *expert inspection*, evaluators—usually usability experts—execute scripted tasks through the target software system or device and determine its conformity to established principles of usability (the "heuristics"). This method is useful when widely recognized usability standards exist or when the goal of the evaluation is very specific, e.g., to improve the accessibility of the software or to eliminate potential patient safety hazards. *Usability experiments* are often used in formative evaluation to comparatively assess multiple design alternatives, or in summative evaluation to correct usability pitfalls before shipping the system/device to the hands of end users. Data collected through usability experiments can be both quantitative (e.g., time for task completion, number of keystrokes and mouse clicks required, and error rates) and qualitative (e.g., participant verbalization expressing their cognitive processes or commenting about the usability issues they encounter). Some usability experiments employ randomized controlled design to maximize the objectivity and generalizability of study results.

Both expert inspection and usability experiments are typically conducted in controlled environments wherein evaluators or test users perform predefined simulation tasks in a manipulated environment void of distractions. These tasks are carefully curated to best represent prospective end users' work, but they are by no means exhaustive. Further, simulation tasks often focus heavily on the user interface (UI) and are designed to assess an individual user working with a computer terminal in silos stripped of the context of a dynamic work setting involving multiple coworkers. As such, these approaches are widely criticized for their lack of consideration of complex task-dependencies in clinical work and the somewhat chaotic nature of clinical work environments ample of interruptions and communication failures.

Field studies conducted to collect *in situ* data describing how end users incorporate the system/device in their everyday job routines have thus become popular in recent years. These studies often involve shadowing clinicians in a medical facility to observe their individual work as well as their interactions with patients and other care providers. They draw upon principles from a variety of scientific fields such as computer-supported cooperative work (CSCW), distributed cognition, and social computing. For non-observable perceptional measures, such as satisfaction, stress, and perceived efficiency gains (and losses), questionnaire surveys and other direct *perception solicitation* methods are widely used (please refer to Chap. 4 in this volume for a detailed review).

While these traditional HCI approaches have great merit and are indispensable in studying and improving usability of software systems and medical devices in healthcare, they have several major limitations in common. First, recruiting research subjects or usability experts is an arduous task, as study participation requires significant time commitments. Second, the sample size of such studies (or size of the expert panel) is often small, constraining the generalization power of their research findings. Third, test users in a controlled environment, or subjects being shadowed by HCI researchers, may exhibit distinctive behaviors deviating from their normal work practice (i.e., the Hawthorne effect). Similarly, self-reported data collected via direct perception solicitation are susceptible to common cognitive biases and recall errors. For example, due to social desirability bias, informants may tend to answer questions in a manner that would be favorably received by others (e.g., to avoid being viewed as lacking competence in adapting to new technologies); or they may assess individual usability items based on their overall impression of the intervention, i.e., the Halo effect. Lastly, existing HCI methods usually produce discrete data representing only a very small fraction of user behaviors of interest, whereas computational ethnographical approaches are able to capture data continuously and at very low costs. For a review of common measurement issues associated with self-reported data, see Ref. [3].

In this chapter, we introduce *computational ethnography*, an emerging family of methods for conducting HCI studies in healthcare, which usually leverages automated and less obtrusive (or unobtrusive) means for collecting *in situ* data reflective of real end users' actual, unaltered behaviors using a software system or a device in real-world settings. These methods are based on the premise that user interactions with modern technologies always leave "digital traces" behind that can be utilized by HCI experts to fully or partially re-enact the activities. Typical examples of such digital traces include browsing history of webpages, keywords typed into a search engine, audit trails recording document access activities in electronic health records, and paging/phone logs stored in telecommunication systems.

In the next section, we will introduce the definition of computational ethnography, common types of digital trace data that are either being routinely collected in a healthcare environment or can be proactively collected by HCI experts, and commonly used analytical approaches for making sense of such data. We will conclude the chapter with two use cases illustrating how this new family of methods has been applied in healthcare to study end users' interactions with technological interventions in their everyday routines.

Computational Ethnography

Definition

The term *ethnography* originates from Greek ἔθνος ethnos ("folk, people, nation") and γράφω grapho ("I write"). It describes a method initially used by social science researchers, cultural anthropologists in particular, to closely examine the meaning in the lives of a cultural group. Researchers conducting ethnographical studies, or *ethnographers*, strive to develop 'thick' descriptions of everyday life and practice through a long-term engagement with the people they study and in the setting where their everyday lives take place. Participant observations and non-participant observations constitute the primary source of ethnographical data, which are often supplemented by other means of data collection such as artifact analysis and formal or informal interviews. Participant and non-participant observations differ on the degree to which researchers become active participants in the lives of the setting, or instead maintain a distance as 'detached' observers.

Ethnographical work by HCI researchers in healthcare produces vivid and nuanced accounts of how different players—clinicians, clerical staff, administrators, patients, and families—engage with technologies both during the early adoption and adaptation phases (the so called "burn-in period") as well as after the system or device has been used on a routine basis. Such work often pays extraordinary attention to the longitudinal and distributed nature of care processes and the complex interplay between people, technology, and the organization. Thus, ethnographical research accounts contain very subtle cultural and social contexts in a healthcare organization (or in a patient community) where technological systems are situated and what their designs ought to be rooted in. Many of the studies conducted in the field of CSCW are of this nature. For a review of these studies, see Ref. [4].

However, the limitations of ethnography are also widely acknowledged. Ethnographical fieldwork is extremely time consuming to conduct, sometimes taking many months, or even years, to complete. The lack of objectivity has always been and continues to be viewed as a threat to the legitimacy of ethnographical studies because generating an interpretive account of the lives of a study setting is inevitably influenced by ethnographers' own personal and professional experiences. This issue is particularly prominent in health sciences where controlled trials producing unambiguous and conclusive results are often deemed as the *de facto* standard of high-quality research. In addition, because of the complexity of medical work, it is often difficult for observers not trained in medicine, or in a particular medical specialty, to be able to understand what they are observing. Further, in modern healthcare organizations, a significant amount of work has become largely invisible or very difficult to observe by ethnographers. Interpersonal communications among healthcare workers for example are increasingly mediated by technologies (e.g., via pager messages or electronic notifications built into an order entry system), and a considerable proportion of clinical work (e.g., documentation) can be now done remotely or even after work.

Nonetheless, the widespread use of information systems and computer-mediated communication technologies in today's highly wired healthcare environments also creates an unprecedented opportunity for collecting ethnographical data through automated and electronic means. In fact, healthcare, perhaps more than any other industry, bears regulatory mandates (e.g., HIPAA[1] and Medicare Conditions of Participation[2] in the US) that require them to truthfully record anything done to the patient, any communications surrounding the care for the patient, and any access to and modifications of the patient's medical records. Failing to do so is associated

---

[1] HIPAA, or the Health Insurance Portability and Accountability Act, defines policies, procedures, and guidelines for maintaining the privacy and security of protected health information as well as outlining offenses and sets civil and criminal penalties for violations.

[2] § 482.24 Condition of Participation: Medical Record Services. http://www.gpo.gov/fdsys/granule/CFR-2011-title42-vol5/CFR-2011-title42-vol5-sec482-24/content-detail.html

with significant financial and legal consequences. As a result, digital traces abound in healthcare organizations, providing an excellent source of data for ethnographers to retroactively reconstruct patient care activities at a fine level of granularity.

Combining the 'thickness' of ethnographical methods with the strength of automated computational approaches is thus a natural next step for HCI researchers. This new way of collecting behavioral and social data not only forms the basis of the computational ethnography methodology described this chapter, but also the emerging field of "computational social science" at large [5, 6]. In the context of this chapter, we define computational ethnography as "a family of computational methods that leverages computer or sensor-based technologies to unobtrusively or nearly unobtrusively record end users' routine, *in situ* activities in health or healthcare related domains for studies of interest to human–computer interaction." Because computational ethnography is based on data automatically captured through technological means, it by nature provides higher objectivity, less intrusion, more inclusiveness (i.e., into spaces and time where/when direct observation by human observers is not possible), and better scalability for data collection, aggregation, and analysis. Note that while recording user interactions with a computer system such as keystrokes [6] and analyzing the behavioral data thus obtained [7] have been a widely used study approach in HCI, unless their data are collected in users' everyday settings via unobtrusive or nearly unobtrusively means (i.e., as opposite to a controlled laboratory environment), such studies do not meet the definition of computational ethnography. Similarly, quantitative observational studies involving independent human observers (e.g., in a time and motion observation) to collect interaction or behavioral data also do not meet the definition of computational ethnography.

Common Sources of Computational Ethnographical Data

As mentioned earlier, in a modern healthcare organization, clinician, staff, and patient activities always leave behind abundant digital traces that can be leveraged to study interesting HCI problems. Such data are already being routinely collected or can be proactively collected by deploying specific tracking devices. In this section, we introduce six sources of computational ethnographical data that have been commonly used in HCI evaluation studies in healthcare.

Computer Logs Most modern computer systems are capable of generating log files for purposes such as helping engineers monitor a system's performance or helping administrators gauge the usage of newly deployed software. In the US, there is a federal mandate by both HIPAA and the HITECH Act[3] demanding all health IT systems have the security auditing capability. For example, the Health IT Certification

---

[3] The Health Information Technology for Economic and Clinical Health Act, or the HITECH Act, sets meaningful use of EHRs as a critical national goal and allocates incentive funds to accelerate their adoption. The HITECH Act contains specific privacy and security requirements, mainly through software certification, to ensure adequate protection of protected health information stored in EHRs.

Program overseen by the Office of the National Coordinator for Health Information Technology (ONC)[4] requires that all electronic health records (EHR) systems certified through the program to implement security audit logs (commonly referred to as audit trails). The certification criteria contain detailed specifications on (1) what constitutes auditable events (e.g., creation, modification, deletion, or printing of electronic health information); (2) metadata that must be recorded for each auditable event (e.g., date, time, patient identification, and user identification); and (3) tamper-resistance measures in place to ensure the auditing function is enabled by default and audit trails are immutable. Having an EHR system equipped with these security-auditing features is a prerequisite to meeting the meaningful use criterion in order to "protect electronic health information created or maintained by the certified EHR technology through the implementation of appropriate technical capabilities." [8] The certification criteria further recommend all EHR systems adopt an American Society for Testing and Materials (ASTM) International standard, ASTM E2147-01,[5] as the format to record and store audit trail data.

Table 6.1 exhibits a sample security audit log. As illustrated in the sample, security log entries contain rich information describing medical work. These log entries not only reveal the occurrence of a clinical event (when, by whom, related to which patient), but also what the event was about (e.g., chart access vs. placing orders) as well as the identifier of the medical record describing the event allowing for further drill-down analyses. In addition, audit trails contain the IP address of the device from which the data access/writing request originated and potentially also geocoding data supplied by mobile devices. Such information can be combined with timestamps to reconstruct the spatiotemporal distribution of clinical work in a medical facility. Audit trail logs thus provide rich sources of data for HCI experts to conduct workflow and temporal rhythm studies, studies on distributed cognition and social information processing, and studies on information and patient handoffs.

Many researchers in fact deem security audit logs a "goldmine" for generating novel insights into healthcare processes and outcomes [9, 10]. For example, Hripcsak et al. used audit logs captured in an EHR system to characterize the amount of time clinicians spent authoring clinical notes and the proportion of such notes that was viewed by others [11]; Adler-Milstein et al. combined self-reported survey data with objectively logged measures (e.g. time after hours on clinic days, time on nonclinic days, and message volume) to study the association between EHR use and clinician burnout [12]; and Holmgren et al. conducted a cross-sectional analysis of log data to compare the EHR burden between US and non-US healthcare systems [13]. In 2019, a National Research Network for EHR Audit Log

---

[4] The Office of the National Coordinator for Health Information Technology (ONC) is the principal federal entity responsible for coordinating nationwide efforts to support the adoption of health IT and the promotion of nationwide health information exchange. It was created in 2004 and is organizationally located within the Office of the Secretary for the U.S. Department of Health and Human Services. http://www.healthit.gov

[5] ASTM E2147-01: Standard Specification for Audit and Disclosure Logs for Use in Health Information Systems. http://www.astm.org/Standards/E2147.htm

Table 6.1 A sample security audit log

TIMESTAMP	EVENT_NAME	EVENT_TYPE	TASK	PARTICIPANT_ID
09/01/2013 07:21:21 UTC	Logon attempt	Security		0
09/01/2013 07:21:22 UTC	Inbox	View list		0
09/01/2013 07:21:45 UTC	Query list	Patient	QUERY read patient list	0
09/01/2013 07:21:48 UTC	Maintain reference data	Organization groups	Tasks that contain only requests that read or query data	0
09/01/2013 07:21:48 UTC	View encounter	Open chart	Patient context	4070370
09/01/2013 07:21:50 UTC	Problems	Read	OUTPUT prompt programs	4070370
09/01/2013 07:21:51 UTC	Query clinical events	Results		4070370
09/01/2013 07:21:51 UTC	Clinical diagnoses	Read	OUTPUT prompt programs	4070370
09/01/2013 07:22:36 UTC	Maintain person	Chart access log	RUN preferences	4070370
09/01/2013 07:22:36 UTC	Flowsheet	View		4070370
09/01/2013 07:22:36 UTC	Maintain person	Chart access log	RUN preferences	4070370
09/01/2013 07:22:36 UTC	Query clinical events	Results	QUERY—clinical event query	4070370
09/01/2013 07:23:02 UTC	Maintain person	Chart access log	RUN preferences	4070370
09/01/2013 07:23:02 UTC	Flowsheet	View		4070370
09/01/2013 07:23:19 UTC	Maintain person	Chart access log	RUN preferences	4070370
09/01/2013 07:23:29 UTC	Maintain clinical document	Attempt to view document		4070370
09/01/2013 07:23:47 UTC	Maintain clinical document	Attempt to view document		/485199
09/01/2013 07:24:53 UTC	Maintain person	Chart access log	RUN preferences	4070370
09/01/2013 07:24:54 UTC	UPDATE orders	Order	10 mg = 1 tab(s), PO, qDay, # 30 tab(s), refill(s) 0	4070370

(continued)

Table 6.1 (continued)

TIMESTAMP	EVENT_NAME	EVENT_TYPE	TASK	PARTICIPANT_ID
09/01/2013 09:00:58 UTC		Order	5 mg = 1 tab(s), PO, qDay, # 30 tab(s), refill(s) 11	4070370
09/01/2013 09:00:59 UTC	Genview	View	IRUN patient list management	4070370
09/01/2013 09:37:40 UTC	Logout attempt	Security		0

Data was formed to stimulate research using such data,[6] which resulted in several recently published papers that proposed common metrics to standardize the measures of logged clinician activites [14]. The value of audit logs is also recognized by the industry. Many EHR vendors now provide built-in tools (e.g., Epic Signal and Cerner LightsOn) to leverage automatically logged data to produce real-time information to inform usage patterns, abnormalities, and performance improvement opportunities. For a review of HCI studies using computer log data, see [15, 16].

A significant limitation of using security audit logs in HCI research is that some transitory screen activities (e.g. user moving a window around to reduce the amount of visual clutter on the screen) are not logged which nevertheless could be of considerable interest to HCI experts. Further, timestamps recorded in a security audit log file only indicate when a clinical action occurred. This information is not adequate to answer important usability questions such as how long it took the user to perform the action (e.g., to fill out a medication ordering form), or if the user chose the optimal options when using the system (since the original clinical context may also be unknown). Additional tools are therefore needed for HCI experts to acquire supplemental data on screen activities, described in the next section.

Screen Activities Screen activities, such as mouse cursor trails, mouse clicks/drags, keystrokes, and window activation and window movements, have been popularly used in HCI research to study user interactions with a software system to detect potential usability pitfalls. Screen activities reveal rich details of user behaviors that may not be otherwise available, e.g., user clicking a "+" sign to expand a tree view to see a full list of medications, or clicking the "Close" button to skip a popup window presenting a computer-generated clinical decision-support reminder. This additional level of detail is very important for HCI research in healthcare because many commercial health IT systems may not log user actions that do not involve direct accesses of or modifications to patient charts.

Screen activities may be recorded as a sequence of screen snapshots or as a video stream. Figure 6.1 illustrates a sample frame from a video clip capturing a user session took place in an outpatient exam room. When a front-mounted camera is

---

[6] https://cliir.ucsf.edu/portfolio/national-research-network-ehr-audit-log-data

6 Computational Ethnography: Automated and Unobtrusive Means for Collecting... 129

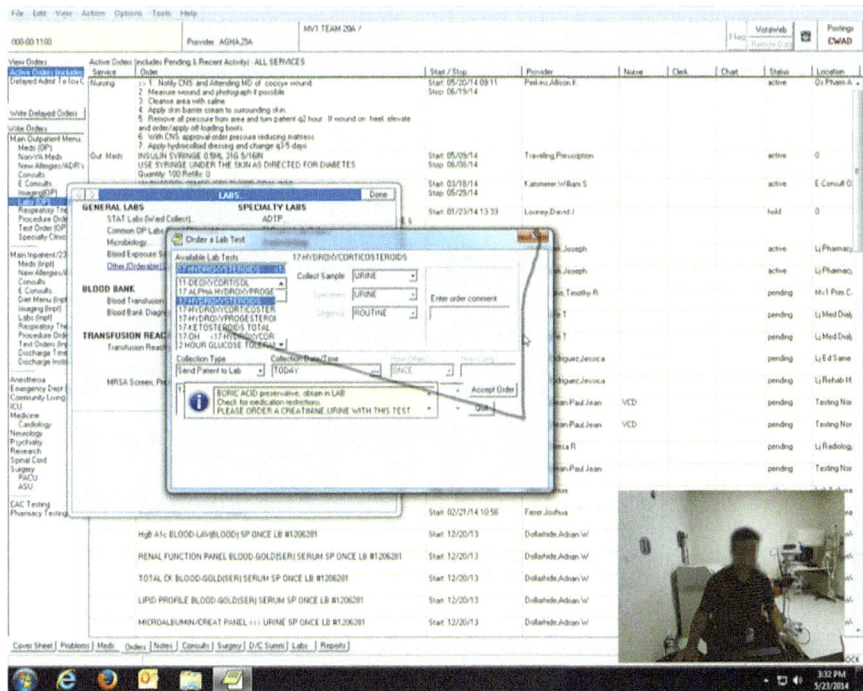

Fig. 6.1 A sample frame from a screen activity video clip recording a clinician interacting with an EHR system. The superimposed dark grey path shows the trail of the mouse cursor over the 1 s prior to the capture of this frame

available, additional contextual video/audio data (shown in the bottom right window) may also be recorded along with screen activities providing an opportunity for HCI experts to study the clinician's (as well as the patient's) facial expressions, body gestures, and conversations between the clinician and the patient.

Screen activities may also be recorded as log data containing a chronological list of user interaction events that can be computationally analyzed. Screen footage and contextual videos, on the other hand, are much harder to analyze which often requires prolonged and laborious manual coding processes. As illustrated in a sample screen activity log shown in Table 6.2, a variety of usability metrics can be readily derived from the structured log data including time efficiency (how much time it takes to complete a given task), operation efficiency (how many mouse clicks or keystrokes it requires to complete a given task), and error rates (e.g., frequency of user clicking a wrong button or the ratio of unnecessary mouse/keyboard activities that did not contribute to the accomplishment of a given task). For example, Magrabi et al. used screen activities to examine how task complexity and interruption affect clinician performance in terms of error rates, resumption lag, and task completion time in creating and updating electronic medication charts [17]. Screen activity logs, especially when combined with other sources of data (e.g., security auditing logs), can also reveal other interaction behaviors of high interest to HCI researchers such as how clinicians copy/paste text from various sources in a an EHR system to construct a narrative note.

Many software tools are available for capturing and analyzing computer screen activities. Morae (TechSmith Corporation, Okemos, MI), for example, is a commercial product widely used in usability studies and market research that allows for observing, recording, and analyzing user interactions with software systems such as websites.[7] Both the video footage shown in Fig. 6.1 and the screen activity log shown in Table 6.2 were generated using Morae. In healthcare, screen activity capturing tools have been developed specifically to work with health IT systems such as EHRs. Turf (an acronym for "Task, User, Representation, Function"), for example, is an EHR usability assessment tool developed at the National Center for Cognitive Informatics and Decision Making funded by the ONC's Strategic Health IT Advanced Research initiative.[8] Turf is an integrated toolkit that allows for screen capturing, UI markups, and heuristic evaluation (e.g., experts can use the system to indicate potential usability issues on a screen and label them as minor, moderate, major or catastrophic). The evaluation criteria incorporated in Turf are based on the National Institute of Standards and Technology's (NIST) EHR usability evaluation protocol, NISTIR 7804.[9]

Eye Tracking Screen activity data capture how users interact with a software system using mouse and keyboard. However, user activities that do not trigger a traceable screen event are not captured. These activities may include, for example, a clinician reading from an EHR system to digest a patient's earlier discharge summary before meeting the patient in an exam room, or examining the content of a computer-generated drug safety alert before acting upon it. Head and eye movements captured through eye-tracking devices can thus become an important source of data enabling HCI experts to study interesting topics such as how clinicians seek information and make sense of a patient case out of a large volume of patient records and whether there is a tendency among clinicians to skip computer-generated advisories without carefully reading them.

An eye-tracking device measures a person's head position (gaze) and eye movements relative to the head that reveal the person's visual and overt attention processes. Modern eye-tracking technologies are often based on optical sensors that capture the vector between the pupil center and the corneal reflections created by casting a beam of infrared or near-infrared non-collimated light on the eye. In HCI, the eye-tracking technique has been commonly used in assessing the usability of websites e.g. to study which portion(s) of the screen that web surfers' attention tends to focus on more often so as to optimize the placement of online advertisements [18]. It has also been used in healthcare particularly in the areas of autism

---

[7] http://www.techsmith.com/morae.html

[8] https://turf.shis.uth.tmc.edu/turfweb/

[9] NISTIR 7804: Technical Evaluation, Testing and Validation of the Usability of Electronic Health Records. http://www.nist.gov/manuscript-publication-search.cfm?pub_id=909701

Table 6.2 A sample screen activity log

ELAPSED_TIME	EVENT	DETAIL	APPLICATION_OWNER	WINDOW_TITTLE	EXTRA
00:13.3	Keystrokes	D (shift)			
00:13.5	Keystrokes	y			
00:13.6	Keystrokes	Backspace			
00:20.4	Mouse clicks	L button down			
00:20.5	Mouse clicks	R button down			
00:20.8	Window/dialog events	Focus	Context	Cut	Ctrl+X
00:21.9	Mouse clicks	L button down		Reminders	
00:34.8	Window/dialog events	Focus		HTN lifestyle education	
00:35.5	Window/dialog events	Move	Reminder resolution: HTN lifestyle education	Reminder resolution: HTN lifestyle education	
00:36.4	Mouse clicks	L button down	Reminder resolution: HTN lifestyle education	Finish	
00:36.6	Window/dialog events	Focus	Sign note		
00:36.6	Mouse clicks	L button down	Sign note	OK	
00:36.7	Window/dialog events	Focus	Order menu		
00:36.9	Mouse clicks	Wheel (−)			

research [19], anxiety and depression [20], and training and assessing the skills of surgeons [21].

Figure 6.2 shows an eye-tracking device mounted below a computer monitor in an outpatient exam room. This configuration is not intrusive and can detect both head and eye movements, and is thus more practical to use in everyday healthcare settings. Eye-tracking data obtained through the device can be synchronized with screen activity recordings to reveal which part of the computer screen the user was looking at moment-by-moment during a use session. The end result can be plotted as heat-maps showing hotspots on an application's UI or eye trails traversing different parts of the screen, as illustrated in Fig. 6.3a, b, respectively. In addition, the eye-tracking data provide hints as to when the user gazes away from the computer to attend to other stimuli in the room, e.g., the patient. This allows HCI experts to study how the presence of computers in an exam room might interfere with patient–provider communications. Many manufactures produce eye-tracking devices and analytical software are produced. Leading vendors include Tobii Technology[10] and SensoMotoric Instruments (SMI).[11]

Motion Capture A considerable body of the HCI literature in healthcare concerns how introduction of computerized systems changes the dynamics of patient–clinician interactions in an exam room. It has been extensively documented that computer use during clinical consultations could be associated with adverse impact such as diminished quality of patient–clinician communications and elevated levels of patient disengagement and dissatisfaction. Some frequently reported reasons include loss of eye contact, rapport, and provision of emotional support; interference with conversations due to the clinician gazing back-and-forth at the computer screen; reduced emphasis on psychosocial questioning and relationship mainte-

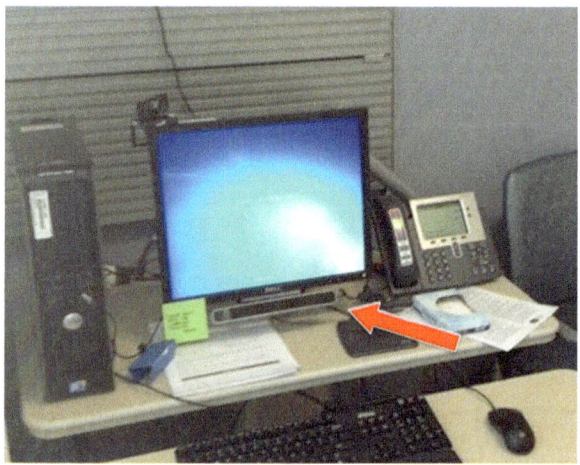

Fig. 6.2 A table-mounted eye tracker in an outpatient exam room

---

[10] http://www.tobii.com/

[11] http://www.smivision.com/

6 Computational Ethnography: Automated and Unobtrusive Means for Collecting...   133

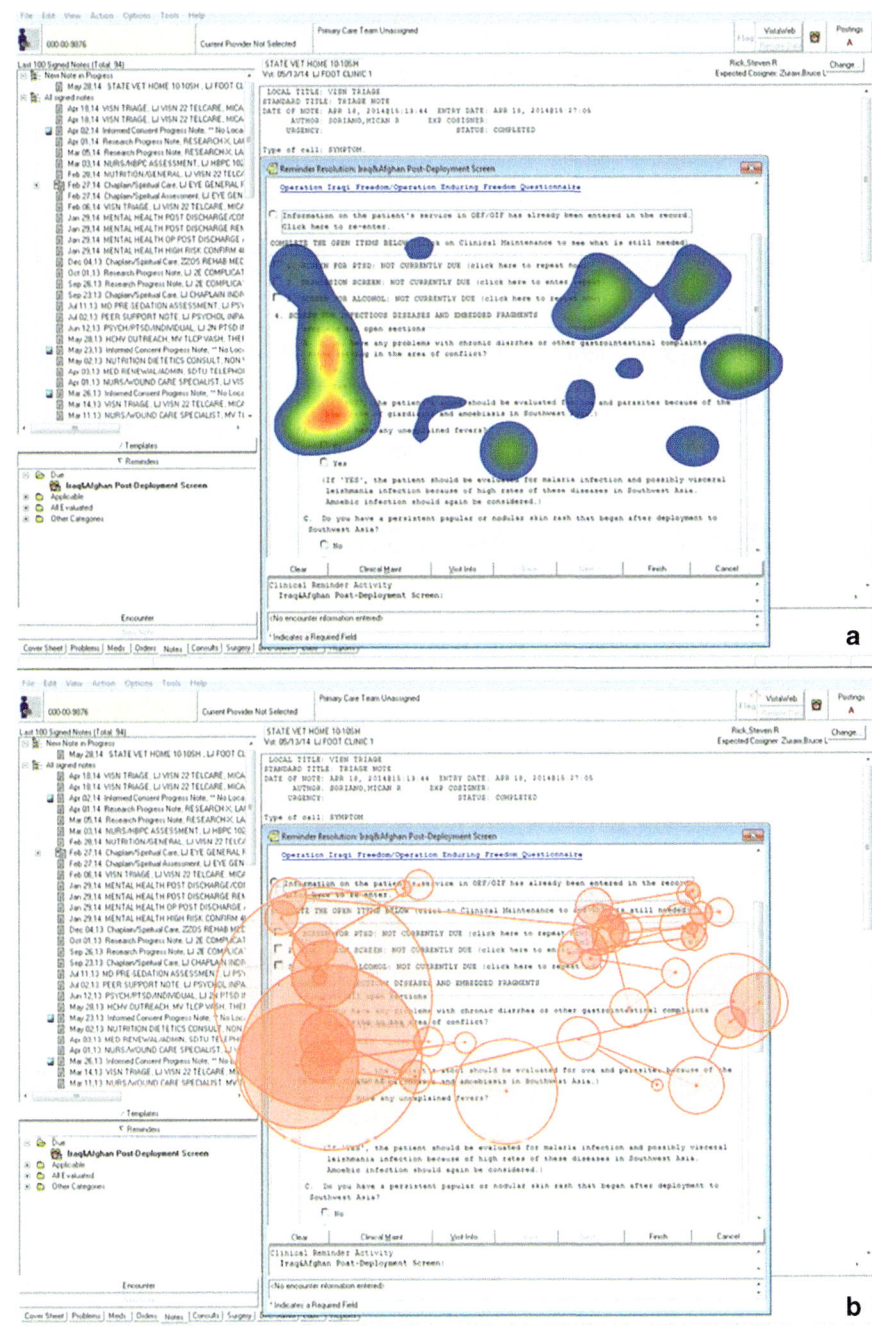

Fig. 6.3 (**a**, **b**) Heat-map and eye trails produced by eye-tracking data

nance; and irrelevant computer-prompted inquiries diluting the focus on the patient's current issues. For a review of these potential issues, see Ref. [22].

Besides the methods for capturing computer activities and eye movements, HCI experts in healthcare are also experimenting with novel sensor-based technologies that allow for automated collection and analysis of additional dimensions of patient–clinician interaction data such as vocalization, body orientation, and body gestures. Microsoft Kinect™,[12] for example, is an affordable yet effective solution that includes an infrared depth sensor for tracking depth data (i.e., participants' distance and angle relative to the position of the camera), body movements (kinetics through motion of body joints e.g. head, should center, shoulder left/right, elbow left/right, wrist left/right, hand left/right, etc.), and head orientation (e.g., pitch, roll, yaw). It also has a built-in microphone array that detects the angle of multiple audio sources which makes it possible to perform automated segmentation of voice data to identify vocalization sequences, clinician's visual attention (EHR vs. patient), as well as characterize turn-talking behaviors in terms of whether the clinician or the patient was talking. Such data can thus enable HCI experts to answer daunting questions e.g. the body language that clinicians use when interacting with patients while simultaneously using computerized systems such as EHRs. Figure 6.4 shows a Kinect mounted above and behind a computer monitor in an outpatient exam room. Figure 6.5 illustrates a sample frame from a depth and skeleton image sequence recorded by Kinect's depth camera.

A distinctive advantage of using sensor-based technologies such as Kinect is that the data collected can be programmatically analyzed eliminating the need to have human coders to manually review hours of video/audio data. Microsoft provides a non-commercial Kinect Software Development Kit (SDK) freely available to HCI experts to develop customized analytical programs to perform post-processing tasks such as background removal, gesture recognition, facial recognition, and voice recognition.[13]

For example, the depth, skeletal, and voice direction data are all recorded as digitized coordinates which can be easily computed to determine the relative positions of the participants in the room (typically a clinician and a patient if it is an outpatient primary care exam room) at each given time during a clinical encounter. This allows HCI experts to automatically segment the progression of a clinical consultation into distinct stages e.g. greetings, physical exam, conversing in seated positions, and patient and/or clinician leaving the room. Nonverbal communications such as head orientation and body gestures can also be automatically recognized and studied, and can be further synchronized with eye-tracking data to precisely profile the clinician's gazing behavior when using the EHR to enter or retrieve information while talking to the patient. Large-scale deep analyses of patient–clinician interactions are thus possible at reasonably costs without involving laborious manual coding processes. For a more in-depth discussion on how to use sensor-based technologies to

---

[12] http://kinectforwindows.org
[13] http://www.microsoft.com/en-us/kinectforwindowsdev/

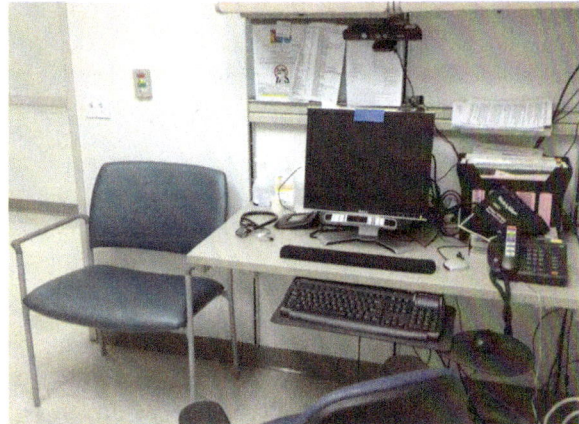

Fig. 6.4 Microsoft Kinect™ installed in an outpatient exam room and monitoring a physician's movements (reproduced from Weibel et al. [23])

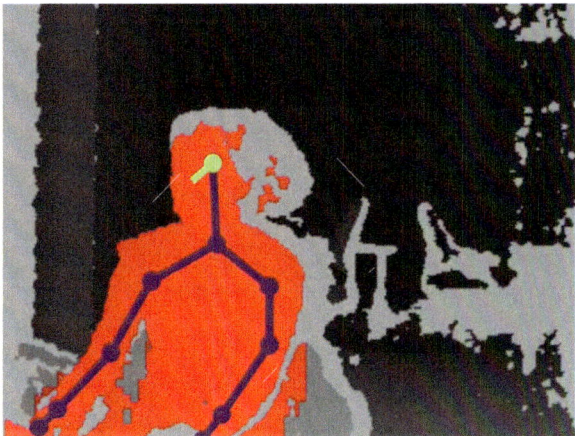

Fig. 6.5 Skeletal and depth data recorded by Kinect. The red overlay indicates that a body has been recognized; the purple dots indicate body joints connected through purple lines; the yellow line indicates the gaze vector as inferred from pitch yaw and roll (reproduced from Weibel et al. [23])

study the dynamics of patient–clinician interactions in exam rooms and potential practical obstacles, see Ref. [23].

Voice Recordings and Clinical Conversation Transcripts The burden of clinical documentation is a major contributing factor of clinician burnout, which has been declared recently as a public health crisis [24]. To alleviate this burden, some hospitals and clinics are starting to implement ambient documentation systems, or "digital scribes," to partially automate the tedious and time-consuming documentation process. This new family of technologies uses automatic speech recognition to transcribe clinical conversations in the exam room or at the bedside, and then uses natural language processing to turn the transcripts into structured or free-text EHR data. Many ambient documentation products have now entered the market, produced by technology giants such as Google [25], Microsoft/Nuance [26], and 3M [27].

A by-product of implementing the ambient documentation technology in healthcare is the voice recordings, as well as the resultant transcripts, that contain rich detail about the information exchange between patients and clinicians and the dynamics of their verbal interactions. Previous studies have used such data to understand clinicians' adherence to evidence-based clinical guidelines [28], prioritization of preventive care services [29], and patient-reported barriers to compliance [30]. Increasingly, HCI researchers also leverage such data to conduct research on topics such as the emotions expressed during the clinical conversation [31] and the conversational flows (e.g. topics and topic turns) [32]. Such studies have the potential to produce valuables insights into improving patient–clinician interactions and communication. The availability of such data may also stimulate computational ethnographic research in additional domains such as clinical workflow, team coordination, and interruptions.

Real-Time Locating Systems (RTLS) Clinicians as well as patients move around constantly in a medical facility to provide/receive care and to interact with other stakeholders (e.g., families, specialists, pharmacists). While the other computational ethnographical methods described in this section help HCI experts examine the interactions between clinicians, patients, and computerized systems, they do not allow for comprehensive collection of motion-location data that may lead into novel insights. For example, with motion-location data, HCI researchers are in a better position to answer questions such as whether the physical layout of an outpatient clinic or an inpatient ward is optimally designed to facilitate patient care delivery, and whether the introduction of health IT systems might result in a reduction of face time among healthcare coworkers. Sensor-based RTLS systems, most commonly based on the radio-frequency identification (RFID) technology,[14] provide a solution to capturing such motion-location data. RFID has a long history of being used in healthcare for supply chain management purposes (e.g., asset tracking of medical devices) and patient safety purposes (e.g., patient identification), and has been increasingly used in HCI studies to determine the whereabouts of clinicians or patients. For a review of applications of RFID in healthcare, see Refs. [33] and [34].

An RFID tag or badge contains an electronic transponder that emits or responds to electromagnetic signals to both identify itself and triangulate its position relative to base stations installed in the environment. The locating precision depends on vendor and configuration, but is generally adequate for studying problems concerned in HCI such as whether two or a group of healthcare providers are in close spatial proximity (e.g., the same room), which provides an opportunity for them to engage in interpersonal communications. Joined with timestamps, the spatiotemporal data collected via an RTLS system allow HCI experts to explore a variety of interesting topics, for example, clinicians' movement patterns, the dynamics of team aggregation and dispersion, and potential workflow deficiencies.

Other Types of Computational Ethnographical Data Besides the six major types of computational ethnographical data discussed in this section, there are also other

---

[14]Wifi, cellular, and ZigBee triangulation technologies have also been developed and used for RTLS.

sources of digital traces that HCI experts may potentially tap into, such as paging/phone logs tracked by telecommunication systems, email messages delivered or received by email servers, internet traffic monitored by proxy servers and firewall systems, and data and metadata collected by barcode scanners and by medical devices e.g. intelligent infusion pumps. Combining these data sources together allows HCI experts to study everyday activities taking place in a healthcare environment at an unprecedented level of comprehensiveness, depth, and accuracy.

Analyzing Computational Ethnographical Data

Coding Computational Ethnographical Data To analyze computational ethnographical data, a coding schema must be first identified or developed for properly labeling and categorizing the events recorded. For example, to make sense of security audit logs, researchers need to first determine the taxonomies used for "event name" and "event type" (see Table 6.1), which can often be found in software documentation or obtained directly from the vendor. Over the years, the HCI and the health informatics research communities have created many task taxonomies to characterize clinicians' work in different care areas or different medical specialties. For example, Tierney et al. developed a clinical task taxonomy comprised of tasks commonly performed by inpatient internists [35] and subsequently adapted it to use in ambulatory primary care settings [36]. Wetterneck et al. developed a comprehensive primary care task list for evaluating clinic visit workflow which incorporates more granular task and task category definitions such as looking up the referral doctor from an EHR system or from a paper chart [37]. Similar taxonomies have been established to characterize the work by anesthesiologists [38], ICU nurses [39], clinicians working on general medicine floors [40], as well as clinical activities specifically related to medication ordering and management [41].

If an HCI study mainly concerns clinicians' documentation behavior, it is advised that the researchers base their analysis on a formal classification of EHR functions and record structures, such as ASTM International's "Standard Practice for Content and Structure of the Electronic Health Record (EHR), ASTM E1384-07,"[15] "Standard Specification for Healthcare Document Formats, E2184-02",[16] or "Data Elements for EHR Documentation" curated by the American Health Information Management Association [42]. These standards define basic functions of EHR systems, common types of clinical documents, and the structure of each document type (e.g., sections and data elements that should be contained in a discharge summary). Using these standards properly can help standardize the conduct and results reporting of documentation behavior research.

---

[15] http://www.astm.org/Standards/E1384.htm
[16] http://www.astm.org/Standards/E2184.htm

Analyzing Computational Ethnographical Data Data collected using computational ethnographical methods can be analyzed in many ways depending on the objective and the context of an HCI study. For example, researchers interested in patient throughput may perform time series analyses to determine the intensity of clinical activities in different units in a hospital during different hours of the day and different days of the year; researchers interested in time efficiency may compute descriptive statistics to determine average turnaround between a medication order is placed and the medication is fulfilled/administered using a new computerized order entry system; and researchers interested in optimizing a UI design may use the amount of eyeball and mouse movements as a surrogate measure of the effectiveness of the organization of information and UI elements on the screen. Error rates, documentation patterns, and formation and dismissal of care teams are also frequently studied research topics [17, 43, 44]. In this section, we describe a few unique analytical approaches that are particularly useful in analyzing computational ethnographical data.

First, *temporal data mining* is commonly used in computational ethnography. This is because computational ethnographical data are always recorded in the form of, or can be easily transposed into, *time-stamped event sequences* exhibiting the temporal (and potentially spatial) distribution of occurrences of a series of events. Because temporal data mining identifies temporal interdependencies between events, this family of methods is ideal for discovering hidden regularities from computational ethnographical data that may have significant clinical or behavioral implications. For example, HCI researchers studying the impact of health IT on clinical workflow may be interested in identifying clinical activities that are usually carried out in a given sequential order to examine whether the design of a health IT system may facilitate or hinder the ordered execution of a series of clinical tasks.

Sequential pattern analysis is one such temporal data mining method for characterizing how interrelated events are chronologically arranged. Sequential pattern analysis was initially developed by Agrawal & Srikant [45] to study customers' shopping behavior, e.g., predicting a customer's future merchandise purchases based on the person's past shopping record. Consider the following three event sequences wherein each symbol representing a clinical activity: *abegcdhf*, *eabhcd*, *abhcdfg*. It can be easily observed that *ab...cd* is a frequently occurring pattern supported by all three sequences. If the implementation of a new health IT system requires *cd* to be performed prior to *ab*, or another task to be performed between *a* and *b* or between *c* and *d*, it is possible that the new system may introduce considerable disruptions to the established workflow as well as clinicians' cognitive processes. For a review of sequential data analysis and temporal mining, see Refs. [46] and [47].

Second, time-stamped events sequences derived from computational ethnographical data can be used for *transition analyses*. For example, from the three sample event sequences above, it can be easily calculated that the probability of observing event *b* following event *a* is 1, and the probabilities of observing *e* and *h* following *b* are 0.25 and 0.5, respectively. This information enables HCI researchers to characterize the nature of task transitions in clinical care. It may also allow HCI researchers to associate 'cost' with each task transition and assess whether the introduction of a new software system might increase or decrease such cost. Here, 'cost' may consist of cognitive load of switching between tasks as well as the physical effort that the task switching may incur. Studying the cost associated with task transitions is important because it has been shown in the cognition literature that frequent task switching is often associated with increased mental burden on the performer (e.g., task prioritizing and task activation). Additionally, switching between tasks that are of distinct natures could result in a higher likelihood of cognitive slips and mistakes; for example, the loss-of-activation error manifesting as forgetting what the preceding task was about in a task execution sequence.

Lastly, transition probabilities hereby obtained allow HCI researchers to conduct Markov chain analysis [48] to determine that in a series of events which event might most likely appear in which step. These Markov chains, based on empirical contexts, may represent activities that a primary care physician performs during an outpatient patient visit or care procedures that a patient must go through before a surgical operation. Such information helps HCI researchers quantify the nature of established workflow in a healthcare environment and design software systems accordingly that best align with such workflow.

Limitation of Computational Ethnography

Comparing to traditional approaches for conducting HCI fieldwork, computational ethnographical methods provide an automated and less intrusive means for HCI researchers to study software systems or medical devices deployed in the field and used in naturalistic settings. However, computational ethnography also has notable shortcomings. A critical limitation of computational ethnographical methods is that while automatically captured digital trace data help HCI researchers tell what happened in the field, they are often inadequate to shed light on why clinicians demonstrated the observed behaviors. Mixed methods, which combine the merits of computational ethnography with qualitative research designs such as interviews, context inquiry and ethnographically based observations, are therefore highly encouraged. Further, computational ethnographical data are not necessarily complete for characterizing clinicians' certain behaviors. For example communication analyses solely based on computer logs (paging/phone, email, messaging, etc.) may fail to consider other important channels of communication among clinicians such as hall way or bedside conversations. Thus, when conducting computational ethnographical investigations, researchers shall be always mindful whether such data are a truly comprehensive reflection of clinicians' work of interest. Lastly, computational ethnographical data may originate from multiple sources posing great challenges to synchronization and integrative analysis. In addition, computational ethnographical data may be originally collected to support operational purposes (e.g., security auditing), rather than research. Preparing such data for research reuse could therefore be resource consuming and may require sophisticated analytical skills.

Case Studies

Understanding Clinicians' Navigation Behavior in EHRS

In their paper "*An Interface-Driven Analysis of User Interactions with an Electronic Health Records System*," Zheng et al. applied the computational ethnographical approach to study primary care physicians' usage behavior of an ambulatory care EHR system [49]. In the study, a homegrown EHR system was reengineered to allow real-time capture of comprehensive UI interaction events such as mouse clicks and keystrokes. These UI interaction events, along with audit trails recording EHR document retrieval, creation, and modification events, provided data for computational ethnographical analyses.

Figure 6.6 illustrates the UI of the EHR system studied. Listed in Table 6.3 are 17 major EHR features provided in the system to allow clinicians to perform various documentation or chart viewing tasks. Based on the digital trace data and time-stamps, event sequences were constructed representing how these 17 EHR features were sequentially accessed, which might represent how the corresponding clinical tasks were sequentially carried out. *HMXAD*, for example, represents a task sequence of "History of Present Illness" (H) → "Medication" (M) → "Physical Examination" (X) → "Assessment & Plan" (A) → "Diagnosis" (D). The empirical study was conducted in an ambulatory primary care clinic and lasted 10 months. Data were recorded in a total of 973 distinct patient encounters seen by 30 resident physicians.

The computational ethnographical data recorded in the empirical study were analyzed using a sequential pattern analysis, which uncovers hidden navigational patterns in the resident physicians' use of the EHR system; and a Markov chain model, which characterizes the sequential dependencies among the 17 EHR features based on transition probabilities. The sequential patterns identified in the study are shown in Table 6.4. These patterns satisfied a minimum support threshold of 15%, i.e., each appeared in at least 15% of the patient encounters studied. As shown in Table 6.4, *ADAD* and *DADA* were the most common recurring feature combinations sequentially carried out, which suggests that when the resident physicians used the EHR system to document or view patient data, they often accessed the "Assessment & Plan" and "Diagnosis" sections of the EHR consecutively, and frequently switched between these two features back and forth. "Medication" and "Order" are another pair of EHR features that appeared to be often used together.

Figure 6.7 illustrates the results obtained from the Markov chain analysis where feature transitions with a probability above 0.5 are highlighted using bold arcs. Prominent transitions can be easily observed from the figure; for example, after a resident physician completed "Physical Examination", the chance that she or he would immediately move on to document "Assessment & Plan" (0.687) is higher than the probabilities of using all other EHR features combined. Similarly, "Assessment & Plan" → "Diagnosis" (0.764) is a frequent task transition, suggesting that immediately after documenting in the "Assessment & Plan" section in the

6 Computational Ethnography: Automated and Unobtrusive Means for Collecting... 141

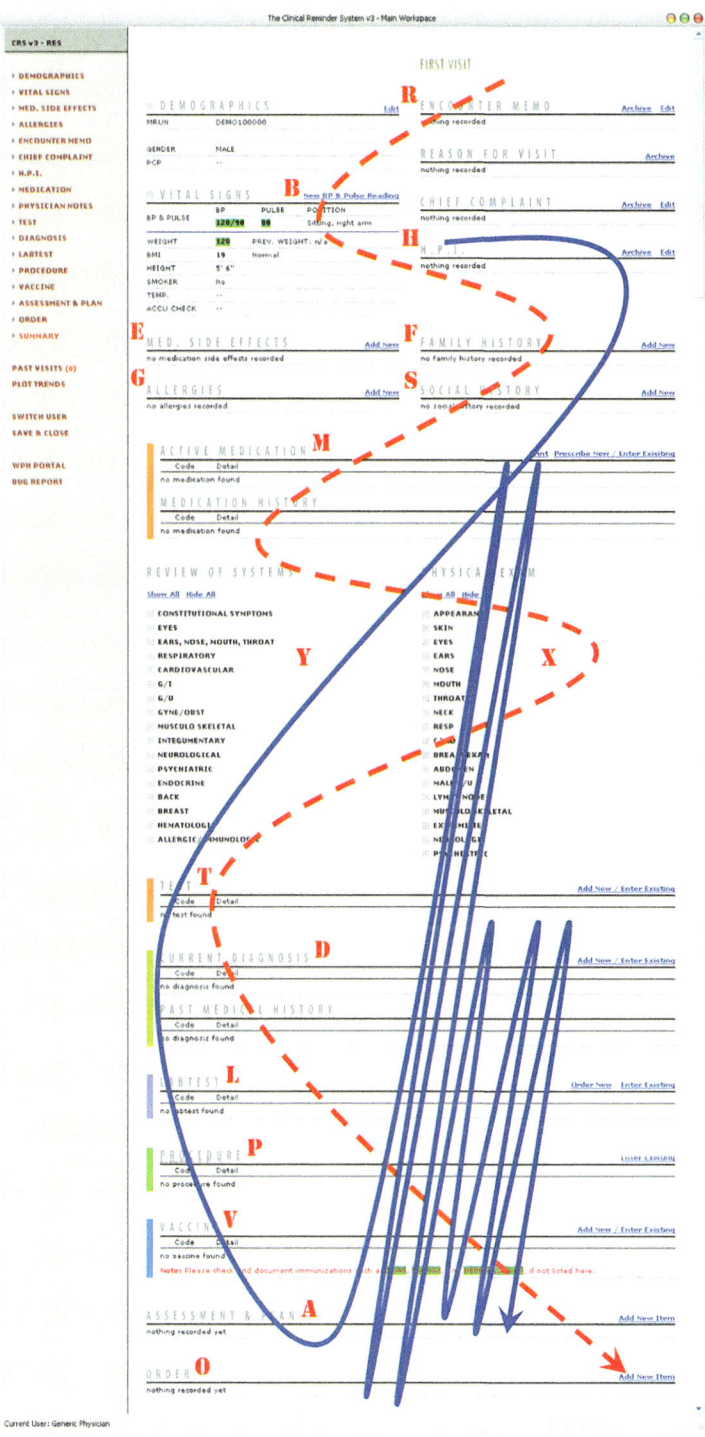

Fig. 6.6 User interface of the EHR system studied in Zheng et al. [49]

Table 6.3 Major EHR features studied

Label	Feature	Label	Feature
A	Assessment & Plan	O	Order
B	Retaking BP	P	Procedure
D	Diagnosis (problem list)	R	EncounteR Memo
E	Medication Side Effects	S	Social History
F	Family History	T	Office Test
G	AllerGies	V	Vaccination
H	History of Present Illness (HPI)	X	Physical EXamination
L	Laboratory Test	Y	Review of SYstems
M	Medication		

Table 6.4 Sequential patterns identified

Pattern	Level of support (%)
ADAD	51.16
DADA	43.97
XADA	40.17
OMOM	32.77
MOMO	29.39
YXAD	21.78
HS	19.03
OL	18.6
OMY	16.7
LO	15.64
HO	15.01

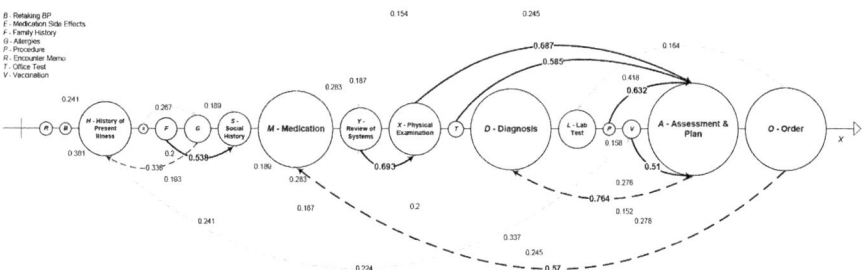

Fig. 6.7 Tasks and task transition probabilities during an outpatient primary care visit (reproduced from Zheng et al. [49]). Size of a node is proportional to the activity's frequency of occurrence as empirically observed. Bold edges: transitions with a probability over 0.5; Dashed edges: task transitions running counter to the anticipated workflow. Transitions with a probability lower than 0.15 are not shown

EHR system, a resident physician would most likely begin working on "Diagnosis." Likewise, "Order" has a high probability of transitioning to "Medication" (0.57), as does "Family History" → "Social History" (0.538).

Figure 6.8 illustrates the Markov chain constructed based on the feature transition probabilities. This information reveals that after a user logged into the EHR system, in which step a particular EHR feature would most likely be accessed. As exhibited in the figure, "History of Present Illness" was usually the first stop after a user started to use the system. Then, the most likely accessed next EHR feature was "Social History," followed by "Assessment & Plan." From Fig. 6.8, it becomes clear how resident physicians in the study practice tended to organize their clinical work chronologically during a typical outpatient primary care encounter.

The results of this computational ethnographical study led to the discovery of the resident physicians' navigational patterns in using the ambulatory care EHR system in the study clinic. This discovery may in turn lead to a better understanding of their cognitive processes when providing patient care. For HCI researchers, this learning may directly inform improvement opportunities to ameliorate the usability of the EHR system, e.g., usability deficiencies may surface if certain UI design of the system might require an excessive number of mouse clicks in order to accomplish frequent task transitions.

For example, the empirical data recorded in this study show that "History of Present Illness" was one of the most frequently used features and was usually accessed immediately after a user logged into the system. This feature should therefore be placed in a distinctive, salient onscreen position in the UI. Further, the study identified several pairs of features (e.g., "Assessment & Plan" ⇄ "Diagnosis" and "Order" ⇄ "Medication") that were often accessed together. This prompts EHR designers to place these features in adjacent locations on the screen, or provide

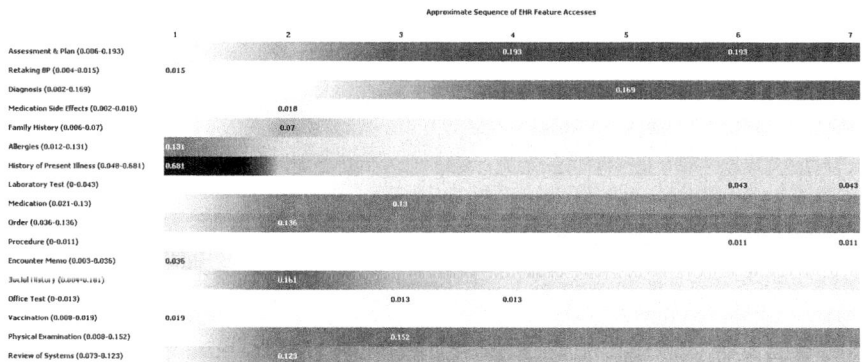

Fig. 6.8 A diagram that visualizes the Markov chain constructed based on transition probabilities (reproduced from Zheng et al. [49]). Gray-scale gradient is proportional to the probabilities of observing a row activity in each of the Markov chain steps. Darker areas indicate higher probabilities. Numbers in parentheses: the range of probabilities of observing an activity in these Markov chain steps; Numeric labels on gray-scale stripes: the maximum probability of observing a row activity

certain navigational aids (e.g. hyperlink shortcuts), to facilitate these frequent feature switches. The result would be a more optimized designs better aligned with clinicians' workflow as well as their mental model of accessing/documenting information and providing patient care.

Analyzing the Dynamics of Provider–Patient Interactions

The second case study, "Interpreter-mediated physician–patient communication: opportunities for multimodal healthcare interfaces," was conducted by Weibel et al. [50]. This study examined physician–patient communications mediated by medical interpreters with patients who have low English proficiency. The fieldwork was conducted at a community health center that provides comprehensive care for low income and multiethnic patient populations. A majority of these patients show limited English proficiency (LEP); most of them require the assistance of an interpreter during physician–patient consultations.

In the study, the researchers analyzed multiparty and multimodal interactions in the exam room from a distributed cognition perspective. The study employed a novel computational ethnographical approach to simultaneously capture multiple data streams to examine physician, patient, and interpreter interactions. This allowed the researchers to investigate beyond speech—what has been traditionally considered the primary modality for communication—to include other types of nonverbal exchanges such as eye contact, gestures, and body orientation.

To capture multiparty multimodal interactions, the study deployed an experimental recording system using two Microsoft Kinects that allowed the capture of body positioning, directional audio, video footage, and depth-imaging of the scene. The analysis leveraged a suite of analysis techniques that the researchers previously developed called ChronoViz (shown in Fig. 6.9),[17] a tool that aids visualization and analysis of multimodal sets of time-coded information with a focus on the analysis of video in combination with other data sources. In this study, ChronoViz was used to facilitate the analysis of simultaneous bodily action, voice, and gaze (head position) of multiple participants [51].

Figure 6.9 also shows the position of patient, doctor, and interpreter in the exam room. The physician and the patient usually sit side-by side. The physician sits in a rolling desk chair, with the EHR directly in front of her on a rolling, height-adjustable platform. The patient sits next to the physician on the front edge of a traditional exam table. The interpreter typically sits in a simple chair backed against the exam room wall, next to the door, approximately 6 ft directly in front of the patient. The empirical study recorded 12 outpatient encounter sessions (half requiring the service of an interpreter). Each generated two video streams, two directional audio streams, two depth data streams, and derived body joint positions (calculated by the Kinect algorithms).

---

[17] http://chronoviz.com/

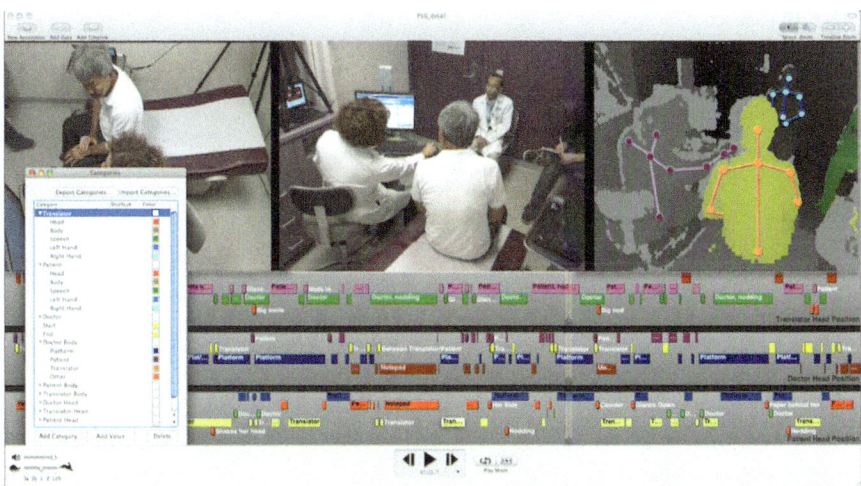

Fig. 6.9 ChronoViz view of Kinect data (reproduced from Weibel et al. [50]). The top half shows video feeds (two video and one depth-image) from two Kinects. The center video and right depth-image show the interpreter facing the physician (left) and the patient (right). The bottom half shows three timelines with annotations of a 5-min medical session indicating information such as who is talking (patient, interpreter, doctor), their body positions, and what they are interacting with

A group of five researchers analyzed the data with the assistance of ChronoViz. Given the richness and complexity of interaction between individuals and with the EHR, as well as the distinct physician–patient interactions while an interpreter was present in the room, two encounters were selected for an in-depth drilldown analysis. One session involved an English-fluent patient; the other involved an LEP patient who required an interpreter. Body position, head position, right and left hand position, and speech instances (not transcriptions of them) of both patient and physician across the entire sessions were coded. Speech, body position, and head position were also annotated for the interpreter in the second session.

The drilldown analysis revealed differing multiparty communication patterns. Not surprisingly, the interpreter functioned as a middleman who spoke directly after both the patient and the physician (Fig. 6.10). This pattern was only interrupted when the interpreter was not able to directly translate the physician or the patient's speech due to usage of other artifacts (e.g., paper, the EHR system). Further, gesture communication patterns differed between the interpreter and non-interpreter sessions. In both sessions, a variety of gesture types were observed, including deictic (e.g. pointing at EHR or paper), iconic (e.g. hand in shape of cyst), and beat gestures (e.g. hand palm up). When the interpreter was not present, the physician's gestures were distributed fairly evenly across the three gesture types; and the patient communicated with more beat gestures (approximately 36% deictic, 10% iconic, 55% beat). The presence of the interpreter radically changed the gesture pattern: the physician used iconic gestures much more often (approximately 31% deictic, 44% iconic, 25% beat), while all of the interpreter's and patient's gestures were iconic (gesture were used exclusively to communicate the shape, size, and location of an injury).

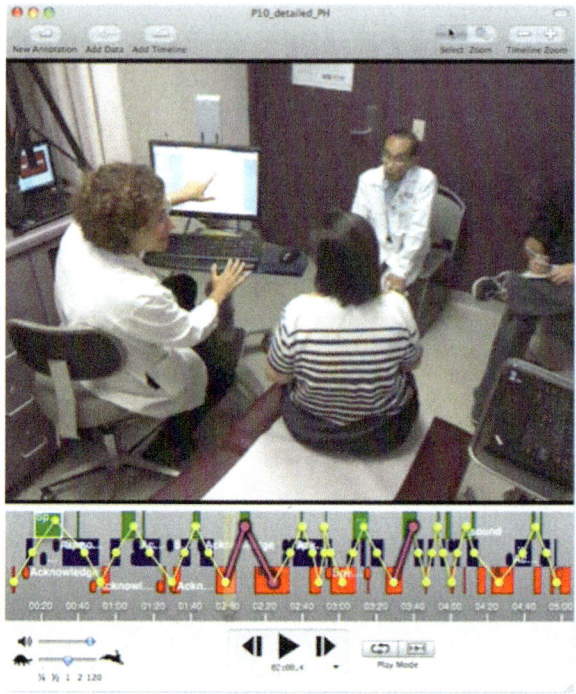

Fig. 6.10 Speech Analysis of an interpreter-mediated communication session (reproduced from Weibel et al. [50]). The timeline displays three levels, each representing the speech of one member of the team: the top line is the patient's speech (green), the middle line is the interpreter's speech (blue), and the lowest line displays the physician's speech (red). A line is superimposed to connect utterances of the three individuals. Yellow lines represent common physician–interpreter–patient interaction patterns; purple lines identify the rare physician–patient interaction patterns

Another key observation from the study is that often one of the parties involved was "left in the dark." The patient often did not understand what the physician was saying and must await the interpreter's translation, and the physician could not understand what the interpreter was saying to the patient nor be sure of translation accuracy. In addition, there were challenges of where to direct attention when various parties were talking. While facial expressions and gesture play a significant in facilitating communication, the patient might be looking at the interpreter when the physician was talking, or the physician at the interpreter when the patient was talking and as a result missed important cues. The communication process was further challenged when the interpreter was left out of the loop because of inability to attend to the EHR display or some other artifact, such as paper. In the study, the physician commonly pointed to the information displayed on the EHR and patients, according to their gestures and body position, suggested that they were also interested in looking at the data. A key problem, however, was that neither the patient nor the interpreter could effectively see the display. This is evident as when the interpreter was present in the room, no pointing gestures to the EHR by the patient or the interpreter were identified from the empirical data. This suggests that the value of using the EHR as a shared communication tool could diminish significantly with LEP patients.

Summary

In summary, comparing to traditional HCI approaches, computational ethnographical methods provide an automated and less obtrusive means for measuring and analyzing the multimodal nature of patient–clinician–computer interactions. Computational ethnography can thus be conducted at an unprecedented level of scale to uncover end users' true, unaltered behaviors interacting with technological systems in healthcare. However, while computational ethnographical data abound in modern healthcare organizations (e.g., routinely tracked audit trails and communication logs), their power for enabling HCI evaluation studies is yet to be fully unleashed. We therefore encourage students, HCI researchers, and healthcare administrators, to carefully consider using computational ethnographical data captured in everyday healthcare settings to generate new knowledge that could inform strategies for improving the usability of technological systems, and ultimately operation efficiency, quality of care, and patient safety.

Acknowledgement We are grateful to Steven Rick who contributed the photos used in this chapter to illustrate computational ethnographical data recording devices deployed in exam rooms.

Discussion Questions

1. The sample audit trail log shown in Table 6.1 exhibits a clinician's use session with an EHR system. In the "PATIENT_ID" column, it can be observed that the clinician worked primarily on patient "4070370" throughout the session but she or he, rather abruptly, viewed a document belonging to patient "7485199" at 07:23:19 UTC.

    (a) What might be the possible explanation(s) of this EHR use behavior? Provide one scenario of "inappropriate" use and one scenario of "beneficial" use.
    (b) How might the EHR system be redesigned to prevent "inappropriate" use, or to facilitate "beneficial" use?
    (c) If the audit trail log were not available, propose an alternative method of recording data that can capture this behavior.

2. Provide an example wherein your everyday activities leave behind some "digital traces" that can be analyzed using computational ethnographical methods.

    (a) Identify the data type that best characterizes these digital traces;
    (b) Propose an analytical method discussed in this chapter to analyze the data;
    (c) Also discuss what potential insights may be drawn from the analysis. These could be insights for better understanding the user behavior or for informing better design of certain technological systems.

References

1. Bloomrosen M, Starren J, Lorenzi NM, Ash JS, Patel VL, Shortliffe EH. Anticipating and addressing the unintended consequences of health IT and policy: a report from the AMIA 2009 Health Policy Meeting. J Am Med Inform Assoc. 2011;18(1):82–90.
2. Kellermann AL, Jones SS. What it will take to achieve the as-yet-unfulfilled promises of health information technology. Health Aff (Millwood). 2013;32(1):63–8.
3. Gonyea RM. Self-reported data in institutional research: review and recommendations. New Dir Inst Res. 2005;127:73–89.
4. Fitzpatrick G, Ellingsen G. A review of 25 years of CSCW research in healthcare: contributions, challenges and future agendas. Comput Supported Coop Work. 2013;22(4–6):609–65.
5. Lazer D, Pentland A, Adamic L, et al. Social science. Computational social science. Science. 2009;323(5915):721–3.
6. Giles J. Computational social science: making the links. Nature. 2012;488(7412):448–50.
7. Card SK, Moran TP, Newell A. The keystroke-level model for user performance time with interactive systems. Commun ACM. 1980;23(7):396–410.
8. Eligible professional meaningful use core measures, measure 14 of 14, stage 1. [cited 2014 May 20]. http://www.cms.gov/Regulations-and-Guidance/Legislation/EHRIncentivePrograms/downloads/15_Core_ProtectElectronicHealthInformation.pdf
9. Adler-Milstein J, Adelman JS, Tai-Seale M, Patel VL, Dymek C. EHR audit logs: a new goldmine for health services research? J Biomed Inform. 2020;101:103343.
10. Kannampallil T, Adler-Milstein J. Using electronic health record audit log data for research: insights from early efforts. J Am Med Inform Assoc. 2022;30(1):167–71.
11. Hripcsak G, Vawdrey DK, Fred MR, Bostwick SB. Use of electronic clinical documentation: time spent and team interactions. J Am Med Inform Assoc. 2011;18(2):112–7.
12. Adler-Milstein J, Zhao W, Willard-Grace R, Knox M, Grumbach K. Electronic health records and burnout: time spent on the electronic health record after hours and message volume associated with exhaustion but not with cynicism among primary care clinicians. J Am Med Inform Assoc. 2020;27(4):531–8.
13. Holmgren AJ, Downing NL, Bates DW, et al. Assessment of electronic health record use between US and non-US health systems. JAMA Intern Med. 2021;181(2):251–9.
14. Sinsky CA, Rule A, Cohen G, et al. Metrics for assessing physician activity using electronic health record log data. J Am Med Inform Assoc. 2020;27(4):639–43.
15. Rule A, Chiang MF, Hribar MR. Using electronic health record audit logs to study clinical activity: a systematic review of aims, measures, and methods. J Am Med Inform Assoc. 2020;27(3):480–90. https://doi.org/10.1093/jamia/ocz196. PMID: 31750912; PMCID: PMC7025338.
16. Rule A, Melnick ER, Apathy NC. Using event logs to observe interactions with electronic health records: an updated scoping review shows increasing use of vendor-derived measures. J Am Med Inform Assoc. 2022;30(1):144–54.
17. Magrabi F, Li SY, Day RO, Coiera E. Errors and electronic prescribing: a controlled laboratory study to examine task complexity and interruption effects. J Am Med Inform Assoc. 2010;17(5):575–83.
18. Poole A, Ball LJ. Eye tracking in human-computer interaction and usability research: current status and future. In: Ghaoui C, editor. Encyclopedia of human-computer interaction. Hershey, PA: Idea Group, Inc.; 2005.
19. Falck-Ytter T, Bölte S, Gredebäck G. Eye tracking in early autism research. J Neurodev Disord. 2013;5(1):28.
20. Armstrong T, Olatunji BO. Eye tracking of attention in the affective disorders: a meta-analytic review and synthesis. Clin Psychol Rev. 2012;32(8):704–23.
21. Tien T, Pucher PH, Sodergren MH, Sriskandarajah K, Yang GZ, Darzi A. Eye tracking for skills assessment and training: a systematic review. J Surg Res. 2014;191(1):169–78.

22. Kazmi Z. Effects of exam room EHR use on doctor-patient communication: a systematic literature review. Inform Prim Care. 2013;21(1):30–9.
23. Weibel N, Rick S, Emmenegger C, Ashfaq S, Calvitti A, Agha Z. LAB-IN-A-BOX: semi-automatic tracking of activity in the medical office. Pers Ubiquit Comput. 2014;19(2):317–34.
24. A crisis in health care: a call to action on physician burnout. [cited 2023 May 9]. https://www.massmed.org/Publications/Research,-Studies,-and-Reports/A--Crisis-in-Health-Care%2D%2DA-Call-to-Action-on%2D%2DPhysician-Burnout/
25. Shafran I, Du N, Tran L, et al. The medical scribe: corpus development and model performance analyses. Paper presented at: Proceedings of the Twelfth Language Resources and Evaluation Conference. 2020. p. 2036–44.
26. Enarvi S, Amoia M, Teba MDA, et al. Generating medical reports from patient-doctor conversations using sequence-to-sequence models. Paper presented at: Proceedings of the First Workshop on Natural Language Processing for Medical Conversations. 2020. p. 22–30.
27. Ambient clinical documentation and virtual assistant solutions. [cited 2023 May 9]. https://www.3m.com/3M/en_US/health-information-systems-us/create-time-to-care/clinician-solutions/virtual-assistant-solutions/
28. Lafata JE, Cooper GS, Divine G, et al. Patient-physician colorectal cancer screening discussions: delivery of the 5A's in practice. Am J Prev Med. 2011;41(5):480–6.
29. Shires DA, Stange KC, Divine G, et al. Prioritization of evidence-based preventive health services during periodic health examinations. Am J Prev Med. 2012;42(2):164–73.
30. Johnson Shen M, Elston Lafata J, D'Agostino TA, Bylund CL. Lower adherence: a description of colorectal cancer screening barrier talk. J Health Commun. 2020;25(1):43–53.
31. Park J, Jindal A, Kuo P, et al. Automated rating of patient and physician emotion in primary care visits. Patient Educ Couns. 2021;104(8):2098–105.
32. Park J, Kotzias D, Kuo P, et al. Detecting conversation topics in primary care office visits from transcripts of patient-provider interactions. J Am Med Inform Assoc. 2019;26(12):1493–504.
33. Wamba SF, Anand A, Carter L. A literature review of RFID-enabled healthcare applications and issues. Int J Inform Manage. 2013;33(5):875–91.
34. Rosen MA, Dietz AS, Yang T, Priebe CE, Pronovost PJ. An integrative framework for sensor-based measurement of teamwork in healthcare. J Am Med Inform Assoc. 2015;22(1):11–8.
35. Tierney WM, Miller ME, Overhage JM, McDonald CJ. Physician inpatient order writing on microcomputer workstations effects on resource utilization. JAMA. 1993;269:379–83.
36. Overhage JM, Perkins S, Tierney WM, McDonald CJ. Controlled trial of direct physician order entry: effects on physicians' time utilization in ambulatory primary care internal medicine practices. J Am Med Inform Assoc. 2001;8(4):361–71.
37. Wetterneck TB, Lapin JA, Krueger DJ, Holman GT, Beasley JW, Karsh BT. Development of a primary care physician task list to evaluate clinic visit workflow. BMJ Qual Saf. 2012;21(1):47–53.
38. Hauschild I, Vitzthum K, Klapp BF, Groneberg DA, Mache S. Time and motion study of anesthesiologists' workflow in German hospitals. Wien Med Wochenschr. 2011;161(17–18):433–40.
39. Douglas S, Cartmill R, Brown R, et al. The work of adult and pediatric intensive care unit nurses. Nurs Res. 2013;62(1):50–8.
40. Westbrook JI, Ampt A. Design, application and testing of the work observation method by activity timing (WOMBAT) to measure clinicians' patterns of work and communication. Int J Med Inform. 2009;78(Suppl 1):S25–33.
41. Westbrook JI, Li L, Georgiou A, Paoloni R, Cullen J. Impact of an electronic medication management system on hospital doctors' and nurses' work: a controlled pre-post, time and motion study. J Am Med Inform Assoc. 2013;20(6):1150–8.
42. Kallem C, Burrington-Brown J, Dinh AK. Data elements for EHR documentation. J AHIMA. 2007;78(7):web extra.

43. Bohnsack KJ, Parker DP, Zheng K. Quantifying temporal documentation patterns in clinician use of AHLTA—the DoD's ambulatory electronic health record. AMIA Annu Symp Proc. 2009;2009:50–4.
44. Vawdrey DK, Wilcox LG, Collins S, et al. Awareness of the care team in electronic health records. Appl Clin Inform. 2011;2(4):395–405.
45. Agrawal R, Srikant R. Mining sequential patterns. Paper presented at: Proceedings of the 11th International Conference on Data Engineering. 1995. p. 3–14.
46. Sanderson PM, Fisher C. Exploratory sequential data analysis: foundations. Hum Comput Interact. 1994;9(3–4):251–317.
47. Laxman S, Sastry PS. A survey of temporal data mining. Sadhana. 2006;31(2):173–98.
48. Grinstead CM, Snell JL. Markov chains. In: Introduction to probability. Providence, RI: American Mathematical Society; 1997. p. 405–70.
49. Zheng K, Padman R, Johnson MP, Diamond HS. An interface-driven analysis of user interactions with an electronic health records system. J Am Med Inform Assoc. 2009;16(2):228–37.
50. Weibel N, Emmenegger C, Lyons J, Dixit R, Hill LL, Hollan JD. Interpreter-mediated physician-patient communication: opportunities for multimodal healthcare interfaces. Paper presented at: Proceedings of the 7th International Conference on Pervasive Computing Technologies for Healthcare (PervasiveHealth '13). 2013. p. 113–20. https://eudl.eu/pdf/10.4108/icst.pervasivehealth.2013.252026
51. Fouse A, Weibel N, Hutchins E, Hollan JD. ChronoViz: a system for supporting navigation of time-coded data. Paper presented at: Proceedings of the 2011 ACM Conference on Human Factors in Computing Systems, Extended Abstracts (CHI EA '11). 2011. p. 299–304.

Further Reading

Adler-Milstein J, Adelman JS, Tai-Seale M, Patel VL, Dymek C. EHR audit logs: a new goldmine for health services research? J Biomed Inform. 2020;101:103343.
Dumais S, Jeffries R, Russell DM, Tang D, Teevan J. Understanding user behavior through log data and analysis. In: Olson JS, Kellogg W, editors. Ways of knowing in HCI. New York: Springer; 2014. p. 349–72.
Laxman S, Sastry PS. A survey of temporal data mining. Sadhana. 2006;31(2):173–98.
Rule A, Melnick ER, Apathy NC. Using event logs to observe interactions with electronic health records: an updated scoping review shows increasing use of vendor-derived measures. J Am Med Inform Assoc. 2022;30(1):144–54.
Sinsky CA, Rule A, Cohen G, et al. Metrics for assessing physician activity using electronic health record log data. J Am Med Inform Assoc. 2020;27(4):639–43.
Weibel N, Emmenegger C, Lyons J, Dixit R, Hill LL, Hollan JD. Interpreter-mediated physician-patient communication: opportunities for multimodal healthcare interfaces. Paper presented at: Proceedings of the 7th International Conference on Pervasive Computing Technologies for Healthcare (PervasiveHealth '13). 2013. p. 113–20. https://eudl.eu/pdf/10.4108/icst.pervasivehealth.2013.252026
Weibel N, Rick S, Emmenegger C, Ashfaq S, Calvitti A, Agha Z. LAB-IN-A-BOX: semi-automatic tracking of activity in the medical office. Pers Ubiquit Comput. 2014;19(2):317–34.
Zheng K, Haftel HM, Hirschl RB, O'Reilly M, Hanauer DA. Quantifying the impact of health IT implementations on clinical workflow: a new methodological perspective. J Am Med Inform Assoc. 2010;17(4):454–61.
Zheng K, Padman R, Johnson MP, Diamond HS. An interface-driven analysis of user interactions with an electronic health records system. J Am Med Inform Assoc. 2009;16(2):228–37.

Chapter 7
Analyzing Video-Based Human-Computer Interaction Data in Healthcare Using a Cognitive-Socio-Technical Framework

Andre W. Kushniruk and Elizabeth M. Borycki

Introduction

The usability of health information systems and technologies has emerged as a critical issue. Globally there are continued reports of health information systems that are difficult to use, that interfere with clinical workflow and that may even be deemed to be unsafe due to poor usability [1–6]. In some cases, end users of these new systems (including physicians, nurses, allied health professionals and patients) have complained about the difficulty in learning how to use them, reported inadvertent changes that the new systems and technologies have imposed on existing health care workflow, and also described a wide range of usability problems. As a result of these concerns, consultants and developers of health information systems and technologies have worked on applying methods from human factors and usability engineering to develop more usable systems. This has included applying design methods such as user-centered design and participatory design [7]. The evaluation of the usability of health information systems and technologies is another area where ideas and methods from human factors have also been applied. Along these lines, usability testing has emerged as one of the main approaches for assessing the usability of information systems and technologies [8, 9]. This approach involves observing and recording end users of system as they interact with the technology to carry out specified tasks. The analysis of this data is critical in being able to identify issues with systems, including usability problems and potential impact on workflow [9–12]. In this chapter we first describe practical approaches to collecting video-based usability data. We then describe methods for analyzing such data using evidence-based coding schemes. The approach described can used in assessing the

---

A. W. Kushniruk (✉) · E. M. Borycki
School of Health Information Science, University of Victoria, Victoria, BC, Canada
e-mail: andrek@uvic.ca

usability of health information systems, as well as evaluating the impact of such systems on cognitive processes involved in healthcare.

Background

In conducting usability testing, the user's interactions with a technology or system are typically observed, recorded and analyzed to identify specific problems and issues [9, 10]. Usability testing has been increasingly employed in the design and deployment of effective and usable health information systems, not only during the design of new systems, but also for the analysis of the impact of implementing commercial vendor-based healthcare systems [9, 13]. Usability testing typically involves the collection of computer screen and audio recordings of users (i.e., usability study participants) as they carry out specific tasks using a technology being evaluated. User interactions with the computer system or technology under study can be captured using continuous screen and audio recordings, using screen recording software [9]. In many studies, participants (e.g., physicians using a new information system who are instructed to carry out a set of tasks) are instructed to "think aloud" or verbalize their thoughts as they carry out tasks using the system or technology under study. In this way, the interaction of the study participant with the information system is recorded in its entirety as a digital movie file, which can be played back for review by analysts or researchers to identify usability issues or problems.

The audio portion of the recordings of study participants can be synchronized with digital video recordings of their actions and actual computer screens, while using the technology under study to carry out the task(s). The audio portion of the video recording can be transcribed and coded, in conjunction with one or more analysts viewing the recorded digital video to identify usability issues (from both the visual and audio data). In the authors' work, the approach to analyzing the verbal protocols (resulting from the audio portion of usability tests) has borrowed from think aloud protocol analysis, as described by Ericsson and Simon [14] and by van Someren, Barnard and Sandberg [15]. The analytic approach has since been applied to the evaluation of users' interactions with a wide range of healthcare information systems and technologies [9, 12].

Observational notes about the user's interactions can also be made during the usability testing. In addition, post-task semi-structured interviews (or standardized usability questionnaires) can be conducted with the participants after usability testing is completed (i.e., immediately after the user has interacted with the system under study). Usability testing has been found to be especially useful for pinpointing specific usability issues and rectifying them [16]. As such they have many advantages over other methods used in isolation, for example administration of usability questionnaires alone [17].

Although a large number of studies have now been reported in the literature that have applied usability testing to evaluate the usability of healthcare information systems and technologies, one of the challenges of this work is the development of effective and practical methods for analyzing such rich qualitative data. The intent is to provide useful results, both for research projects and also for implementation projects having the objective of improving the health information technology products being developed and deployed. There are a wide range of approaches to coding and analyzing video data that results from usability testing. Coding typically involves analyzing the content of digital video recordings of end users to identify themes in the data that may indicate specific usability issues or problems. These include inductive approaches such as grounded theory, where codes are not predefined, but rather are inductively developed from examining the data itself, as in a qualitative analysis approach known as grounded theory [18]. On the other hand, analytic approaches using coding may include pre-existing codes (deductive approaches including model-based coding) that may be used to identify usability problems from the data (e.g., specific usability problems such as navigation errors). In this chapter we focus on an approach that borrows from both perspectives, where we describe the development of a set of codes to analyze data. The approach also allows for (and does not preclude) identification of new and emergent themes and codes (i.e., codes not previously discussed in the literature). Indeed, the identification of new themes ultimately adds to the refinement and extension of deductive coding schemes as will be described from our work over time [19]. However, the development of principled coding schemes does help to streamline and facilitate the process of coding video data emerging from usability testing of healthcare systems and applications.

The approach to analyzing and coding usability data described in this chapter emerged from extensive work conducted by the authors in designing and evaluating health information technologies. The overall approach involved the development of a coding system that contains a number of well-defined codes or categories that can guide the analyst, when viewing recordings of user interactions to identify usability issues. These codes contained in the coding system emerged from a number of sources, including an examination of coding categories that have been developed from the human-computer interaction (HCI) literature for conducting usability inspections (a quite different purpose as this does not involve observing users), categories emerging from examination of evidence-based research publications on usability in healthcare [20, 21], as well as from experience in video coding usability data in a variety of usability studies [9, 13]. For example, this has included: (a) creating video coding categories borrowed from work in the cognitive analysis of information seeking, medical decision making and reasoning [22–26], (b) categories that have been adapted from Nielsen's heuristics (used for heuristic evaluation) that we have modified for use as video coding categories [8, 9], (c) creating categories from research on evidence-based user interface guidelines [20, 21, 27] and (d) using categories that have emerged from our own prior work from conducting many different usability studies over time [9–13]. This chapter will focus on qualitative analysis of usability data using such a system of coding, however, we will begin with a brief discussion of the methods used to collect video-based usability data as a precursor to our discussion of how to code and analyze such data. We will then touch on some basic quantitative measures that can be obtained from analysis of such video-based data before proceeding to a full discussion of the coding system we have developed for qualitatively analyzing human-computer interaction in healthcare.

Collecting Video-Based Usability Data

Digital video recordings of user interactions with information systems and technologies usability can provide a rich source of data in human factors studies. This type of data can be collected in a variety of ways and both the collection and analysis of this data has become increasingly simplified over the years with advances in technology.

One approach that has been employed involves having representative users of a system interact with that system to carry our representative tasks. The approach is based on a method called task analysis, which has been used in many areas of human factors research and has an extensive history of use in the human factors literature [28, 29]. For example in conducting usability testing of a new electronic health record system used by clinicians, this may involve creating a set of representative tasks (e.g., entering new patient information, looking up medications administered etc.). Then a number of representative users (e.g., physicians) would be recorded as they carry out tasks using the technology. In a usability test, representative users (i.e., the physician users) would be observed and their interactions and verbalizations recorded. The recording of users carrying out tasks, can be achieved using a number of recording approaches and technologies. Cognitive task analysis extends this approach by also focusing on the cognitive processes involved in carrying out the task, including reasoning and decision making processes and the knowledge and strategies that completing the task requires [30–32].

In the simplest case only the computer screens that the user interacts with need to be recorded, and this can be done by installing freely available screen recording software on the device (e.g., desk-top computer, laptop or mobile phone) that the user is interacting with (in carrying out the tasks) [9]. Many computers now have this recording software built in, for example Quicktime® on Macintosh® computers. Such screen recording software allows for the creation of digital movie files that result from recording users interacting with that device or computer. The recording allows for input from the computer's or device's microphone, resulting in a digital movie that records the full user interaction with the technology, including all the screens along with user verbalizations, which can be immediately played back for review and analysis. Other screen recording software are available free or for a nominal charge (e.g., Hypercam®, which can be rapidly installed on most PCs) and can be readily downloaded and installed on the computer or device to be used in the usability testing. When the study participants begin working on a task, the screen recording software is turned on, resulting in the creation a digital movie file. This provides inputs into the type of analysis described in this chapter.

In some studies, external video recording of participants' physical actions and activities may also need to be collected (in addition to recording only computer screen interaction). For example, studies of how a computer system affects doctor-patient interviews in a clinic also typically require a second external video view (e.g., which could simply involve using a video camera on a tripod, or a ceiling mounted camera focused on the participant user) to record physical actions or record how the clinician interacts with the computer system under study in their physical environment. However, for many studies a simple set up with the recording of screens on the user's computer will suffice. In any case, the coding system described in this paper can be applied to a range of data collection approaches, as it can be applied to a variety of video recordings of user interactions collected during usability testing.

Usability testing can also involve collecting "think aloud" data, when recording the user interacting with a system or technology under study [9]. This essentially adds an audio track to the video recording of what participants are doing as they interact with the information system or technology. This typically involves instructing the participants to "think aloud" or "verbalize" their thoughts while carrying out tasks using the system [9]. In this way, what the user verbalizes during the testing can be linked in time to what they are actually doing using the computer, making for a complete and integrated record of the user interaction, including what screens they are interacting with, what they are clicking on as well as what they are thinking [9, 10].

In recent years usability testing has involved the remote collection of usability data, using any number of commonly used video conferencing tools (e.g., Zoom® or Webex®) For example, using Zoom® for conducting usability testing remotely, allows the usability testing session to be simply run as a zoom meeting. The remote participant is first asked to share their screen (using Zoom®'s screen sharing function). The remote participant in the testing is then asked to access the application under study (e.g., an electronic health record system) on their computer with screen sharing, allowing the remote experimenter/researcher to see the participant's screens (as the user interacts with the system or application under study). The participant is then instructed to use the system under study to carry out one or more tasks, which is recorded at the researcher's end, resulting in a movie capture of the entire user interaction. Just as in the face-to-face scenario, participants are typically asked to carry out a set of pre-specified tasks (e.g., look up patient information, enter information about a patient into the system, etc.) and they may also be instructed to "think aloud" or verbalize their thoughts while doing the tasks. This is all recorded using the web-conferencing tool's record function, resulting in a digital movie file of the remote users' interaction and verbalizations. Many web conferencing tools also provide transcription software built in (e.g., Zoom's live transcript function) that will allow for the audio portion of the digital movie file (i.e., the participant's thinking aloud) to be automatically transcribed (which will be useful in analyzing this data as described in a subsequent section of this chapter). This automated transcription can also be a time saving, although it often does require checking of the accuracy of the automated transcription.

The overall approach described above for collecting and analyzing usability data has been termed "low-cost rapid usability testing" as the equipment and software are now low cost and readily available [33–35]. This is in contrast to set ups that involve expensive fixed usability laboratories. The advantage of the low-cost approach is that it can be taken into virtually any setting and lends itself to more ecologically valid data collection and analysis. The approach can be rapidly applied to collecting rich video-based data that contains data from the recording of user screens, as well as verbalizations of user participants, which can be subsequently coded for analyzing human-computer interaction at multiple levels, as will be described later in this chapter.

Analyzing Video-Based Usability Data

The effective analysis of data resulting from usability testing (i.e., digital video and audio recordings of user interactions) is a critical part of the process. Methods used for analyzing this type of recorded data from usability testing may range from informal approaches consisting of simply playing back recorded user interactions of interest to system designers (to inform developers about user problems—what Mann et al refer to as "pragmatic" objectives [36]). On the other hand, the methods may also include more formalized scientific and academic analysis, with the objective of adding to the body of scientific research about usability (although these different objectives are not mutually exclusive [36]).

Simply viewing selected video recordings of interesting user interactions and showing them to designers, developers and decision makers can provide important visual feedback to those developing systems and technologies. This will cue them to where specific system improvements are needed and can be of critical importance for improving communication with developers (as they may be removed from seeing the actual use of their products in real world contexts). There is often a disconnection between the designers of systems and their end users and presenting video recordings of user interactions to developers can help bridge this gap (i.e., the gap or "gulf" that often exists between designer and users, which has been described by Norman in his work on user-centered design [37]). From our experience, simply presenting developers with such visual evidence (i.e., by watching users interact with systems or user interfaces) can be very powerful for motivating programmers to make changes to improve systems or user interfaces from the users' perspective. Thus video-based usability data alone (i.e., screen and audio recordings of users), even with simple forms of analysis, can constitute a powerful form of visual evidence and feedback about the usability of health information systems and technologies.

More formalized methods are needed for more rigorous analysis. This work includes the application of evidence-based coding schemes, as will be described in this chapter. A range of quantitative and qualitative approaches to analysis can also be applied to analyzing usability data and many studies employ a mixed-method approach, where both types of analysis are conducted. Quantitative approaches can include collecting metrics on the number of errors participants make in carrying out tasks during a usability testing session, as well as the time taken by users to complete tasks (which can be obtained from the digital video recording of the participants' interactions). It should be noted that measures such as time can be recorded by observers of usability testing studies as participants carry out tasks requested of them and there are a range of automated tools and logging software for collecting such data (see [38] for details). Specific quantitative measures that can be made to characterize user interactions include the following:

- Time to complete each task
- Number and percentage of tasks completed correctly
- Number and percentage of tasks completed incorrectly
- Time required to access information in online help
- Total number of errors
- Time needed to recover from errors
- Total number of usability issues
- Total number of incorrect menu choices
- Total number of incorrect icons selected
- Total number of user actions to complete task
- Total number of user comments
- Number of user comments by type

There are a number of considerations that need to be taken into account when quantifying the user experience. For example, in order to measure task success (e.g., number and percentage of tasks completed correctly) it is necessary that the task be well defined and there be a clear and correct way to do the task. Tasks could include for example, successfully documenting administration of a medication into a medication administration system, or correctly responding to an alert in a decision support application. Success measures (which can be assessed from viewing recordings of user interactions) can also be considered in terms of leves—e.g., complete success in doing the task, partial success (e.g., requiring some assistance from the test monitor) and failure. Measures of time can be calculated exactly from replaying digital video recordings of users, but automated tools may also be useful for measuring time on task as well. Measuring errors requires comparison of the user's actions with correct actions or outcomes for each specific task (e.g., responding appropriately to an alert indicating a patient has a drug allergy in testing a medication administration system). In addition to applying purely quantitative approaches, over the past decade the authors have focused on developing qualitative methods for identifying and coding usability problems, which will be the focus of the remainder of this chapter.

Towards A Theoretical Framework for Analyzing Usability Data

There are a variety of qualitative approaches to analyzing usability testing data. In this chapter we describe an approach that is part of what the authors have termed low-cost rapid usability engineering [33]. This approach involves several phases of analysis and draws on methods for coding and analyzing video-based usability data. Such coding schemes and systems can be used to guide the detailed analyses of data from usability testing and can be focused at a number of levels ranging from analyzing the impact of healthcare technologies at the cognitive level, to assessing their impacts on workflow and organizational practices, as will be detailed.

The authors have also drawn on studies of medical reasoning, information seeking and decision making to extend coding schemes for usability data. For example, the authors have developed an overall coding system, consisting of several other schemes that can be modified for use in studying health professionals' interactions with information systems and technologies [39–41]. Theoretical perspectives from the general area of human-computer interaction were also found to have considerable relevance for analyzing video data from usability testing. For example, work based on human information processing theory [42] has lead to studies in numerous domains of study where think aloud protocols are collected concurrently with study participants carrying out a task. This has allowed researchers to identify the cognitive steps needed to solve a problem or complete a task using the technology under study. Categories borrowed from heuristic evaluation, developed Jacob Nielsen [8] can also be adopted and modified for use in analyzing video data. In addition, we found that Lewis and Norman's concepts of user slips and mistakes could similarly be used in video coding and analysis, especially when looking for potential safety issues with technology [43].

To guide our analysis of usability data the authors have developed a conceptual framework that considers human-computer interaction at multiple levels (see Fig. 7.1). The cognitive socio-technical framework, which emerged from our work in human factors in healthcare, considers user interaction with technologies at multiple levels [44]. In this chapter we present a modified version this framework that can be applied to assisting in conceptualizing, designing and implementing coding schemes for analyzing human computer interaction.

The first level of analysis (Level 1) in Fig. 7.1 we refer to as the "Individual Level" of human-computer interaction. At Level 1 the focus of the analysis is on the individual user interacting with an individual system or user interface. At this level ergonomic issues and surface level aspects of usability are most salient and an important focus on coding is at evaluating if the system or user interface features allow the user to complete tasks using a system in isolation (i.e., identifying surface level usability issues). At Level 1, coding of human-computer interaction can also include consideration of aspects of design, such as how well the screen is laid out, how navigational cues are organized, how menus and interface features are perceived and used, and other surface level usability issues arise.

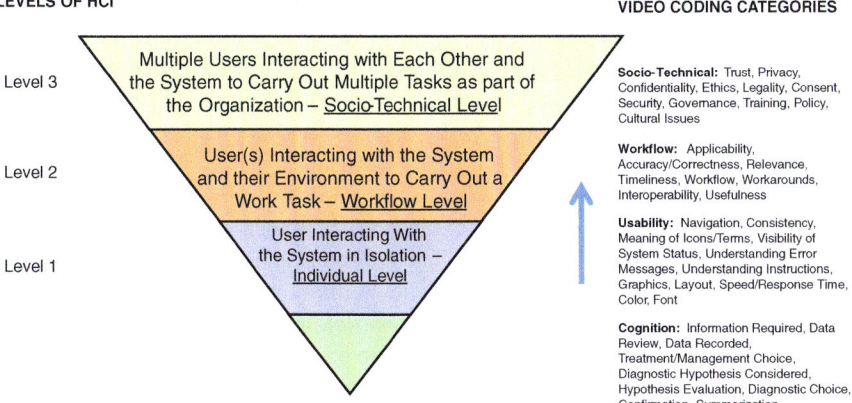

Fig. 7.1 Cognitive-socio-technical levels of video-based coding

Coding at Level 1 of human-computer interaction can include consideration of the cognitive aspects of the user interaction, such as ability of the individual user to seek information, understand and comprehend system operation and use the system in basic information seeking, reasoning and decision making tasks [45]. This is the level that corresponds conceptually to the level of the human information processing model—a well known model and influential of human-computer interaction that appeared early on and that has been considered highly valued in the field of human-computer interaction since its inception [43]. Some cognitive aspects of the user interaction that may be of interest to the evaluator at this level include how the system may impact an individual's information seeking, decision making and reasoning when operating the system to help them with a task (e.g., making a diagnosis while using a complex system such as an EHR).

At Level 2, the focus is on analysis of the workflow involved in the user interaction. The focus of this level is analysis of the user interacting with the system to carry out specific work tasks, which may involve multiple participants as well as complex work activities. This level we have labelled the "Workflow Level" focuses on the impact of the system or interface on work activities in work settings (e.g., clinics, hospitals etc.) that involves multiple participants and systems. This includes assessing how the system under study affects complex activities involved in patient and health care. At this level, issues come into play related to impact of technology upon communication of health professionals and their integration with other systems in clinical environments. Analysis at this level includes a focus on how the technology impacts work efficiency and effectiveness in carrying out real-world tasks. This typically involves multiple participants and multiple systems in complex healthcare settings and contexts. This level of human-computer interaction corresponds to the distributed cognition model, another influential perspective on human-computer interaction that emerged to take into account the real-world complexities and interactions amongst multiple systems and users of those systems in carrying out work tasks. This approach essentially aims to describe how information processing and decision making is distributed amongst multiple people, systems and technological representations and how these are all integrated in performing work activities [46–48]. In healthcare this would include, for example, study of the use of a system such as an electronic health record by a physician while interviewing and interacting with patients and other health professionals in a busy clinical setting.

At Level 3 (labelled the "Socio-Technical Level") the focus is on aspects of user interaction related to social, policy or organizational aspects of technology use. This includes human-computer interaction related to social and organizational aspects of technology design and use [49–51]. This level may impact policy on technology implementations, ethics and confidentiality, as well as considering communication and coordination issues across larger healthcare organizational boundaries and settings. User issues and concerns may include those around policies related to increasing user trust and the confidentiality of information (e.g., concerns about who will see data entered into a patient portal and how that information will ultimately be used and accessed) across different healthcare settings and organizations. The evaluation of systems at this level can include assessment of their impact on social structures, social dynamics, perceptions of personal control and safety as well as human factors issues around technology policy and planning.

The cognitive-socio-technical model grew from a conceptual approach to human factors that considers the integration of both cognitive and socio-technical approaches to assessing the impact of information systems [44]. The approach has been applied in a range of studies for helping to define the level of user interaction involved in evaluating and understanding human-computer interaction [44]. This approach has involved mapping different types of evaluative methods to the levels described above, from the level of the individual user interacting with a system in isolation, to the level of considering how the technology is used to carry out work activities, and finally to the level of studying the impact of systems on organizational aspects of its use and deployment.

The example coding schemes presented in this chapter are organized around the different three level model described above. The schemes evolved from the authors' earliest work in this area through to our subsequent work in areas related to studying the links between usability and technology-induced error in healthcare technology as well as the application of methods for evaluating the impact of systems on reasoning and decision making [52, 53]. Our earliest work focused on the Level 1 aspects of human-computer interaction. This was followed by a range of studies that focussed additionally on assessing the impact of healthcare systems on work activities and workflow as the technologies that we studied began to be deployed on a large scale in healthcare organizations (Level 2 coding categories). Subsequently, much of our recent work has focussed on aspects that may be considered belonging to this socio-technical level (Level 3). This has lead to the development of a set of new coding categories and schemes.

As will be shown, the codes can be used to tag and identify sections of video and audio log files that can be characterized by the categories. The codes are given in Tables 7.1, 7.2, 7.3, 7.4, and 7.5, along with the codes themselves capitalized along

Table 7.1 Level 1 HCI—usability codes

Code	Code definition	Example
NAVIGATION	Coded when a review of the video data indicates the user has problems moving through a system or user interface.	e.g., A physician using an electronic health record system (EHR) cannot backtrack to a screen with patient allergy information [39].
CONSISTENCY	Coded when a review of the video indicates the user has problems due to a lack of consistency in the user interface.	e.g., The way a user enters month, day and year in a system has a different order in two parts of that system [39].
MEANING OF ICONS/TERMS	Coded when a review of the video data indicates the user does not understand language or labels used in the interface.	e.g., A user of a decision support system does not realize that a button labelled "best practice advisory" contains drug alerting information [39].
VISIBILITY OF SYSTEM STATUS	Coded when a review of the video data indicates the user does not know what the system is doing.	e.g., A nurse does not know if a medication administration system is not working, or if it just taking time processing, as there no indication in the interface of what the system is doing [39].
UNDERSTANDING ERROR MESSAGES	Coded when a review of the video data indicates the user does not understand meaning of error messages.	e.g., A pharmacist using a medication administration system receives a computer message "Error 102" and has no idea of what it means [39].
UNDERSTANDING INSTRUCTIONS	Coded when a review of the video data indicates the user does not understand user instructions.	e.g., A patient user of a personal health record (PHR) system does not understand the instructions for entering data into the PHR [39].
GRAPHICS	Coded when a review of the video data indicates there are issues with graphics.	e.g., The data values in a graph or table in a personal health record are not understandable as they are too close together on a graph [39].
LAYOUT	Coded when a review of the video data indicates there are problems with the layout of screens or information on those screens.	e.g., The summary screen for patient data is crowded and difficult to scroll through [39].
SPEED/RESPONSE TIME	Coded when a review of the video data indicates the system is slow or response time is an issue.	e.g., Users feel the system it taking too long to respond to their inputs [39].

(continued)

Table 7.1 (continued)

Code	Code definition	Example
COLOR	Coded when a review of the video data indicates the user does not like color or color schemes used in the interface.	e.g., Users comment that they do not like the use of colors in an electronic health record (EHR) [39].
FONT	Coded when a review of the video data indicates the font is too small or not readable.	e.g., A nurse cannot see the decimal point in a drug dosage presented on the screen of a medication administration system [39].

Table 7.2 Level 1 HCI codes—cognitive codes

Code	Code definition	Example
INFORMATION REQUIRED	Coded for when information is required or requested when using a system.	e.g., A physician while using a system to record patient data asks the patient about the history of their medication use [40].
DATA REVIEW	Coded when the user reviews data.	e.g., A pharmacist reviews data entered into a pharmacy information system [40].
DATA RECORDED	Coded when data is recorded into a system.	e.g., A nurse enters patient blood pressure information into an EHR [40].
COMPARISON	Coded for when there is a choice being made (e.g., between diagnoses or treatments).	e.g., A physician compares two different possible diagnoses for a condition while using a EHR [40].
TREATMENT/ MANAGEMENT CHOICE	Coded when a treatment or management choice is made.	e.g., A physician makes a choice about a specific treatment or procedure [40].
DIAGNOSTIC HYPOTHESIS CONSIDERED	Coded when a diagnostic hypothesis is considered.	e.g., A diagnostic hypothesis is considered by a health professional [40].
HYPOTHESIS EVALUATION	Coded when a diagnostic hypothesis is evaluated against evidence.	e.g., A diagnostic hypothesis is being considered in light of new clinical evidence about a patient [40].
DIAGNOSTIC CHOICE	Coded for when a diagnostic choice is made.	e.g., A physician makes a choice about a diagnosis for a patient while using a HER [40].
CONFIRMATION	Coded for when a diagnosis is confirmed.	e.g., A physician confirms a diagnosis with the arrival of key diagnostic imaging [40].
SUMMARIZATION	Coded for when information is summarized.	e.g., A nurse summarizes patient information while using a nursing station [40].

Table 7.3 Level 2 workflow codes

Usefulness Code	Code definition	Example
APPLICABILITY	Coded when a review of the video data indicates that information presented is not applicable to real healthcare practice or cases encountered.	e.g., A recommendation from a clinical decision support tool is ignored by the end user (a health professional) as the user does not feel it is advice applicable to his/her patient [39].
ACCURACY/ CORRECTNESS	Coded when review of data or user comments indicates information or advice provided by system is not correct or accurate.	e.g., The user of an eHealth health promotion application feels that the educational advice provided by the app is not correct [39].
RELEVANCE	Coded when a review of the video data or user comments indicate information presented by a system is not relevant to their carrying out their task.	e.g., Educational information is provided by a system that the user does not feel is relevant to their clinical task [39].
TIMELINESS	Coded when a review of the video data or user comments indicate that information is not timely.	e.g., A decision support system offers advice to the user about what medications to order, but the advice only comes after the physician has already ordered the medication [39].
WORKFLOW	Coded when a review of video data or comments indicates unexpected impact of the system on work activities.	e.g., Users of a new system indicate that the system requires that they spend more time to the same activities, as compared to when they used paper records [39].
WORKAROUNDS	Coded when the user is not using the approach to carrying out work that is recommended by the healthcare organization. These can be sub-coded as NEGATIVE (e.g., use of incorrect, suboptimal or dangerous approaches), NEUTRAL (i.e., no impact on safety) or POSITIVE (i.e., increases safety).	e.g., A user of a system is routinely by-passing alerts integrated into and electronic health record system (in order to save time that would have been spent to attend to and process the alerts) [39].

(continued)

Table 7.3 (continued)

Usefulness Code	Code definition	Example
INTEROPERABILITY	Coded when a review of the video data or comments indicate that there are issues with communication of information	e.g., A system requires a user to enter basic patient data or demographics that must be re-entered when they invoke another system (i.e., lack of interoperability) [39].
USEFULNESS	Coded when the user specifically comments about usefulness of the system or technology. (This code can also be qualified as being POSITIVE or as being NEGATIVE, depending on whether the user finds the system/technology useful or not.	e.g., A patient indicates that they find a mobile health application is very useful for helping them to monitor their condition [39].

with their definitions, thus forming what we refer to as a *coding dictionary*. This coding dictionary is used by an analyst when analyzing, reviewing and annotating video data, as will be described later in this chapter. A description of the codes in this chapter will be followed by examples of their application.

Individual Level (Level 1) Human-Computer Interaction Codes

Level 1 usability codes can be used to assist researchers in the analysis of basic human-computer interaction, with a focus on individual interaction with a health information system or technology. This includes considering both surface level usability issues as users interact with systems, as well as assessing the impact of systems on cognitive processes involved in using a technology and solving problems with that technology. Level 1 codes of human-computer interaction can be broken down into two main categories: (1) codes dealing with basic aspects of usability and ergonomics at the level of the individual computer user, and (2) codes dealing with cognitive aspects of the use of the technology to solve problems (e.g., using the technology to assist in solve problems involved in reasoning or decision making).

Table 7.1 lists codes that we have developed that focus on aspects of the user interface and the user-system interaction at the basic level of human-computer interaction involving the individual user interacting with a system or technology. These codes include categories developed for other purposes (e.g., modified from questionnaires, heuristic evaluation and cognitive research, but adapted to coding video-based usability data). The codes were reviewed by a panel of human factors experts and refined iteratively. The sources used to develop the codes included: (1) categories that were initially developed to guide usability inspections, such as usability heuristics, (2) categories that emerged from design and evaluation guidelines, (3)

Table 7.4 Level 3 socio-technical codes

TRUST	Coded when the user comments about trust issues or trust in using a system.	e.g., a pharmacist indicates that the medication list in a pharmacy system is likely to be incomplete or inaccurate and so is deemed untrustworthy by the pharmacist [41].
PRIVACY	Coded when the user comments about concepts related to privacy in using a system.	e.g., A patient user of a health portal is concerned that the information they enter about sexual history will not be private and then fails to enter that information into the portal [41].
CONDIFENTIALITY	Coded when the user comments about issues or concerns around confidentiality of information in using a system.	e.g., A health professional is concerned that the report they are entering into a EHR may not be stored in a confidential way [41].
ETHICS	Coded when the user comments about issues or concerns around ethical issue of technology or information use.	e.g., A patient user is concerned about the ethical use of a new AI applications in terms of its impact on society [41].
LEGALITY	Coded when the user comments about issues or concerns around legal issues in using an information technology.	e.g., A physician is concerned about using medical dictation software due to the legal implications of an error in transcription made by the system [41].
CONSENT	Coded when the user comments about issues or concerns around consent when using a system.	e.g., A physician finds the process embedded in a health information exchange is burdensome for consenting patients to allow for data access [41].
SECURITY	Coded when the user comments about security concerns or issues (or when the video indicates user problems around security).	e.g., A health information system is not fully utilized as users often forget usernames and passwords but the password recovery process is difficult (requiring tech staff intervention) [41].
GOVERNANCE	Coded when the user comments about governance issues related to use of a technology.	e.g., Due to lack of governance, a system that allows for standardized medical forms to be exchanged fails as different sites are using different versions of the forms (and this is noted by the user) [41].
TRAINING	Coded when the user comments about issues or ideas related to training required for effective use of a technology or system.	e.g., A decision support system is deployed in a hospital, but users indicate that it was not accompanied by training on how to use it and so it remains unused [41].

(continued)

Table 7.4 (continued)

POLICY	Coded when the user comments about issues of use of a technology related to policy.	e.g., A clinical user complains about the policies related to requirements to use only electronic versions of reports [41].
CULTURAL ISSUES	Coded when the user comments about cultural issues or concerns related to use of a technology or user interface.	e.g., A user of a patient facing application from a minority group comments on the issue that the user interface is only in English [41].

Table 7.5 Safety codes: definitions and examples

Safety Code	Code definition	Example
SLIP	Coded when a review of the video data indicates the user has made a mistake but corrects the mistake.	e.g., A physician entered a wrong dosage for a medication but corrects it before the system writes the information to its database [4].
MISTAKE	Coded when a review of the data indicates the user has made a mistake that is not corrected.	e.g., A physician misreads information on the screen about when to give a medication but has no idea that a mistake has been made (i.e., does not correct it) [4].

categories that emerged from numerous studies conducted by the authors, and (4) categories from the field of medical cognition (that deal with coding for reasoning and decision making processes). In our work, codes developed from these categories were incorporated into a coding scheme for use in coding video based usability data.

In Table 7.1, Level 1 codes related to usability are defined, along with an example of the application of each code (which are based on real examples from studies we have conducted). The codes essentially form a coding dictionary that can be used by analysts or researchers coding video-based usability data. In doing so, the analyst reviews the digital video of the user interaction, consults the code definition, and notes in a log file instances where each type of usability problem occurs [9]. Examples of when each of the codes is used is given in the right hand column of Table 7.1 and can be used to guide the analyst when deciding on which code to assign to a specific issue or problem (as will be described in the next section).

Table 7.2 presents codes related to cognitive aspects of use of information technology. For example, codes are listed in the table for identifying when a user of a system requires further information for problem solving, reviews data and makes a decision when using a computer system [9, 23].

Example of Video Coding

To illustrate how the above codes can be used to aid in analysis, we provide an excerpt of a coded transcript from a physician's interaction with an EHR that was designed to provide evidence-based clinical decision support (by automatically presenting the physician with guidance in the form of best practice advisories). Fig. 7.2 gives a section of a coded log of user interactions with this system. This is an excerpt from a study where physicians interacted with an EHR system that included clinical decision support. The participants were instructed to "think aloud" as they interacted with the system and this was recorded on the audio track, while the user interactions with the computer and computer screens were recorded as digital video.

00:01:25 Subject open up the category "family history" in the electronic health record
"I am opening up the information about the past medical history for this patient and I am looking to see if there is a family history of cancer"
[**COGNITIVE CODE - DATA REVIEW** (EHR) - family history of cancer]

"I see that the patient's mother and uncle died of pancreatic cancer so I am wondering if the patient might have cancer or some genetic predisposition"
[**COGNITIVE CODE - DIAGNOSTIC HYPOTHESIS CONSIDERED** – cancer, cause genetic]

"I would like to know if the patient has symptoms consistent with this particular type of cancer"
[**COGNITIVE CODE - INFORMATION REQUIRED** – symptoms of patient]

00:02:25 Subject scrolls up and down current screen
"But I don't know how to get to the screen with the lab results"
[**USABILITY CODE - NAVIGATION PROBLEM** – can't find lab results tab]

00:02:45 Subject notices an alert at top of the screen but does not know what it means
"I just noticed a yellow pop up at the top of the screen with BPA written on it, but I don't know what BPA means"

[**USABILITY CODE – MEANING OF LABELS PROBLEM** – does not know what the label "BPA" on the alert means – which refers to "Best Practice Advisories"]
"I find this distracting as it has interfered with my train of thought about what I was looking up"

[**USABILITY CODE – INTERFERENCE WITH WORK PROCESS** – alert distracting]
"I just clicked on the button with BPA written on it and it is telling me there is a risk the patient has high blood pressure. I would now like to know if this has anything to do with the patient's current chief complaint"

[**COGNITIVE CODE – GOAL FORMED** – determine if information in the alert is related to the chief complaint for the current visit]
"Now I'll now go to look up those values"

[**COGNITIVE CODE - INFORMATION REQUIRED** – lookup blood pressure]

Fig. 7.2 Example of a coded excerpt

The log file in Fig. 7.2 was initially created from a verbatim transcription of the audio portion of the usability testing session (i.e., the participant's "thinking aloud") and opened up as a Microsoft Word® file (which we refer to a log file). This file initially contains the verbatim transcription of the audio from the recorded interaction. The text in the file is then segmented into short sections or paragraphs (that reflect natural pauses in speech). The analysts then review the corresponding sections of the digital video recording (of computer screens with the audio recording of the participant). In doing so, the following is added directly into the log file: (a) time stamps for key events that are observed from watching the video, (b) annotations for key events that occur in the user-system interaction, and (c) codes that represent themes in the data (and that come from the coding schemes presented in this chapter).

In the resultant log file shown in Fig. 7.2, the participant's verbalizations are given in quotations and the log file has also been annotated with time stamps and marked up in italics with annotations to indicate what actions the user is doing on the computer (obtained from viewing the recording and adding time stamps and annotations directly to the log file) [9]. Codes (from the above coding scheme) have been added to the log file and are indicated in capitals in boldface in square brackets.

The above example illustrates Level 1 coding of human-computer interaction for both the cognitive aspects of the interaction, as well as usability issues. It also illustrates how the codes related to the two can be interleaved in the transcript and the interaction itself. This reflects how the participant alternates between dealing with usability issues (such as problems navigating through the system) and considerations related to medical decision making. This allows for elucidating the impact of system design (e.g., how the screen is laid out, where to find information in the system, such as lab results, and how the interaction is designed etc.) with decision making and clinical reasoning processes. In the example, the participant had issues in finding key information needed to make an informed diagnosis. This approach also allows the researcher to quantify and statistically relate aspects of reasoning and decision making with features related to the user interface and usability (e.g., features such as prominence of alerts, labelling of screen items, screen design etc.) [53].

Workflow Level (Level 2) Codes

The fit of the design of a health information system with the work of the human user is intended to support is critically important in healthcare. This includes determining how well the system supports the flow and sequencing of processes and tasks involved in complex health related work, referred to as system workflow [44]. Processes supported by technology in healthcare include many examples, from systems that support the interaction of clinicians with patients (e.g., EHRs) to systems that provide detailed guidance and instruction (e.g., forms of clinical decision support and some artificial intelligence (AI) applications for supporting areas such as complex treatment planning). At this level we can ask does the system provide the right information at the time it is needed by the clinician or other end user, is the content and advice provided by the system relevant to dealing with patient cases, and does the system fit within the desired workflow of the human users? Codes used for video analysis at this level focus on how well a system or user interface supports real work activities, in real or realistic (e.g., clinical simulations) contexts of use [10, 54].

"Usefulness codes" (see Table 7.3) are used to describe issues regarding the usefulness of the user interface or system being evaluated from analyzing the data. At the workflow level, the usefulness of the content of health information systems is extremely important to end users and can be differentiated from usability problems (e.g., a system may be usable, but contain data or information that is not deemed useful to a healthcare worker in carrying out work tasks). Furthermore, health professional and patient users are highly sensitive to the content they are provided via technology as well as how and when that content is provided—e.g., its reliability, relevance, timeliness etc. Table 7.3 gives the code definitions associated with Level 2 workflow analysis, along with examples of the application of each code listed.

Socio-Technical Level (Level 3) Codes

At Level 3 (the socio-technical level) theoretical perspectives from the growing body of research in socio-technical aspects of human factors are leveraged. Sociotechnical theories and approaches emerged from the management and engineering literatures [44, 49–51]. They form the basis for research in health informatics that focuses on adoption issues at the social and community levels. This has included research into how systems are adopted, propagated as well as how technologies may be used in ways never considered by their designers [49–51]. Sittig and Singh describe an eight-dimensional model for studying health information technology as complex adaptive systems [51]. This approach takes into consideration aspects of health information system design and implementation related to workflow and communication, organizational policies and procedures, as well as technical aspects related to the user interface, hardware and software [51]. Coding categories related to socio-technical issues and concerns are becoming increasingly important as health information technology begins to touch many aspects of our lives from the individual to the community and beyond. Research has indicated that there are a number of unintended consequences of implementation of technology and these are also considered at this level [55]. This includes issues related to privacy, confidentiality and the perceived impact of health systems on healthcare communication, communities and the daily lives of health professionals, patients and citizens (see Table 7.4). This level has considerable importance in understanding how technologies that might otherwise be deemed as being useful and usable, may still fail to be adopted or used as intended in healthcare.

Case Study Example: Extending and Applying the Approach to the Study of System Safety

Poor usability of healthcare information systems has been linked to medical error and increased likelihood of mistakes made by users of such systems. Since 2004 a number of publications appeared showing how human-computer interaction problems could lead to error and how user interfaces could be analyzed to identify usability problems related to medical error. In response to this issue, researchers have begun to conduct studies that examine the relationship of usability problems to what is now termed "technology-induced error". Technology-induced errors are errors that may arise from the design, implementation or use of technology [4–6]. They are often not detected until systems are in use in complex healthcare settings and contexts. Safety codes are used to identify and tag such errors made by users when analyzing data [4].

As an example of how the approach described in the chapter is extensible and can be customized to specific areas and emerging areas of study we provide an example. In this example, codes described above can be enhanced with the addition of codes related to the emerging area of health information technology safety. Table 7.5 gives additional safety and technology-induced error codes along with an example of the application of each of the codes.

Coded interaction can include identification of codes related to both basic level 1 human-computer interaction usability codes, as well as codes related to identification of possible safety issues (i.e., slips and mistakes). This approach, as described by the work by Kushniruk et al., examined the statistical relationship between surface level usability problems with the occurrence of medication error in using a prescription writing application [4]. From that work the coding approach allowed for collection of quantitative data about a number of usability problems in relation to a number of medication errors committed by physicians during clinical simulations. It was found that serious usability problems were highly correlated with medication entry errors.

To illustrate analysis of video-based usability data (and the application of the coding scheme described above) the authors provide an illustrative excerpt in Fig. 7.3 to show how the coding scheme described above can be applied to the analysis of a user's (i.e., a physician's) interaction with a new medication administration system (with codes given in bold).

In this example, it should be noted that an actual error in entering a medication correctly occurred and corresponded to the occurrence of a usability problem (as identified from the coding). This approach to coding allows for the occurrence of user errors in interacting with a system to be analyzed in relation to the occurrence of usability issues (see [4] for details). In this way serious usability problems associated with increased likelihood of medication error can be located and corrected.

00:00:00 *Start of testing session – user is given instructions to enter the medication "Doxepin"*

"I am waiting for the medication entry screen to appear, I have clicked what I think is the enter medication icon, but I am not sure"

MEANING OF ICONS/TERMS PROBLEM

00:00:45 *Medication entry screen comes up*

"Ok, it finally came up, but it seems like it took forever"

SPEED/RESPONSE TIME PROBLEM

00:00:48

"I am not sure what to click on now, as I don't follow the instructions on the screen"

UNDERSTANDING INSTRUCTIONS PROBLEM

00:01:05 *Participant clicks on "enter medication" button and begins to enter medication name into the text box that appears*

"Ok, here we go, the patient in your scenario has back pain and I am going to prescribe him the medication Darvon, which I sometimes prescribe for this problem"

00:01:30 *The system responds with names of medications that start with the letter "D" and user scans the list*

00:01:35 "Ok I will select from this list, but my eyesight is getting poor and this font is too small"

FONT PROBLEM

00:01:45 *User highlights and selects the medication "Digoxin" from the list displayed*

MISTAKE – WRONG MEDICATION ENTERED – "Digoxin entered instead of Doxepin"

Fig. 7.3 Example of a coded excerpt from a usability testing session showing usability problems and an associated safety issue (i.e., a coded error in entering a medication)

The Phases of Video-Based Coding of Usability Data

There a number of phases the authors have employed in conducting video-based analyses and coding resulting from usability testing. These are described below:

Phase 1—Transcription and Log File Creation
As noted above, the data obtained from usability testing typically includes screen recordings (of the user's interactions with a health information system or technology), along with the audio recordings of their verbalizations. The analyst begins analysis by having the audio portion of the interaction simply transcribed in its entirely. This leads to the creation of a log file (the file contains the text of user and test monitor verbalizations), which may consist of a word processing file containing the transcription of the user's verbalizations.

Phase 2—Annotation (Video Coding)
In the annotation phase of analysis, the analyst(s) plays back and reviews the digital video recording of the user's interactions from the usability testing, while annotating the file containing the transcribed audio recordings. To do this, the analyst marks up the log file (resulting from the transcription phase) with annotations and time stamps (obtained from watching the video recording) to indicate key user actions (e.g., entering a new function in a system, or exiting the program), key system responses (e.g., system crash), or other interesting aspects of the user-system interaction. These annotations can be entered directly into the log file of user verbalizations at the appropriate point in the audio transcriptions.

In addition to annotating the log file with notes about user-system interactions of interest (e.g., what the user is doing, such as clicking on a menu item), in the annotation phase the data can be coded for specific usability problems and issues. Here, a coding scheme (such as those described in this chapter) can be applied to guide the analysis. In addition, to marking up and coding the video data using pre-defined categories or codes, problems or issues may be identified that were not predicted by analysts (and were not contained in any coding scheme), which we refer to as "emergent" issues or problems.

Phase 3—Summarization
In this phase, the transcribed, annotated and coded log files (from each user-system interaction) are analyzed to create a summary of usability problems, usefulness concerns or issues, and safety problems both within and across users. The number of user problems, their severity, and their potential impact can be tabulated. The number of users who had a particular problem can also be taken into account when summarizing usability data. The summary can be used for providing input to system developers and implementers as well as providing a basis for technical and academic reports about types of healthcare information applications.

After completing analysis of usability data a report is typically compiled that can be used by designers, developers, healthcare IT staff or management. The specific focus of the report summarizing the usability data will depend on who the target audience is, and whether the study was conducted for pragmatic reasons (e.g., improving a user interface prior to releasing the system in a hospital), or academic reasons (e.g., understanding the relation between usability and cognitive aspects of system use) [36]. It has been demonstrated that application of the approach described in this paper can lead to a considerable return on investment by allowing for early identification of usability problems that could otherwise result in serious safety or implementation failures if left undetected [56].

Use of Video Analysis Tools and Automated Coding Research

The analysis of video data obtained from the usability testing does not necessitate use of complex qualitative coding software, as it may simply involve opening up the file obtained from transcription of user interactions (i.e., an initial log file) and then observing the video of the user interaction (e.g., a screen capture file with the audio track giving user verbalizations) and marking up the log file with annotations and codes (as illustrated in the above example). There are however, a number of tools available that can facilitate the coding process. Using the approach described above we have employed tools such as Transana®, f4®, f5®, NVivo, ATLAS.ti® and MAXQDA® to facilitate coding and analysis. Such tools allow for opening up the log file containing transcripts in one window of the tool, and then opening up the file containing the digital movie file of user interactions in another window. Codes can be dropped into the log file from a pre-determined menu of codes (entered by the experimenter) as outlined earlier in this paper. Time stamps can be automatically entered into the log file as well. In addition, a number of qualitative tools which have been used for coding of qualitative data now offer the ability to allow for the same functionality as Transana® by allowing for watching video files while entering codes and annotations (e.g., NVivo® and other such tools). An advantage of using such tools is that they may greatly facilitate the summarization phase of analysis, by automatically tallying up the number of codes and presenting distributions of codes over time. In addition, such tools can facilitate the process of obtaining inter-rater reliability where the same sections of the log file can be coded by more than one analyst and then compared for consistency statistically, using statistics such as Cohen's kappa coefficient (see van Someren [15] for details on interrater reliability for measuring the degree of agreement among multiple analysts when coding transcripts).

However, such tools do require analyst time to learn how they operate and how to use the analysis software. In recent developments some of these tools (such as NVivo®) have begun to incorporate machine learning technology leading to semi-automated coding of transcripts that can be obtained from usability testing [57, 58]. We have employed such tools for analyzing textual documents and audio-recorded interviews. This can save time in the pre-processing of the verbal parts of a recorded session. The automated analysis of the video portion from recordings of end users (e.g., screens) is more difficult to achieve and is still experimental. However, the application of coding schemes described in this chapter speeds the process of analysis and the authors are currently working on development of tools to fully automate the coding process, using the categories presented in this chapter.

Experiences to Date and Future Directions

Over the past several decades the authors have worked on evaluating a wide range of health information systems using approaches based on variations of the methods for data collection and analysis described in this chapter. This work initially began with analyzing data from think-aloud studies of users interacting with electronic health record systems and prototypes [12] and then began to extend to the study of health information systems in real or highly realistic settings [13, 59]. This has included study of systems such as decision support tools, clinical guidelines and medication administration systems for assessing both their usability and their impact on patient safety (i.e., the extent to which they are able to decrease medication error, as well as identifying any potential negative unintended consequences—i.e., sources of technology-induced error). For example, in a study of clinical guidelines embedded in a commercial electronic record system, a modified version of the coding scheme in this paper was used to identify problems related both to usability (e.g., identifying issues such as understanding labels on pop-up menus) and usefulness (e.g., issues around lack of user confidence in certain recommendations provided by the system) [13]. Based on the findings from the usability testing and clinical simulations conducted in this study, both the guidelines and the user interface were modified, which lead to improved user uptake of the guideline recommendations overall.

In another line of studies, a modified version of the coding scheme described in this paper was used to code both physician and pharmacist interactions with medication reconciliation software. Using the coding approach, major differences were identified between the type of usability problems that participants of the two groups encountered, as well as differences in how they incorporated the tool into their workflow. Based on the results the user interface of the tool was modified and a training program initiated for users of the different user groups [60]. In addition, the approach has also been used to evaluate the impact of hybrid environments (containing both paper and electronic resources) on novice nurse information seeking [26] and on nurse tele-health decision making [61].

We have also conducted work that has evaluated the cost effectiveness of applying a rapid usability engineering approach, which has included the coding of video data as described in this paper. The results from that study indicate that conducting usability engineering work by using predetermined coding schemes (like the one described in this chapter) can lead to reductions in coding time, leading to a decrease in the cost of doing usability testing while yielding a higher return on investment for carrying out usability tests [56].

Conclusions

The analysis of data emerging from usability testing is important in assessing the usability of health care information systems and technologies. Simply providing visual evidence of usability issues by playing back recorded videos to system developers and designers can on its own provide useful information for improving health information systems and technologies. In addition, as shown in this chapter, the data from usability testing can also be more formally analyzed in order to provide very specific information about usability problems and issues. This information can be used by system designers and developers to improve the usability of the health information systems and technologies. This level of feedback can be achieved by applying principled coding schemes in analyzing video-based usability data. The coding schemes presented in this chapter were developed to suit the analysis for a wide range of health information systems. The categories and approaches described in this paper have proven generalizable enough to have been employed on a wide range of published projects that involved collection and analysis of data from usability studies conducted in hospitals, clinics and even patient homes. The approach provides a simplified methodology for coding usability problems that can be modified and extended for different types of system and technologies.

Discussion Questions
1. Why is the analysis of video-based HCI data important for usability research and practice?
2. What are the main practical ways for collecting video-based data from usability tests?
3. What are the main approaches to analyzing video-based usability data?
4. How can surface level usability problems be identified from digital recordings of user interactions?
5. How can the impact of health information systems and technologies be characterized in terms of their effect on cognition, including information seeking, reasoning, and decision making?
6. What are the main approaches to coding video-based usability data to assess impact of systems and technology on work activities in healthcare?
7. Why is development of evidence-based coding schemes important in usability engineering in healthcare?

References

1. Kellermann AL, Jones SS. What it will take to achieve the as-yet-unfulfilled promises of health information technology. Health Aff (Millwood). 2013;32(1):63–8. https://doi.org/10.1377/hlthaff.2012.0693.
2. Koppel R, Metlay JP, Cohen A, et al. Role of computerized physician order entry systems in facilitating medication errors. JAMA. 2005;293(10):1197–203.

3. Hettinger AZ, Melnick ER, Ratwani RM. Advancing electronic health record vendor usability maturity: Progress and next steps. J Am Med Inform Assoc. 2021;28(5):1029–31.
4. Kushniruk AW, Triola MM, Borycki EM, Stein B, Kannry JL. Technology induced error and usability: the relationship between usability problems and prescription errors when using a handheld application. Int J Med Inform. 2005;74(7–8):519–26. https://doi.org/10.1016/j.ijmedinf.2005.01.003.
5. Borycki EM, Kushniruk AW. Where do technology-induced errors come from? Towards a model for conceptualizing and diagnosing errors caused by technology. In: Borycki EM, Kushniruk AW, editors. Human, social, and organizational aspects of health information systems. Hershey, PA: IGI Global Books; 2008.
6. Borycki E, Kushniruk A. Identifying and preventing technology-induced error using simulations: application of usability engineering techniques. Healthc Q. 2005;8(Sp):99–105. https://doi.org/10.12927/hcq..17673.
7. Kushniruk A, Nøhr C. Participatory design, user involvement and health IT evaluation. Stud Health Technol Inform. 2016;222:139–51.
8. Nielsen J. Usability engineering. New York: Elsevier; 1994.
9. Kushniruk AW, Patel VL. Cognitive and usability engineering methods for the evaluation of clinical information systems. J Biomed Inform. 2004;37(1):56–76.
10. Kushniruk A, Borycki E, Kuwata S, Kannry J. Predicting changes in workflow resulting from healthcare information systems: ensuring the safety of healthcare. Healthc Q. 2006;9(Sp):114–8. https://doi.org/10.12927/hcq..18469.
11. Kushniruk AW, Patel VL. Cognitive computer-based video analysis: its application in assessing the usability of medical systems. Medinfo. 1995;8(Pt 2):1566–9.
12. Kushniruk AW, Kaufman DR, Patel VL, Lévesque Y, Lottin P. Assessment of a computerized patient record system: a cognitive approach to evaluating medical technology. MD Comput. 1996;13((5):406–15.
13. Li AC, Kannry JL, Kushniruk A, et al. Integrating usability testing and think-aloud protocol analysis with "near-live" clinical simulations in evaluating clinical decision support. Int J Med Inform. 2012;81(11):761–72. https://doi.org/10.1016/j.ijmedinf.2012.02.009.
14. Ericsson KA. Protocol analysis. In: Bechtel W, Graham G, editors. A companion to cognitive science. Blackwell; 2017. p. 425–32.
15. Van Someren M, Barnard YF, Sandberg J. The think aloud method: a practical approach to modelling cognitive. London: Academic Press; 1994. p. 29–41.
16. Jaspers MW, Steen T, van den Bos C, Geenen M. The think aloud method: a guide to user interface design. Int J Med Inform. 2004;73(11–12):781–95. https://doi.org/10.1016/j.ijmedinf.2004.08.003.
17. Kushniruk AW. Analysis of complex decision-making processes in health care: cognitive approaches to health informatics. J Biomed Inform. 2001;34(5):365–76.
18. Strauss A, Corbin J. Basics of qualitative research, vol. 15. Newbury Park, CA: Sage; 1990.
19. Hsieh HF, Shannon SE. Three approaches to qualitative content analysis. Qual Health Res. 2005;15(9):1277–88.
20. Carvalho CJ, Borycki EM, Kushniruk A. Ensuring the safety of health information systems: using heuristics for patient safety. Healthc Q. 2009;12(Sp):49–54. https://doi.org/10.12927/hcq.2009.20966.
21. Carvalho CJ, Borycki EM, Kushniruk AW. Using heuristic evaluations to assess the safety of health information systems. Stud Health Technol Inform. 2009;143:297–301.
22. Hassebrock F, Prietula MJ. A protocol-based coding scheme for the analysis of medical reasoning. Int J Man-Mach Stud. 1992;37(5):613–52.
23. Patel VL, Kushniruk AW, Yang S, Yale JF. Impact of a computer-based patient record system on data collection, knowledge organization, and reasoning. J Am Med Inform Assoc. 2000;7(6):569–85.

24. Borycki EM, Lemieux-Charles L, Nagle L, Eysenbach G. Evaluating the impact of hybrid electronic-paper environments upon novice nurse information seeking. Methods Inf Med. 2009;48(02):137–43.
25. Borycki EM, Lemieux-Charles L, Nagle L, Eysenbach G. Novice nurse information needs in paper and hybrid electronic-paper environments: a qualitative analysis. Stud Health Technol Inform. 2009;150:913–7.
26. Borycki EM, Lemieux-Charles L. Does a hybrid electronic-paper environment impact on health professional information seeking? Stud Health Technol Inform. 2008;136:505–10.
27. U.S. Department of Health and Human Services. Research-based web design and usability guidelines. 2006 [cited 2016 Jul 1]. Available from: http://guidelines.usability.gov/
28. Diaper D, Stanton N, editors. The handbook of task analysis for human-computer interaction. New York: CRC Press; 2004.
29. Annett J, Stanton NA, editors. Task analysis. CRC Press; 2000.
30. Schraagen JM, Chipman SF, Shalin VL, editors. Cognitive task analysis. Psychology Press; 2000.
31. Clark RE, Feldon DF, Van Merrienboer JJ, Yates KA, Early S. Cognitive task analysis. In: Handbook of research on educational communications and technology. Routledge; 2008. p. 577–93.
32. Wei J, Salvendy G. The cognitive task analysis methods for job and task design: review and reappraisal. Behav Inform Technol. 2004;23(4):273–99.
33. Kushniruk AW, Borycki EM. Low-cost rapid usability engineering: designing and customizing usable healthcare information systems. Healthc Q. 2006;9(4):98–100, 102.
34. Kushniruk AW, Borycki EM. Integrating low-cost rapid usability testing into agile system development of healthcare IT: a methodological perspective. Stud Health Technol Inform. 2015;210:200–4.
35. Kushniruk AW, Borycki EM, Kuwata S, Watanabe H. Using a low-cost simulation approach for assessing the impact of a medication administration system on workflow. Stud Health Technol Inform. 2008;136:567.
36. Mann DM, Chokshi SK, Kushniruk A. Bridging the gap between academic research and pragmatic needs in usability: a hybrid approach to usability evaluation of health care information systems. JMIR Hum Factors. 2018;5(4):e10721. https://doi.org/10.2196/10721.
37. Norman DA. Cognitive artifacts. In: Carroll JM, editor. Designing interaction: psychology at the human-computer interface. Cambridge: Cambridge University Press; 1991. p. 17–38.
38. Albert B, Tullis T, Tedesco D. Beyond the usability lab: conducting large-scale online user experience studies. Morgan Kaufmann; 2009.
39. Kushniruk AW, Borycki EM. Development of a video coding scheme for analyzing the usability and usefulness of health information systems. Stud Health Technol Inform. 2015;218:68–73.
40. Kushniruk AW, Monkman H, Kitson N, Borycki EM. Development of a video coding scheme for understanding human-computer interaction and clinical decision making. Stud Health Technol Inform. 2019;265:80–5. https://doi.org/10.3233/SHTI190142.
41. Kushniruk A, Borycki E, Kitson N, Kannry J. Development of a video coding scheme focused on socio-technical aspects of human-computer interaction in healthcare. Stud Health Technol Inform. 2019;257:236–43.
42. Card SK, Moran TP, Newell A. The psychology of human-computer interaction. Hillsdale, NJ: Lawrence Erlbaum Associates, Inc; 1983.
43. Lewis C, Norman DA. Designing for error. In: Readings in human–computer interaction. Morgan Kaufmann; 1995. p. 686–97.
44. Borycki EM, Kushniruk AW. Towards an integrative cognitive-socio-technical approach in health informatics: analyzing technology-induced error involving health information systems to improve patient safety. Open Med Inform J. 2010;4:181–7. https://doi.org/10.2174/1874431101004010181.
45. Patel VL, Kushniruk AW. Understanding, navigating and communicating knowledge: issues and challenges. Methods Inf Med. 1998;37(4–5):460–70.

46. Hutchins E. Cognition in the wild. MIT press; 1995.
47. Zhang J, Patel VL. Distributed cognition, representation, and affordance. Pragmat Cogn. 2006;14(2):333–41.
48. Perry M. Distributed cognition. In: HCI models, theories, and frameworks: toward a multidisciplinary science. Morgan Kaufmann; 2003. p. 193–223.
49. Baxter G, Sommerville I. Socio-technical systems: from design methods to systems engineering. Interact Comput. 2011;23(1):4–17.
50. Aarts J, Callen J, Coiera E, Westbrook J. Information technology in health care: socio-technical approaches. Int J Med Inform. 2010;79(6):389–90.
51. Sittig D, Singh H. An eight-dimension sociotechnical model for studying health information technology in complex adaptive healthcare systems. In: Cognitive informatics for biomedicine: human compute interaction in healthcare. Springer; 2015. p 81–109.
52. Borycki EM, Kushniruk AW, Bellwood P, Brender J. Technology-induced errors. The current use of frameworks and models from the biomedical and life sciences literatures. Methods Inf Med. 2012;51(2):95–103. https://doi.org/10.3414/ME11-02-0009.
53. Kushniruk A, Triola M, Stein B, Borycki E, Kannry J. The relationship of usability to medical error: an evaluation of errors associated with usability problems in the use of a handheld application for prescribing medications. Stud Health Technol Inform. 2004;107(Pt 2):1073–6.
54. Borycki EM, Kushniruk AW, Kuwata S, Kannry J. Engineering the electronic health record for safety: a multi-level video-based approach to diagnosing and preventing technology-induced error arising from usability problems. Stud Health Technol Inform. 2011;166:197–205.
55. Campbell EM, Sittig DF, Ash JS, Guappone KP, Dykstra RH. Types of unintended consequences related to computerized provider order entry. J Am Med Inform Assoc. 2006;13(5):547–56.
56. Baylis TB, Kushniruk AW, Borycki EM. Low-cost rapid usability testing for health information systems: is it worth the effort? Stud Health Technol Inform. 2012;180:363–7.
57. Borycki EM, Farghali A, Kushniruk AW. Do health technology safety issues vary by vendor? Stud Health Technol Inform. 2022;295:345–9. https://doi.org/10.3233/SHTI220734.
58. Borycki EM, Farghali A, Kushniruk AW. Integrating human patterns of qualitative coding with machine learning: a pilot study involving technology-induced error incident reports. Stud Health Technol Inform. 2022;295:276–80. https://doi.org/10.3233/SHTI220716.
59. Kushniruk A, Nohr C, Jensen S, Borycki EM. From usability testing to clinical simulations: bringing context into the design and evaluation of usable and safe health information technologies. Contribution of the IMIA human factors engineering for healthcare informatics working group. Yearb Med Inform. 2013;8:78–85.
60. Boockvar KS, Santos SL, Kushniruk A, Johnson C, Nebeker JR. Medication reconciliation: barriers and facilitators from the perspectives of resident physicians and pharmacists. J Hosp Med. 2011;6(6):329–37. https://doi.org/10.1002/jhm.891.
61. Hall SA, Kushniruk AW, Borycki EM. Usability analysis of the tele-nursing call management software at HealthLink BC. Stud Health Technol Inform. 2011;164:208–12.

Further Reading

Kushniruk AW, Borycki EM. Development of a video coding scheme for analyzing the usability and usefulness of health information systems. Stud Health Technol Inform. 2015;218:68–73.

Kushniruk AW, Monkman H, Kitson N, Borycki EM. Development of a video coding scheme for understanding human-computer interaction and clinical decision making. Stud Health Technol Inform. 2019;265:80–5. https://doi.org/10.3233/SHTI190142.

Kushniruk AW, Patel VL. Cognitive and usability engineering methods for the evaluation of clinical information systems. J Biomed Inform. 2004;37(1):56–76.

Lazar J, Feng JH, Hochheiser H. Research methods in human-computer interaction. Morgan Kaufmann; 2017.

Patel VL, Arocha JF, Kaufman DR. A primer on aspects of cognition for medical informatics. J Am Med Inform Assoc. 2001;8(4):324–43.

Chapter 8
A Cognitive Approach to Understanding and Mitigating a Pernicious Infodemic

David R. Kaufman and Tonya N. Taylor

Introduction

> We live in an age of misinformation—an age of spin, marketing, and downright lies. [1]

The COVID-19 pandemic inexorably changed the world that we live in, with likely health, social, economic, and political repercussions for decades. The pandemic's sudden emergence, significant uncertainty, and unclear public health messaging led to an information vacuum [2]. This resulted in widespread confusion and misunderstandings, eroding the credibility of public institutions, and diminishing trust in public health measures [3]. Such shortcomings provided fertile ground for the spread of misinformation. We can define health "misinformation" as claims not supported by conventional scientific evidence, regardless of their intent [4]. Disinformation is a type of misinformation that is distinguished by the deliberate intent to deceive or mislead [5]. An "infodemic" is a term used to describe an overwhelming amount of information, including misinformation and disinformation, related to a specific topic or event [5]. The term is often employed in the context of a crisis, particularly public health emergencies like the COVID-19 pandemic. During an infodemic, rapidly circulating accurate and inaccurate information can make it difficult for individuals and organizations to discern what is true from falsehoods. The deluge of information can exacerbate anxieties, lead to poor decision-making, and undermine efforts to manage the crisis effectively [6]. The term

D. R. Kaufman (✉) · T. N. Taylor
Health Informatics Program, School of Health Professions, SUNY Downstate Health Sciences University, Brooklyn, NY, USA

Department of Medicine, Division of Infectious Disease, and Special Treatment and Research (STAR), SUNY Downstate Health Sciences University, Brooklyn, NY, USA
e-mail: david.kaufman@downstate.edu

© The Author(s), under exclusive license to Springer Nature Switzerland AG 2024
A. W. Kushniruk et al. (eds.), *Human Computer Interaction in Healthcare*, Cognitive Informatics in Biomedicine and Healthcare, https://doi.org/10.1007/978-3-031-69947-4_8

infodemic underscores the challenges posed by excess information and the urgent need for reliable, verified data during critical events.

In this chapter, we first situate the problem in relation to the discipline of human-computer interaction. Following this introduction, we turn our attention to delineating various forms of inaccurate health-related information. In the section, we expand on the case of fake news in the context of diabetes and anti-vaxxer conspiracy theories. Next, the chapter discusses the role of xenophobia in the propagation and amplification of disinformation. The subsequent section scrutinizes the distinct influence exerted by various social media platforms on the spread of misinformation. We then investigate what makes individuals susceptible to false health information, considering social, cultural, and cognitive determinants. The last section assesses the range of strategies implemented to mitigate the adverse effects of misinformation.

Social Media, Health Information and Human-Computer Interaction

The dissemination of fallacious health information is far from a new phenomenon. Federal regulation concerning the safety and efficacy of drugs was not instituted in the United States until 1906, as per the U.S. Food and Drug Administration. Prior to this time, numerous newspaper advertisements and itinerant salespeople promoted questionable remedies as cure-alls. The COVID-19 infodemic, consisting of a rapid diffusion of credible information and highly politicized misinformation, has had lethal consequences [7]. Social media platforms were the primary accelerant for disseminating misinformation and fake news because they are accessible and allow anyone to participate in public discourse.

As of July 2023, social media is used by around 4.88 billion people, or over 60% of the world's population. The average social media user spends 2.5 h a day online, using platforms for messaging, engaging in discourse, and sharing original and published or previously posted content [8]. Users typically visit an average of 6.7 different social platforms each month.

Social media platforms cultivate the process of information democratization in which everyone can generate content with no intermediary to check or confirm authenticity or accuracy [9]. We now understand that this democratization has the unintended consequence of empowering skeptics and individuals with financial or political agendas to amplify the spread of dangerous misinformation. The inherent ease of sharing information on these platforms allows one to quickly reach large audiences and spread their messages.

Health misinformation is inextricably linked to a politicized complex ecology that was most evident during the COVID-19 pandemic. With escalating mortality rates and economic jeopardy [10], online extremists recalibrated their conspiracy narratives to align with current political events (2020 Presidential election), thereby attracting a new cadre of followers [11]. Using machine learning models, Velazquez and colleagues demonstrate that harmful disinformation and misinformation related to COVID-19—encompassing racism, xenophobia, and anti-science beliefs—form an interconnected landscape of online extremism and animosity proliferated rapidly, eluding social media platforms' regulatory mechanisms [12]. Attempts to moderate platforms and mitigate disinformation resulted in clashes with commercial incentives and ideological goals to preserve free speech. For example, when Elon Musk acquired Twitter (now known as X), he removed moderating mechanisms and policies regarding hate speech, resulting in large spikes in racist, antisemitic, and homophobic content [13]. The Anti-Defamation League quickly challenged Musk's politically-driven choices for echoing antisemitic tropes attacking George Soros, the Jewish megadonor and supporter of progressive causes [14]. We expand on the issue of xenophobia in a subsequent section.

Conversely, information democratization can also be beneficial; for example, it is instrumental to applications of consumer health informatics, especially patient support groups that offer a podium for those afflicted with particular conditions to share information [15]. There is evidence to support the notion that social media platforms can be harnessed effectively to promote beneficial health practices and align with broader public health objectives [16]. During the pandemic, prominent infectious disease prevention specialists used social media platforms to counter the wave of harmful COVID-19 misinformation and disinformation.

Research indicates that social media can enhance individual well-being by expanding access to health-related information and providing channels for social support [17]. Social media can augment health promotion efforts by extending reach, reducing costs, and facilitating the delivery of interactive or tailored messages [18]. The discipline of human-computer interaction (HCI) can help us navigate the perilous terrain of misinformation and conspiracy theories by providing insight into the user experience and leveraging tools to fashion solutions and mitigate problems. Historically, HCI has had a narrow focus on the design and usability of computing systems [18]. Today, the scope is much broader, encompassing the theory, research, and practice of designing user experiences across a wide array of technologies, systems, and products [19]. The breadth of HCI in healthcare currently encompasses the full range of systems, applications, and user experiences across healthcare providers, patients, and health consumers.

The discipline of computer-supported cooperative work (CSCW) [20], an adjacent field to HCI, has focused for decades on social and cognitive behavior and how different media and tools support and sometimes impede collaborative efforts in work contexts across various domains, including healthcare. However, the focus in CSCW research has been largely on the work of healthcare professionals as opposed to patients and consumers. In recent years, HCI research on social media has grown considerably, focusing on interactions and phenomena related to user experience, user behavior patterns, attitudes, decision-making, community discourse, and design [21]. Misinformation has become a focal public concern, increasingly drawing HCI investigators' attention [22].

Conceptualizing False Information

The term "fake news" is a rhetorical and discursive strategy to undermine and discount any opposing or competing opinions or facts held by the mainstream media, or other perceived political or ideological adversaries [3]. The term, made popular by Donald Trump, is now commonly used in everyday parlance, but there are important distinctions between fake news and misinformation and disinformation [6]. Previous studies have found that the coexistence of terms like misinformation, disinformation, rumors, fake news, misleading information, and hoaxes has contributed to a lack of conceptual clarity. Li and colleagues conducted an extensive literature review on health misinformation and social media and used this information to crystallize a typology of misleading health information [22]. Cinelli et al., similarly scrutinized commonly used definitions for misinformation in empirical research [23]. In this section, we draw liberally on their work, exploring and delineating the boundaries between these concepts (Table 8.1) [26].

Wardle and Derakhshan classified misinformation into two categories [26]: (1) false connection (which describes the headlines, visuals, or captions do not support the content) and (2) misleading content (which describes using information in a misleading way to frame a problem or characterize an individual). They similarly categorized disinformation into four types: (1) false context, which involves presenting authentic content within misleading contextual information; (2) imposter content, defined as the act of impersonating legitimate sources; (3) manipulated content, which entails altering authentic information or imagery to deceive; and (4) fabricated content, characterized by the creation of entirely false content designed to deceive and cause harm. Alex Jones' malicious lie that the Sandy Hook massacre was a hoax is a classic example of disinformation and fabricated content [27–29]. The hoax perpetrated by Jones served to undermine the "establishment narrative" or mainstream reporting of 26 deaths, including 20 children, in the minds of followers and caused them to act with malice towards the victims [30].

Fake news stories routinely flood social media, such as the "Pizzagate" fake news/conspiracy story that resulted in potential violence. According to Tandoc et al., on December 4, 2016, a man carrying an assault rifle walked into a pizza restaurant in Washington, DC, intent on "self-investigating" whether the restaurant was the headquarters of an underground child sex ring allegedly run by then-presidential candidate Hillary Clinton and her former campaign manager, John Podesta [31]. In the process of his "self-investigation," he fired several shots into the ceiling of the restaurant. It was just one of the several threats to the pizzeria after the news report spread through social media sites, such as Facebook, Reddit, and Twitter." This man's rationale for his actions was influenced by his consumption of fake news stories on right-wing blogs and social media [31].

In most cases, fake news mimics the appearance and structure of legitimate journalism, from website design and article formatting to the inclusion of photo attributions [31]. This veneer of legitimacy allows fake news to assume a certain level of credibility, making it difficult to distinguish from real news. Waszak et al. [32]

Table 8.1 Explanation of analytic terms used concerning the spread of incorrect information

Concept	Explanations
Misinformation	Misinformation pertains to information that is inaccurate, false, or misleading and does not accurately represent either the factual situation or the genuine intentions of the communicator. This definition holds irrespective of whether such information is disseminated with the intent to deceive.
Disinformation	Disinformation involves the intentional dissemination of false or misleading information for the purpose of deception. Disinformation is a specialized form of misinformation, distinguished by the deliberate intent to deceive or mislead. It points to people being disinformed by malicious actors.
Mal-information	True information, but used to inflict harm on a person, organization, or country. For example, this includes efforts to reveal a person's sexual orientation or something about their private lives with the intent to harm or discredit them. It may be a precursor to a broader act of deception or malice [22].
Fake news	Misinformation mimics the characteristics of traditional news media and is purported to be conveyed by an authoritative source. It can be in the form of "clickbait," which refers to misleading headlines and thumbnails of content on the web that tend to be fake stories with catchy headlines aimed at enticing the reader to click on a link [24].
Conspiracy theories	These theories include unsubstantiated and often implausible beliefs that involve the role of a malevolent force in plotting major events. Suspicions that powerful people or organizations secretly carry out sinister plans by deceiving the public. For example, one that gained some currency was the idea that Bill Gates arranged for microchips to be secretly implanted in humans via vaccine doses.
Rumor	Rumor refers to unconfirmed bits of information.
Satire and parody	Clever satire, such as reports from the Onion, can seem very real, even if they have an absurd quality. Satirist Andy Borowitz labels his column "Satire from the Borowitz Report" because it is presented as a news report. After hearing that it was the primary news source for many watchers, John Stewart would point out that the Daily News was a comedy show rather than a news program.
Outdated information	Outdated information may have been communicated through official channels. The information had been revised, but people continued to use the old information. For example, the initial belief that COVID-19 was transmitted primarily by touching surfaces could lead to arguments that masking was unnecessary.
Infodemic motifs	These involve a mixture of misinformation and folk medicine common to many countries (chicken soup as a sure or rest as a cure for anything). Arkhipova and Brodie describe an anti-vaccine anecdote from Russia: "—they put Lucifer's gene inside it. Everybody who got the vaccine starts to hate God [25]. Better stay home and drink hot tea; this is a good prevention against COVID." This statement combines fragments of misinformation with common folk wisdom to make the argument against vaccines more plausible. This is akin to repurposing old folk tales towards particular ends, and no doubt resonates differently in different cultures.

describe three categories of fake medical news: (1) fabricated news that refers to completely fictitious information about medical facts, (2) manipulated news that leverages true basic information but false conclusions, and (3) advertisement news that refers to stories to criticize conventional therapies and advertise products.

A common feature of fake or disinformation news sites is that they follow a "fabricated legitimacy" template [33] by mimicking legitimate news sources to create the illusion of credibility [28], employing a process of strategic presentation of fake content. They employ a similar presentation style, such as using familiar fonts and colors to authentic their fake news [34]. Fake news sites also tend to cover topics addressed by mainstream media but misrepresent and sensationalize certain facts [31]; for example, "Pope Francis shocks world: endorses Donald Trump for President." Allcott and Gentzkow [34] estimated that fabricated news relating to Donald Trump was shared 30 million times on Facebook, while those relating to Hillary Clinton were shared only eight million times. It was reported that perhaps as much as 50% of readers accepted these stories at face value [34]. Fake news often contains profanities and is designed to elicit more positive and negative affect to elicit an emotional response [35].

Fake News: The Case of Diabetes

According to the Center for Disease Control, more than 37 million people in the United States have diabetes, and one in five don't know it [36]. Diabetes is the eighth leading cause of death. Over the past two decades, the incidence of adult diabetes diagnoses has more than doubled, a trend that parallels the aging of the American population and increasing rates of overweight and obesity. The American Diabetes Association (ADA) states that lifestyle changes such as diet, exercise, stress management, and medical interventions can frequently prevent, delay, or even induce remission in type 2 diabetes [37]. However, the condition is generally not regarded as curable or reversible.

Keselman and colleagues analyzed 25 type 2 diabetes sites and videos that made claims about curing diabetes [38]. They found that most pages either explicitly promised or strongly hinted at a high likelihood of full recovery. Some expressed a very high level of certainty: "If you follow our recommendations to the letter, we guarantee that you will eventually be able to throw your medication away and never need it again!" Only a single article, authored by a registered dietitian, discussed what it meant by diabetes reversal, explaining how remission is more accurate than cure.

Keselman and colleagues also found that many sites criticized mainstream healthcare practices while also selling commercial products like dietary supplements or books [38]. Of these sites critical of mainstream healthcare practices, 13 suggested malicious intent or conspiracy by various establishment agents. Pharmaceutical companies received the greatest amount of criticism. For example, one page stated that "the pharmaceutical industry is a gigantic machine which has to sustain itself" and asked, "why would these companies be at all interested in truly reversing diabetes? How would that benefit them financially?" Another wrote, "Most big pharma companies don't know how to reverse your diabetes." The critiques aimed at established healthcare systems are concerning because they undermine the credibility of evidence-based care while promoting alternative methods as primary solutions instead of complementary ones. These critical websites must balance their criticisms of established healthcare systems while valuing science and evidence-based practices by selectively citing certain studies to bolster their claims.

Following Waszak et al.'s categories, most websites in Keselman and colleagues' study could be classified as advertisement news and manipulated news [32]. They embraced kernels of truth but used medical facts selectively to support unwarranted conclusions. We observed that the language used on some of these sites featured emotionally charged personal quotes that strained credulity. Using a multipronged approach of discounting credible medical institutions, fabricating emotional appeals, and tactics to foster empathy with the reader ("we are just like you") is an effective strategy for getting social media consumers to believe misinformation and disinformation.

Anti-Vaxxer Conspiracy Theories

Vaccines have long been the target of conspiracy theorists [39]. In 2018, Heidi Larson (WHO vaccine initiative) predicted that "the deluge of conflicting information, misinformation and manipulated information on social media" would impede global vaccine efforts [40]. Social media has been a primary source for disseminating many anti-vax conspiracies. Antivaccine advocates have a significant presence on social media [39]. For example, as many as 50% of tweets about vaccination contain antivaccine beliefs [41]. These conspiracies can have real-world consequences. Vaccine-hesitant parents are likelier to have faith in the Internet for information and less likely to trust healthcare providers and public health experts [42]. Exposure to the vaccine debate often suggests that there is no scientific consensus, thus reducing confidence in vaccination [43]. In other words, science remains equivocal, and the health decision remains a matter of personal choice. Evidence suggests that false vaccine narrative across platforms tends to drive hesitancy, making it more difficult to the public health strategies needed to drive collective behavioral changes [44]. Such information can stoke pre-existing fears, seeding doubt and cynicism over new vaccines, and can limit public uptake of COVID-19 vaccines. Loomba and colleagues demonstrated that exposure to false information can reduce intent by more than 6% in both UK and US sample populations [44]. Scientific-sounding statements such as "the vaccine will literally alter your DNA" had the greatest negative impact on the intent to vaccinate.

Although they may stretch the bounds of credulity, conspiracy theories may be more elaborate, involving a constellation of beliefs, and may cohere better than other forms of misinformation/disinformation. They include unsubstantiated and often implausible beliefs that involve the role of a malevolent force in plotting major events. Suspicions that powerful people or organizations secretly carry out sinister plans by deceiving the public. The theories assert that people in the seat of power (e.g., senior government officials or corporate leaders) are covertly executing malevolent schemes while misleading the general populace.

The "Disinformation Dozen" comprises 12 prominent purveyors of anti-vaccine misinformation concerning COVID-19 vaccines [45]. They were identified based on their large followings, the substantial volume of anti-vaccine content they produce, or the swift growth of their social media accounts over the past 2 months. An analysis of a representative sample of anti-vaccine content shared or posted on Facebook and Twitter from February 1 to March 16, 2021, reveals that 65% of such content can be attributed to these 12 individuals [45]. Despite frequent violations of the terms of service for Facebook, Instagram, and Twitter, most members of the Disinformation Dozen remain active on all three platforms [45]. At the same time, only three have been fully removed from a single platform.

Naomi Wolf was a highly respected author and one of the leading voices of the feminist movement [46]. She completed a Doctor of Philosophy degree in English literature from Oxford University. Several years before the pandemic, she embraced conspiracy theories. Although not one of the Disinformation Dozen, Wolf had emerged as a significant disseminator of alarming misinformation, nearly doubling her Twitter following from the previous year (2019–2020) to 138,000 [47]. She was banned from Twitter in April 2021 because of her anti-vaccine conspiracy theories [48]. Wolf characterized actions taken by health authorities to manage the virus as part of a nefarious scheme. These alleged schemes were aimed at objectives such as harvesting our DNA, causing illness, sterilization, infant mortality, invasive tracking, emotional desensitization of children, subversion of the U.S. Constitution, and weakening Western power [47]. Wolf also posited that the virus and the vaccines might serve as biological weapons, potentially targeting politicians for assassination [47]. She has written, "Local leaders are dying too," adding, "This is why I fear this is an attack. The dosages differ." She further compared Anthony Fauci, then the U.S. National Institute of Allergy and Infectious Diseases director, to Satan and labeled efforts to correct vaccine misinformation as "demonic." [48].

Wolf is a gifted writer with a clear and compelling dystopian message that we are teetering on the brink of disaster; "a world managed by machines and mediated via digital interfaces; a world predicated on cruelty, without human empathy as an organizing principle; a world in which national boundaries, cultures, and languages are drained of meaning, in which institutions embody only the goals of distant metanational oligarchs, a world organized for the benefit of massive pharmaceutical companies, a few global tech giants and technocrats, and a tyrannical superpower that is our deadly adversary (p. 11)." [49] The widespread online myth suggesting a link between vaccines and infertility had a particularly detrimental impact in the digital sphere focused on women's wellness [47]. One influencer, who declared a passion for "womb health," warned her audience to maintain distance from individuals who had received the vaccine [47]. In response to these claims, a private school in Florida even went so far as to prohibit vaccinated teachers from entering classrooms, citing concerns over vaccine "shedding" [50]. An investigative report by NPR, supported by specialized data analysts, found that much of this misinformation could be traced back to Naomi Wolf [47].

There is evidence to suggest that even when individuals are skeptical of anti-vaccination content, exposure to such narratives may still instill uncertainties regarding the safety and efficacy of vaccines and create suspicion about the intentions of those responsible for their production and distribution [45]. Conspiracy theories are often well-formed arguments put forth by individuals who should have credibility. They play to the individual's fear of the unknown, suspicions about technology and lack of trust in institutions. They can increase vaccine hesitancy and have a disruptive impact on public health initiatives [44].

Governmental responses in certain states have echoed the vaccine-hesitant and even anti-vaxxers in policy formulation. In 2021, Under Governor Ron DeSantis, Florida became the only state to recommend against vaccinating children and signed a bill prohibiting businesses from discriminating based on vaccination status or requiring face masks [51]. In the fall of 2023, Florida's Surgeon General, Dr. Joseph Ladapo, warned healthy adults under the age of 65 against taking a new COVID-19 booster, contradicting the Centers for Disease Control (CDC) and Food and Drug Administration(FDA) recommendations [52].

Xenophobia and Health Misinformation from AIDS to COVID-19

> There is a virus, which is not new, potentiating the effects of the pandemic of the new coronavirus, the infectious agent of xenophobia. [53]

Long before the advent of social media, history is replete with examples of how health misinformation was intricately intertwined with hate propaganda. Historically, pandemics and the spread of infectious diseases have been associated with elevated levels of prejudice, racial discrimination, and xenophobia [54]. The worldwide proliferation of the Human Immunodeficiency Virus (HIV) virus that causes AIDS was accompanied by misinformation or disinformation fueled by racial, homophobic, and xenophobic bias and blame [55]. The late Dr. Jonathan Mann, the founder of the WHO Global Program on AIDS, recognized that the blame and vilification of those infected undermined the "social, cultural, economic, and political responses to AIDS," which he described as being "integral to the global AIDS challenge as the disease itself [56]."

Throughout history, a recurring interpretive framework ascribes the cause of plagues, contagions, and deadly diseases to entities outside the communal or national identity (e.g., foreigners, immigrants, or socially marginalized groups). The Athenian plague, the fourteenth-century Bubonic plague, the influenza pandemic in 1918, and the cholera outbreak in the United States in 1832 scapegoated Jews and social outsiders [57, 58]. In 1348, as the plague neared the territories of the

German Empire, authorities and religious figures propagated baseless rumors claiming that Jews had tainted water supplies to infect Christians. Thousands of Jews were executed by burning, tortured into confessions, and had their assets seized leading to widespread persecution in over 300 communities [53].

At the beginning of the AIDS pandemic, much like the onset of COVID-19, countries that were heavily affected by the rapid diffusion of HIV initially attributed the crisis to those groups perceived as societal 'others,' that included (but were not limited to): Africans or Black immigrants and marginalized communities (e.g., homosexuals and substance users) [59]. Racist beliefs about African and Asian primitiveness quickly attributed the pandemic's origins to the seemingly "exotic" food culture that includes wildlife trade and consumption that exacerbated global discrimination against Africans and Asians during the AIDS and COVID-19 pandemics, respectively [60, 61]. Individuals from countries severely impacted by AIDS, like Uganda, faced detainment at airports or visa denials. African students in Russia and China were compelled to depart due to escalating hostilities fueled by infection fears.

As health agencies scrambled to address the global proliferation of COVID-19, they encountered the challenge of combating misinformation and conspiracy theories related to the virus [54]. Much of this misinformation was framed in racially charged language, specifically concerning the virus's origins and the attribution of responsibility for its spread. This contributed to the formation of associated conspiracy theories. Racially motivated scapegoating the use of derogatory language such as the "China Virus" or "Kung Flu" in public and political discourse effectively shifted the blame onto China [62]. A study using Crowdtangle, a search platform that enables the monitoring of hashtags or keywords across Facebook, Instagram, and Twitter, revealed that from February 2020 to March 2021, the term "Chinese virus" appeared in 43,779 Facebook posts, garnering a total of 3,535,409 interactions [63]. In addition, there was a 900% increase in hate speech on Twitter directed towards China and the Chinese and a 200% increase in traffic to hate sites and specific posts against Asians [63].

This precipitated a surge in anti-Asian hate crimes globally [64]. Dow and colleagues argue that as online communities reinforce conspiracy theories, they give rise to social norms that translate these beliefs into tangible actions [65]. These real-world activities are subsequently shared on social media platforms, where they undergo further reinforcement and amplification, perpetuating a cyclical pattern.

Divergent Mediation Across Social Media Platforms

> Misinformation is worse than an epidemic: It spreads at the speed of light throughout the globe and can prove deadly when it reinforces misplaced personal bias against all trustworthy evidence.—Marcia McNutt, President of the National Academy of Sciences of the United States (2021)

Billions of users engage in Online Health Information (OHI) seeking on diverse digital media platforms, including traditional online news outlets, social media platforms like Facebook, Twitter, and Instagram, and mobile social networking applications such as WhatsApp and WeChat. Live streaming services, including YouTube Now, Facebook Live, TikTok Live, and Instagram Live, are growing in popularity. The platforms vary along different dimensions, including their reach level, audience, and means of engaging users (Table 8.2).

Table 8.2 Social media platforms, monthly users and modes of engagement

Social media platform	Monthly active users[a]	Modes of engagement
Facebook	2.989 billion	Facebook employs a range of modes of engagement, including status updates, photo and video sharing, comments, reactions, and messaging. Users can also join and participate in groups, pages, and events, which enable them to connect with others who share their interests or are part of their communities.
X (formerly known as Twitter)	564 million	Tweets are posts limited to 280 characters. Users can also share photos and videos, like and retweet other users' tweets, and reply to tweets to start conversations.
Instagram	2 billion	Photo and video sharing platforms, and their primary mode of engagement, is through visual content. Users can like and comment on posts, send direct messages, and use Instagram Stories and Reels to create and share short-form content.
TikTok	1.081 billion adults	Short-form video-sharing platform and its primary mode of engagement is through creating and sharing short videos. Users can like, comment, share videos, follow creators and hashtags, and participate in challenges and trends.
YouTube	2.527 billion	Videos engage its audience through various tools such as the likes/dislikes system, a comments section, and a subscribe button for channel support. Additional features like Community Tabs, live stream Super Chats, and YouTube Shorts offer specialized forms of interaction. These tools facilitate everything from passive approval to active discussion and financial contributions, fostering a multifaceted social experience on the platform.
Reddit	430 million users	Social news aggregation and discussion platform, and its primary mode of engagement is through user generated content and discussions. Users can submit and upvote/downvote content, comment on posts, and participate in communities based on specific topics or interests.
Gab	3.7 million users	Gab fosters user engagement through features like posts, comments, upvotes, and downvotes. It allows users to follow one another and has a direct messaging system for private conversations. Gab aims to promote free speech and offers a space primarily for users who seek an alternative to mainstream social media platforms.

[a]All monthly user statistics were drawn from Data Reportal Global Media Statistics (https://datareportal.com/social-media-users). Gab statistics [66] drew on different reporting services and is best viewed as an approximation. The reason for its inclusion is the impact this smaller site had on spreading misinformation and xenophobia

Unfortunately, most of these social media platforms lack gatekeepers or trusted entities to verify the accuracy of information. While firsthand experiences of patients on social media platforms may offer useful perspectives on prevention or treatment, the lack of endorsement by medical authorities contributes to an unpredictable mixture of accurate and erroneous health information.

A study by Fondazione Bruno Kessler [67] scrutinized over 100 million tweets, using computational capture and analytic methods, about COVID-19 and concluded that upwards of 40% featured information from untrustworthy sources, with 42% of the posts emanating from bots, or a computer program that simulates human activity for a user or other program. Similarly, Lee et al. [68] surveyed 1049 South Korean adults and found that approximately 68% of adults had encountered COVID-19-related disinformation via social networking services or instant messaging platforms.

Social media platforms are designed to capture and maintain users' attention, as this directly influences advertising revenue. HCI principles are often employed to make platforms addictive and engaging. However, this attention-driven design can prioritize sensational or emotionally charged content, including health misinformation, to keep users engaged [69]. The larger social media platforms have billions or hundreds of millions of monthly users. A 2023 Pew Internet survey found that 44% of the population in the United States gets their news from Facebook [70]. A pivotal factor in disseminating misinformation is how social media platforms obfuscate the origins of the content [31]. Social media platforms amplify the impact of the "bandwagon heuristic," using visible popularity metrics, such as likes, shares, and comments [31]. This is a phenomenon whereby the rate of uptake of beliefs and trends increases with respect to the proportion of others who have already done so. When a post garners such engagement, it captures more attention and becomes increasingly susceptible to further interactions, thereby entering a self-perpetuating cycle of popularity and a desire to stay on the bandwagon. According to Tandoc et al. [31], this cyclical nature of social media engagement facilitates the dissemination of unverified information, further complicating the landscape of public knowledge and discourse.

Platforms like YouTube and X (formerly known as Twitter) offer unparalleled access to a vast array of content, but they also serve as conduits for amplifying rumors and dubious information [23]. Algorithms, designed to align with users' preferences and attitudes, act as intermediaries in content promotion and information dissemination. This departure from traditional news models has profound implications, significantly affecting the shaping of social perceptions, narrative framing, and political communication, particularly in the context of contentious issues. Additionally, users often gravitate towards information that aligns with their preexisting worldviews while disregarding dissenting perspectives (Confirmation bias), forming polarized communities centered around shared narratives. In an environment characterized by such high levels of polarization, misinformation finds fertile ground for rapid proliferation.

Gab is a lesser-known social networking platform that promotes itself as a platform committed to the principles of free speech and positions itself as an alternative to mainstream social media platforms like Facebook and Twitter, which it accuses of censoring conservative voices and perspectives. Gab has attracted a user base that includes various groups, among them free speech advocates, conservatives, libertarians, and far-right users [64]. One of the distinct characteristics of Gab is its more lenient content moderation policies compared to mainstream platforms, which has led it to be criticized for being a haven for hate speech, extremist ideologies, and disinformation [71].

Dow and colleagues suggest individuals are often ensnared in homogeneous informational echo chambers with members with congruent interests and beliefs [65]. Within these communities, social reinforcement mechanisms, such as shared posts, likes, and followers, establish a perpetuating feedback loop. This loop encourages heightened engagement among ideologically similar individuals and fosters social cohesion, particularly among those inclined toward conspiracy theories.

Di Domenico and colleagues systematically reviewed studies on fake news and identified important themes and patterns regarding spread conditions [33]. They argue that fake news spreads freely and widely because of four features or characteristics; the first feature is low barriers to entry. Creating an account on social media is free, and improving an account's popularity to amplify the effects of the posted content has a relatively low cost. The second characteristic pertains to the structure of information on social media. It is delivered in brief, fragmented units, a phenomenon referred to as 'thin slices' [34], making it challenging for users to assess the content's reliability. In this context, headlines are crafted to capture immediate attention; the greater the user engagement with a post, measured by likes, comments, or shares, the more likely it is to be featured prominently in news feeds. The third characteristic is social media polarization, earlier referred to as the creation of homogeneous informational echo chambers. Individuals confined to these online communities are generally exposed solely to information confirming their beliefs, even when such information includes intentionally false claims. Personalization algorithms contribute to forming these echo chambers, thereby creating environments conducive to the proliferation of disinformation across these platforms [34]. The fourth feature is that social media becomes the primary or sole source of information. These platforms started as a means to connect with their friends, but it has morphed into platforms where users create, consume, and exchange different types of information, including fake news [33].

In a comprehensive analysis of 1225 instances of fabricated news stories related to COVID-19, Naeem and his team discovered that social media platforms were responsible for disseminating over half of these false narratives [72]. Vosoughi et al. examined more than 126,000 online news stories distributed on Twitter between 2006 and 2017. Deceptive information, rumors, and hoaxes diffused significantly farther, faster, and more broadly than information deemed to be reliable and accurate [73].

Using these data, Naeem and collaborators identified three categories of COVID-19-related misinformation: (a) Erroneous assertions, such as claims that houseflies or mosquitoes could transmit the virus; (b) Conspiracy theories, which include speculations about the relationship between 5G networks and the coronavirus. (c) Unfounded health treatments, like the notion that a colloidal silver solution could remedy the virus.

Misleading statements that downplayed the severity of COVID-19, such as 'it's akin to the flu' or that the reported death tolls were grossly inflated, gained traction on social media [74]. Promoting pseudoscientific treatments like Ivermectin, an antiparasitic medication commonly used in veterinary practice, further muddied the waters. Loomba et al. carried out a randomized controlled trial in both the UK and the USA to assess the impact of exposure to online misinformation related to COVID-19 vaccines on individuals' intentions to get vaccinated [44] The study employed a pre-and-post exposure design, along with a questionnaire, to evaluate the causal effect of encountering online misinformation about COVID-19 and vaccines on the willingness to receive a COVID-19 vaccine, in comparison to exposure to factual information. They found that exposure to false information as of September 2020 led to more than a 6% reduction in the intent to get vaccinated among sample populations in the U.K. and the U.S. Statements that wore the guise of scientific credibility, such as 'the vaccine will alter your DNA,' were found to have the most deleterious impact.

Agents of Disinformation

Both humans and automated agents, known as bots, can spread misinformation and disinformation. Human agents can be classified into two distinct groups: malicious and benign [33]. Malicious users willingly spread disinformation, knowing that the information is false. Human agents can be paid actors or advocates for a particular cause, such as anti-vaccination. Their objective is to sew discord and confusion, which can be deeply consequential in healthcare.

In contrast, benign users share misinformation without knowing the information is false. Benign users may have sincere intentions, for example, to warn people against taking medication they believe to be ineffective. In addition, Benign users may be motivated by affirmative comments in the homogeneous informational echo chamber, such as likes or shares that serve as a self-propagating mechanism.

Social media platforms use content-recommendation algorithms that prioritize content based on user preferences and attitudes. Unfortunately, these algorithms often amplify popular posts to boost user engagement without evaluating the quality or integrity of the content [67]. Troll farms or organized groups deliberately posting contentious material on social networks, have garnered significant reach through platform algorithms. For example, Facebook's engagement-oriented algorithms facilitated Eastern European disinformation campaigns to reach approximately half of the American populace prior to the 2020 presidential election [75]. These troll farms collectively reached a monthly audience of 140 million U.S. users and 360 million global users weekly. Often, these troll farms act as state actors or "cyber troops," described as "teams affiliated with governments, militaries, or political parties aimed at manipulating public opinion on social media" [76]. Since 2010, numerous countries have utilized cyber troops to shape public opinion domestically and internationally.

Software bots are automated tools or scripts that can perform monotonous tasks [77]. However, these bots also function as instruments for disseminating disinformation or executing denial-of-service attacks on networked systems. Remarkably, about 94% of websites have experienced a bot attack [78]. These malicious bots, constituting 26% of all internet traffic, are becoming increasingly sophisticated at mimicking human interactions, making them challenging to identify and block. They enable a wide range of malicious activities, from website and app attacks to API incursions [78]. In 2022, automated internet traffic, commonly known as bots, constituted 47.4% of all online activity, marking a 5.1% increase from the previous year's 42.3%; within this automated traffic, malicious or "bad" bots accounted for 30.2%, up 2.5% from 27.7% in 2021 [78].

Meanwhile, human-generated traffic experienced a notable decline, dropping 5.1% from 57.7% in 2021 to 52.6% in 2022 [78]. According to Imperva's data from the past year [78], 27% of all recorded attacks were attributable to bad bots engaging in business logic abuse. An additional 26% were linked to other forms of automated threats. According to an Imperva Cyber Security report, there has been a staggering 372% increase in malicious bot traffic on healthcare websites since September 2020, with one bot observed making up to 12,000 vaccine appointment requests per hour [78]. Bots have significantly altered the landscape of social media. They create illusions of widespread popularity and endorsement while magnifying certain topics' significance [65]. Such bots effectively propagate conspiracy theories and generate the false perception that misleading information enjoys broad support.

Predisposition to Believe in Disinformation: Social, Cultural and Cognitive Factors

> "As a rule, people don't want to spread false content," he said. "But at a time like this, when people are worried about the virus, headlines like 'Vitamin C Cures Covid' or 'It's All a Hoax' tend to travel widely" [79]

How does disinformation endure in the individual's and in collective mind after the false narrative has been thoroughly corrected and debunked [80]. In 1998, a discredited study published in The Lancet falsely asserted a link between the measles, mumps, and rubella (MMR) vaccine and an increased risk of autism in children [81]. This erroneous claim offered a rudimentary, causal explanation for the onset of autism, contributing to widespread skepticism about childhood vaccine safety, which is a belief held by as many as 33 million Americans [82]. Despite concerted efforts by governmental, scientific, and media institutions to debunk this misinformation [83], public acceptance of false narratives persists. This persistence of continuing to endorse known false information has been associated with a rise in outbreaks of infectious diseases that are preventable with vaccines, such as measles [84]. In times of crisis, conspiracy theories become prevalent, often fulfilling the need for certainty and a sense of control [85]. Anti-science and anti-vaccination disinformation during the COVID-19 pandemic severely hampered the uptake of COVID-19 vaccines, undermining public health efforts to quell the pandemic [86]. This aligns with findings that individuals are likely to gravitate towards online communities that promote scientifically unfounded theories on subjects like vaccines, climate change, and genetically modified food [87].

Many Americans continue to doubt vaccines' safety and effectiveness despite the data and reassurance provided by the CDC, health professionals, and federal and local governments [80]. Keselman and colleagues surveyed the impact of cognitive and cultural factors on attitudes towards vaccinations in general and specific attitudes towards the COVID-19 vaccines [88]. Those factors explored included information literacy, science literacy, attitudes toward science, interpersonal trust, trust in public health institutions, political ideology, and religiosity. Information literacy refers to a set of skills to locate, select, evaluate, and use information efficiently for various purposes [16]. They found that multiple factors shaped general vaccination attitudes. The most significant factors were attitudes toward science and trust in public health institutions. Information literacy, science literacy, and religiosity had a moderate impact. When focusing on attitudes toward COVID-19 vaccines, trust in public health institutions again stood out as the most pivotal factor, followed to a lesser extent by general interpersonal trust, political ideology, and attitudes toward science. Among all the factors examined, public health trust influenced actual COVID-19 vaccination uptake the most. Persuading the public about the safety and efficacy of COVID-19 vaccines remains a formidable challenge for public health authorities. This study emphasizes the critical role of fostering trust in scientific and public health institutions in overcoming this hurdle.

The COVID-19 pandemic is disproportionately affecting ethnic minority communities, thereby amplifying pre-existing inequalities in healthcare access and treatment [89–91]. Data from the COVID States project indicate that, in 2020, African Americans, Hispanics, and Asian Americans all held a greater number of COVID-19 misperceptions relative to non-Hispanic White Americans [92]. Purveyors of vaccine-related misinformation have strategically targeted Black people with inaccurate information to encourage support for the antivaccination cause [91]. These discrepancies have largely persisted within the domain of COVID-19 vaccines [93].

Disparities in susceptibility to misinformation faced by racial and ethnic minority communities are intertwined with medical mistrust, historical inequity, mistreatment, and ongoing systemic and structural barriers [89]. Because of such earned mistrust, timely and accurate health information may fail to connect meaningfully with marginalized communities, deepening social inequities in access to health information and the ability to detect and fend off misinformation. Political ideology and partisan affiliation also powerfully influence individuals' susceptibility to misinformation. Politically conservative individuals are more likely to hold COVID-19 misperceptions than their moderate and liberal counterparts [92]. This finding is consistent with research finding political conservatism associated with individual characteristics that could foster vulnerability to misinformation, such as close-mindedness, intolerance of ambiguity, and homogeneous social networks [94]. In other issue domains, one might find different correlations between political ideology and individuals' susceptibility to misinformation. For example, inequality-driven mistrust contributed to the embrace of misinformation among potentially liberal-leaning Black populations and others regarding the HIV virus and its origins [95].

Racial undertones in certain COVID-19 conspiracy theories are likely to trigger specific racial attitudes and identities, primarily racial resentment and white identity among white populations [54]. Racial resentment is commonly interpreted as a blend of negative feelings toward Black individuals and the belief that they do not adhere to traditional American values. Farhart and Chen argue that these racial perspectives are susceptible to activation by the prevailing social and political climate [54]. As such, they contribute to the endorsement of COVID-19 conspiracy theories, especially when those theories contain explicit racial elements. They found that the construct white identity significantly influences the endorsement of COVID-19 conspiracy theories and adherence to preventive health measures. This emphasizes the pandemic's role as an event that threatens identity, especially for white individuals who were generally more advantaged under the societal norms that existed before the pandemic.

Conversely, the dynamics of racial animus operate distinctly. Individuals harboring racial resentment are notably less inclined to adopt protective behaviors [54]. Intriguingly, these racial attitudes become influential in endorsing conspiracy theories only when those theories are articulated in racial terms. Specifically, when a foreign entity is implicated in the conspiracy theory, individuals with racial resentment are more likely to endorse it.

Trust in science is a complex multidimensional construct. For example, one may believe in the work of science and the scientific method but be wary of scientists [96]. Individuals may regard scientists as experts yet perceive them as emotionally detached and not dedicated to addressing issues relevant to their local communities. In a 2019 study conducted by Pew Research that surveyed a substantial number of U.S. adults, 63% expressed confidence that the scientific method generally yields accurate results [97]. Conversely, 35% believed that the scientific method could be manipulated to support any conclusion desired by the researcher. When public trust in science is anchored in an overly simplistic understanding of the scientific process, the stage is set for potential disillusionment [96]. People with such limited views often expect science to deliver unequivocal answers and become disenchanted when it fails to provide exact predictions or there is no consensus among experts. The presence of scientific debate may be misconstrued as an indicator of the field's unreliability and fallibility. Parties with vested interests exploit this unrealistic vision of science on this naive perception of science, emphasizing uncertainties and divergent opinions on specific issues as a strategy to sway public sentiment regarding broader areas of study [96]. The message conveyed is that scientists can't be trusted.

There are a range of cognitive explanations to account for susceptibility to misinformation and disinformation. Susmann and Wegener explored the role of the continued influence effect (CIE) that purports that the impact of misinformation endures because it provides a measure of coherence with their worldview/mental model or explanation for how the world works [80]. When certain facts or realities conflict with our worldview, we experience cognitive dissonance or incoherence. If a piece of misinformation is central to one's worldview, retracting this misinformation creates a causal gap in the worldview/model, leaving it unclear how initial causes led to outcomes [98]. Susmann and Wegener experimentally demonstrated that a causally incomplete worldview/model (based on the retraction of erroneous information) elicited a sense of psychological discomfort [80]. This may cause the individual to retain fragments or some enduring belief in the discounted model despite knowing that some facts are incorrect. There is an implicit commitment to maintain some coherence in one's causal account or worldview/mental model, even if that means not letting go of information known to be inaccurate. We see this play out in the political arena, where individuals continue to cling to the notion that the 2020 presidential election was stolen despite knowing that the evidence shows to the contrary.

Humans respond to existential threats by compensatory mechanisms that restore psychological equilibrium [99]. The pandemic has disrupted lives on a massive scale, and we cannot discount this fact as an explanatory force. For more than 2 years, people have been living with a lot of uncertainty, causing increased anxiety and irrational thinking [100]. These conditions have made spreading false information, conspiracy theories, and blame on immigrants easier [65]. Many studies have looked at why people think in biased or irrational ways. This is best exemplified by the heuristic and biases program pioneered by Tversky and Kahneman [101]. This program has informed cognitive theories that endeavor to explain external conditions that lead to receptivity to disinformation, conspiracy theories, and the psychological states that predispose individuals to process information selectively.

Dow et al. propose a comprehensive framework explaining why the pandemic's social and cognitive disruptions have made some individuals susceptible to harmful conspiracy theories [65]. The disorienting effects of lockdowns, business shutdowns, and mask mandates contributed to feelings of loss of control or reduced personal agency. The 25% surge in internet use following lockdown measures [102] suggests that people turned to social media as a coping mechanism to regain some semblance of control [65]. While the pandemic undermined traditional social interactions and heightened loneliness and isolation, engagement on social media platforms enabled many to fulfill their basic needs for social connection and belonging [65].

Kahneman and Tversky's [101] seminal heuristics and biases program partly gave rise to interesting new lines of research investigating how social beliefs inform science-related decisions. The notion that belief in false political news is primarily fueled by partisanship is widely supported [103]. Such beliefs can influence individuals to heed or disregard evidence in science-related decisions. A study by Zhao et al. established a link between people's media preferences and their pandemic-related behaviors in the United States [104]. For example, individuals who viewed Fox News as a reliable source than mainstream media were more likely to engage in risky behaviors and less likely to take preventive measures against COVID-19, such as wearing face masks [96].

Kahan introduces the concept of "Identity Protective Cognition" (IPC) as a mechanism to explain this phenomenon. IPC suggests that people are inclined to selectively embrace or reject information based on whether it aligns with their group's prevailing beliefs [95]. This aligns with findings that individuals will likely gravitate towards online communities promoting scientifically unfounded theories on subjects like vaccines. It may also suggest that those with a strong sense of white identity may be partial to conspiracy theories that blame outsiders or foreigners. Kahan's review of diverse research on scientific decision-making [103] indicated that individuals process information to reinforce beliefs consistent with their identity rather than striving for factual accuracy. For issues like fracking or climate change, responses can be anticipated based on one's position on the liberal-conservative spectrum. However, political orientation seems to have less impact on beliefs for less politically charged topics, such as genetically modified food.

Pennycook and his colleagues challenge the notion that Identity Protective Cognition (IPC) is the primary cognitive framework for susceptibility to fake news [105, 106]. They base their argument on Kahneman's dual-process theory [107], which differentiates between System 1 and System 2 thinking. The two systems capture an essential difference between cognitive processes that seem automatic, for example, involving pattern recognition and those processes that engage more in the way of cognitive resources. System 1 thinking is quick, intuitive, and requires minimal cognitive effort, for example, finding one's car in a parking lot. System 2 thinking is deliberate, analytical, and cognitively demanding. System 2 thinking would be invoked in any sort of problem-solving or decision-making process. In their research, Pennycook and Rand used the Cognitive Reflection Test (CRT) to assess an individual's inclination toward analytical thinking [106]. They presented participants with 15 accurate and 15 fake news headlines, categorized as Democrat-consistent, Republican-consistent, or politically neutral. Their findings revealed a positive correlation between a predisposition to analytical thinking and the ability to distinguish between genuine and fake news. Interestingly, the political alignment of the headlines did not significantly influence these outcomes.

Pennycook and Rand argue that susceptibility to fake news is more likely attributed to inattentive System 1 thinking than to politically biased reasoning [106]. However, it is crucial to acknowledge that these experimental findings require validation in real-world scenarios. It is plausible that both IPC mechanisms and lazy System 1 thinking could make individuals prone to misinformation. Furthermore, deeper personal involvement in controversy may activate IPC-like reasoning when assessing the truthfulness of a claim.

In summary, there are many explanations as to why an individual would be vulnerable to misinformation. Social, cultural and cognitive factors all likely play a significant role in their processing of information.

Mitigating Misinformation Madness

> [T]he basic issues involved in presenting information on the internet have changed little since Gutenberg first pulled the lever on his printing press... there are standards by which to judge the quality of editorial content, to differentiate author from shill, editorial from advertising, education from promotion, evidence from opinion, science from hype. [108]

Fast forwarding approximately a quarter of a century, it is imperative to recognize that social media has fundamentally transformed the domain of health information dissemination. The statement above, published in the American Medical Association's flagship journal, suggests an earnest agreement between producers and consumers of health information. Yet, as elaborated in this chapter, the landscape teems with malevolent entities and well-intentioned but misinformed individuals who disseminate disinformation that can proliferate with alarming rapidity. There have been numerous efforts to mitigate the spread of disinformation. In this section, we consider the prospects of developing more enlightened citizens who are more information literate and also possess greater degrees of science literacy. We briefly discuss various cognitive and behavioral initiatives. Finally, we consider efforts by social media platforms to contain the spread of disinformation.

In the first decade of the World Wide Web's existence, various approaches have been proposed to address the quality of health information, ranging from purely human-driven solutions to entirely machine-based methods [16]. The DISCERN instrument emerged from a comprehensive collaboration involving a diverse array of information users, including physicians, librarians, health communicators, patient support group representatives, individuals from the medical publishing sector, medical journalists, and researchers. The initial impetus of developing the DISCERN instrument was to assist healthcare professionals and patients in evaluating the quality of written information about health treatments [16].

The instrument, which can serve as both a benchmark and a checklist for content developers, has 15 discrete criteria for users to assess websites and uses a 5-point Likert scale (1 indicates "Serious or extensive shortcomings," to 5, signifying "Minimal shortcomings"). For healthcare providers, it offers a framework for selecting patient educational content. For consumers and patients, it serves as a decision-support tool. Some of the questions include: *Are the aims clear? Does the publication achieve its aims? Is it relevant? Is it clear what sources of information were used to compile the publication (other than the author or producer)? Is it clear when the information used or reported in the publication was produced? Is it balanced and unbiased? Does it refer to areas of uncertainty?* As indicated by the criteria outlined above, the DISCERN instrument can aid a health consumer in making informed decisions regarding medical content on a website [16]. While it may not be directly applicable to brief social media communications, like tweets or Facebook posts, consider a scenario where an individual possesses a certain level of information literacy and has internalized these questions. The supposition is that such knowledge would be valuable in forming assessments about a message and its originator.

Guyatt and colleagues coined the term "evidence-based medicine" or EBM, which he defines as "the conscientious, explicit, and judicious use of current best [research-based] evidence in making decisions about the care of individual patients" [109]. This was viewed as the standard for practice and decision-making by healthcare providers [4]. We can't expect the exact same standard for laypeople as health professionals. Then the question is what the minimum level of scientific knowledge necessary. To address the question of what general knowledge in science the public should possess, science education has introduced the concept of science literacy, which consists of multiple components [110]. These components of science literacy can be represented as follows: Knowledge of science (knowledge of facts, laws, and theories), Knowledge about science (knowledge about scientific methods), and Attitudes toward science (attitudes toward the role of science in society and about the scientists' intentions).

Individuals with limited scientific understanding are susceptible to belief systems that could result in less-than-ideal decision-making and poor outcomes [4]. Lacking a solid knowledge base, such individuals have no inherent reason to favor biological explanations for health and disease. The dilemma is that high school and even introductory college biology classes do not prepare individuals to grapple with issues such as the appropriate treatment and other health issues. Health science education classes that employ concepts from the biological sciences to health issues may provide a foundation for evaluating health information and making sound decisions.

Understanding of science encompasses familiarity with the methods, tools, and principles employed to generate scientific knowledge [4]. Scientific inquiry involves skill sets related to data collection, such as designing experiments, planning observations, and gathering measurements. Mastering scientific inquiry, students become acquainted with sampling methods, sample size considerations, measurement accuracy, and variable control. On the other hand, scientific explanation entails synthesizing collected data with pre-existing knowledge to draw informed conclusions. This stage utilizes the findings from the inquiry process to achieve the objectives of scientific investigations.

Another element increasingly highlighted in science education is understanding the Nature of Science (NOS) as a collective enterprise [4]. These principles involve understanding that science is a human endeavor to obtain knowledge about natural phenomena. This endeavor is based on empirical evidence and generates dynamic and self-correcting knowledge, open to revisions based on new emerging evidence. It is an inherently imperfect and iterative process. When confronted with a novel and deeply consequential problem like COVID-19, science can seem chaotic, uncertain, and without answers to address the deadly pandemic. On the other hand, disinformation can be very easy to comprehend and has a certain seductive appeal, especially when it plays to one's bias. Understanding science as an iterative, imperfect process may serve to mitigate the acceptance of disinformation and conspiracy theories.

Zhao et al. reviewed efforts at misinformation correction through behavioral and cognitive change [90]. Growing concerns about the prevalence and impact of misinformation have spurred efforts to identify and evaluate strategies for correction. Notable examples of such corrective approaches include fact-checking [111], news literacy programs [112] and nudges toward accuracy [113]. The evidence from various contexts suggests that corrective messaging can be effective. However, the effectiveness of such corrections in fully neutralizing the impact of misinformation remains questionable. A recent meta-analysis focused on interventions to counter COVID-19 misinformation included 16 studies involving 33,378 participants [114]. Although the mean effect size indicated a positive but not statistically significant, a closer examination of individual studies revealed modest and mixed effect sizes. Some patterns emerged from moderation analysis, suggesting that factors such as high issue involvement, attitude-based outcomes, and text-based correction messages yielded larger effect sizes. Behavioral and cognitive interventions show some promise, but research is still at a relatively early stage.

Numerous online tools aimed at combating misinformation have been devised [115]. These range from educational resources and bot-detection software to algorithms for detecting misinformation, propagation models, and credibility assessments. Some tools employ statistical patterns and machine-learning algorithms for operation, while others rely on non-automated approaches like crowdsourcing or manual fact-checking [115]. Social media platforms attempt to thwart conspiracy theorists and demagogues.

Before Elon Musk's involvement, platforms like Facebook, YouTube, and Twitter (now X) had consistently thwarted numerous covert yet highly orchestrated "information operations [116]." These operations are frequently deployed by politicians, advocacy groups, and foreign entities to disseminate discord and misinformation. Unfortunately, these platforms have been less stringent in dealing with "superspreaders," who operate openly [116]. Much of the harm and misinformation is not disseminated by anonymous bots but by well-known, often verified, users. These individuals commonly include influencers, public figures, politicians, or celebrities who may be monetizing their reach, advocating a political stance, promoting a cause, or opposing vaccines. Platforms are often hesitant to remove such users because their large following equates to significant engagement, generating substantial advertising revenue for the platforms [116]. Rather than taking more stringent measures, most major social media platforms predominantly rely on fact-checking services. As an illustrative example, Facebook forwards its most popular and broadly circulated posts to one of its 90 international fact-checking partners for assessment. Posts deemed false or misleading by these organizations are subsequently labeled accordingly and deprioritized in Facebook's news feed to reduce their visibility to users [116].

In recent years, algorithms have been incorporated into fact-checking pipelines. They are used to flag previously fact-checked misinformation and suggest which trending claims should be prioritized for fact-checking—a paradigm [117]. It is a useful but imperfect process [116]. Platforms such as Facebook and Twitter have had greater success in flagging and removing hate speech [63].

A recurring theme in this paper is the interplay between xenophobia and the spread and magnification of misinformation. The serious risks associated with the pandemic, compounded by societal uncertainty and perceived loss of freedoms, have fueled hate speech and conspiratorial narratives on a global scale. Political leaders and public influencers have either spearheaded these movements or, at the very least, tacitly supported them. Such dynamics pose a significant challenge to initiatives aimed at curtailing the proliferation and acceptance of false information.

To conquer the misinfodemic, a multifaceted strategy will be necessary. Individuals need to be better equipped with literacy tools to process health information strategically. Technological advances in flagging and removing false information are necessary for the solution. Social media platforms try to balance allowing individuals to express themselves freely and vigorously moderating malevolent posts containing fraudulent information and hate speech.

Conclusions

Social media will continue to be the primary vehicle for spreading misinformation or disinformation. Public health must develop new strategies to counterbalance the harmful impact of health-related misinformation and disinformation through these unregulated and unchecked platforms. Psychosocial or cognitive approaches are critical to understanding why individuals intentionally or unintentionally gravitate towards misinformation and disinformation, conspiratorial thinking, and skepticism towards science, medicine, healthcare systems, government institutions (i.e., the CDC, NIH) and adjacent health-related entities (e.g., Big Pharma, the World Health Organization). More research is needed to understand further the complex interplay between cognitive, social, and cultural factors that make individuals receptive to embracing misinformation and disinformation. We should also continue to explore cognitive and HCI approaches to better understand and diminish the impact of disinformation on social media. The **pernicious** COVID-19 **Infodemic** revealed how dangerous misinformation and disinformation can be during a public health crisis by fostering uncertainty and skepticism in scientific evidence-based best practices and policies, resulting in high levels of anxiety, paranoia, and delusional thinking.

Discussion Questions
1. Why is health misinformation and disinformation an important issue in relation to the delivery of healthcare and as a matter of public health?
2. Explain how social media has amplified the spread of health misinformation.
3. What are some of the distinctions between the different forms of false information and why is it important to understand them?
4. What is the relationship between xenophobia, racism, and the spread of conspiracy theories?
5. What are some of the factors that predispose individuals and groups to be receptive to disinformation?
6. What are some of the strategies we can use to mitigate misinformation and reduce the harm caused by them?

References

1. O'Connor C, Weatherall JO. The misinformation age: how false beliefs spread. Yale University Press; 2019.
2. Escandón K, et al. COVID-19 false dichotomies and a comprehensive review of the evidence regarding public health, COVID-19 symptomatology, SARS-CoV-2 transmission, mask wearing, and reinfection. BMC Infect Dis. 2021;21(1):1–47.
3. Wang Y, Thier K, Nan X. Defining health misinformation. In: Keselman A, Arnott Smith C, Wilson AJ, editors. Combating online health misinformation: a professional's guide to helping the public. Rowman & Littlefield; 2022. p. 3–16.
4. Keselman A. The case of everyday science. In: Keselman A, Arnott Smith C, Wilson AJ, editors. Combating online health misinformation: a professional's guide to helping the public. Rowman & Littlefield; 2022. p. 91.
5. World Health Organization. Novel coronavirus(2019-nCoV) situation report - 13. 2020.
6. Kaufman DR, Jumbo AE, Taylor TN. The ecology of online health information and COVID-19 misinformation. In: Keselman A, Arnott Smith C, Wilson AJ, editors. Combating online health misinformation: a professional's guide to helping the public. Rowman & Littlefield; 2022. p. 17.
7. Ghebreyesus TA. Munich security conference. In: World Health Organization newsletter. WHO; 2020.
8. DATAREPORTAL. Overview of social media use. In: Global social media statistics; 2023.
9. Di Sotto S, Viviani M. Health misinformation detection in the social web: an overview and a data science approach. Int J Environ Res Public Health. 2022;19(4):2173.
10. Lwin MO, et al. Global sentiments surrounding the COVID-19 pandemic on Twitter: analysis of Twitter trends. JMIR Public Health Surveill. 2020;6(2):e19447.
11. Restrepo NJ, Larson H. Mainstreaming of conspiracy theories and misinformation. arXiv preprint arXiv:2102.02382. 2021.
12. Velásquez N, et al. Hate multiverse spreads malicious COVID-19 content online beyond individual platform control. arXiv preprint arXiv:2004.00673. 2020.
13. Hickey D, et al. Auditing Elon Musk's impact on hate speech and bots. Paper presented at: Proceedings of the international AAAI conference on web and social media. 2023.
14. Israel S. Musk defames the ADL. The Hill. 2023.
15. Jimison HB, et al. The role of human computer interaction in consumer health applications: current state, challenges and the future. In: Patel VL, Kannampallil TG, Kaufman DR, editors. Cognitive informatics for biomedicine: human computer interaction in healthcare; 2015. p. 259–78.
16. Arnott Smith C, Keselman A. Consumer health informatics: enabling digital health for everyone. Chapman and Hall/CRC; 2020.
17. Moorhead SA, et al. A new dimension of health care: systematic review of the uses, benefits, and limitations of social media for health communication. J Med Internet Res. 2013;15(4):e1933.
18. Chou WS, et al. Web 2.0 for health promotion: reviewing the current evidence. Am J Public Health. 2013;103(1):e9–e18.
19. Preece J, Sharp H, Rogers Y. Interaction design beyond human-computer interaction. Wiley; 2019.
20. Dourish P, Bellotti V. Awareness and coordination in shared workspaces. Paper presented at: Proceedings of the 1992 ACM Conference on Computer-supported Cooperative Work. 1992.
21. Shibuya Y, Hamm A, Pargman TC. Mapping HCI research methods for studying social media interaction: a systematic literature review. Comput Hum Behav. 2022;129:107131.
22. Li Y-J, et al. Health misinformation on social media: a systematic literature review and future research directions. AIS Trans Hum-Comput Interact. 2022;14(2):116–49.
23. Cinelli M, et al. The COVID-19 social media infodemic. Sci Rep. 2020;10(1):1–10.

24. Zannettou S, et al. The web of false information: rumors, fake news, hoaxes, clickbait, and various other shenanigans. J Data Inf Qual (JDIQ). 2019;11(3):1–37.
25. Arkhipova A, Brodie I. Flies in the ointment. In: Keselman A, Arnott Smith C, Wilson AJ, editors. Combating online health misinformation: a professional's guide to helping the public. Rowman & Littlefield; 2022. p. 45.
26. Wardle C, Derakhshan H. Information disorder: Toward an interdisciplinary framework for research and policymaking, vol. 27. Council of Europe Strasbourg; 2017.
27. Swire-Thompson B, Lazer D. Public health and online misinformation: challenges and recommendations. Annu Rev Public Health. 2020;41(1):433–51.
28. Lazer DM, et al. The science of fake news. Science. 2018;359(6380):1094–6.
29. Caramancion KM An exploration of disinformation as a cybersecurity threat. Paper presented at: 2020 3rd International Conference on Information and Computer Technologies (ICICT). IEEE; 2020.
30. Williamson E. Here's what Jones has said about Sandy Hook. New York Times. 2022.
31. Tandoc EC Jr, Lim ZW, Ling R. Defining "fake news": a typology of scholarly definitions. Digit Journal. 2018;6(2):137–53.
32. Waszak PM, Kasprzycka-Waszak W, Kubanek A. The spread of medical fake news in social media–the pilot quantitative study. Health Policy Technol. 2018;7(2):115–8.
33. Di Domenico G, et al. Fake news, social media and marketing: a systematic review. J Bus Res. 2021;124:329–41.
34. Allcott H, Gentzkow M. Social media and fake news in the 2016 election. J Econ Perspect. 2017;31(2):211–36.
35. Asubiaro TV, Rubin VL. Comparing features of fabricated and legitimate political news in digital environments (2016-2017). Proc Assoc Inf Sci Technol. 2018;55(1):747–50.
36. Center for Disease Control and Prevention. Diabetes fast facts. 2023. Available from: https://www.cdc.gov/diabetes/basics/quick-facts.html
37. American Diabetes Association. Get smart about risks and diabetes prevention. [cited 2024 Jun 7]. Available from: https://diabetes.org/about-diabetes/diabetes-prevention
38. Keselman A, et al. Evaluating the quality of health information in a changing digital ecosystem. J Med Internet Res. 2019;21(2):e11129.
39. Broniatowski DA, et al. Weaponized health communication: Twitter bots and Russian trolls amplify the vaccine debate. Am J Public Health. 2018;108(10):1378–84.
40. Larson HJ. The biggest pandemic risk? Viral misinformation. Nature. 2018;562(7726):309–10.
41. Betsch C, et al. Opportunities and challenges of Web 2.0 for vaccination decisions. Vaccine. 2012;30(25):3727–33.
42. Jones AM, et al. Parents' source of vaccine information and impact on vaccine attitudes, beliefs, and nonmedical exemptions. Adv Prev Med. 2012;2012:1–8.
43. Witteman HO, Zikmund-Fisher BJ. The defining characteristics of Web 2.0 and their potential influence in the online vaccination debate. Vaccine. 2012;30(25):3734–40.
44. Loomba S, et al. Measuring the impact of COVID-19 vaccine misinformation on vaccination intent in the UK and USA. Nat Hum Behav. 2021;5(3):337–48.
45. The Center for Countering Digital Hate. The disinformation dozen: why platforms must act on twelve leading online anti-Vaxxers. Center for Countering Digital Hate Ltd.; 2021.
46. Wikipedia. Naomi Wolf. 2023. Available from: https://en.wikipedia.org/wiki/Naomi_Wolf
47. Klein N. Doppelganger: a trip into the mirror world. New York: Farrar, Straus and Giroux; 2023.
48. BBC News. Covid: Twitter suspends Naomi Wolf after tweeting anti-vaccine misinformation. 2021 Jun 6 [cited 2024 Jun 15]. Available from: https://www.bbc.com/news/world-us-canada-57374241
49. Wolf N. The bodies of others: the new authoritarians, COVID-19 and the war against the human. All Seasons Press; 2022.
50. Wadman M. Florida private school threatens jobs of teachers who seek COVID-19 vaccines. Science. 2021. Internet.

51. Governor of Florida. Governor Ron DeSantis signs legislation to protect Florida jobs. 2021.
52. Sarkissian A. Florida surgeon general rejects FDA guidance, urges people under 65 not to get covid booster. Politico. 2023.
53. Silva HM. The xenophobia virus and the COVID-19 pandemic. Ethique Sante. 2021;18(2):102–6.
54. Farhart CE, Chen PG. Racialized pandemic: the effect of racial attitudes on COVID-19 conspiracy theory beliefs. Front Polit Sci. 2022;4:648061.
55. Farmer P. Infections and inequalities: the modern plagues. Univ of California Press; 2001.
56. Mann JM. Statement at an informal briefing on AIDS to the 42nd session of the United Nations General Assembly. J R Stat Soc Ser A (Stat Soc). 1988;151(1):131–6.
57. Dionne KY, Turkmen FF. The politics of pandemic othering: putting COVID-19 in global and historical context. Int Organ. 2020;74(S1):E213–30.
58. Markel H, Stern AM. The foreignness of germs: the persistent association of immigrants and disease in American society. Milbank Q. 2002;80(4):757–88.
59. Royles D. Why black AIDS history matters. In: Black perspectives. Internet: African American Intellectual History Society; 2022.
60. Hirsch VM, et al. An African primate lentivirus (SIVsm) closely related to HIV-2. Nature. 1989;339(6223):389–92.
61. King MT, et al. Rumor, Chinese diets, and COVID-19: questions and answers about Chinese food and eating habits. Gastron J Food Stud. 2021;21(1):77–82.
62. Walker D, Daniel Anders A. "China Virus" and "Kung-Flu": a critical race case study of Asian American journalists' experiences during COVID-19. Cult Stud Crit Methodol. 2022;22(1):76–88.
63. Perez AL. The "hate speech" policies of major platforms during the COVID-19 pandemic. UNESCO; 2021. p. 32.
64. Gover AR, Harper SB, Langton L. Anti-Asian hate crime during the COVID-19 pandemic: exploring the reproduction of inequality. Am J Crim Justice. 2020;45:647–67.
65. Dow BJ, et al. The COVID-19 pandemic and the search for structure: social media and conspiracy theories. Soc Personal Psychol Compass. 2021;15(9):e12636.
66. Goodwin J. Gab: everything you need to know about the fast-growing, controversial social network. CNN.COM. 2021.
67. Lupi V. COVID-19 and fake news in the social media Bruno Kessler Foundation. Fondazione Bruno Kessler; 2020.
68. Lee JJ, et al. Associations between COVID-19 misinformation exposure and belief with COVID-19 knowledge and preventive behaviors: cross-sectional online study. J Med Internet Res. 2020;22(11):e22205.
69. The U.S. Surgeon General's Advisory on Building a Healthy Information Environment. Confronting health misinformation. Human Health and Services; 2021. Internet.
70. Gottfried J, Shearer E. News use across social media platforms 2016. Pew Research Center; 2016.
71. Kennedy B, et al. Introducing the Gab Hate Corpus: defining and applying hate-based rhetoric to social media posts at scale. Lang Resour Eval. 2022;56:79–108.
72. Naeem SB, Bhatti R, Khan A. An exploration of how fake news is taking over social media and putting public health at risk. Health Info Libr J. 2021;38(2):143–9.
73. Vosoughi S, Roy D, Aral S. The spread of true and false news online. Science. 2018;359(6380):1146–51.
74. Kotseva B, et al. Trend analysis of COVID-19 mis/disinformation narratives-a 3-year study. PLoS One. 2023;18(11):e0291423.
75. Hao K. Troll farms reached 140 million Americans a month on Facebook before 2020 election, internal report shows. MIT Technology Review. 2021 Sep 16.
76. Bradshaw S, Howard P. Troops, trolls and troublemakers: a global inventory of organized social media manipulation. In: Computational propaganda research project. Oxford Internet Institute; 2017.

77. Eslahi M, Salleh R, Anuar NB. Bots and botnets: an overview of characteristics, detection and challenges. Paper presented at: 2012 IEEE International Conference on Control System, Computing and Engineering. IEEE; 2012.
78. Imperva. Imperva bad bot report 2023. 2023.
79. Carey B. A theory about conspiracy theories. New York Times. 2020.
80. Susmann MW, Wegener DT. The role of discomfort in the continued influence effect of misinformation. Mem Cognit. 2022;50(2):435–48.
81. Rao TS, Andrade C. The MMR vaccine and autism: sensation, refutation, retraction, and fraud. Indian J Psychiatry. 2011;53(2):95–6.
82. Reinhart R. Fewer in US continue to see vaccines as important. Gallup; 2020.
83. Kata A. A postmodern Pandora's box: anti-vaccination misinformation on the internet. Vaccine. 2010;28(7):1709–16.
84. Smith CA, Keselman A. Consumer health informatics: enabling digital health for everyone. Chapman & Hall/CRC Press; 2021.
85. Keselman A, Smith CA, Wilson AJ. Combating online health misinformation: a professional's guide to helping the public. Rowman & Littlefield; 2022.
86. Cornwall W. Officials gird for a war on vaccine misinformation. Science. 2020;369(6499):14–5.
87. Hmielowski JD, et al. An attack on science? Media use, trust in scientists, and perceptions of global warming. Public Underst Sci. 2014;23(7):866–83.
88. Keselman A, et al. Cognitive and cultural factors that affect general vaccination and COVID-19 vaccination attitudes. Vaccine. 2022;11(1):94.
89. Krishnan L, Ogunwole SM, Cooper LA. Historical insights on coronavirus disease 2019 (COVID-19), the 1918 influenza pandemic, and racial disparities: illuminating a path forward. Ann Intern Med. 2020;173(6):474–81.
90. Zhao X, et al. Openness to change among COVID misinformation endorsers: associations with social demographic characteristics and information source usage. Soc Sci Med. 2023;335:116233.
91. Southwell BG, et al. Health misinformation exposure and health disparities: observations and opportunities. Annu Rev Public Health. 2023;44:113–30.
92. Druckman JN, et al. The role of race, religion, and partisanship in misperceptions about COVID-19. Group Process Intergroup Relat. 2021;24(4):638–57.
93. Ognyanova K, et al. Covid-19 vaccine misinformation trends (No. 82), the Covid States Project: a 50-state covid-19 survey. The Covid States Project. 2022.
94. Jost JT, et al. Ideological asymmetries in conformity, desire for shared reality, and the spread of misinformation. Curr Opin Psychol. 2018;23:77–83.
95. Jaiswal J, LoSchiavo C, Perlman DC. Disinformation, misinformation and inequality-driven mistrust in the time of COVID-19: lessons unlearned from AIDS denialism. AIDS Behav. 2020;24:2776–80.
96. Keselman A, Wilson AJ. An examination of the multiple dimensions of public trust in science as health misinformation roadblocks. In: Keselman A, Arnott Smith C, Wilson AJ, editors. Combating online health misinformation: a professional's guide to helping the public. Rowman & Littlefield; 2022. p. 105.
97. Funk C. Key findings about Americans' confidence in science and their views on scientists' role in society. Pew Research Center; 2020.
98. Hamby A, Ecker U, Brinberg D. How stories in memory perpetuate the continued influence of false information. J Consum Psychol. 2020;30(2):240–59.
99. Simchon A, et al. Beyond doubt in a dangerous world: the effect of existential threats on the certitude of societal discourse. J Exp Soc Psychol. 2021;97:104221.
100. Grimes DR. Medical disinformation and the unviable nature of COVID-19 conspiracy theories. PLoS One. 2021;16(3):e0245900.
101. Kahneman D, Slovic P, Tversky A. Judgment under uncertainty: heuristics and biases. Cambridge University Press; 1982.

102. Rizzo L, Click S. How COVID-19 changed Americans' internet habits. Wall Street Journal. 2020.
103. Kahan DM. Misconceptions, misinformation, and the logic of identity-protective cognition. In: Cultural cognition project working paper 2017. Yale Law School; 2017.
104. Zhao Y, Da J, Yan J. Detecting health misinformation in online health communities: incorporating behavioral features into machine learning based approaches. Inf Process Manag. 2021;58(1):102390.
105. Pennycook G, et al. Fighting COVID-19 misinformation on social media: experimental evidence for a scalable accuracy-nudge intervention. Psychol Sci. 2020;31(7):770–80.
106. Pennycook G, Rand DG. Lazy, not biased: susceptibility to partisan fake news is better explained by lack of reasoning than by motivated reasoning. Cognition. 2019;188:39–50.
107. Kahneman D. Thinking, fast and slow. New York: Macmillan; 2011.
108. Silberg WM, Lundberg GD, Musacchio RA. Assessing, controlling, and assuring the quality of medical information on the internet: caveant lector et viewor—let the reader and viewer beware. JAMA. 1997;277(15):1244–5.
109. Guyatt G, et al. Evidence-based medicine: a new approach to teaching the practice of medicine. JAMA. 1992;268(17):2420–5.
110. Bybee R, McCrae B, Laurie R. PISA 2006: an assessment of scientific literacy. J Res Sci Teach. 2009;46(8):865–83.
111. Nyhan B, et al. Taking fact-checks literally but not seriously? The effects of journalistic fact-checking on factual beliefs and candidate favorability. Polit Behav. 2020;42:939–60.
112. Vraga EK, Bode L, Tully M. Creating news literacy messages to enhance expert corrections of misinformation on Twitter. Commun Res. 2022;49(2):245–67.
113. Pennycook G, et al. Shifting attention to accuracy can reduce misinformation online. Nature. 2021;592(7855):590–5.
114. Janmohamed K, et al. Interventions to mitigate COVID-19 misinformation: a systematic review and meta-analysis. J Health Commun. 2021;26(12):846–57.
115. Czerniak K, et al. A scoping review of digital health interventions for combating COVID-19 misinformation and disinformation. J Am Med Inform Assoc. 2023;30(4):752–60.
116. Waldrop MM. How to mitigate misinformation. Proc Natl Acad Sci. 2023;120(36):e2314143120.
117. Neumann T, Wolczynski N. Does AI-assisted fact-checking disproportionately benefit majority groups online? Paper presented at: Proceedings of the 2023 ACM Conference on Fairness, Accountability, and Transparency. 2023.

Further Reading

Keselman A, Smith CA, Wilson AJ. Combating online health misinformation: a professional's guide to helping the public. Rowman & Littlefield; 2022.
Klein N. Doppelganger: a trip into the mirror world. New York: Farrar, Straus and Giroux; 2023.
Li Y-J, et al. Health misinformation on social media: a systematic literature review and future research directions. AIS Trans Hum-Comput Interact. 2022;14(2):116–49.
Southwell BG, et al. Health misinformation exposure and health disparities: observations and opportunities. Annu Rev. Public Health. 2023;44:113–30.

Chapter 9
Visual Analytics: Leveraging Cognitive Principles to Accelerate Biomedical Discoveries

Suresh K. Bhavnani

Introduction

The *Open Science* movement (e.g., data from NIH-funded studies being made publicly available), combined with access to electronic health records, in addition to rapid advances in the development of inexpensive high throughput technologies (e.g., multiplex assays for measuring whole genome data across many patients) has resulted in vast digital resources accessible by both scientists and the lay public [1]. However, the sheer magnitude of such resources far exceeds our cognitive abilities to exploit them for the prevention, diagnosis, and treatment of diseases. For example, translational teams consisting of biologists, clinicians, and epidemiologists increasingly need to integrate and comprehend the relationships among large and disparate types of information including molecular, biochemical, and environmental variables, with the goal of comprehending complex phenomena such as heterogeneities and corresponding pathways underlying different diseases.

One approach to integrate and comprehend such vast and disparate information is through methods being developed in the field of visual analytics. This chapter begins by presenting an overview of the evolving theoretical foundations for visual analytics, and the cognitive and task-based motivations to use methods from this field to help comprehend complex biomedical data. Next, the chapter provides a brief overview of visual analytical applications in the biomedical domain, with a demonstration of how to use one of the most advanced forms of visual analytics called networks, which are particularly useful for analyzing complex molecular and

---

S. K. Bhavnani (✉)
Department of Biostatistics and Data Science, School of Public and Population Health,
Institute for Translational Sciences, University of Texas Medical Branch,
Galveston, TX, USA
e-mail: subhavna@utmb.edu

© The Author(s), under exclusive license to Springer Nature
Switzerland AG 2024
A. W. Kushniruk et al. (eds.), *Human Computer Interaction in Healthcare*,
Cognitive Informatics in Biomedicine and Healthcare,
https://doi.org/10.1007/978-3-031-69947-4_9

clinical data. These analyses reveal the strengths and limitations of network analysis, which are critical for its practical use to analyze ever increasing and complex biomedical data. The chapter concludes with theoretical, applied, and pedagogical hurdles that need to be addressed through future research which will enable visual analytics to fully realize its potential in accelerating biomedical discoveries.

Visual Analytics: Theoretical Foundations[1]

Visual analytics is defined as the science of analytical reasoning, facilitated by interactive visual interfaces [3]. The primary goal of visual analytics is to augment cognitive reasoning by translating symbolic data (e.g., numbers in a spreadsheet) into *visualizations* (e.g., a scatter plot) which can be manipulated through *interaction* (e.g., highlight only some data points in the scatter plot). As discussed below, visualizations, and interaction with those visualizations, are powerful for helping analysts comprehend complex relationships in biomedical data because of the nature of human cognition, and the nature of tasks performed by analysts.

Why Do Visualizations Matter?

Visualizations of data are often powerful because they leverage the massively parallel architecture of the human visual system consisting of the eye and the visual cortex of the brain [4]. This parallel cognitive architecture enables the rapid comprehension of multiple graphical relationships simultaneously, which often leads to insights about relationships in complex data such as similarities, trends, and anomalies [3]. For example, Fig. 9.1a shows a spreadsheet representing the systolic blood pressure of patients before and after taking a drug. The task of determining which of the two conditions have more patients with systolic >140 is time consuming and error prone because the analyst has to compare the number in each cell with 140, remember the result of each comparison, and then make a final count to determine which column has a higher number of patients with systolic >140. Such symbolic processing is serial in nature, and therefore highly dependent on the number of data points, which when large can quickly overwhelm an analyst.

In contrast, as shown in Fig. 9.1b, if all cells in the spreadsheet with values >140 are colored red, the resulting visual representation enables processing of red cells in each column to be conducted in parallel, resulting in a more rapid determination that the left column has more red cells compared to the right column. Such parallel processing is independent of the number of cells, and therefore scales up well to

---

[1] Portions of this section appeared in Bhavnani et al. [2]. With kind permission from Springer Science+Business Media.

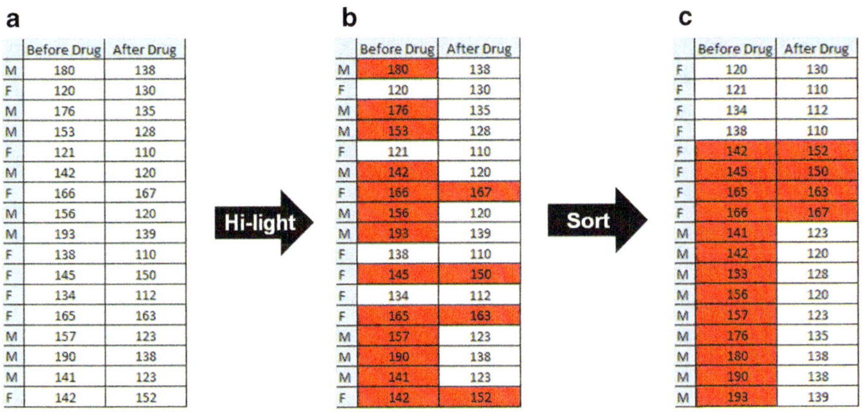

Fig. 9.1 An example of how symbolic data in a spreadsheet (**a**) when converted into a visual representation (**b**) leverages the parallel processing abilities of the visual cortex which enables faster comprehension of patterns in the data. Because visual processing is parallel in nature, it scales to handle large amounts of data. When the same data is sorted by sex (**c**), the visual representation reveals yet another pattern demonstrating how interaction with the data is a critical aspect of visual analytics, and can guide the verification of the patterns using the appropriate quantitative measures

large amounts of data. Data visualizations therefore help to shift processing from the slower symbolic processing areas of the human brain, to the faster graphical parallel processing of the visual cortex enabling detection of patterns in large and complex biomedical data sets. Furthermore, by externalizing key aspects of the task, the representation in Fig. 9.1b shifts information from an internal to an external representation, making other tasks such as counting the number of patients with systolic >140 in each column much easier [5].

Unfortunately, not all data visualizations are effective in augmenting cognition. For example, a road map pointing south is not effective for a driver who is facing north because it requires a mental rotation of the map before it can be useful for navigation. Similarly, an organizational chart of employee names and their locations laid out in a hierarchy based on seniority is not very useful if the task is to determine patterns related to the geographical distribution of the employees. Finally, if a chart has an incorrect or missing legend and axes labels, the visualization is difficult to comprehend because it cannot be mapped to concepts in the data. Therefore visualizations need to be aligned with mental representations of the user [6], tasks [7], and data, before those visualizations can be effective in augmenting cognition.

Why Does Interactivity Matter?

While static visualizations of data can be powerful if they are aligned with mental representations, tasks, and data, they are often insufficient for comprehending complex data. This is because data analysis typically requires many different tasks performed on the same data such as discovery, inspection, confirmation, and explanation [8], each requiring different transformations of the data. For example, if the task in Fig. 9.1b is to understand the relationship of the drug to sex, then the data can be sorted based on sex. As shown, interaction with the data through such sorting reveals that the drug has no effect on females (low values remain low, and high values remain high), whereas it has a dramatic effect on lowering systolic values in males (all high values become low). Therefore, while it is well accepted that interactivity is crucial for the use of most computer systems, interaction with data visualizations can help to reveal relationships that are otherwise hidden when using a single representation of the data.

Interactivity is also critical when analysis is done in teams consisting of different disciplines, where each member often requires a different representation of the same data. For example, a molecular biologist might be interested in which genes are co-expressed across patients, whereas a clinician might be interested in the clinical characteristics of patients with similar gene profiles, and later how they integrate with the molecular information. To address these changes in task and mental representation, visualizations require interactivity or the ability to transform parts, or the entire visual representation.

Theories Related to Visual Analytics

Although the field of visual analytics has drawn on theories and heuristics from different disciplines such as cognitive psychology, computer science, and graphic design, the development of theories and taxonomies for visual analytics are still in early stages of development [3]. For example, there are a number of attempts to classify visual analytical representations [9, 10], and interaction intents at different levels of granularities [11, 12].

One attempt to classify visual analytical representations groups them into (1) time series (e.g., line graphs showing how the expression of different genes change over time), (2) statistical distributions (e.g., box-and-whisker plots), (3) maps (e.g., pie charts showing percentages of different races at different city locations on the US map), (4) hierarchies (e.g., top-down tree showing the management structure of an organization), and networks (e.g., a social network of how friends connect to other friends such as on Facebook). Once these visualizations are generated, they are considered visual analytical if they enable interaction directly or indirectly with part, or all of the information being represented. Examples for such interactivity include transforming a top-down tree into a circular tree, coloring nodes in the tree based on specific properties such as sex, or dragging a node in the tree to swap its location with another sibling node.

Similarly, there have been several attempts to classify interactions with visualizations at different levels of granularity. For example, Amar et al. [11] proposed eight low-level interaction intents: retrieve value, filter, compute derived value, find extremum, sort, determine range, characterize distribution, find anomalies, and cluster and correlate. In contrast, Yi et al. [12] proposed six higher level interaction intents typically used: select, explore, reconfigure, encode, abstract/elaborate, filter and connect.

While the above classifications of visual analytical representations and interaction with them are useful as check lists for building effective visual analytical systems, they do not provide an integrated understanding of how they work together to enable analytical reasoning, a primary goal of visual analytics. To address this gap, Liu and Stasko [13] proposed a framework which integrates visual representation, interaction, and analytical reasoning. The framework specifies that central to reasoning with an external visual analytical representation (e.g., the table in Fig. 9.1b) is a *mental model* which is an analog of the external representation stored in working memory, and which is "runnable" to enable reasoning of the data and relationships. This is achieved by creating a mental model in working memory which is a "collage" of some or all of the structural, semantic, and elemental details present in the visual representation, in addition to other information from long term memory relevant to the task. For example as shown in Fig. 9.1b, an analyst conducting the task of determining which of the two columns have more patients with systolic >140 might construct a mental model in working memory consisting of two columns with cells colored red and white, but excluding elements such as the numbers in the cells. Similar to the speed of accessing information stored in the memory of a computer versus from disk, a mental model stored in the brain's working memory can be used to rapidly achieve tasks such as determining which of the two columns have more red cells, or even determining that the first column has approximately three times more red cells compared to the second column.

The framework further specifies that because working memory has size constraints, a mental model can typically contain only some of the information present in the external visualization at any given time. Therefore, when the task changes, it motivates a tight interactive coupling between the internal mental model and the external visual representation, through which new information is extracted from the existing state of the visualization or from long term memory, irrelevant information in the mental model is discarded to make room for new information, the external visual representation itself is transformed to reveal new relationships, or the conceptual information is externalized onto the visual representation to enable future tasks. For example, when the task described in Fig. 9.1 involves exploring or determining the relationship of systolic blood pressure to sex, then a tight coupling between the internal and external representations is triggered enabling the extraction of sex-related information and its relationship to systolic blood pressure. This can be done either by extracting the information from the current representation (requiring often costly mental manipulations) to identify patterns, or by transforming the external representation through manipulations such as sorting (requiring relatively cheaper physical actions) to reveal new relationships, which are then immediately available for internal reasoning tasks such as determining inequalities between the columns. Furthermore, information about the current or previous task such as a discovered pattern can be externalized onto the visual representation through annotations, and therefore freeing up working memory for subsequent tasks.

The framework proposes that the coupling of internal and external representations can be characterized by three interacting goals: (1) *External anchoring* or the process of connecting conceptual structures (e.g., systolic blood pressure > 140) to material elements of the visualization (red colored cells), (2) *Information foraging* or the process of exploring the external visual representation through extraction (e.g., counting the red cells related to female patients) or through transformation (e.g., sorting) of the representation, and (3) *Cognitive offloading* or the process of transferring a conceptual structure onto the visual representation to reduce working memory demands (e.g., encircling or annotating in Fig. 9.1c all female patients who have systolic >140 before and after taking the drug).

While the above integrated framework of visual representation, interaction, and analytical reasoning still needs to be elaborated into a theory and tested through predictive models, it provides a first step into how the critical concepts of visual analytics could be working together to enable analytical reasoning, leading to implications for the design and evaluation of effective visual analytical systems.

Finally, it is important to note that visual analytics has considerable overlap with the fields of scientific visualization (focused on modeling real-world geometric structures such as earthquakes), and information visualization (focused on modeling abstract data structures such as relationships). However, as described above, visual analytics places a large emphasis on approaches that facilitate reasoning and making sense of complex information individually and in groups [3].

Visual Analytics: Biomedical Applications

The use of visual analytical representations is increasingly becoming pervasive in the biomedical domain. The selection of visual analytical representations is highly dependent on the users of the information and their goals, which can be classified in the following two broad categories:

Information Consumers

The primary goal of information consumers is to make biomedical information actionable in terms of directly affecting change in health-related behaviors. An important class of information consumers is patients and care providers whose primary goal is to track and modify personal health and life style behaviors through the use of biomedical and social data. For example, the website *PatientsLikeMe* [14] enables users to input health and lifestyle variables of specific individuals. This information is displayed using visual analytical representations such as longitudinal charts and graphs which can be modified to display different granularities of data. Users can also find patients who are similar to their profile, and learn about their real-world experiences of dealing with their diseases, with the goal of improving the quality of life for themselves or for those they provide care. Similarly, personal and wearable activity monitors (e.g., fitbit) have been developed to motivate behavior change such as weight loss by monitoring how many steps a user has taken on a particular day, and displaying that information on a smart phone using visualizations such as a progress bar and the recommended target. Such information can be shared with other users in a social network to provide additional motivation through competition.

Another important class of information consumers consists of healthcare providers such as physicians and first-responders whose primary goal is to make healthcare decisions relevant to specific patients and situations by extracting relevant information from databases such as electronic health records. For example, the Twinlist system [15] was developed to reconcile multiple lists of drugs (e.g., from the hospital records versus what the patient reports taking) associated with a patient by graphically displaying what is similar and different among the different lists. The goal of this prototype was to enable caregivers to rapidly reconcile contradictory information with the goal of reducing errors in treatment.

A third class of information consumers consists of policy makers from federal and state agencies whose primary goal is to make policy decisions based on public health information. For example, the Centers of Disease Control provides interactive maps showing the incidence of different disease outbreaks across the US [16], with the goal of enabling faster response.

Given that the primary goal of information consumers is to make specific forms of biomedical information actionable, an active area of research is to determine which visual analytical representations are appropriate for which classes of users and goals, and to design and evaluate systems which are easy to learn, and intuitive to use [17]. For example, while interactive time series, maps, and hierarchies when designed carefully are considered easy to comprehend and to interact with, other representations such as networks with more than a few dozen nodes are considered more difficult to comprehend and tend to be avoided as representations for information consumers.

Information Analysts

In contrast to information consumers, the primary goal of information analysts in academic and industrial settings is to make contributions to biomedical scientific knowledge. While the goal of all biomedical information users is to ultimately improve health outcomes, the process of reaching that long-term goal is achieved by information analysts through progressive contributions to scientific knowledge. An important class of information analysts consists of biologists and bioinformaticians whose primary goal is to decipher the biological mechanisms involved in different diseases. For example, biologists often use network visualization and analysis tools like Cytoscape [18] to comprehend complex disease-protein associations [19] with the goal of deciphering the functions and pathways related to proteins of interest.

A second class of information analysts consists of clinical researchers and medical informaticians whose primary goal is to develop new methods to improve patient treatment by analyzing the relationship between clinical variables and outcomes. For example, networks visualizations have been used to analyze Medicare claims from more than 30 million patients, which enabled researchers to infer patterns in the progression of different diseases [20]. One of the their observations was that that highly connected nodes in the network had high lethality implying that patients with such diseases are more likely to have an advanced stage of disease.

A third class of information analysis consists of epidemiologists whose primary goal is to analyze public health information. For example as shown in Fig. 9.2, Christakis and Fowler [21], found that the flu infection in a social network consisting of Harvard students peaked 2 weeks earlier compared to a random set of students from the same population. Such advanced warning could be effective for planning immunizations during outbreaks of infectious diseases.

An active area of visual analytics research is to develop new approaches that integrate molecular, clinical, and epidemiological information, in a single representation. For example, translational scientists working in teams have used network visualization and analyses to integrate molecular and clinical information with the goal of inferring heterogeneity in asthma, and the respective biological mechanisms (e.g., Bhavnani et al. [2]).

Given the importance of networks for the analysis and presentation of complex relationships in a wide range of data types, and because it is one of the most advanced form of visual analytics, the rest of this chapter focuses on providing a

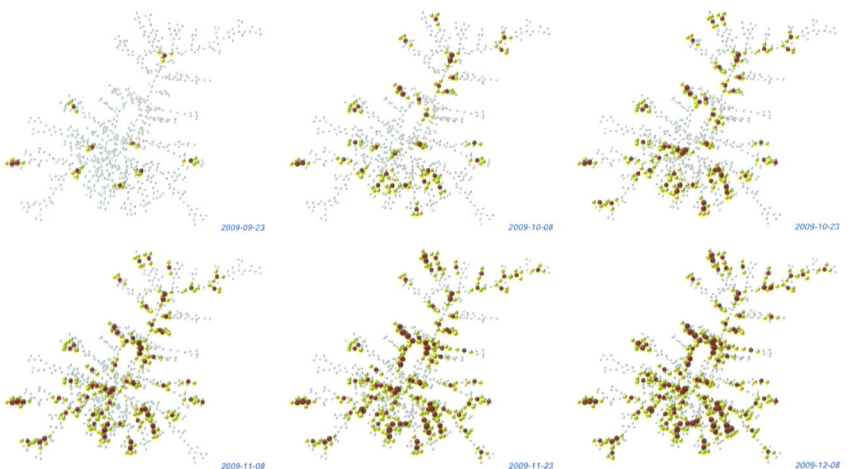

Fig. 9.2 Progression of the flu infection through a social network of students from Harvard University [21]. The red nodes represent infected students, the yellow nodes represent friends of infected students, and the edges connecting the nodes represent self-reported friendship links. Reprinted under Creative Commons license originally published in PLOS One [21]

concrete understanding of this approach as applied to the integrative analysis of molecular and clinical information.

Network Analysis: Making Discoveries in Complex Biomedical Data[2]

Networks [23] are an effective representation for analyzing biomedical data because they enable an interactive visualization of complex associations. Furthermore, because they are based on a graph representation, they also enable the quantitative verification of the patterns that become salient through the visualization. Networks are increasingly being used to analyze a wide range of molecular measurements related to gene regulation [24], disease-gene associations [25], and disease-protein associations [19]. A network (also called a graph) consists of a set of nodes, connected in pairs by edges; nodes represent one or more types of entities (e.g., patients or genes). Edges between nodes represent a specific relationship between the entities (e.g., a patient has a particular gene expression[3] value). Figure 9.3 shows a

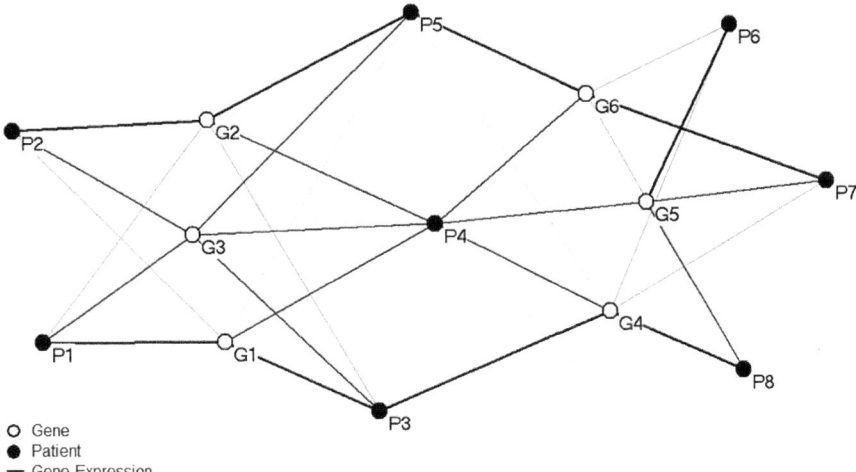

Fig. 9.3 A sample bipartite network where edges exist only between two different types of nodes. In this case, nodes represent either patients (black) or genes (white), and edges connecting the two represent gene expression

---

[2] Portions of this section appeared in Bhavnani et al. [22].

[3] Gene expression is the process by which the information in a gene is translated into a gene product such as a protein which can be involved in biological processes like inflammation during an infection.

sample bipartite network where edges exist only between different types of entities [23], in this case between patients and genes.[4]

Network analysis of biomedical data typically consists of three steps: (1) **exploratory visual analysis** to identify emergent bipartite relationships such as between patients and genes; (2) **quantitative analysis** through the use of methods suggested by the emergent visual patterns; (3) **inference** of the biological mechanisms involved across different emergent sub-phenotypes. This three-step method used across several studies [8, 26, 27] have revealed complex but comprehensible visual patterns, each prompting the use of quantitative methods that make the appropriate assumptions about the underlying data, which in turn led to inferences about the biomarkers and underlying mechanisms involved. Each of the three steps of this method is described below, followed by its application to analyze a data set of subjects and gene expressions.

Exploratory Visual Analysis

Network analysis typically begins by transforming symbolic data into graphical elements in a network. To achieve this, the analyst needs to decide which *entities* in the data represent the nodes in the network, in addition to how other useful information can be mapped onto the node's shape, color, and size. Similarly, the analyst needs to decide which *relationships* between the entities in the data are represented by the edges in the network, in addition to how to map other useful information to the edge's thickness, color, and style. These selections are made based on an understanding of the kinds of relationships that need to be explored, and is often an iterative process based on an understanding of the domain and the nature of the data being processed.

Once the symbolic data has been mapped to graphical elements, the resulting network is laid out so the nodes and edges can be visualized. The layout of nodes in a network can be done where either the distance between nodes has no meaning (e.g., nodes laid out randomly or along a geometric shape such as a line or circle), or where the distance between nodes represents a relationship such as similarity (e.g., similar cytokine expression profiles). Layouts where distance has meaning are typically generated through force-directed layout algorithms. For example, the application of the *Kamada-Kawai* [28] layout algorithm to a network results in nodes with a similar pattern of connecting edge weights to be pulled together, and those with different patterns to be pushed apart.

Figures 9.4, 9.5, 9.6, and 9.7 show the steps that were used to generate a bipartite network of 101 subjects and 18 genes, data which is described in more detail in the original study [29]. The 101 subjects consisted of 28 influenza (flu), and 51

---

[4] Researchers have explored a wide range of network types including unipartite, directed, dynamic, and networks laid out in three dimensions to analyze complex data. As this wide range is beyond the scope of this chapter, we suggest other excellent sources [23] for such information.

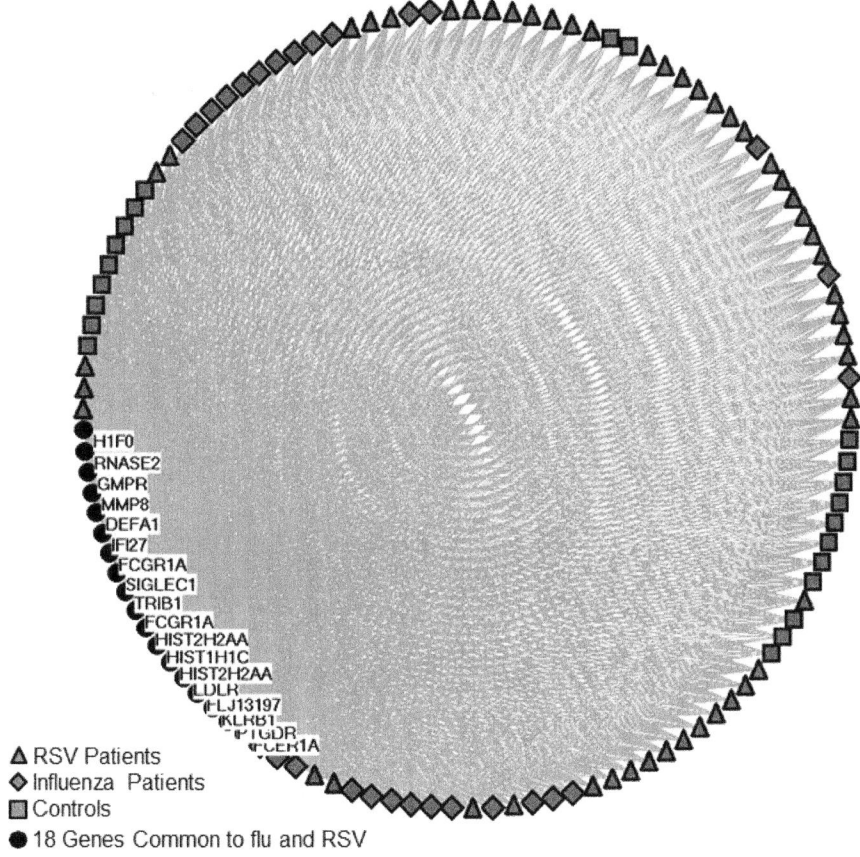

Fig. 9.4 A bipartite network showing subject nodes (RSV patients = triangles, flu patients = diamonds, and controls = squares) and gene nodes (black circles) connected in pairs by edges, which represent normalized gene expression. Patient and gene nodes were separately grouped and randomly laid out equidistantly around a circle

respiratory syncytial virus (RSV) cases, and 22 age, sex, and race matched healthy controls. The 18 genes were highly significant, differentially-expressed genes that were common to both infections. The goal of this analysis was to identify subgroups of cases that had different molecular profiles and therefore could suggest sub-phenotypes that require different treatments. Figure 9.4 shows how the three types of subjects were represented as RSV (gray triangles), flu (gray diamonds), and controls (gray squares), and the genes were represented as circular black nodes. Furthermore, normalized gene expression values were represented as edges connecting each subject to each gene. These nodes were laid out equidistantly around a circle. Figure 9.5 shows the same network but where the edge thicknesses are proportional to the normalized gene expression values. Therefore, thicker edges

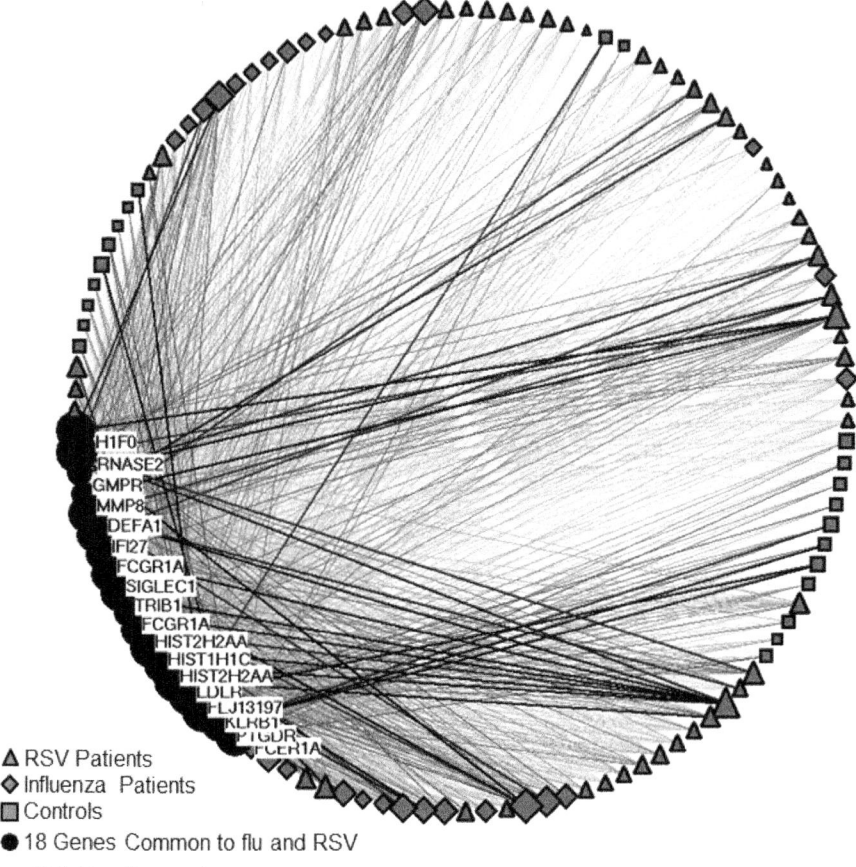

Fig. 9.5 The same network as in Fig. 9.4 but where edge thickness is proportional to the normalized gene expression value and the size of each node is proportional to the total expression values of the connecting edges. Thick edges represent higher gene expression values compared to thin edges. Similarly, larger subject nodes have higher aggregate gene expression values compared to smaller patient nodes

represent higher gene expression values as compared to the thinner edges. Furthermore, the size of the node was made proportional to the total expression value of the connecting edges. Therefore, larger patient nodes have overall higher aggregate gene expression values compared to smaller patient nodes.

Although the patients, genes, and the gene expression have been visually represented, the distances between the nodes have no meaning. To better comprehend the data, the subjects that have higher expression value for a particular gene should be spatially closer to that gene compared to those that have lower gene expressions. This approach of using short distances between entities to show similarity, and long distances between entities to show dissimilarity is typical across clustering

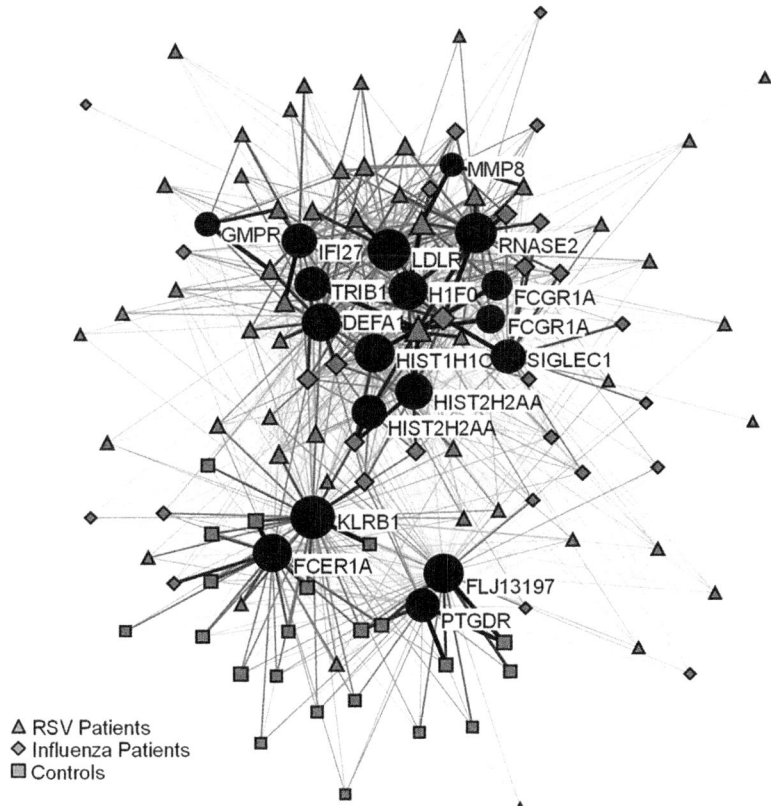

Fig. 9.6 Application of *Kamada-Kawai*, a force-directed algorithm, to the circular layout. The algorithm pulls nodes with similar gene expression patterns closer together while pushing apart those with dissimilar expression patterns. The layout of the network suggested the existence of distinct subject and gene clusters, and revealed inter-cluster relationships such as how the subject clusters express particular gene clusters. However, quantitative methods must be used to identify cluster boundaries

algorithms. As shown in Fig. 9.6 and previously reported [22], application of the forced-directed algorithm Kamada-Kawai to the circular layout results in nodes that have a similar pattern of gene expression to be pulled together, and those that are not similar to be pushed apart.

The resulting layout suggests that there exist distinct clusters of subjects and genes. As shown in Fig. 9.6, the subjects had a complex but understandable topology consisting of a majority of the cases (triangles and diamonds) on the top cluster which had a preferential expression of the top 14 genes, and a majority of the controls (squares) at the bottom of the network which had preferential expression of the bottom four genes. In addition, the cases on the top had a core-periphery topology, where there were some cases with high overall gene expression in the center, and many patients with low overall gene expression in the periphery. Finally, there were

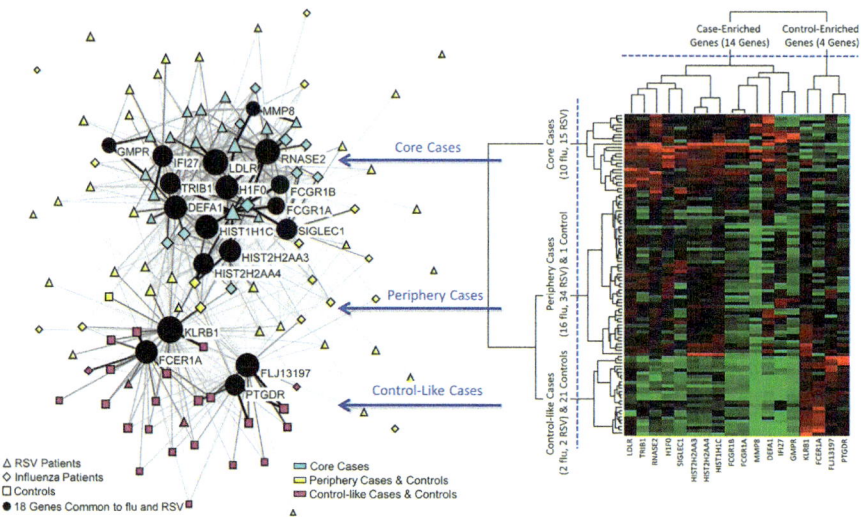

Fig. 9.7 A heatmap with dendrogram generated through hierarchical clustering helped to identify the boundaries of three subject clusters, which were superimposed onto the network shown in Fig. 9.3 using colored nodes to denote cluster membership. The network also shows the relationship of the subject clusters to the top gene cluster consisting of 11 genes, and bottom gene cluster consisting of four genes. Reprinted by permission from the American Medical Informatics Association [22]

four cases (triangles and diamonds) that were clustered with the controls at the bottom of the network.

While the network layout suggests the existence of distinct clusters, it is not designed to reveal the members of each cluster. We therefore need to use quantitative methods that are explicitly designed to identify the boundaries of clusters based on a multivariate analysis of the data.

Quantitative Verification

There exist a wide range of quantitative methods to verify patterns discovered through network visualization methods. While in principle any statistical method can be used to quantitatively analyze a pattern observed in a network, many patterns are often analyzed using graph-based methods [23] that specialize in analyzing complex relationships. For example, *degree assortativity* measures whether one type of nodes in a network which have high weighted degree (e.g., subjects that have large nodes in Fig. 9.6), are preferentially connected to another type of nodes that have high degree (e.g., genes that have large nodes in Fig. 9.6), or vice versa.

Another approach that can be used to verify patterns in a network is hierarchical clustering [30]. This unsupervised learning method attempts to identify the number and boundary of clusters in the data. For example, hierarchical clustering can be used to identify clusters of patients based on their relationship to genes, or clusters of genes based on their relationship to patients. The method begins by putting each node in a separate cluster, and then progressively joins nodes that are most similar based on their relationship to connected nodes. This progressive grouping generates a tree structure called a *dendrogram*, where distances between subsequent layers of the tree represent the strength of dissimilarity between the respective clusters; the larger the distance between two subsequent layers, the stronger the clustering. Analysts therefore determine the number and membership of the clusters by identifying relatively large breaks between the layers in the dendrogram.

Given the wide range of quantitative methods available, the patterns in the network are used to guide the selection of the appropriate method. For example, if distinct clusters do not exist in a network, then it is not appropriate to apply a clustering algorithm to the network. This approach of selecting methods based on the inspection of the data is similar to how statisticians determine whether to use parametric or non-parametric inferential methods based on the underlying distribution of the data.

Because the network in Fig. 9.6 suggested the existence of distinct clusters, hierarchical clustering was used to identify the boundary and members of the clusters. As shown in Fig. 9.7b, the horizontal dendrogram represents the gene clusters, the vertical dendrogram represents the patient clusters, and the colored cells represent normalized gene expression ranging from green (0) to red (1). The dendrograms shows a clear break at two clusters for the genes, and three clusters for subjects (as shown by the corresponding blue dotted lines across each dendrogram).

While there may be clear breaks in the dendrograms, the overall pattern could have occurred by random chance. Patterns discovered in networks, and subsequently the dendrograms, are therefore, tested for statistical significance. One approach to do this is to compare the patterns in the data to random permutations of the network.

To test whether there were significant breaks in the dendrogram (denoting the existence of distinct clusters), the variance, skewness, and kurtosis of the dissimilarities (generated by the hierarchical clustering algorithm) in the flu/RSV network were compared to 1000 random permutations of the data. For each network permutation, the number of nodes and the number of edges connected to each node, in addition to the edge weight distribution of subjects were preserved when analyzing the gene dendrogram, and vice versa. Significant breaks in the subject or gene dendrograms would result in a significantly larger variance, skewness, and kurtosis of the dissimilarity measures, compared to the same measures generated from the random networks. As previously reported [22] the results showed the clusteredness of the subjects in the network was significant as measured by the variance of the dissimilarities (flu/RSV = 2.75, Random-Mean = 0.88, $p < .001$ two-tailed test), skewness of the distribution of dissimilarities (flu/RSV = 5.55, Random-Mean = 3.94, $p < .001$ two-tailed test), and kurtosis of the distribution of dissimilarities (flu/RSV = 38.69, Random-Mean = 25.03, $p < .001$ two-tailed test).

The same approach was used to test the clusteredness of the gene clusters. The results showed that the gene clustering was also significant when compared to 1000 random networks based on variance of the dissimilarities (flu/RSV = 2.91, Random-Mean = 0.24, $p < .001$ two-tailed test), skewness of the distribution of dissimilarities (flu/RSV = 2.01, Random-Mean = 0.80, $p < .001$ two-tailed test), and kurtosis of the distribution of dissimilarities (flu/RSV = 7.81, Random-Mean = 3.16, $p < .001$ two-tailed test).

To understand why the subjects and genes were clustered, and how they related to each other, the cluster memberships were superimposed onto the network. As shown in Fig. 9.7a, the subject nodes were colored (blue, yellow, and pink) to denote their membership in three separate clusters referred to as core cases, periphery cases, and control-like cases. Furthermore, the 14 genes on the top, and the four genes at the bottom also formed distinct clusters, but because they were easy to distinguish by their spatial separation, they were kept black to reduce visual complexity.

As shown in Fig. 9.6, in addition to the above clustering, the core cases appeared to have higher overall gene expression (based on their size which is proportional to the sum of their edge weights) compared to the periphery cases. This pattern was quantitatively verified by comparing the weighted degree centrality (sum of edge weights) of the core cases to those of the periphery cases. This can be done with well-known statistical tests such as the Mann Whitney U test, a non-parametric test, which can be used to determine if the median of a variable is significantly different across two groups.

The results showed that the core cases (Median = 4.55) were significantly different ($U = 49.00$, $p < .001$, two-tailed test) compared to the periphery cases (Median = 2.52) verifying that the overall gene expression of the patients in the core was higher compared to those in the periphery. Furthermore, the median gene expression of the 14 genes across the 25 core cases (Median = 4.22) was significantly higher ($U = 16$, $p < .001$, two-tailed test) compared to the 50 periphery cases (Median = 1.95). This pattern can also be seen in the high expression values (shown in mostly red cells) in the upper left-hand corner of the heatmap in Fig. 9.7b. Finally, there was no significant difference ($\chi^2(2, N = 79) = 0.86$, $p = 0.652$) in the proportion of flu vs. RSV patients across the three case clusters, suggesting that the gene-based clustering was common across both types of infection.

The above results of the cluster analysis superimposed over the network, in addition to quantitative analysis of gene expression across the clusters enabled the identification of three potential sub-phenotypes: (1) **core cases** who had a significantly higher gene expression of the top cluster of 14 genes, (2) **periphery cases** that had a medium expression of the top 14 genes, and (3) **control-like cases** whose profiles were similar to the controls with high expression of the bottom cluster four genes. These three sub-phenotypes were common across both infections.

Inference of Sub-Phenotypes and Biological Mechanisms

While the visual and quantitative analysis helped to reveal patterns in the data, the ultimate goal of the network analysis is to infer the biological mechanisms involved, and the emergent sub-phenotypes in the data. This inferential step requires an integrated understanding of the molecular and clinical variables.

One approach to conduct such an integrated analysis, is to analyze how the patients in each emergent cluster (based on molecular profiles), differ in their clinical variables. As the primary data included disease severity of each patient [29], we used the Mann Whitney U test to analyze if the core and periphery cases were significantly different in their disease severity. The test revealed that the disease severity of core cases (Median = 7) was significantly higher ($U = 261.50$, $p < .001$, two-tailed test) compared to periphery cases (Median = 2). This result suggested a significant association between the high gene expression of the 14 top genes in the core-cases, and higher disease severity.

The bipartite visualization and quantitative verifications therefore revealed not only sub-phenotypes based on the molecular profiles, but also how they related to clinical variables, which enabled the domain experts to infer three possible sub-phenotypes and their potential pathways [22].

1. The **core cases** have significantly higher expression of 14 up-regulated genes, which included four histone genes, four genes with to date have unknown function in antiviral response, and six immune-related genes each of which has a well-known non-overlapping antiviral function. An Ingenuity Pathway Analysis [31] of the 14 genes suggested an indirect but strong interferon signature including TNFα and IL-6 cytokines involved in antiviral and innate inflammatory responses. Because the core cases also had a significantly higher disease severity score, they represent a distinct at-risk sub-phenotype that are hyper responsive to pathways targeted to viral clearance, and possibly carry a risk for long-term epithelial cell damage.
2. The **periphery cases** have a medium expression of all 18 genes and therefore suggest a second subphenotype with a subdued anti-viral response relative to the above hyperresponders.
3. The **control-like cases** have a high expression of four down-regulated genes, and low expression of the 14 up regulated genes, and therefore mirror the expression patterns in uninfected controls. The results therefore suggest that the down-regulation of these four genes indicates a "protective" phenotype making them similar to the uninfected controls. Existing literature on these genes provide some confirmatory evidence. While the exact role of the high-affinity receptor which binds to the constant portion of IgE (FcER1) is unknown in viral pathogenesis, SNPs included on this gene have been shown to be associated with severe RSV disease [32]. Additionally, KLRB1, which has been shown to have inhibitory functions on natural killer (NK) cells [33] was downregulated, suggesting an enhanced antiviral response in patients resembling the immune response of controls. Finally, PTGDR a receptor important in mast cell function

was downregulated, but the exact role of this receptor in viral infection is still unknown. Overall, control-like cases suggests a third subphenotype which have a "just enough" response to the virus, without overt stimulation of virally induced genes, and therefore potentially with reduced bystander damage.

One might argue that the above result could also be the result of the progression of infection over time. For example, the core cases could be at the peak of infection, the periphery cases could be later in the infection, and the control-like cases could be recovering from the infection. However, an additional analysis revealed that the three case clusters were not significantly different ($H(2, N = 79) = 2.56, p = 0.278$) in time of sample collection after hospitalization. There is of course the possibility that the children were infected at very different times before hospitalization, but controlling such a variable is practically impossible in the analysis of naturally infected humans. Therefore, we provide two explanations for why sample collection time is probably not an adequate explanation for the results: (1) Because all case samples were collected from patients that were hospitalized indicating severe illness, a resolution of such severity in the short time window of 42–72 h is unlikely to occur. (2) The gene expression changes in the PBMCs of the patients suggest a specific induced innate immune response (e.g., Toll-like receptor) to viruses. Such signaling pathways (which induce interferon secretion and contribute to anti-viral immunity) last several days which exceeds the sample collection time window in this study. We therefore propose that the three case clusters are more likely the result of inherent host differences in anti-viral responses, and therefore represent distinct sub-phenotypes.

Informed by these underlying molecular processes, the network analysis of subjects and genes therefore helped to infer not only the sub-phenotypes, but also the possible mechanisms involved, and which sub-phenotypes had a high risk of developing severe complications. The results therefore provided data-driven hypotheses of sub-phenotypes and their mechanisms which can be validated in future research with other datasets. Such analysis therefore could lead to future treatments that are targeted to specific sub-phenotypes, and is therefore an important step towards personalized medicine.

Strengths and Limitations of Network Analysis[5]

Network analysis has several strengths and limitations, whose understanding can lead to informed uses of the method, appropriate interpretation of the results, and insights for future enhancements and complementary methods.

---

[5] Portions of this section appeared in Bhavnani et al. [2]. With kind permission from Springer Science+Business Media.

Strengths

Network visualization and analysis provide four distinct strengths for enabling rapid discovery of patterns in complex biomedical data.

1. **Provides Integrative Visualizations.** Because networks are based on graph theory, they provide a tight integration between visual and quantitative analysis. For example as shown in the Fig. 9.7a, networks enable the integrative visualization of multiple raw values (e.g., subject-gene associations, gene expression values, subject phenotype), aggregated values (e.g., sum of gene values), and emergent global patterns (e.g., clusters) in a single representation. This uniform visual representation leverages the parallel processing power of the visual cortex enabling the comprehension of complex multivariate, quantitative relationships.
2. **Guides Quantitative Analysis.** Networks do not require *a priori* assumptions about the relationship of nodes within the data, in contrast to hierarchical clustering or k-means which assume the data is hierarchically organized or contain disjoint clusters, respectively. Instead, by using a simple pairwise representation of nodes and edges, network layouts enable the identification of multiple structures (e.g., hierarchical, disjoint, overlapping, nested) in a single representation [34]. Therefore, while layout algorithms such as Kamada-Kawai depend on the force-directed assumption and its implementation, such algorithms are viewed as less biased for data exploration because they do not impose a particular cluster structure on the data, often leading to the identification of more complex structures in the data [26]. The overall approach therefore enables a more informed selection of quantitative methods to verify the patterns in the data.
3. **Enables Pathway Inference through Co-occurrence.** Network layouts such as the one shown in Fig. 9.7a, preserve highly-correlated variables (such as genes) and display them through clustering. Furthermore, the bipartite network representation enables the comprehension of inter-cluster relationships such as between variable (e.g., genes) clusters and subject clusters. These features provide important clues to domain experts about the pathways that involve those variables. This is in contrast to many supervised learning methods which drop highly correlated variables in an attempt to identify a small number of variables that together can explain the maximum amount of variance in the data. While this approach is powerful for developing predictive models, the reduction in variables could limit the inference of biological pathways involved in the disease.
4. **Accelerates Discovery through Interactivity.** Networks enable high interactivity enabling the rapid modification of the visual representation to match the changing task and representation needs of analysts during the analysis process. For example, nodes that represent patients in a network can be interactively colored or reshaped to represent different variables such as sex and race, enabling the discovery of how they relate to the rest of the network.

Limitations

Networks have three important limitations that are important to understand for their current use, and need to be addressed in future research.

1. **Constrains Number of Node Properties.** While node shape, color and size can represent different variables, there is a limit on the number of variables that can be simultaneously represented. Furthermore, a visual representation can get overloaded with too many colors and shapes, which can mask rather than reveal important patterns in the data. Therefore, while networks can reveal complex multivariate patterns in the data based on a few variables, they often require complimentary visual analytical representations such as Circos ideograms [35, 36] to explore data that is high-dimensional (e.g., large number of attributes related to entities such as subjects in the network).
2. **Requires Advanced Computational Skills.** While networks provide a rich vocabulary of graphical elements to represent data, their design and use requires iterative refinement based on an understanding of the domain, knowledge of graphic design and cognitive heuristics, and the use of complex interfaces that are designed for those facile in computation. This combination of knowledge required to conduct network analyses makes domain experts dependent on network analysts to generate and refine the representations, which can limit the rapid exploration and interpretation of complex data.
3. **Lacks Systematic Approaches for Finding Structure in Hairballs.** While network layout algorithms are designed to reveal complex and unbiased patterns in multivariate data, they often fail to show any patterns in the data resulting in what is colloquially called a "hairball". In such cases, the nodes appear to be randomly laid out providing little guidance for how to proceed with the analysis. While network applications offer many interactive methods to filter data such as by dropping edges and nodes based on different thresholds, many of these methods are arbitrary and therefore unjustifiable to use when searching for patterns especially in important domains such as biomedicine. There is therefore a need to develop more systematic and defensible methods to find hidden patterns in network hairballs.

Future Directions in Network Analysis of Biomedical Data

The limitations of networks discussed above motivate future research with the goal of overcoming theoretical, practical, and pedagogical hurdles. **Theoretically**, we need better frameworks that tightly integrate existing theories from cognition, mathematics, and graphic design. Such theories can help predict for example which combination of visual representations can together help researchers to best comprehend patterns in different types of data such as genes versus cytokines. Furthermore, given that many network layouts show no structure, future algorithms should attempt to integrate different methods from machine learning to enable the discovery of hidden patterns. These research directions could enable the rapid discovery of patterns in the age of big data and translational medicine. **Practically**, visual analytical tools tend to be designed for analysts, often requiring substantial programming to make a dataset ready for visualization, and therefore limiting the use of the methods to only a few biologists and physicians. This hurdle motivates the need for tools that enable biologists and physicians to explore data on their own so that they can better leverage their domain knowledge in interpreting the patterns in the data. Of course such patterns need to be statistically verified by subsequent analyses, but currently such analysis is done mostly by analysts who could miss important associations due to the lack of domain knowledge. **Pedagogically** there needs to be a concerted effort to train the next generation of biomedical informaticians for developing and using novel visual analytical approaches, and to train biologists and physicians on how to make important biomedical discoveries in visual analytical representations of their data. Such advances should enable visual analytics to fully realize its potential to accelerate discoveries in increasingly complex and big biomedical data.

Recent Developments in the Identification and Interpretation of Biclusters

Although clustering methods like hierarchical clustering and k-means are widely used, they have critical limitations including the requirement of inputting user-selected parameters (e.g., similarity measures and the number of expected clusters), in addition to the lack of a quantitative measure to describe the quality of the clustering (critical for measuring the statistical significance of the clustering). More recently machine learning methods have attempted to address the above limitations by automatically identifying *biclusters* of patients and their characteristics simultaneously through the use of an algorithm called bicluster modularity maximization [37–39]. This algorithm provides a quantitative measure for the quality of the biclustering called bicluster modularity, which can be used to determine if the biclustering is significant with respect to a distribution of the same measure generated from random permutations of the network.

While the above approach automatically identifies the number and members of biclusters in large networks, the biclusters are often too overlapped when visualized using conventional force-directed algorithms, and are therefore difficult for domain experts to interpret their clinical utility. To address this gap, a more recent algorithm called *ExplodeLayout* [40, 41] combines results from bicluster modularity maximization with force-directed algorithm in two steps: (1) lay out the nodes and edges of the network using a conventional force-directed algorithm, and (2) "explode" or move the nodes and edges within the bicluster by radiating them as a unit away from the center of the network, until there is a minimal overlap between the biclusters.

This algorithm therefore preserves the relative distances between nodes within each bicluster (generated by the force-directed algorithm) to preserve their original associations, but stretches the distances between the biclusters to reduce their overlap and improve their interpretability. The above approach of using bicluster modularity maximization in combination with *ExplodeLayout* has been used successfully to quantitatively identify and interpret biclusters in a wide range of datasets [37, 42–47], and is currently being used to integrate them with other machine learning methods with the goal of translating them into the design of clinical decision-support systems [47]. The code for the bicluster modularity maximization and *ExplodeLayout* is publicly available [48, 49], and has been downloaded worldwide [50].

Acknowledgements I thank Shyam Visweswaran, Rohit Divekar, Bryant Dang, and Weibin Zhang for their contributions to this chapter. This research was supported in part by NIH UL1 TR001439 UTMB CTSA, the Institute for Human Infections and Immunity at UTMB, the Rising STARs Award from University of Texas Systems, and NIH AIM-AHEAD #1OT2OD032581-02-293 and CDC/NIOSH #R21OH009441-01A2.

Discussion Questions
1. Why are visualizations and interactivity critical in making discoveries in complex biomedical data?
2. What are the strengths and limitations of networks, and how can future research fully exploit the strengths, and overcome the limitations?

References

1. Molloy JC. The Open Knowledge Foundation: open data means better science. PLoS Biol. 2011;9:e1001195.
2. Bhavnani SK, Drake JA, Divekar R. The role of visual analytics in asthma phenotyping and biomarker discovery. In: Brasier A, editor. Heterogeneity in asthma. Springer; 2014b. p. 289–305.
3. Thomas JJ, Cook KA. Illuminating the path: the R&D agenda for visual analytics. National Visualization and Analytics Center; 2005.
4. Card S, Mackinlay JD, Shneiderman B. Readings in information visualization: using vision to think. San Francisco: Morgan Kaufmann Publishers; 1999.
5. Zhang J, Norman DA. Representations in distributed cognitive tasks. Cogn Sci. 1994;18:87–122.
6. Tversky B, Morrison JB, Betrancourt M. Animation: can it facilitate? Int J Hum-Comput Stud. 2002;57:247–62.
7. Norman D. Things that make us smart. New York: Doubleday/Currency; 1993.
8. Bhavnani SK, Bellala G, Victor S, et al. The role of complementary bipartite visual analytical representations in the analysis of SNPs: a case study in ancestral informative markers. J Am Med Inform Assoc. 2012;19:e5–e12.
9. Heer J, Bostock M, Ogievetsky V. A tour through the visualization zoo. Commun ACM. 2010;53:59–67.
10. Shneiderman B. The eyes have it: a task by data type taxonomy for information visualization. Paper presented at: Proceedings 1996 IEEE Symposium on Visual Languages. IEEE; 1996. p. 336–43.

11. Amar R, Eagan J, Stasko J. Low-level components of analytic activity in information visualization. Paper presented at: Proceedings of IEEE InfoVis '05, Minneapolis, MN, October 2005. p. 111–7.
12. Yi JS, Kang YA, Stasko J, et al. Toward a deeper understanding of the role of interaction in information visualization. IEEE Trans Vis Comput Graph. 2007;13:1224–31.
13. Liu Z, Stasko JT. Mental models, visual reasoning and interaction in information visualization: a top-down perspective. IEEE Trans Vis Comput Graph. 2010;16(6):999–1008.
14. PatientsLikeMe. 2014 Apr 28. Available from: http://www.patientslikeme.com/
15. Plaisant C, Chao T, Wu J, et al. Twinlist: novel user interface designs for medication reconciliation. AMIA Annu Symp Proc. 2013;2013:1150–9.
16. Centers for Disease Control and Prevention. Interactive atlas of heart disease and stroke. 2014 Apr 28. Available from: http://nccd.cdc.gov/DHDSPAtlas/#
17. Shneiderman B, Plaisant C, Hesse BW. Improving healthcare with interactive visualization. Computer. 2013;46:58–66.
18. Cytoscape. 2014 Apr 28. Available from: http://www.cytoscape.org/
19. Ideker T, Sharan R. Protein networks in disease. Genome Res. 2008;18:644–52.
20. Hidalgo CA, Blumm N, Barabási A-L, Christakis NA. A dynamic network approach for the study of human phenotypes. PLoS Comput Biol. 2009;5(4):e1000353.
21. Christakis NA, Fowler JH. Social network sensors for early detection of contagious outbreaks. PLoS One. 2010;5(9):e12948.
22. Bhavnani SK, Dang B, Caro M, et al. Heterogeneity within and across pediatric pulmonary infections: from bipartite networks to at-risk subphenotypes. AMIA Jt Summits Transl Sci Proc. 2014a;2014:29–34.
23. Newman MEJ. Networks: an introduction. Oxford University Press; 2010.
24. Albert RK. Boolean modeling of genetic regulatory networks. Lect Notes Phys. 2004;650:459–81.
25. Goh K, Cusick M, Valle D, et al. The human disease network. Proc Natl Acad Sci USA. 2007;104:8685–90.
26. Bhavnani SK, Bellala G, Ganesan A, et al. The nested structure of cancer symptoms: implications for analyzing co-occurrence and managing symptoms. Methods Inf Med. 2010;49:581–91.
27. Bhavnani SK, Victor S, Calhoun WJ, et al. How cytokines co-occur across asthma patients: from bipartite network analysis to a molecular-based classification. J Biomed Inform. 2011b;44:S24–30.
28. Kamada T, Kawai S. An algorithm for drawing general undirected graphs. Inf Process Lett. 1989;31:7–15.
29. Ioannidis I, McNally B, Willette M, et al. Plasticity and virus specificity of the airway epithelial cell immune response during respiratory virus infection. J Virol. 2012;86(10):5422–36.
30. Johnson RA, Wichern DW. Applied mutlivariate statistical analysis. Prentice-Hall; 1998.
31. Ingenuity. 2014 Apr 28. Available from: http://www.ingenuity.com/products/ipa
32. Janssen R, Bont L, Siezen CL, et al. Genetic susceptibility to respiratory syncytial virus bronchiolitis is predominantly associated with innate immune genes. J Infect Dis. 2007;196(6):826–34.
33. Pozo D, Valés-Gómez M, Mavaddat N, Williamson SC, Chisholm SE, Reyburn H. CD161 (human NKR-P1A) signaling in NK cells involves the activation of acid sphingomyelinase. J Immunol. 2006;176(4):2397–406.
34. Nooy W, Mrvar A, Batagelj V. Exploratory social network analysis with Pajek. Cambridge University Press; 2005.
35. Bhavnani SK, Pillai R, Calhoun WJ, et al. How circos ideograms complement networks: a case study in asthma. AMIA Jt Summits Transl Sci Proc. 2011a.
36. Krzywinski M, Schein J, Birol I, et al. Circos: an information aesthetic for comparative genomics. Genome Res. 2009;19:1639–45.
37. Bhavnani SK, Dang B, Penton R, et al. How high-risk comorbidities co-occur in readmitted patients with hip fracture: big data visual analytical approach. JMIR Med Inform. 2020;8(10):e13567. https://doi.org/10.2196/13567.

38. Chauhan R, Ravi J, Datta P, et al. Reconstruction and topological characterization of the sigma factor regulatory network of Mycobacterium tuberculosis. Nat Commun. 2016;7:11062. https://doi.org/10.1038/ncomms11062.
39. Treviño S, Nyberg A, Del Genio CI, Bassler KE. Fast and accurate determination of modularity and its effect size. J Stat Mech Theory Exp. 2015;2015(2):P02003. https://doi.org/10.1088/1742-5468/2015/02/p02003.
40. Bhavnani SK, Chen T, Ayyaswamy A, et al. Enabling comprehension of patient subgroups and characteristics in large bipartite networks: implications for precision medicine. AMIA Jt Summits Transl Sci Proc. 2017;2017:21–9.
41. Dang B, Chen T, Bassler KE, Bhavnani SK. ExplodeLayout: enhancing the comprehension of large and dense networks. AMIA Jt Summits Transl Sci Proc. 2016.
42. Bhavnani SK, Dang B, Bellala G, et al. Unlocking proteomic heterogeneity in complex diseases through visual analytics. Proteomics. 2015;15(8):1405–18. https://doi.org/10.1002/pmic.201400451.
43. Bhavnani SK, Dang B, Kilaru V, et al. Methylation differences reveal heterogeneity in preterm pathophysiology: results from bipartite network analyses. J Perinat Med. 2018;46(5):509–21. https://doi.org/10.1515/jpm-2017-0126.
44. Bhavnani SK, Kummerfeld E, Zhang W, et al. Heterogeneity in COVID-19 patients at multiple levels of granularity: from biclusters to clinical interventions. AMIA Jt Summits Transl Sci Proc. 2021;2021:112–21.
45. Bhavnani SK, Zhang W, Bao D, et al. Subtyping social determinants of health in all of us: opportunities and challenges in integrating multiple datatypes for precision medicine. MedRxiv (preprint). 2023. Available from: https://www.medrxiv.org/content/10.1101/2023.01.27.23285125v2.full.pdf
46. Bhavnani SK, Zhang W, Hatch S, Urban RJ, Tignanelli C. Identification of symptom-based phenotypes in PASC patients through bipartite network analysis: implications for patient triage and precision treatment strategies. J Clin Transl Sci. 2022a;6(Suppl 1):68.
47. Bhavnani SK, Zhang W, Visweswaran S, Raji M, Kuo YF. A framework for modeling and interpreting patient subgroups applied to hospital readmission: visual analytical approach. JMIR Med Inform. 2022b;10(12):e37239. https://doi.org/10.2196/37239.
48. Bhavnani SK, Zhang W. ExplodeLayout: CRAN R package. 2022. Available from: https://cran.r-project.org/web/packages/ExplodeLayout/index.html
49. Chen T, Zhang W, Bhavnani S. BipartiteModularityMaximization: CRAN R Package. 2022.
50. DataScienceMeta. CRAN R packages by number of downloads. 2023. Available from: http://www.datasciencemeta.com/rpackages

Further Reading

Card S, Mackinlay JD, Shneiderman B. Readings in information visualization: using vision to think. San Francisco: Morgan Kaufmann Publishers; 1999.
Newman MEJ. Networks: an introduction. Oxford University Press; 2010.
Thomas JJ, Cook KA, Cook KA. Illuminating the path: the R&D agenda for visual analytics. National Visualization and Analytics Center; 2005.
Tufte ER. The visual display of quantitative information. Chesire, CT: Graphics Press; 1983.

Part III
Design

Chapter 10
User-Centered Design and Evaluation of Health Information Systems: A Rapid Usability Engineering Approach

Andre W. Kushniruk, Helen Monkman, Elizabeth M. Borycki, and Joseph Kannry

Introduction

Designing useful and usable health information systems continues to be a major challenge [1–6]. There are numerous reports of clinical information systems that have failed to be fully used by clinicians, deemed to be unusable by end users or do not fit the workflow of the healthcare settings where they are deployed. In addition to this, it has been recognized that poorly designed health information systems can increase cognitive load and negatively impact workflow, which may affect cognitive processes involved in clinical decision making and reasoning [7, 9]. In addition, poorly designed systems and user interfaces may pose significant hazards to patient safety, in some cases, leading to technology-induced errors [1–4, 11]. In this chapter, we describe approaches for the design and evaluation of user interfaces for health information systems based on methods from the usability engineering literature that have been adapted for the design and evaluation of health information systems. These approaches can be applied to identify usability issues as well as used to assess the impact of systems on human cognitive processes. The intent of the work is to develop more usable health information systems and applications that effectively facilitate human information processing, reasoning and decision making. Several examples involving the application of user centered design (UCD) approaches will be described, including the application of rapid low-cost usability engineering methods and the use of clinical simulations. Challenges in designing

---

A. W. Kushniruk (✉) · H. Monkman · E. M. Borycki
School of Health Information Science, University of Victoria, Victoria, BC, Canada
e-mail: andrek@uvic.ca

J. Kannry
Department of Medicine, Icahn School of Medicine at Mount Sinai, New York, NY, USA

and deploying usable interfaces for clinical information systems will be considered. The content of this chapter should be of interest to a wide audience, ranging from those who design and evaluate health information systems, to end users of such systems (i.e., doctors, nurses, and patients) who would like an appreciation of how system usability can be assessed and improved in their organization and homes.

Usability can be defined as a measure of use and ease of system use in terms of the following dimensions: (1) effectiveness, (2) efficiency, (3) learnability, (4) safety, and (5) enjoyability [5]. User experience refers to the whole set of a user's experience with a technology, including the user's expectations, perceptions, feelings about and interactions with that technology. Usability engineering involves the application of scientific methods for the evaluation of usability of information systems in order to assess the usability of systems and to ultimately improve overall user experience with that technology [5]. Usability engineering methods can be applied throughout system development process, from early system prototyping to system deployment and post-implementation [6–10]. Usability engineering emerged as a field of study in the 1980s and aims to improve the usability of existing or proposed user interfaces, feeding recommendations back to designers. Initially, the field emerged from the disciplines of Computer Science and Psychology, but has now led to the development and training of professional practitioners, who work in the area of usability engineering and apply methods such as usability testing and usability inspection.

As will be described, usability engineering methods involve two main approaches: (1) usability testing, where users of systems or user interfaces are observed (and typically recorded) as they interact with the system under study to carry out tasks, and (2) usability inspection methods, which involve trained usability analysts systematically "stepping through" a user interface or system, comparing it against a set of usability principles and noting usability problems [8]. We argue that UCD in conjunction with rapid usability evaluation is more likely to lead to systems that are both useful and usable [11]. In addition, an in-depth focus on better understanding the information needs and cognitive processes of end users of health information systems and the impact of technologies on human information processing is needed. This includes the study of how such technology can impact clinician reasoning and decision making [6, 7].

We begin with a discussion of a topic central to effective design and evaluation of health information systems, namely the incorporation of user input into the design and refinement of clinical information systems through UCD. Closely related to this is a discussion of the application of methods that have emerged from the field of usability engineering that can be employed in conjunction with UCD in order to develop and test systems. As will be described, such approaches can be applied at a low cost in settings ranging from fixed usability laboratories to real-world settings and contexts. They can also be applied to assess both user information needs and impact of technology on clinical reasoning and decision making [2, 6, 7]. Extension of the approaches involving the use of clinical simulations will be described along with the importance of applying usability engineering methods to ensure system safety.

In addition, in this chapter we discuss how the approach can be used to assess the impact of systems on usability problems, but also how the methods can be applied to evaluate the impact of technology on health professional cognitive processes, including reasoning and decision making processes. The intent is to develop systems and applications that more closely fit with the thought and work processes of their users. This includes better understanding the interaction of end users with systems over time as they adapt to using technology in their work. There are numerous challenges in successfully implementing health information technology in healthcare. Understanding the impact of new technology on cognitive and social processes is important as the technology may change the way clinical users reason, make decisions and interact with others. In this chapter the methods described have been applied to evaluate the usability of health information systems as well as for assessing their impact on cognitive and work processes [6, 7, 9].

Assessing Information Needs and User Cognitive Requirements

UCD has been defined as "a multi-disciplinary design approach based on active involvement of users for a clear understanding of the user and task requirements, and the iteration of design and evaluation" [12]. UCD aims to develop systems that are useful and usable by applying tenets of human factors (i.e., to enhance human capabilities and overcome human limitations) to the design of products and systems to promote user acceptance and adoption [13, 14]. UCD specialists aspire to design systems that accommodate users' characteristics, limits, tasks and workflows [15]. Rather than strictly relying on input from system designers, UCD enlists users as participants to help inform their design solutions. Additionally, UCD encompasses the philosophies and methodologies whereby design is guided by observing, working with and studying users and their requirements [13]. Methods of user involvement can vary from consulting with end users to analyzing their interactions with systems and information needs in detail [16]. Gould and Lewis proposed three principles for UCD: (1) focus early on users and their tasks, (2) conduct empirical evaluation and measurement, and (3) apply iterative design processes [17]. Thus, UCD involves collection of data from users and its transformation to design solutions for improving the usefulness and usability of products.

Traditionally, system designers expected users to align with how a system operated. In contrast, system development guided by user input increases the likelihood that the resulting systems will be easy to learn, minimize errors, and will also increase user productivity, acceptance and satisfaction. However, failing to incorporate iterative and ongoing user feedback in the design process can result in a lack of alignment between user needs and system capabilities. There are a number of advantages to involving users during system development. Identifying user needs early in the design phase is imperative to designing systems that meet user specifications and to keep project costs to a minimum [15]. The costs associated with making system changes escalate as system development progresses. Moreover, failing to adequately consider users in the design process often requires system redesign, which is both costly and time-consuming [15]. The financial benefits of user involvement include increased adoption and user productivity, and decreased training and user support costs. In considering aggregated evidence from increased user involvement in ethnographic, qualitative and quantitative studies, the following benefits have been reported: (1) more accurate user requirements, (2) minimization of superfluous functionality, and (3) improved user acceptance of systems [18]. Thus, it has been argued that it is financially prudent to adopt good design principles and incorporate user exemplars to identify any design and usability issues early on in the development process.

Several challenges offset the benefits of user involvement. For one, methods that include users in an integral way can be more time consuming and expensive than developing a system with limited user input [18]. Recruiting participants may be a more time consuming process in itself. It can be difficult to select the ideal users to participate in system development. Users need to be representative of the prospective user group(s); this may require a number of participants with different disciplinary backgrounds (e.g., medicine, nursing, or pharmacy) and specialties (e.g., general medicine, cardiology, or surgery) [19]. Ideally, users selected for participation should be able to articulate the needs and requirements of representative end users, not just themselves. That is, there may be considerable individual variability in user needs, and this should be reflected in the resultant system. In addition, it may be difficult to attain consensus amongst the users [18].

There are a variety of approaches for increasing user involvement [20] during system design (e.g., ethnography, contextual design, user-centered design, participatory design) (see [18] for comparison among methods). The emphasis of UCD is on understanding user needs. This includes understanding what tasks they undertake, how they solve problems and how they represent and process information. UCD methods include cognitive task analysis, prototyping and usability evaluations [18]. Cognitive task analysis, which is employed in the methods described in this chapter, focuses not only analyzing and understanding user actions in carrying out work tasks, but also on describing and understanding users' mental activity in carrying out tasks, and the knowledge and representations that underlie the observed behaviors and decisions [7].

UCD is inherently guided by user goals; that is, the emergent system should be developed driven by what users need to accomplish [21]. Assessing user needs and obtaining feedback from users for the design of clinical information systems can be challenging in clinical settings for a number of reasons: (1) healthcare is a complex domain, (2) there may be many classes of users for a particular clinical information system, (3) users may have varied healthcare and IT backgrounds, (4) workflow must be carefully considered in addition to more static elements of system user interfaces, and (5) the context of use of systems can vary considerably.

In 2012, Kushniruk and Turner proposed a three-dimensional model (known as the User-Task-Context matrix) to aid in the planning for end user involvement in designing and testing information systems [19]. The model can be used to both capture design requirements and also provide a basis for setting up specific usability tests to ensure a partially or fully completed system meets clinical user needs. The approach can be used to drive both the development of use case scenarios for use in scenario-based design of healthcare information systems, as well as for summative testing of systems once they are implemented [19, 21]. The model has three dimensions to guide requirements gathering and specification:

- The **User Dimension**—e.g., user experience, age, gender, profession, education, job level, e-health literacy level etc.
- The **Task Dimension**—e.g., specific function of tasks, task complexity, expected successful completion and error rates etc.
- The **Context Dimension**—e.g., the physical location of use, urgency, uncertainty, time constraints, organizational goals etc.

For example, along the **User Dimension**, the different classes of users a system in healthcare (e.g., physicians, pharmacists, nurses, patients etc.) are delineated along with their attributes (e.g., level of experience/expertise, age range). A number of cognitive aspects of the user come into play when characterizing classes of users, including their level of knowledge and expertise, health literacy as well as e-health literacy levels. Along the **Task Dimension**, the various tasks and the attributes of those tasks are defined for each class of user (e.g., tasks such as using an electronic health record system to access health data). These tasks can be used to drive usability testing scenarios. The combination of User and Task dimensions made up a model known in the software industry as the User-Task Matrix for specifying user requirements [22]. In our work in healthcare contexts, it became apparent that a third dimension, the **Context Dimension**, is also needed when designing health information systems. This perspective is consistent with work from the sociotechnical design literature for healthcare IT development (where the role of social context is emphasized) and can help provide an explicit model of context in relation to user types and users' tasks. Context refers to the healthcare setting or environment into which healthcare IT will be deployed. As an illustration, the User-Task-Context model can be used to consider under what conditions a new speech recognition/dictation system would likely be effective for physicians dictating reports while using an electronic health record system (i.e., the **Task**). The effectiveness of the component can be shown to vary considerably even when considering the same class of users, depending on whether the speech recognition component is deployed in a quiet office setting or in a noisy clinic (i.e., the **Context**). Thus, the success or failure of health information systems and technologies is related to adequate consideration of all three dimensions when designing and implementing them.

In our work developing requirements, application of this model has proven useful for activities ranging from creation of system requirements during early requirements analysis, to generation of use cases (which describe in detail the scenarios involved in specific uses of the system) used in system design. They can also be used in the generation of scenarios that can be used to drive later usability testing. The system development life cycle (SDLC) provides a useful formal framework for considering where this type of user modeling can be applied and consists of the following phases: (1) the Planning Phase, where the initial planning of the system development is initiated, (2) the Analysis Phase, where there is a focus on requirements gathering, (3) the Design Phase, where detailed architectural blueprints for the system are developed, (4) the Implementation phase, where the system is programmed, and (5) the Support Phase, where the system is in use [23]. In the context of the SDLC, the User-Task-Context approach to modelling is useful at a number of stages including early in Planning and Analysis phases to specify user requirements, during the Design Phase to drive refinement of use cases, and during the Implementation Phase, to provide those testing a system with a list of users and tasks for target testing.

Low-Cost Rapid Usability Engineering in Health Informatics

In this section, we describe methods collectively known as rapid low-cost usability engineering methods designed to be used for analyzing user interactions with health information systems, which can be an integral part of UCD in healthcare [11, 24]. As will be shown, the methods can be employed during UCD, and also upon completion of a clinical information system during its deployment phase (i.e., during the support phase of the traditional SDLC).

Usability testing involves observing representative users of a system (e.g., physicians, nurses, or patients) while they use a system or user interface to carry out representative tasks (e.g., entering medications into a clinical information system) [7, 8]. Observing users typically involves video recording user interactions, on-screen actions and verbalizations using verbal protocol analysis, which is a psychological method that involves eliciting verbal reports from participants as they solve tasks. These reports can then be analyzed to identify cognitive processes [7]. Use of verbal protocol analysis is also key to understanding not only the user's physical actions (such as clicking on user interface items) but also their underlying thinking processes while using the technology under study. This involves instructing users to "think aloud" and verbalize their thoughts while interacting with a system under study, providing a rich recording of both computer actions and participants' thinking processes [7]. Such data can be transcribed and coded to identify usability problems and issues [7]. Usability testing methods have been employed widely in the design and evaluation of a range of health information systems over the past several decades. Usability testing methods can be used along the entire SDLC and the focus of the testing will depend on the stage of development of the system [25].

A variety of usability engineering methods have evolved in response to advances in technology. For example, free or low-cost screen recording software and built-in microphones on computers and smart devices have enabled "low-cost rapid usability testing" to become more widely applied [26]. The goal of this method is to provide an informative usability test that is efficient and cost effective. Moreover, low-cost rapid usability testing is not limited to the confines of a laboratory setting.

Rather, by employing low-cost portable methods that can be taken directly into settings like operating rooms or clinics, the approach allows for what we have referred to as "in-situ" usability testing. Such testing has the advantage of having greater fidelity than laboratory-based usability testing. Such testing can also vary in terms of whether the experimenter exerts control over the study, or allows the users' interactions to be more naturalistic, which allows for a range of study types. It also is arguably far less expensive, since if the testing can be taken into real settings after hours or when available, then the cost of the testing can be reduced [26]. Regardless of whether usability testing is conducted in a laboratory setting or in a real clinical environment, there are a number of steps that need to be considered in setting up such testing. Kushniruk and colleagues have previously outlined the stages of this approach [7]:

1. Identification of test objectives
2. Selection of participants (e.g., 10–20 representative system users)
3. Selection of representative experimental tasks (involving the computer system under study)
4. Selection of an evaluation environment (e.g., fixed usability laboratory versus remote or real-world setting)
5. Observation and recording of users' interaction with the health information system
6. Analysis of usability data (i.e., coding of screen and/or video recordings and audio transcripts to identify usability issues and impact of systems)
7. Translating findings and feedback into suggestions for system improvement

Evaluating System Impact on Reasoning and Decision Making

An important aspect of evaluating health information systems in terms of their use and usability in healthcare is the need to assess their impact on end user cognitive processes, including the clinical reasoning and decision making processes of users of the technology. To assess impact of health information systems on cognitive processes, a number of variations of rapid usability testing can be applied, as described in this section.

In a series of studies, conducted by Patel and colleagues, a modified version of the basic usability testing paradigm was employed in order to identify how differences in system and user design impact knowledge representation and clinical reasoning processes [6, 60]. In one such study the impact of using an electronic health record system (EHR) was assessed by recording participants (physicians) in two experimental conditions [60]. In one condition, study participants interacted with the EHR in isolation while "thinking aloud" using a modified usability testing procedure. In a second condition the participants were asked to interact with the EHR while they interviewed a "simulated patient", which was an actor playing the role of a patient using a pre-determined script (this approach is now known as a clinical simulation, and will be described below) [60]. The task given to the clinician participants was to interview the patient, and enter patient data and diagnoses into the EHR. By varying the complexity of the simulated cases and by recording users (i.e., physicians who had received the new EHR) over time, it was found that the design of the user interface had a profound impact on how information from the doctor-patient interview was represented and stored in the EHR system, as well as the order and nature of the questions posed by the clinician to the patient.

In addition to the above results, it was found that the design and layout of information categories on the computer screen had an important impact on what and how much patient data was entered into the system, in turn having an impact on the decision making processes of the clinicians [6, 60]. In the simulated patient condition (i.e., where the physician used the EHR during patient encounters) it was further found that the flow of questioning of the simulated patient was to a large extent driven by the workflow embedded in the EHR (i.e., what sequence of screens appeared when using the EHR and how that information was laid out and organized). It was found that the system could lead the physicians to what was termed "screen driven" behavior, where the information on the screen in the system dictated their questioning, rather than following their preferred way of interviewing [6]. This effect of using the system in turn was shown to have important impact on the physician's reasoning processes and pattern (as compared to how they interviewed patients without the system), ultimately affected their decision making, and in some cases making expert clinicians appear to reverting to a less than expert level [60]. In addition, over time it was found that physicians using the EHR system had to adapt their style considerably to the system, in some cases modifying the system using its customization capability (i.e., modifying information on its screens) in order to lead to a human-machine interaction style that they felt was more natural and conducive to supporting their reasoning and decision making style [6, 60].

Subsequent to these initial studies of the impact, further evaluations have indicated that the design of the user interface of complex healthcare systems can have a profound impact on not only usability, but also the safety of systems such as medication administration applications. In one study it was found that the presence of specific usability problems were statistically related to different types of cognitive errors in entering medications when using a handheld application, where a range of mistakes were identified that were related to specific usability issues [41]. More recent work applied the usability engineering approach to analysis of integration of clinical guidelines into a commercial EHR deployed in a large hospital setting [40]. This study found that ordering of screens imposed by a decision support tool could have a profound impact on clinician workflow and decision making. This work also indicated that prior to deploying such systems hospital-wide, cognitive studies of user interaction are recommended [40].

Low-Cost Rapid Usability Engineering in Practice

The low-cost rapid usability engineering method has been shown to drastically reduce development costs, as it can provide useful feedback into streamlining and optimizing the design of health information technology. In one study, adopting this method resulted in an estimated cost savings between 36.5% and 78.5% [68]. Costs associated with design changes are much less expensive to fix if discovered early in the SDLC. For example, identifying a usability problem or error early in the design phase may require minimal effort to fix. However, once a system is deployed, even minimal changes may be impossible or prohibitively expensive. Furthermore, mitigating errors before deploying the system reduces the potential of technology-induced errors (i.e., errors resulting from the use of an information system that may be caused from poor usability or from interactions with a system in a real setting) which in some cases are costly to address from a systems and human perspective in terms of patient safety [28]. Low-cost rapid usability engineering minimizes the probability of requiring a system re-design. As such, the approach has been recommended for use to mitigate the risk of lack of user adoption, often associated with large-scale implementations of systems such as EHRs. Along these lines it has been argued that the method should be considered for application by management of organizations responsible for implementing large scale IT projects [27]. In addition to this, the method is appealing as it is both efficient and inexpensive to employ [68]. Currently, the required apparatus for conducting such studies (i.e., the screen of a device, screen recording software, and microphone) is embedded in most laptops and therefore a usability test can be conducted anywhere [26]. The low-cost rapid usability engineering approach can also be conducted remotely by employing commonly available web-conferencing and screen sharing software to remotely view and record the screens and audio of subjects performing tasks during usability testing remotely [29, 51, 52].

In considering at what points in the SDLC that low-cost rapid usability engineering can be applied, the literature indicates that such testing can be carried out at various stages [7]. For example, in the early development of the user interface for an electronic health record (EHR) system (e.g., during the Analysis and Design phases), early prototypical designs can be analyzed by having representative users (e.g., physicians and nurses) comment on, and interact with partially functioning mock-ups and prototypes in order to determine the most effective interface. In addition, continual usability testing throughout the Implementation Phase is recommended as the feedback gained from end users can be used to refine the system/user interface. Finally, upon delivery of a clinical information system within an institution, the application of low-cost rapid usability engineering is highly recommended in order to ensure that systems that are beginning to be deployed are both safe and effective for end users.

An important aspect of conducting effective usability tests is the delineation of the following: (1) user classes (i.e., who are the different users or potential users of the system being designed and have they all been defined and characterized?), (2) the tasks the system will be designed to support (e.g., what tasks will the system be used for?), and (3) the context in which the system will be deployed (where will the system be implemented?). As such, the User-Task-Context model described in the previous section can be used to decide what users, tasks and situational contexts can drive usability testing.

Using Low-Cost Rapid Usability Engineering in Conjunction with Rapid Prototyping

Rapid prototyping uses models (ranging from paper mock-ups and wireframe models to partially functioning systems) to illustrate/simulate system functionality [23]. These models depict different options about how the system *could* operate in order to gain insight and feedback from users without investing substantial time and resources in system design. This may also involve cognitive task analysis, where participants (i.e., potential end users) are asked to interact and comment on rapidly developed prototype designs in the context of solving specific tasks while "thinking aloud". For example, Axure (www.axure.com) software can be used to develop interactive wireframe mock-ups without writing any code. Other related software allows designers to upload screenshots or sketches and then asks users to do a task, pick from a selection or give feedback. This can include collection of a variety of data on how the users interacted with the prototype screens (e.g., "heat maps" of user clicks, accuracy of user clicks, how long users took to click). Thus, a range of software tools can facilitate the development of prototypes quickly and these potential design solutions can be compared and evaluated by users.

Rapid prototyping focuses on key system functionality, and thus minimizes the time invested in system design prior to gaining user feedback about critical aspects of the system or user interface design. Rapid prototyping can be integrated into UCD by allowing for continual input from users into system design. Moreover, rapid prototyping can be used to investigate specific system components independently. Developing components in parallel allows for the progression of other components to continue despite barriers impeding the development of specific components. Furthermore, several different solutions can be evaluated to discern the best solution before considerable investment in designing the actual system. Additionally, different ways of integrating components can be explored to determine which combinations are most successful. Thus, rapid prototyping integrates users' choice and feedback about how a system will operate with minimal expenses. Kushniruk [23] outlines the process of incorporating rapid prototyping into system design. The flowchart in Fig. 10.1 depicts the iterative nature of rapid prototyping to refine the solution and ensure that user requirements are met by subjecting the prototypes to usability evaluations before a final solution is implemented. In Fig. 10.1, the box in the flowchart corresponding to "Prototype Testing (Usability Testing)" is a time point where low-cost rapid usability testing methods can be applied.

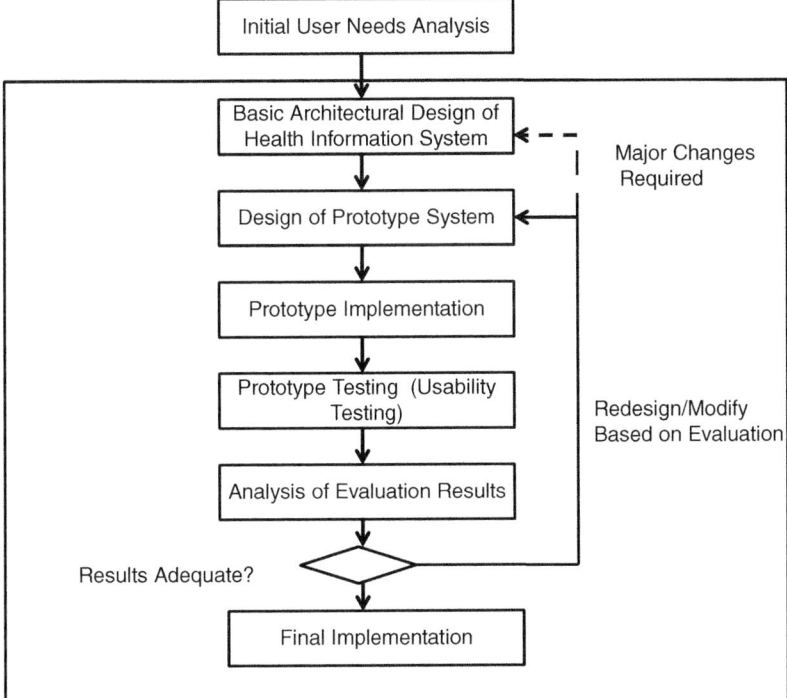

Fig. 10.1 Systems development based on prototyping and iterative usability testing

In addition, application of usability inspection methods, such as heuristic evaluation [8, 30–32] and cognitive walkthroughs [6] are potential techniques for evaluating the usability of prototypes. These methods do not involve observing users but rather having one or more expert analysts "stepping through" and methodically comparing the interface design against design guidelines in the case of heuristic evaluation [8]. In the case of cognitive walkthrough this involves "inspecting" areas where users might be expected to have problems by identifying user goals, actions, and system responses [33]. Hybrid usability inspection methods have also emerged, including one such approach that combines heuristic evaluation and the cognitive walkthrough [69]. However, it should be noted that during prototyping and health information system development there is no substitute for actually observing users' interactions with a technology under study, which will form the focus of this chapter. Observational methods, such as usability testing, are needed in order to gain an in-depth understanding of usability and workflow problems, as well as assessing potential impact of systems on cognition, reasoning and decision making. Such methods can also be used to identify specific user issues that need to be corrected before system release.

The adoption of rapid prototyping techniques in health information system design (in conjunction with usability testing) has been shown to improve the usability and usefulness of these systems while simultaneously minimizing development costs. Rapid prototyping fosters inexpensive exploration and refinement of models before a system is developed. Thus, more options are available for users to assess. In addition to *what* users are testing during system development, advancements in *how* usability tests are conducted have been made. For example, rapid approaches are now being used that can practically be incorporated within iterative prototyping cycles to feed information back into design based on analysis of user interactions with systems.

Use of Clinical Simulations in System Design and Evaluation

Clinical simulations represent a development that follows logically from usability testing methods and can be practically employed during UCD [27]. As described above, usability testing can be characterized as involving observation of *representative users* of a system being observed/recorded while they carry out *representative tasks* (using a system being evaluated). Clinical simulations extend the realism of testing by also carrying out evaluation in *representative contexts* of use (i.e., representative settings, environments or contexts that are typical of where the system being designed or developed will ultimately be deployed). Examples of clinical simulations include work conducted in the evaluation of the impact of EHRs on clinical reasoning and decision making (described above in section—"Evaluating System Impact on Reasoning and Decision Making"). In these studies, participants (i.e., clinicians) are observed and recorded as they are asked to carry out representative work tasks. In work by Patel and colleagues this has involved having physicians interview simulated patients (i.e., actors using a patient script) while using a system such as an EHR to record the information in [6, 60]. The resultant recordings can then be analyzed to identify impact of the system on information gathering, reasoning and decision making under realistic conditions of use of the system.

In addition, clinical simulations have been used in studies of medication administration systems in order to assess the impact of different system designs on usability and patient safety [34]. In a series of studies conducted "in-situ" in a hospital setting, realistic clinical situations were set up by using hospital rooms "after hours", where the system was to be deployed [11, 35]. This approach included using mannequins (i.e., life size physical representations of the human body used in health professional education) in place of patients, as the simulations were to include not only use of computer systems in the room, but also physical interactions such as hanging intravenous bags and ergonomic aspects of the room layout (i.e., where the computer is located). This reduced the cost of setting up in-situ testing, as the hospital room was already in place along with integration with other hospital systems and technologies. The advantages include not only a reduction in cost, but also the fidelity or realism of the study was increased as the setting mirrored the actual location where the medication administration would be implemented. It also included testing the human-computer interaction involving integration with other technologies already in the hospital such as bar code scanning technology.

For this study, a User-Task-Context approach was used to brainstorm a set of users, representative tasks and contexts of use that ranged from using the system to administer routine medications, through to complex medical regimes. In addition, scenarios were also created that included physical interruptions and unexpected emergency conditions. Representative users included 16 health professionals (physicians and nurses) that were recruited to participate in one-hour sessions, where they interacted with the new system to carry out the set of representative medication administration tasks. Recording of the tasks involved installing screen recording software (e.g., Hypercam®) on the computer the participants used to access the medication administration system. This allowed for recording of all user interactions with the medication administration system. In addition, a camcorder was used to obtain a wide-angle view of the physical interactions of the participants with the system and other technologies in the room (see Fig. 10.2).

Video analysis of the screen recordings in conjunction with audio recordings of users interacting in the task and external video views were integrated using Adobe® Premiere video editing software. During the analysis of the data, users' interactions were coded for: (a) usability problems in using the medication administration system, (b) ergonomic issues, and (c) issues in the integration of differing technologies (e.g., medication administration system with bar coding). The coding methodology

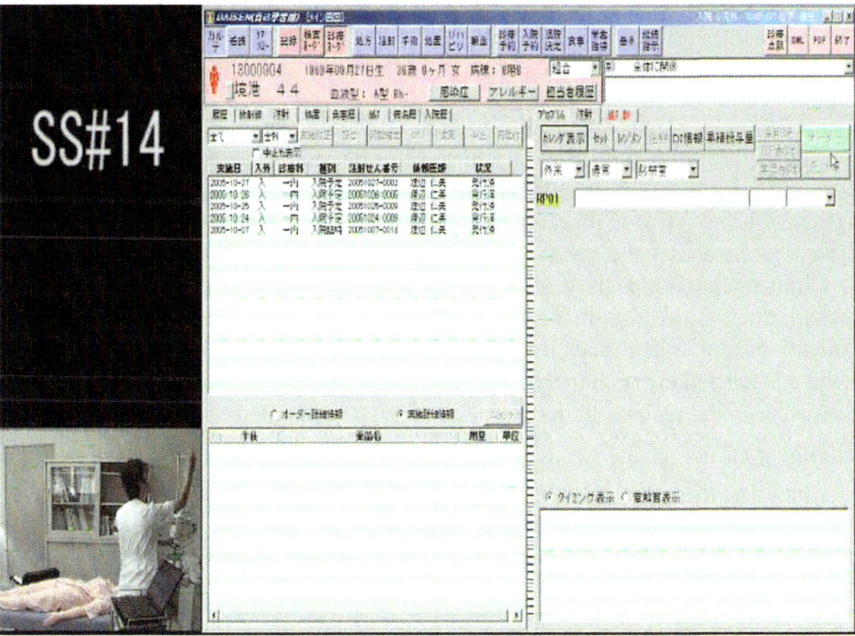

Fig. 10.2 External video view and screen view of user interactions with a medication administration system

used was modified and adapted from that first described by Kushniruk and Patel and involved first transcribing all audio recordings and then observing the video and screen recordings. This results in creation of an annotated log file of verbalizations and actions for each participant observed [7]. The interactions were coded for time taken to complete tasks and subtasks (e.g., verifying patients, reviewing medication orders, entering administration information) as well as for problems and issues encountered using the system. In addition, a post-task audio-recorded semi-structured interview was conducted to ask each participant about his or her experience in using the system. The results indicated that for routine medication administration, the system operated safely and was deemed to be usable, when simple lists of medications were to be administered. However, as the complexity of the tasks increased it was found that the rigidity of the system locked the user into a workflow sequence, which although it supported safety in some contexts (in not allowing for any deviation from a specified workflow) the change in workflow did pose potential safety risks (e.g., when emergency and time limited conditions were simulated). Specifically, when a simulated emergency occurred there was not enough time for all steps to be completed in sequence (as guided by the system) and there was a need for emergency override capability. As a result of this study, such an emergency override capability was included in the system design prior to widespread release [11, 35].

Carrying out system evaluation in-situ can increase the fidelity of testing while at the same time reducing costs. Another cost-effective approach involves integrating clinical simulations into the operations of simulation laboratories that are becoming increasingly commonly used for medical and nursing education purposes. An example of this is the IDX laboratory that was established in Copenhagen [36]. The laboratory was initially used for medical and nursing education purposes (i.e., computer controlled mannequins are used for training students), but was expanded for use in testing the usability and safety of clinical information systems. In addition, it has been used for installing candidate clinical information systems for testing those systems during a regional procurement process having the objective of selecting a system that matched the needs of users in the Copenhagen region.

Clinical simulations have fewer potential risks, offer more experimental control and are often more cost effective than testing a health information system with real patients once a system goes live. In conducting such simulations, it is valuable to build unexpected events into the simulations that emulate uncommon circumstances that occur in the real world during UCD [36]. For example:

- How does the health information system react if the user is called for an emergency and there is a delayed period of non-interaction?
- What happens in the event of a power failure?
- How does the system behave if two users are trying to modify the same patient chart at the same time?

In-situ testing can be undertaken prior to implementation to minimize the potential risks of the introduction of healthcare IT. This is also a prudent approach for deployment of new electronic systems in healthcare. Specifically, a gradual roll-out of new healthcare IT enables the system to be tested and limits the potential impact of technology-induced errors, whereas a "big bang" deployment of health IT has an increased potential to compromise patient safety. Further, testing should be done on a regular basis, not just at the time of deployment. Users may only find issues with the IT after months of use when they become familiar with it. Alternatively, the healthcare environment itself may evolve and may need adjustments in the health information system to accommodate these changes [36].

Clinical simulations have a number of limitations and may involve some logistical challenges. For example, although clinical simulations conducted in-situ can be cost-effective (as they do not require trying to recreate real environments) they do require permission and access to real local environments (e.g., hospital rooms) in order to carry out simulation studies (typically when such environments are not being used for patient care, such as after hours). On the other hand, conducting clinical simulations in fixed laboratories does not require such permission. However, such fixed laboratories can be expensive to build and require expertise in running the equipment. The cost may be leveraged by developing facilities for testing information systems within simulation laboratories that may already be in place for training healthcare professionals.

A Layered Approach to Evaluating Health Information Systems

Thorough testing is a critical component for revealing the possible usability and system safety issues. As such, the Institute of Medicine argued "it is critical to test health IT during *all stages* of development to determine whether user requirements have been translated into software that actually does what the user wants" [37]. An effective approach to improving patient safety requires continuous testing [36]. In addition, it is recommended that the fidelity of the testing environment should be gradually increased from low fidelity (e.g., an office laboratory), to medium fidelity (e.g., clinical simulation), to high fidelity (e.g., in-situ) [23]. It is important to investigate the system in a variety of settings to reveal as many potential problems and shortcomings as possible.

In applying usability engineering in health informatics, system testing should include a focus on the examination of the single user and system in detail (Level 1 in Fig. 10.3). From a theoretical perspective, this level can be seen as corresponding to the Human Information Processor model, which views user interactions with information systems as involving two "information processors": the human end user and the computer system [38]. At this level of testing, surface level usability problems (e.g., navigational problems, user interface consistency problems) can be readily detected. An additional focus at this level are cognitive aspects of human-computer interaction, including assessment of the impact of user interface and system design on individual clinical reasoning processes, as described above [6, 7, 60].

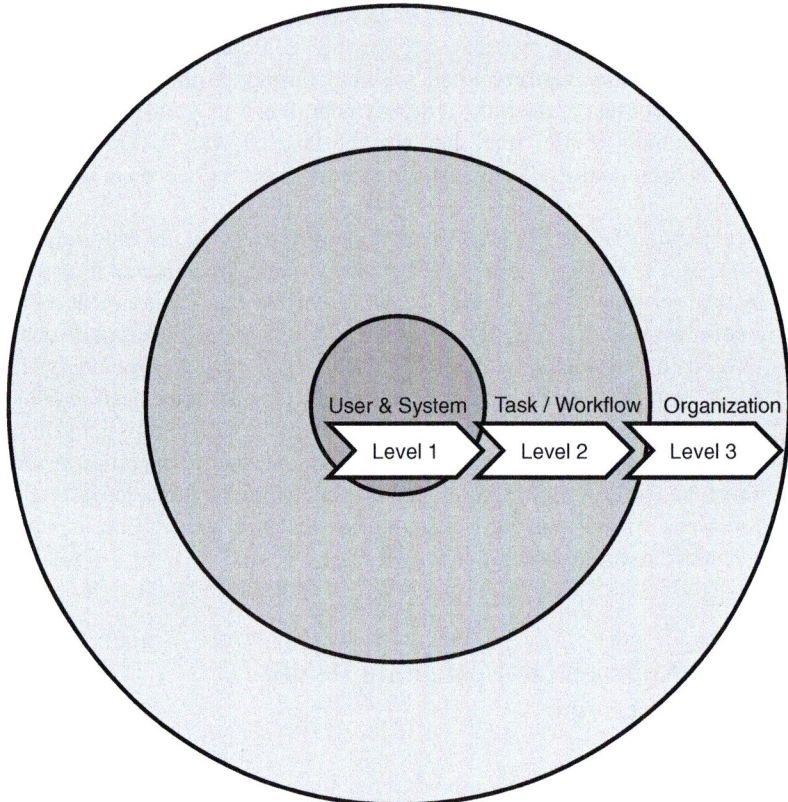

Fig. 10.3 Depiction of a layered approach to clinical information system evaluation

This analysis can then be followed by evaluation of use of the system in carrying out work tasks (Level 2). At this level, issues involving workflow inefficiencies and potential safety problems when using the system to carry out work tasks can often be detected. Assessment of the impact of using a health information system on medical processes and workflow can be critical in order to assess the usability of systems and to identify areas where the system or user interface need to be modified to accommodate to an effective and supportive workflow.

Finally, consideration of use of the system within the complex organizational setting is needed (Level 3). From a theoretical perspective, these last two levels can be construed as being at the level of distributed cognition—that is, cognition that is distributed amongst multiple agents, including various computer systems, people and representations [9]. This multi-layered approach to considering testing for usability and safety borrows from the three layers of human-computer interaction as described by Eason [39] and expanded on by Kushniruk and Borycki in the context of healthcare IT [2].

Case Study Example: Multi-Level Usability Analysis of Clinical Decision Support

In our work, we have applied such a layered approach to organizing and conducting evaluations and analyses of clinical information systems. For example, in work conducted by Li and colleagues, clinical guidelines designed for incorporation into a commercial electronic health record (EHR) system were tested using this multi-layered approach prior to being released within a large healthcare organization [40]. In the first phase of testing, physicians interacted with the initial prototype of the guideline design in isolation using a "traditional" laboratory-style usability testing approach that involved asking subjects to "think aloud". Based on this analysis, a variety of surface level usability problems were identified (with this level of analysis corresponding to Level 1 of Fig. 10.3). In this study the experimenters presented participant users (eight physicians) with two hypothetical patient cases using the electronic health record implemented at the hospital—one for strep throat and one for pneumonia. Participants were instructed to use the electronic health record and follow a scripted navigation that was designed to trigger the decision support tool under study (which provided evidenced-based guidelines and alerts to physician users about patient conditions). Usability testing was initially conducted where the physician participants were asked to "think aloud" and their interactions with the electronic health record were digitally recorded (using freely available screen recording software). The data from this initial level of testing were analyzed to identify surface level usability problems and inefficiencies, which ranged from navigational issues to lack of visibility of the alerts. Subsequent modifications were then made based on the analysis of the usability data. A video coding scheme was employed to identify usability problems and issues at a detailed level including identifying the specific screens and interactions where usability problems occurred. The scheme applied can used to also identify the impact of the system on clinician workflow, decision making and reasoning processes (see the chapter in this edition authored by Kushniruk and Borycki on video coding of usability data for details on the video coding process).

After refining the system based on the first phase of the study, a second phase of testing was subsequently conducted which involved observing physicians interacting with the guidelines embedded in the EHR while interviewing a "digital" patient (a video clip of a patient designed to elicit the physician's preferred way of interacting with the guidelines). This phase included a clinical simulation, and corresponds to Level 2 of the layers described above (i.e., using the system to carry out a work task involving not only the computer, but one or more other active participants). Based on results from this testing it was found that the guidelines often triggered at points during user interaction that interfered with the physicians' desired workflow and decision making processes, requiring further refinement of the guidelines and the interaction with the physician users.

In a third and final layer of testing, corresponding to Level 3 (i.e., analysis of a system in a socially complex setting or environment), physicians' interaction with the guidelines were recorded for a limited number of live patient interactions before deploying the system more widely ("in-situ" testing). After optimizing their design, the integrated system was released on a large scale across the hospital setting, which was attributed to the detailed levels of usability analyses that were conducted prior to release. From a subsequent clinical trial, it was found the guidelines were readily adopted by end users throughout the institution. In summary, the approach essentially moves from the artificial to the more realistic, naturalistic setting in sequence (see Fig. 10.4).

The example described above was significant in that it demonstrated that usability analyses could be practically conducted using a multi-layered approach that examined different types and levels of interactions with users prior to widespread release of a new clinical system. It should also be noted that the entire process of conducting usability analyses was conducted alongside the actual implementation of the integrated EHR-guideline system within a period of a few months, which corresponded to the actual development timeline and process.

Implications of User-Centered Design for Improved Usability and System Safety

A major concern with serious usability problems or issues is that they may lead to medical error [41]. For example, if the layout of information on the screens of an electronic health record make it difficult for users to locate key information (e.g., a patient's drug allergies), then it becomes more likely that such information might not be accounted for when prescribing new medications (potentially leading to adverse drug events). Furthermore, healthcare can be characterized by contextual conditions that might cause errors, including high workloads, poor interface designs, stressful and fast-paced environments, and user fatigue [42]. User interfaces that are poorly organized and that contain too much information may lead to high levels of cognitive load, and the application of user-centered design methods are essential in order to identify where a system or user interface is detrimentally affected the cognitive processes of the end user. Thus, it is important to employ UCD coupled with usability engineering methods as a means to improve system usability and patient safety in healthcare. However, healthcare systems pose unique challenges for UCD because situations are dynamic and tasks fluctuate according to circumstances [32,

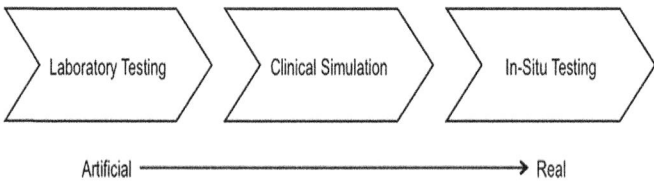

Fig. 10.4 Continuum of studies to ensure system safety prior to release

43]. That is, not all patients can be treated the same way or will have the same outcomes for any given treatment. Furthermore, human error in healthcare (that could be a result of poor user interface design) can result in serious medical error [11]. Recent research has indicated that the deployment of new health information systems has the potential to introduce technology-induced errors [11, 32]. Having increased input from healthcare providers during design and development improves the likelihood that new systems will maximize efficiency, minimize errors, and be compatible with their workflow. Further, given that healthcare is always in flux, it is imperative that systems are flexible so they can adapt to the needs and challenges of any situation.

The Institute of Medicine's report entitled *Health IT and Patient Safety: Building Safer Systems for Better Care* has indicated the need for greater emphasis on testing with end users in the design process (i.e., a user-centered design). Improved usability (e.g., easy navigation, simple intuitive data displays) was identified as being important for improving health IT safety [37]. However, successful and safe system development rests on the realization that UCD and application of user testing is a continuous process and not just a singular phase at a particular stage of health IT development. UCD methods in conjunction with usability engineering should be applied throughout system development, and may involve not only usability testing, but also use of in-situ clinical simulations and observation of naturalistic use of systems to ensure system usability and safety [36].

In order to increase safety of systems, a number of standards have also emerged for the design of user interfaces, including some that are general, and others that are specific to health IT. For example, the National Institute of Standards and Technology in the United States has developed the Common Industry Specification for Usability [44], which can be used to guide system development. Other guidelines have been developed around the area of designing more usable user interfaces for web accessible systems [45]. In health informatics, examples of user interface guidelines include work towards developing a common user interface for EHR systems (MCUI, 2014). In addition, this has led to more specific guidelines to help in designing and assessing user interfaces involving medications or devices, such as the United Kingdom's National Health Services design for patient safety guidelines [46]. By providing more standards and well thought out guidelines to aid in design and evaluation of clinical information systems, it is expected that the potential for technology-induced error will be reduced and the learning time for mastering the use of systems will also be reduced [47].

Emerging Trends: Towards Remote and Large-Scale Usability Studies

There are a number of emerging directions and trends in usability engineering for supporting improved design of health information systems. As discussed in this chapter, an improved understanding of system and user interface design on the cognitive processes of the end user and their work activities is essential. As illustrated in a number of studies described above, the design and organization of information contained in systems can have a subtle yet profound impact on the style and accuracy of clinical reasoning. Thus, assessing the impact of system design on optimizing clinician reasoning and decision making is an important area for further work and has remained to be more fully explored. Furthermore, the assessment of the impact of systems on workflow and work activities has become another issue that will require application of methods such as those described in this chapter. In this chapter it has been shown that methods used for conducting traditional usability testing can be extended to clinical simulation methods that can reveal the impact and consequences (both intended and unintended) of different system designs on critical healthcare activities and work processes.

Another important trend involves conducting online usability testing and data collection remotely. Along these lines, the term "televaluation" has been used to describe "virtual" usability engineering [48]. Using this approach, system users and experimenters can be located anywhere in the world, making it readily feasible and reducing costs associated with transporting users or testers to fixed locations to carry out usability evaluations. This may involve remotely recording users interacting with systems by using remote screen monitoring and Web conferencing tools with screen sharing capabilities e.g., Zoom®, Webex® and many other such tools commonly used today. Such remote testing can be carried out simply and inexpensively using remote screen sharing where the user's screens and audio (from the remote location) are seen by the experimenter on their computer (and can be recorded in their entirety). Moreover, variations in usability testing approaches also now allow for remote automated and simultaneous testing of a system in an array of different environments. Thus, usability issues that may only arise in specific environments can be identified early in the design phase. Furthermore, by removing the physical presence of a researcher, and any external equipment, it is less likely that participants will be affected by their participation in an experiment. Remote usability testing can involve remotely "recording all human–computer interaction (i.e., video recording all computer screens) and audio-recording all subject verbalizations as they interact with systems" [48]. The findings from such remote virtual usability testing can include: (1) suggestions by users for improvements to both the user interface and system functionality, (2) identification of usability problems such as lack of consistency in interface operations, and (3) quantitative measurements including time for task completion and system response times. This data can be used to create suggestions to improve health information systems' design to enhance the interface and functionality, ameliorate usability issues and reduce the time to complete tasks. Remote usability testing has the advantage of allowing for flexibility in conducting usability studies and collecting data [49, 50]. This includes flexibility in setting test times and the ability to conduct usability tests with many users from many locations, which otherwise would be impossible or prohibitively expensive to carry out, allowing for increased user participation [51].

In addition to a move towards remote usability testing, there are a range of approaches to conducting larger scale automated usability studies [52, 53]. This can involve creation of online usability testing scenarios that can be deployed remotely to participants using automated scripts (without requiring the presence of an experimenter, either physical or virtual) allowing for collection of usability data from a much larger number of participants than is possible with traditional usability testing methods. For example, using tools such as UserZoom® automated testing tasks can be created that can be deployed automatically administered to large numbers of users remotely [53]. For example, screens can be designed to allow users to explore a new user interface, allow users to try out new features or rate the usability of health information systems or different user interface designs remotely. Such studies can allow for tracking of user actions as well as collecting open ended responses (using open ended text boxes), rating scales, as well as clickstream tracking data on user performance (e.g., time to completion of tasks, errors etc.) in carrying out tasks. This data can be statistically analyzed to determine user preferences and collect usage data for optimizing user interface designs and system usability, which can involve descriptive, non-parametric and inferential statistical methods (e.g., for comparing user reactions to one or more different user interface designs) [54]. In addition, online usability questionnaires (which can include open ended text box questions as well as typical likert scales) can be deployed to a large number of users remotely using tools such as SurveyMonkey®. In health informatics, a notable example is of a study carried out in Finland where online questionnaires have been deployed via email to thousands of physicians to assess the usability of electronic health records in that country [55]. The information gained from this survey has been fed back to inform decision makers regarding the state of usability of electronic health records and usability of vendor products at regional as well as national levels.

Along these lines, in healthcare an approach known as the "Virtual Usability Laboratory" (VuLab) was piloted to allow for both remote data collection and collation of large amounts of user tracking data, subjective questionnaire and automated interview data and other forms of both quantitative and qualitative data that can be automatically collected from any number of users of a system remotely. To aid researchers and developers in analyzing this type of data the VuLab also contained automated tools for data analysis and summarization of usability data collected remotely. The approach was used to evaluate use of clinical guidelines in Canada, and feedback from this study has been used to refine both content and sequencing of clinical guidelines as well as health related content targeted to patients [29].

It should be noted that although automated usability studies (using remote large scale data collection) and smaller scale laboratory based studies have been shown to capture similar types of information about usability, there are differences in the results from both [56]. Kushniruk et al. have argued that in health informatics the results from these different methods can be quite complementary. For example, some studies may begin with in-depth smaller scale laboratory based evaluation and be followed by large scale usability studies to examine the generalizability of findings from smaller scale laboratory-based studies [36]. Another approach is to conduct large scale studies (e.g., using automated scripts or online usability surveys) to identify general areas to be examined in greater depth using laboratory-based usability testing. When the objective of the studies is to assess the impact of health information technology on human cognition, including impact on cognitive processes such as clinical reasoning and decision making, automated large-scale studies can provide useful information. However, they typically do not substitute for in-depth usability testing and clinical simulations (involving a smaller number of participants studies in laboratory or near live settings studied in more detail) [6, 40, 60].

An area of future research from a practical perspective includes development of rapid and automated or semi-automated methods to speed up analyses of usability data. In order for usability engineering methods (such as those described in this chapter) to be employed more widely, this is perhaps one of the greatest challenges. Methodological approaches such as low-cost rapid usability engineering [24] and IDA (Instant Data Analysis) [57] are attempts at reducing schedule and cost barriers to application of usability testing in system design and deployment. Other approaches to increasing the speed of usability analyses for incorporation into rapid prototyping include the work of Duman and Salzman in the development of the Rapid Iterative Test and Evaluation (RITE) method. The RITE method argues for continually repeating the same evaluation tasks and redesigning until the problems have been fixed or until there are no more resources [58]. The RUE (Rapid Usability Evaluation) method also attempts to reduce the time required to complete the appropriate sections of the testing method [59]. Although these approaches attempt to speed up time and lessen resources needed for user testing, rapid and agile application of usability testing in the design and deployment of many health information systems has not yet become the norm. However, with methodological advances including potential for automation of both testing and analysis processes, the situation may gradually improve. Along these lines, the authors have conducted research in applying machine-learning methods to auto-code much of the analysis of usability reports, along with work on the extension of the approach to automated coding of video-based usability data to identify usability problems [61]. In addition, new methods and frameworks will be needed for studying the impact of health information technologies involving artificial intelligence applications as they will provide new challenges and need for new frameworks for evaluation of their impact at multiple levels, from the cognitive to the social [62–64]. In addition, the emergence of a range of new information systems and technologies for use directly by patients poses a number of unique challenges and opportunities for designing and conducting both in-depth as well as large-scale usability studies [65, 66].

Conclusion

The usability of healthcare information systems depends on improved input from users in the design and implementation phases of the SDLC. In this chapter, we have discussed approaches to UCD that incorporate key elements from usability engineering. The application of these approaches is necessary for not only ensuring the usability of clinical information systems, but also their safety. Furthermore, the methods can be extended to assess not only the impact of system design on surface level usability, but also the impact of the systems we design on clinician cognitive processes, including knowledge organization, reasoning and decision making, as well as assessing their impact on work activities and processes. It should be noted that the approaches described in this chapter have also begun to be used in the selection and procurement of clinical information systems that better match user needs in healthcare settings, as a way to test out and evaluate candidate systems during the selection process [67]. In addition, the extension of usability testing to clinical simulations and naturalistic in-situ approaches is leading to new ways of evaluating systems in order to identify and prevent both usability errors and safety hazards. Along these lines, application of methods that can be applied to assess the impact of systems on user cognition, including their reasoning and decision making processes, will be critical.

A key aspect of more widely introducing these methods into health IT and health informatics is that of reducing the cost and effort required to apply usability engineering in healthcare. Along these lines, research has already begun to indicate that the effort in terms of cost and manpower to apply the methods described in this chapter is well worth the effort in terms of return on investment [68]. It can be concluded that critical comparison of methodological approaches is essential for determination of the most appropriate and practical methods for carrying out usability engineering in healthcare, given the specific objectives of the study. This will continue to be the case into the future as new variations on usability engineering emerge, along with the appearance of new types of health information technologies, including advanced information systems and applications of artificial intelligence.

Discussion Questions
1. What are the essential characteristics of user-centered design (UCD)?
2. What are the issues and challenges in applying UCD in healthcare IT design?
3. What are some of the main issues in understanding and representing user needs as a basis for designing healthcare systems?
4. How can the impacts of systems on essential cognitive processes of users be assessed and why is this critical?
5. How can usability testing methods be practically applied in UCD and rapid prototyping?
6. How do clinical simulations extend usability testing approaches?
7. What are the advantages and disadvantages of remote usability engineering methods and large scale usability studies?

References

1. Beuscart-Zéphir MC, Pelayo S, Anceaux F, Meaux JJ, Degroisse M, Degoulet P. Impact of CPOE on doctor–nurse cooperation for the medication ordering and administration process. Int J Med Inform. 2005;74(7–8):629–41.
2. Kushniruk AW, Borycki EM, editors. Human, social, and organizational aspects of health information systems. IGI Global; 2008.
3. Koppel R, Metlay JP, Cohen A, et al. Role of computerized physician order entry systems in facilitating medication errors. JAMA. 2005;293(10):1197–203.
4. Borycki E, Dexheimer JW, Hullin Lucay Cossio C, et al. Methods for addressing technology-induced errors: the current state. Yearb Med Inform. 2016;25(01):30–40. https://doi.org/10.15265/IY-2016-029.
5. Preece J, Sharp H, Rogers Y. Interaction design: beyond human-computer interaction. Wiley; 2015.
6. Kushniruk AW, Kaufman DR, Patel VL, Lévesque Y, Lottin P. Assessment of a computerized patient record system: a cognitive approach to evaluating medical technology. MD Comput. 1996;13(5):406–15.
7. Kushniruk AW, Patel VL. Cognitive and usability engineering methods for the evaluation of clinical information systems. J Biomed Inform. 2004;37(1):56–76.
8. Nielsen J. Usability engineering. Morgan Kaufmann; 1994.
9. Patel VL, Kaufman DR. Cognitive science and biomedical informatics. In: Biomedical informatics: computer applications in health care and biomedicine. London: Springer London; 2013. p. 109–48.
10. Kaufman DR, Patel VL, Hilliman C, et al. Usability in the real world: assessing medical information technologies in patients' homes. J Biomed Inform. 2003;36(1–2):45–60.
11. Borycki E, Kushniruk A, Nohr C, et al. Usability methods for ensuring health information technology safety: evidence-based approaches contribution of the IMIA working group health informatics for patient safety. Yearb Med Inform. 2013;22(01):20–7.
12. Mao JY, Vredenburg K, Smith PW, Carey T. The state of user-centered design practice. Commun ACM. 2005;48(3):105–9.
13. Karat J. Evolving the scope of user-centered design. Commun ACM. 1997;40(7):33–8.
14. Rouse WB. Design for success: a human-centered approach to designing successful products and systems. New York: Wiley-Interscience; 1991. 270 pp.
15. Johnson CM, Johnson TR, Zhang J. A user-centered framework for redesigning health care interfaces. J Biomed Inform. 2005;38(1):75–87.
16. Damodaran L. User involvement in the systems design process-a practical guide for users. Behav Inform Technol. 1996;15(6):363–77.
17. Gould JD, Lewis C. Designing for usability: key principles and what designers think. Commun ACM. 1985;28(3):300–11.
18. Kujala S. User involvement: a review of the benefits and challenges. Behav Inform Technol. 2003;22(1):1–6.
19. Kushniruk A, Turner P. A framework for user involvement and context in the design and development of safe e-Health systems. In: Quality of life through quality of information. IOS Press; 2012. p. 353–7.
20. Saffer D. Designing for interaction: creating smart applications and clever devices. New Riders; 2007.
21. Rosson MB, Carroll JM. Narrowing the specification-implementation gap in scenario-based design. In: Scenario-based design: envisioning work and technology in system development. New York: Wiley; 1995. p. 247–78.
22. Hackos JT, Redish J. User and task analysis for interface design. New York: Wiley; 1998.
23. Kushniruk A. Evaluation in the design of health information systems: application of approaches emerging from usability engineering. Comput Biol Med. 2002;32(3):141–9.

24. Kushniruk AW, Borycki EM, Kuwata S, Watanabe H. Using a low-cost simulation approach for assessing the impact of a medication administration system on workflow. Stud Health Technol Inform. 2008;136:567.
25. Kannampallil TG, Abraham J. Evaluation of health information technology: methods, frameworks and challenges. In: Cognitive informatics for biomedicine: human computer interaction in healthcare. Springer; 2015. p. 81–109.
26. Kushniruk AW, Borycki EM. Low-cost rapid usability engineering: designing and customizing usable healthcare information systems. Healthc Q. 2006;9(4):98–100, 102.
27. Kushniruk AW, Borycki EM. Human factors in healthcare IT: management considerations and trends. Healthc Manage Forum. 2023;36(2):72–8.
28. Borycki E, Keay E. Methods to assess the safety of health information systems. Healthc Q. 2010;13(Sp):47–52.
29. Kushniruk A, Owston R, Ho F, et al. Design of the VULab: a quantitative and qualitative tool for analyzing use of on-line health information resources. Paper presented at: Proceedings of ITCH. 2007.
30. Nielsen J. Usability inspection methods. Paper presented at: Conference on Human Factors in Computing Systems, 1994 Apr 28. p. 413–4.
31. Zhang J, Johnson TR, Patel VL, Paige DL, Kubose T. Using usability heuristics to evaluate patient safety of medical devices. J Biomed Inform. 2003;36(1–2):23–30.
32. Carvalho CJ, Borycki EM, Kushniruk A. Ensuring the safety of health information systems: using heuristics for patient safety. Healthc Q. 2009;12:49–54.
33. Wharton C. The cognitive walkthrough method: a practitioner's guide. In: Usability inspection Methods. New York: Wiley; 1994. p. 105–40.
34. Borycki EM, Kushniruk AW, Kuwata S, Kannry J. Engineering the electronic health record for safety: a multi-level video-based approach to diagnosing and preventing technology-induced error arising from usability problems. Stud Health Technol Inform. 2011;166:197–205.
35. Kushniruk A, Borycki E, Kuwata S, Kannry J. Predicting changes in workflow resulting from healthcare information systems: ensuring the safety of healthcare. Healthc Q. 2006;9(Sp):114–8.
36. Kushniruk A, Nohr C, Jensen S, Borycki EM. From usability testing to clinical simulations: bringing context into the design and evaluation of usable and safe health information technologies. Yearb Med Inform. 2013;22(01):78–85.
37. Institute of Medicine (U.S.). Committee on Patient Safety and Health Information Technology. Health IT and patient safety: building safer systems for better care. Washington, DC: National Academies Press; 2012.
38. Newell A, Simon HA. Human problem solving. Englewood Cliffs, NJ: Prentice-hall; 1972.
39. Eason KD. Ergonomic perspectives on advances in human-computer interaction. Ergonomics. 1991;34(6):721–41.
40. Li AC, Kannry JL, Kushniruk A, et al. Integrating usability testing and think-aloud protocol analysis with "near-live" clinical simulations in evaluating clinical decision support. Int J Med Inform. 2012;81(11):761–72.
41. Kushniruk AW, Triola MM, Borycki EM, Stein B, Kannry JL. Technology induced error and usability: the relationship between usability problems and prescription errors when using a handheld application. Int J Med Inform. 2005;74(7–8):519–26.
42. Reason J. Understanding adverse events: human factors. Qual Health Care. 1995;4(2):80–9.
43. Carayon P, editor. Handbook of human factors and ergonomics in health care and patient safety. CRC press; 2016.
44. NISTR. Common industry specification for usability requirements 2007 – NISTIR 7432. Available from: http://zing.ncsl.nist.gov/iusr/documents/CISU-R-IR7432.pdf
45. Usabilility.gov. Improving the user experience. Available from: http://guidelines.usability.gov/
46. NHS. Design for patient safety guidelines. Available from: http://www.nrls.npsa.nhs.uk/resources/collections/design-for-patient-safety/

47. Kushniruk AW, Bates DW, Bainbridge M, Househ MS, Borycki EM. National efforts to improve health information system safety in Canada, The United States of America and England. Int J Med Inform. 2013;82(5):e149–60.
48. Kushniruk AW, Patel C, Patel VL, Cimino JJ. 'Televaluation'of clinical information systems: an integrative approach to assessing web-based systems. Int J Med Inform. 2001;61(1):45–70.
49. Andreasen MS, Nielsen HV, Schrøder SO, Stage J. What happened to remote usability testing? An empirical study of three methods. Paper presented at: Proceedings of the SIGCHI Conference on Human Factors in Computing Systems, 2007 Apr 29. p. 1405–14.
50. Hill JR, Brown JC, Campbell NL, Holden RJ. Usability-in-place—remote usability testing methods for homebound older adults: rapid literature review. JMIR Form Res. 2021;5(11):e26181.
51. Sherwin LB, Yevu-Johnson J, Matteson-Kome M, Bechtold M, Reeder B. Remote usability testing to facilitate the continuation of research. Stud Health Technol Inform. 2022;290:424–7.
52. Kushniruk A, Kaipio J, Nieminen M, et al. Human factors in the large: experiences from Denmark, Finland and Canada in moving towards regional and national evaluations of health information system usability. Yearb Med Inform. 2014;23(01):67–81.
53. Albert B, Tullis T, Tedesco D. Beyond the usability lab: conducting large-scale online user experience studies. Morgan Kaufmann; 2009.
54. Fritz M, Berger PD. Improving the user experience through practical data analytics: gain meaningful insight and increase your bottom line. Morgan Kaufmann; 2015.
55. Kaipio J, Lääveri T, Hyppönen H, et al. Usability problems do not heal by themselves: national survey on physicians' experiences with EHRs in Finland. Int J Med Inform. 2017;97:266–81.
56. Tullis T, Fleischman S, McNulty M, Cianchette C, Bergel M. An empirical comparison of lab and remote usability testing of web sites. Paper presented at: Usability Professionals Association Conference, 2002 Jul.
57. Kjeldskov J, Skov MB, Stage J. Instant data analysis: conducting usability evaluations in a day. Paper presented at: Proceedings of the Third Nordic Conference on Human-Computer Interaction, 2004 Oct 23. p. 233–40.
58. Dumas JS, Salzman MC. Usability assessment methods. Rev Hum Factors Ergon. 2006;2(1):109–40.
59. Russ AL, Baker DA, Fahner WJ, et al. A rapid usability evaluation (RUE) method for health information technology. AMIA Annu Symp Proc. 2010;2010:702–6.
60. Patel VL, Kushniruk AW, Yang S, Yale JF. Impact of a computer-based patient record system on data collection, knowledge organization, and reasoning. J Am Med Inform Assoc. 2000;7(6):569–85.
61. Borycki EM, Farghali A, Kushniruk AW. Integrating human patterns of qualitative coding with machine learning: a pilot study involving technology-induced error incident reports. Stud Health Technol Inform. 2022;295:276–80.
62. Shneiderman B. Human-centered AI. Oxford University Press; 2022.
63. Kushniruk A, Borycki E. The human factors of artificial intelligence–where are we now and where are we headed? Lessons learned from AI in healthcare. In: AI and society. Chapman and Hall/CRC; 2022. p. 3–16.
64. Kushniruk A, Borycki E. The human factors of AI in healthcare: recurrent issues, future challenges and ways forward. In: Multiple perspectives on artificial intelligence in healthcare: opportunities and challenges. Cham: Springer; 2021. p. 3–12.
65. Cimino JJ, Patel VL, Kushniruk AW. The patient clinical information system (PatCIS): technical solutions for and experience with giving patients access to their electronic medical records. Int J Med Inform. 2002;68(1–3):113–27.
66. Holden RJ, Cornet VP, Valdez RS. Patient ergonomics: 10-year mapping review of patient-centered human factors. Appl Ergon. 2020;82:102972.
67. Kushniruk A, Beuscart-Zéphir MC, Grzes A, Borycki E, Watbled L, Kannry J. Increasing the safety of healthcare information systems through improved procurement: toward a framework for selection of safe healthcare systems. Healthc Q. 2010;13(Sp):53–8.

68. Baylis TB, Kushniruk AW, Borycki EM. Low-cost rapid usability testing for health information systems: is it worth the effort? Stud Health Technol Inform. 2012;180:363–7.
69. Kushniruk AW, Monkman H, Tuden D, Bellwood P, Borycki EM. Integrating heuristic evaluation with cognitive walkthrough: development of a hybrid usability inspection method. Stud Health Technol Inform. 2015;208:221–5.

Further Reading

Albert W, Tullis T. Measuring the user experience. San Francisco: Morgan Kaufmann; 2010.

Albert B, Tullis T, Tedesco D. Beyond the usability lab: conducting large-scale online user experience studies. Morgan Kaufmann; 2009.

Borycki E, Kushniruk A, Nohr C, et al. Usability methods for ensuring health information technology safety: evidence-based approaches contribution of the IMIA working group health informatics for patient safety. Yearb Med Inform. 2013;22(01):20–7.

Fritz M, Berger PD. Improving the user experience through practical data analytics: gain meaningful insight and increase your bottom line. Morgan Kaufmann; 2015.

Kuniavsky M. Observing the user experience: a practitioner's guide to user research. Elsevier; 2003.

Kushniruk A. Evaluation in the design of health information systems: application of approaches emerging from usability engineering. Comput Biol Med. 2002;32(3):141–9.

Kushniruk A, Nohr C, Jensen S, Borycki EM. From usability testing to clinical simulations: bringing context into the design and evaluation of usable and safe health information technologies. Yearb Med Inform. 2013;22(01):78–85.

Kushniruk AW, Patel VL. Cognitive and usability engineering methods for the evaluation of clinical information systems. J Biomed Inform. 2004;37(1):56–76.

Patel VL, Kushniruk AW, Yang S, Yale JF. Impact of a computer-based patient record system on data collection, knowledge organization, and reasoning. J Am Med Inform Assoc. 2000;7(6):569–85.

Rogers Y, Sharp H, Preece J. Interaction design: beyond human-computer interaction. Wiley; 2023.

Chapter 11
Human Factors and Design for Supporting Healthcare Teams

Charlotte Tang, Yan Xiao, Yunan Chen, and Paul N. Gorman

Introduction

Healthcare today is a team sport, no longer dominated by the vision of a single nurse or doctor interacting with a patient. Rather, modern healthcare occurs through a coordinated action of many individuals, possessing diverse skills and expertise, sometimes collocated but often distributed in time and space. Obvious examples of healthcare teams include a surgical team performing an operation, emergency department (ED) personnel stabilizing a trauma patient, a "code team" responding to in-hospital cardiac arrest, and daily bedside rounds by multi-disciplinary teams in an intensive care unit. Less obvious are examples of health professional communication and collaboration that do not occur face-to-face. For example, a nurse may notice unexpected symptoms in her patient during night-shift, contact a pharmacist to learn this is a medication side effect, pass this information on verbally at shift report so other nurses can monitor the effects, record the information in the medical record for all clinicians to be aware, and perhaps add a paper or electronic "post-it" note for the physician, suggesting a change of the medication order at morning rounds long after the night-shift nurse has left.

C. Tang (✉)
University of Michigan-Flint, Flint, MI, USA
e-mail: tcharlot@umich.edu

Y. Xiao
University of Texas at Arlington, Arlington, TX, USA

Y. Chen
University of California, Irvine, CA, USA

P. N. Gorman
Oregon Health & Science University, Portland, OR, USA

© The Author(s), under exclusive license to Springer Nature
Switzerland AG 2024
A. W. Kushniruk et al. (eds.), *Human Computer Interaction in Healthcare*,
Cognitive Informatics in Biomedicine and Healthcare,
https://doi.org/10.1007/978-3-031-69947-4_11

In these contexts, electronic health records (EHR) and other health information technologies (health IT) can function in ways that support healthcare teams, becoming a routine part of healthcare delivery and changing the ways teams work, communicate and collaborate. Outside the hospital, consumer-centered health IT such as patient portals and personal health records (PHR) can enable individuals to become more effectively engaged in their care, sharing information and communicating with multiple members of the healthcare team. In this chapter, we review healthcare teams, key concepts and theories of teamwork, and present two case studies on teamwork in healthcare.

Diversity of Healthcare Teams

In team research literature, an often adopted definition of a team is "*a distinguishable set of two or more people who interact dynamically, interdependently, and adaptively toward a common and valued goal/object/mission, who have each been assigned specific roles or functions to perform, and who have a limited life span of membership*" ([1], p. 4). This definition goes beyond mere affiliation, emphasizing common goals and specific role assignments. In healthcare, role assignments may be perceived differently by different parties or may at times be unclear. For example, a surgeon, a nurse, and a patient may identify team membership or roles and responsibilities differently, and changing conditions and personnel in attendance may make assignments less clear and require re-negotiation. Table 11.1 lists several key characteristics of healthcare teams with examples.

It is important to recognize that a great variety of teams exist in healthcare, with varying degrees of shared objectives, clarity of role specifications, and interdependencies. For example, ED care is characterized by unpredictable and changing

Table 11.1 Key characteristics of healthcare teams

Healthcare team characteristics	Examples
Multidisciplinary	Multidisciplinary rounds in pediatric intensive care unit (Fig. 11.3)
Dynamic team formation, composition, and role assignment, blurry role differentiation	Ad hoc medical teams formed in ED to stabilize trauma patients (Fig. 11.2)
Distributed or collocated teams, or a combination	Multidisciplinary Medical Team (MMT) meetings with remote consultation with specialists; telemedicine
Coordination needed for continuous coverage	Shift handovers in inpatient care; patient transfer to ICU for close monitoring
May be defined by profession, discipline, physical location, temporal shift, patient needs, etc.	Pharmacists vs. radiologists; outpatient unit vs. ICU; day nurses vs. night nurses
Communication mediated through cognitive artifacts	EHR for physicians and nurses to communicate; whiteboard for residents' patient assignment; intercom for broadcasting within a medical unit

combinations of patient care needs, sometimes shifting abruptly from low-demand to highly complex and urgent. In response, ED teams tend to be highly adaptive and ephemeral, changing in composition, roles, and assignments based on shifting requirements of a fluctuating group of patients and care issues. Intensive care units (ICUs) also exhibit such ad hoc, self-assembling teams, which then dissolve once conditions have stabilized. For ICU teamwork, strategy and goal formulation were the most common team tasks, and the level of teamwork was significantly associated with ICU patient outcomes, as found in a systematic review [2]. By contrast, other healthcare contexts are characterized by stable, well-defined teams, for example, a cardiac surgery suite where a small and select group of surgeons, nurses, surgical technicians, perfusionists, and anesthesiologists work together frequently, developing well defined roles and responsibilities, and familiar communication patterns often used measures for patient safety [3].

A review of teamwork in healthcare [4] used the concept of "organizational shell" to understand various types of teams in healthcare in terms of how an organization provides a structural context for the functioning of a team. A team may find a strong infrastructure ("organizational shell") with explicit requirements on personnel with respect to training, skills, knowledge, certification, and privileges; well thought-out structures for team tasks such as protocols, standardized operating procedures; and well-designed technology support. Such a strong organizational shell reduces coordination needs [5]. In many healthcare settings, work demands may be less predictable or work systems less well designed. In these cases, team membership and task assignments may be less clear, work practices become adaptive, and workarounds become common. Such fluid behavioral norms and authority arrangements render it difficult to make general statements about healthcare teams independent of the care context and the degree to which an "organizational shell" exists.

In addition to the role that an "organizational shell" may provide, multiple factors contribute to effective team functioning in healthcare, including prior education, training, and experience, professional group influences, regulatory policies, and cultural norms [5]. As a result, team roles, expectations, and lines of authority are sustained across contexts and organizations, exhibiting what amounts to interoperability of health professionals as they move across organizational contexts.

Characteristics of Healthcare Teams

Xiao et al. [4] highlight several features commonly found in healthcare teams, two of which are very relevant to the design of health IT. First, team composition changes, depending on settings and needs, or simply over time. A family physician may work with different supporting staff in her clinic to address varying issues and patient care needs. A nurse often must contact different physicians at different times of the day when making referral appointments for a patient so that her routine practices are not impacted. Hospital staff such as interns and residents in training, hospitalist physicians, or surgical specialists may rotate on and off duty over a short cycle time, resulting in fluctuating configurations of staff and a high degree of adaptability by team members [3]. Moreover, team composition can change as a function of a patient's illness and treatment trajectory, when the needs of a patient change. Health IT can thus play important roles in enabling team members to see which care clinicians have participated in the care of a patient and in providing up-to-date information on the roles of each team member in relation to a patient.

Second, the delineation of responsibility and the communication structure in healthcare teams may become unclear across temporal or functional boundaries. Individual patients, particularly in hospital settings, require participation by changing groups of health professionals, with cross-coverage responsibilities over nights or weekends and other changes to work and personnel arrangements. In military settings, a designated and clear structure for communication and role differentiation can reduce the overhead of communication and negotiation [6], a principle that may be applied in healthcare settings as well.

Definition of teams can have profound implications for how health IT should be designed to enhance team communication and collaboration. For example, teams may be defined by profession and discipline, by physical or temporal context, or by emerging patient needs. Examples of professional or disciplinary teams include (a) surgeons who share the care of patients who have had surgery, (b) nurses who share responsibility for care of patients on a nursing unit, or (c) physical therapists who share responsibility for therapy needs of patients distributed throughout the hospital. Examples of contextually defined teams include the multidisciplinary team responsible for patients in a specific location such as an operating room or emergency department, or those responsible for care over a specific period of time such as the night shift. Examples of teams defined by emerging care needs include the ad hoc, self-assembling teams that form and dissolve in response to emergent needs in an intensive care unit or delivery room.

These forms of team definition and composition have implications for the processes and artifacts or tools used for communication and collaboration. To illustrate, a surgical resident may consider the attending surgeons and surgical residents on his/her surgical service as his/her team, sharing responsibility for the preoperative and postoperative care of patients receiving surgery from a member of their group. Such a group will typically have routines for group discussion to share patient information and care plans (during "rounds"), as well as shared cognitive artifacts (either paper or electronic) for recording and transferring this information within the group. These routines and artifacts support transfer of information, collective management of responsibility, and shared situation awareness that enable them to achieve the shared goal of caring for all the patients on their service throughout the day, ideally with processes that are robust to disruptions in availability and responsibility, such as when members of the team are unexpectedly called to or are delayed in the operating room, requiring others on the team to shift roles and responsibilities.

By contrast, multidisciplinary teams that are defined by context often have distinct routines or work processes for working together such as multidisciplinary rounds, and informal rules for turn-taking in discourse, as well as separate artifacts, such as whiteboards or printed lists, that support the somewhat different work that is accomplished in a multidisciplinary context.

Team composition and function may not be perceived in the same way by all members. As an example, the clinicians and staff who provide care to a patient often have defined roles and common goals, even though the patient may never think of them as comprising a team. At the same time, the patient's family and loved ones may play significant roles in the determination and delivery of care, even though the clinician may be unaware of this. In designing health IT, it may thus be constructive to consider the entire group of healthcare professionals and family members as a team.

When healthcare teams working together to care for an individual patient are not located together in the same place at the same time, the need for technologies to support their interaction is especially great. In these cases communication among team members in healthcare must be mediated by appropriate technologies, such as fax machines and increasingly through the EHR, whether by use of a common EHR system or through development of mechanisms for interoperability. As such, the design of health IT has direct impact on how team members "*interact dynamically, interdependently, and adaptively*" ([1], p. 4). Healthcare teams during the COVID-19 pandemic used health IT extensively to cope with social distancing requirements, such as adapting team huddles and other team activities to be temporally and spatially distributed [7]. Inadequate understanding of how teams coordinate has resulted in suboptimal patient care (e.g., [8, 9]). Two examples are communication of medication orders and use of bar code medication administration systems (BCMA). With communication of medication orders, a physician may assume an order, once entered, will be acted upon immediately by the pharmacist or nurse, when in fact, many EHR implementations require the nurse to log in and specifically look for new orders. With BCMA systems, a nurse may assume the system checks the identity of the medication and of the patient, when in fact some systems do not confirm the identity of the patient [10]. Similar "illusion of communication" leads to many incidences of communication breakdowns [9]. Therefore, some hospitals have developed policies, for example for physicians to talk directly with nurses when time-sensitive orders are placed on EHR, so that harmful delays can be avoided.

Teamwork in Healthcare Practices

Healthcare work can be highly dynamic, requiring intense, often multidisciplinary, collaboration. Patient care teams often consist of a large number of personnel ranging from clinicians, e.g., doctors, nurses, and pharmacists, to non-clinical members, e.g., unit coordinators, administrative staff, and those responsible for equipment supply and maintenance, [11, 12]. These team members may be co-located, such as those in emergency care or during a routine family doctor visit [13, 14], but more often, they are distributed over different spatial locations [8, 15]. This is particularly the case for patients with complex or multiple illnesses who require coordinated care from different specialists, each contributing to the treatment plan. Although health IT such as the EHR can help facilitate communication between distributed collaborators, the need for clinicians to move between distributed locations while conducting medical work has been found to be indispensable [15, 16]. In addition, hospital work is typically under "continuous coverage" [17] in order to offer around-the clock patient care. Thus, temporal coordination of work among team members must be carefully maintained [18, 19]. Taken together, these collaboration challenges increase the risk of communication breakdowns and can negatively impact the quality of patient care if they are not properly considered and addressed [20–25].

Healthcare work is often considered information work such that collaborative work relies on a variety of information media, such as verbal exchange, paper, and display media [26–31]. In particular, paper artifacts are often used to record and track a work plan, as a bedside information source, opportune notepad, and tool for information transfer within and across shifts [32, 33]. In addition, patients' medical records are instrumental in supporting collaborative practices, acting as a "collection and distributing device" [34] that constitutes and mediates social relations and interrelated patient care tasks. The medical records also serve as a communication vehicle, linking heterogeneous health professionals and mediating much of the healthcare system [35].

Team Effectiveness

Hackman [36] considers team effectiveness as a combination of team performance (a reflection of individual and team-level teamwork when working towards a shared goal), team functioning (how a team performs on a daily basis with regard to teamwork and taskwork), and team viability (future prediction of team functioning). In the U.S. alone, 134 million adverse events take place in hospitals leading to 2.6 million deaths annually [37], imposing serious patient safety challenges. While poor team functioning has been found to be a critical factor for adverse events in patient safety [38], role clarity among healthcare providers can improve team functioning [39, 40], which in turn can result in better outcomes for patients, providers, and healthcare systems [41–43]. On the other hand, team training has been identified to be essential for improving team performance. Thus there has been an increasing interest worldwide in finding ways to improve team performance and team functioning [44]. A recent systematic review showed the promising role of brief team interventions on team functioning in acute care in-patient settings and a clear need for studies to investigate how short team interventions can improve role clarity and team functioning among healthcare teams that involve patients and families in other settings [45]. Given the frequent, dynamic changes in healthcare team membership due to rotations and shift changes, it is thus imperative for healthcare teams to improve on communication and to have clear roles of team members, including those of patients and families.

Burnout in Healthcare Providers

Burnout among healthcare providers has been a universal phenomenon that unfolds over time due to the complex, dynamic, and demanding work environment. It affects not only healthcare providers but also their patients and more broadly the healthcare system [46]. This phenomenon is characterized by emotional exhaustion (feelings of being over-extended or drained), depersonalization (having negative, even hostile attitudes and detached feelings towards patients), and a diminished sense of personal accomplishment (feeling incompetent and inefficient at work) [47].

Healthcare teams interact with human health and illness, and high levels of uncertainty everyday. When caring for complex patient cases and supporting their families, healthcare teams are inherently disposed to higher risk of burnout. As such, 25–60% of physicians across various specialties experienced exhaustion [48–50]. Thus, it is important to recognize and address the consequences of burnout in healthcare teams so that the detriments on healthcare providers, patients and their families, and healthcare system at large can be mitigated.

While burnout affects every profession, frontline healthcare teams were found to be particularly prone to burnout. A survey conducted between 2011 and 2014 found an increase of U.S. physicians reporting at least one symptom of burnout from 45.5% in 2011 to 54.4% in 2014. In contrast, their satisfaction with work-life balance had declined from 48.5% in 2011 to 40.9% in 2014 [51]. Another survey conducted in August–November 2014 by Tawfik et al. [52] found similar result on U.S. physicians reporting symptoms of fatigue (54.3%). It also reported excessive fatigue (32.8%), a significant medical error in the past 3 months (10.5%), recent suicidal thoughts (6.5%), and poor or failing patient safety rating (3.9%). Burnout can also lead to increased stress, disruptive behavior, mood disorders, and depression [53, 54]. In fact, physicians were found to be at a much higher risk of suicide compared to the general population: 28–40 vs. 12.3 per 100,000 [55]. Yet, burnout is not limited to physicians. Forty-three percent of nurses working in U.S. hospitals experience symptoms of emotional exhaustion [18]. Depersonalization among nurses was found to be associated with increased self-reported adverse events [56]. In particular, burnout has been found to be detrimental to healthcare team communication which in turn could lead to diminished team efficacy [57]. Moreover, physicians in training, residents, of all specialties reported an overall 69% burnout rate [58] and more than 50% of medical students in U.S. experience burnout symptoms [59].

Not only does exhaustion affect one's well-being and patient care, but it can also adversely impact the health care system since a healthcare provider suffering from burnout is less productive, deliver poorer patient care, jeopardize patient safety, and may even quit or retire early [60–63]. For example, a physician's departure will require additional administrative costs in replacing the trained healthcare provider, reduced quality, diminished productivity, and lower morale among healthcare providers in the organization [64]. Thus, burnout can have substantial economic impact on the healthcare system.

Key Concepts and Theories for Team Performance

Sociotechnical Aspects of Teamwork

Previous studies on healthcare teamwork investigated a variety of sociotechnical issues, e.g., mobility [15, 16, 65], temporality [18, 26, 66], coordinating artifacts [15, 27], communication channels [24, 67, 68], and richness of information [69–72]. From these studies, we have gained considerable insights into the processes and challenges for achieving effective collaboration in healthcare.

Dynamic Communication Behaviors

Effective communication is essential for successful teamwork. In medical settings, communication is ubiquitous and accounts for a substantial portion of daily routines, including interactions and information sharing in varying contexts, across temporal and spatial dimensions [15, 73, 74]. Communication failure among clinicians, however, has been frequently found to contribute to preventable adverse events [68].

Face-to-face communication offers a richer communication experience, providing paralinguistic and nonverbal information in addition to the words themselves, and likely offers the best quality and spectrum of communication [31, 75–77]. Furthermore, colocation of healthcare work permits indirect and informal communication [78], enhancing situational awareness among members of the group in a manner similar to more formalized coordination mechanisms such as "voice loops" [79]. The mobile and dynamic nature of medical work presents challenges to effective communication. Artifacts such as whiteboards and bulletin boards, used both synchronously and asynchronously, provide a flexible shared workspace that facilitates joint discussion and provide shared and persistent information display [31, 80], promoting awareness and coordination of ongoing activities [26, 31].

In hospitals especially, healthcare work is peripatetic: it is necessary for patients, health professionals, and equipment to move among spatially distributed "work centers" (e.g. emergency department, imaging suite, operating room, intensive care unit) each with specialized personnel and equipment. Mobility is therefore crucial, for people, equipment, and the health IT that connects them. Thus, Bardram and Bossen [15] regarded medical work as *mobility work* because mobility is often required to bring together "*the right configuration of people, resources, knowledge and place in order to carry out tasks*". Although mobility itself does not usually accomplish any concrete tasks, without mobility, many tasks cannot be fulfilled. In particular, mobility enables distributed collaborators to conduct rich face-to-face communication, and to access information artifacts such as large whiteboards located in different units in order to achieve effective patient care.

Meanwhile, communication across temporal boundaries such as work shifts is essential to ensure continuity of monitoring, diagnosis, and treatment regimes.

Staggers and Jennings [81] investigated nursing shift report in seven medical and surgical units to identify the content and context of information exchange across nursing shifts. Their findings aligned with the results of a systematic review of studies on nursing and physician handovers [82], which revealed that there were many types and situational varieties of handovers and shift handovers and concluded these could be better supported by an EHR system if a standardized set of key information was exchanged in a structured manner.

In addition, medical team members such as physicians, nurses, and pharmacists typically have different temporal work routines and shift cycles, increasing the challenges of coordinating team activities [66]. Breakdowns in communication between teams have been found to contribute to many adverse events. For example, Horwitz et al. [23], examining adverse events at the transition from ED to in-hospital care found that "communication failure at some point of care was central to most" reported errors. As an example, an investigation into the amputation of a patient's wrong leg revealed an inadvertent communication error during shift report [83]. More recent research on patient handover between medical units in the same hospital revealed a variety of communication challenges that involved competing departmental goals, resources, and teams. This sometimes led to limited information sharing between departments. For example, a department may conceal bed availability information from other departments so that they can make their own decisions on bed assignments, which not only affected the inter-departmental coordination but also mitigated the organizational efficiency [8, 84].

Medical Records for Supporting Collaborative Work

Amongst the diversity of coordination artifacts and mechanisms used in healthcare work, patient medical records are the fundamental information infrastructure enabling collaboration across time and space. Medical records are not merely a documentation tool for patient's health conditions [85], but also an information collection and distribution device that connects interrelated patient care tasks and social relations in a clinical environment. For instance, while a surgical team interacts face-to-face inside an operating room, team members also communicate through clinical notes in the patient's medical record when working independently on different threads of patient care activities.

In recent years, EHR systems have been widely implemented to replace paper medical records in clinical settings. The benefits of EHR systems include improvements in accessibility, patient safety, accountability, and cost-savings [70, 86]. However, the design of these systems has largely focused on EHR systems as an information storage and retrieval tool for administrative, research, and legal usage [87], with little attention to how the EHR can support communication, coordination, and collaboration of healthcare teams [88, 89]. Many prior studies reported cases in which poorly designed health IT systems have led to unintended negative consequences after deployment, including dissatisfaction, adoption failures, inefficiencies, and even increased medical errors [90–93]. These studies suggest that health

IT systems do not properly support communication and coordination activities in team-based health care.

In contrast, properly designed and implemented health IT solutions have the potential to support collaboration among a variety of stakeholders, from patients to clinicians, individuals to institutions, and policymakers at all levels. In recent years, through government programs and incentives, the EHR and other health IT have become virtually universal, making it critically important and timely to address these issues resulting from the complex interplay among human, organizational, and technological systems in healthcare.

(a) Relational Coordination and Social Interaction in Teamwork

The dynamic and often urgent nature of healthcare work amplifies the need for effective coordination of interdependent work tasks. In this respect, interpersonal communication and relationships have been found to facilitate work coordination [94], as evidenced in the reduction of adverse events such as hospital-acquired infections and medication errors [95]. Specifically, work coordination in healthcare settings requires frequent communication of accurate and timely information, and can be enhanced through relationships via shared goals, shared knowledge, and mutual respect. Such relational coordination is particularly instrumental in healthcare settings as patients' illness trajectories are often associated with a high degree of uncertainty. For example, when a patient's condition unexpectedly becomes unstable, effective communication and efficient work coordination among relevant healthcare team members would be critical for addressing the unexpected emergency. Coordination among team members can be more effective if positive interpersonal relationships exist [76, 94, 96–99].

Interpersonal relationships are often achieved through informal social interactions, which are generally characterized by being impromptu, brief and context-rich, and often involve small groups of people triggered by their proximity ([99]; [97]). These informal social interactions are important for articulating work among team members and coordinating shared resources for collaboration ([100]; [101]). Yet, as healthcare work becomes more fragmented and time-pressured, clinicians less frequently find time to interact socially with their colleagues during their shift [33]. This may be made worse by health IT because systems may hinder articulation work and social interactions [102]. For example, physical interaction through circulation of paper charts and paper prescriptions among team members allows impromptu interpersonal interactions [103], while a shift to greater use of EHR is often coupled with time spent in isolation at the computer [104], reducing mobility [105], and hindering interpersonal communication [33].

(b) Formal and Informal Work

The use of technology in healthcare settings has been criticized for a tendency toward "formalizing" work practices, such as increasing the structuralization of information representation, and making work processes standardized and rigid [102, 106, 107]. Therefore, team members may have to rely on informal practices to leverage the flexible and spontaneous aspects of collaborative work [97, 99, 108–110]. Informal practices identified in the literature include impromptu human interactions and the use of tools outside of the central system, [97, 99, 109, 110] such as face to face conversations, instant messaging, and text messaging which overcome the rigidity and formality of EHR systems [11, 111, 112].

In practice, clinicians frequently adopt informal workarounds beyond the standard operations of health applications and health IT [113, 114] in order to circumvent problems that emerge when a newly deployed IT system disrupts workflows and interferes with task performance or goal attainment [115, 116]. These workarounds can be new or reconfigured tools, artifacts, or ways of interacting with an EHR system [9, 33, 90, 92, 117]. Well-documented examples of workarounds are the use of "*scraps*" or "*paper notes*" [20, 33, 93, 118, 119] and clinicians' avoidance of documenting social-psycho-emotional information in EHRs [120, 121].

In healthcare settings, organizational culture and policy determine the kind of information an artifact should contain and who may view or alter this information. Some information artifacts are meant to be maintained permanently as the official legal record of care. Other information artifacts are created for temporary and informal use, to mediate work processes [122] or transmit sensitive information [120], only to be disposed of afterwards. Clinicians often use a variety of informal, sometimes individualized information tools to represent information in ways that support specific tasks, in addition to the official, archival EHR record. Temporary storage on paper or personal computing devices may be used to gather fragments of information found in different information systems or in fragmented locations within a single EHR. Portable and temporary forms of information may support tasks and work activities or to support certain activities that EHRs fail to support. These informal artifacts have been pervasively used by clinicians and play a vital role in coordinating healthcare work [32, 33, 93, 118, 119, 123].

Previous studies also found that clinicians often chose to refrain from entering social-psycho-emotional information regarding a patient's care in EHR systems, as this type of subjective information often conflicts with the objective and factual requirements of EHR-based formal documentation ([120]; [124]; [121]). Thus informal artifacts such as the "kardex" are frequently used for sharing work-related information including subjective patient care information during shift transitions ([118]; [122]; [119]; [93]; [33]) and they carry flexible and work-in-progress notes that are not ready to be documented in archival format in the EHR ([20]; [117]; [33]).

(c) Visible and Invisible Work
Current health IT is primarily designed for performing explicit, visible tasks and supporting visible roles, but healthcare work also involves important but less visible roles and tasks [125]. The concept of visible and invisible shares some similarities to the front-stage-back-stage concept; an explication of the latter is presented in the second case study at the end of the chapter. Examples of invisible tasks include those performed by nurses to conduct comfort work [12] and secretaries to

coordinate patient transfer [126, 127]. These tasks are not recorded, thus become invisible, in patient medical records, but these invisible tasks are important, and often indispensible, for work accomplishment. However invisible work has been overlooked in the design of many IT systems [128].

Thus, the design of complex collaborative systems should recognize and represent all invisible roles, tasks, and processes in the collaboration process [129, 130]. This goal of making work visible is difficult to achieve, however, with EHR designs that are focused primarily on explicit tasks and documentation. For example, non-clinical or unlicensed staff in hospitals and clinics such as clerical personnel, social workers and case managers, or medical assistants often remain invisible in systems, and the critical roles they play in providing and coordinating care may not be taken into account in the IT infrastructure [125–127]. Other important work processes are also neglected. In particular, EHRs often display aggregated tasks without showing and tracking the multiplicity of individual work tasks involved [20]. The lack of a systems-level representation of these invisible but critical steps can result in serious collaboration breakdowns.

Furthermore, system design has to balance visibility and invisibility among different team members so that individuals will not be overwhelmed by specific details that are not related to their work [128], e.g., keeping backstage work invisible and providing different levels of granularity to different roles. Yet, current EHRs sometimes present the exact same view to team members with different information and communication needs, e.g., physicians and nurses likely require and use information differently but the information display in current EHRs are typically the same [117]. Finally, given the life-critical, and often time-constrained nature of healthcare work, maintaining a good balance between visible and invisible work is crucial to collaborative work supported by the central information infrastructure.

Supporting Team Collaboration with New Technologies

Research on collaborative work in healthcare investigates how current practices are conducted in specific settings or examines the impact of new technologies in supporting collaborative work *in situ*. These studies have often led to new implications for supporting collaborative work practices or insights for improving current health IT. In this section, we briefly review new technologies developed in supporting collaborative work in healthcare. Of special note, there are only a handful of studies that actually designed and deployed new technologies for real use, which is largely due to the high threshold of safety control and regulations in healthcare settings. Current and future studies on health IT during the COVID-19 pandemic will likely generate new insight on socio-technological requirements during rapidly changing work patterns while health IT infrastructure itself tends to be rigidly configured [7].

Technology for Supporting Distributed Communication in Healthcare

Collaborative healthcare practices often require that workers have timely access to people, information, and resources [15]. However, competing tasks as well as spatial and temporal distribution of team members create barriers or delays in communication. Mobile wearable communication devices (e.g., Vocera) provide voice-operating connectivity for ad hoc communication among team members that can improve communication and reduce their spatial movements [131, 132]. In particular, such devices allow clinicians to continue with a current task while communicating with team members about other patients or tasks, improving the efficiency and the quality of patient care [132]. Similarly, Richardson and Ash [105] found that the use of hands-free communication devices in clinical settings provided clinicians with better communication access and also better control over the information they could access.

Technologies for Supporting Coordination in Medical Work

Other than supporting point-to-point direct communication, technologies have also been developed to support social awareness that underpins collaborative work. In particular, Bardram and Hansen [133] developed the AWARE architecture that offered a platform for supporting context-mediated social awareness for mobile and distributed teams. AwarePhone was a context-aware technology designed to support awareness among hospital clinicians and AwareMedia was developed on a large interactive display that supports social, spatial, and temporal awareness with a shared messaging system [134]. In recent years, chat apps have become very popular and have found their way into various hospital settings across the globe [135]. For example, WhatsApp has become an important tool within the organizational communication ecosystem in a large multi-specialty hospital in India because of its ease of use and rich features (e.g., photo sharing). The chat app helped reinforce communication on both the organizational and local work practices, and bridge across shift boundaries [136]. These technologies provided new ways for promoting awareness in hospital work and their deployment showed promising results in enhancing communication.

Moreover, supporting the coordination of actual work tasks among collaborators is crucial for team-based practices, and a special challenge when task scheduling must be dynamically changing in response to changing needs. For example, surgical operations require careful planning of resources and personnel including the operating room, equipment, specialized surgeons, anesthesiologists, and nurses, taking account of their availability, schedule, and constraints. In fact, coordination and scheduling are often tightly coupled and are necessary for achieving collaborative healthcare work. However in practice, these tasks are non-trivial and often challenging as resource optimization, a key goal for hospital efficiency, must be balanced against changing patient care needs and competing demands on personnel [137]. Thus, a variety of new technologies such as electronic whiteboards and scheduling systems have been developed and deployed to facilitate the coordination of team-based activities. For example, a study conducted in an emergency department found that the use of an electronic whiteboard improved work efficiency and communication quality among clinicians [138]. Wong et al. [139] conducted a survey and found that 71% of the respondents considered that the whiteboard helped improve their team-based communication and 62% agreed that they were able to retrieve patients' medical information faster with the whiteboard. Moreover, a prototypical Patient Scheduler deployed in a surgical unit was also found to help facilitate patient scheduling, and temporal coordination of the collaborative work and allocation of resources in the hospital [26].

Technology for Supporting Information Access

Most modern healthcare settings are equipped with an EHR system to facilitate the retrieval and use of medical information for improving the quality of patient care. Mobile devices have been introduced to supporting flexible bedside access to the EHR and other information, including tablets [140, 141] and computers-on-wheels [33]. Though potentially helpful, challenges have been documented including mechanical flaws and perceived intrusiveness into the nurse-patient relationship as the nurse shifted focus to the computer screen (Fig. 11.1) [33]. The nurses were also found to continue to use paper notes that they had always created and used for their shift work despite the availability of the mobile computers-on-wheels intended for information access at bedside.

Based on their longitudinal field studies in a hospital including the computers-on-wheels study previously described, Tang and Carpendale [143] developed a prototype technology that made use of digital pen and paper that allowed nurses to

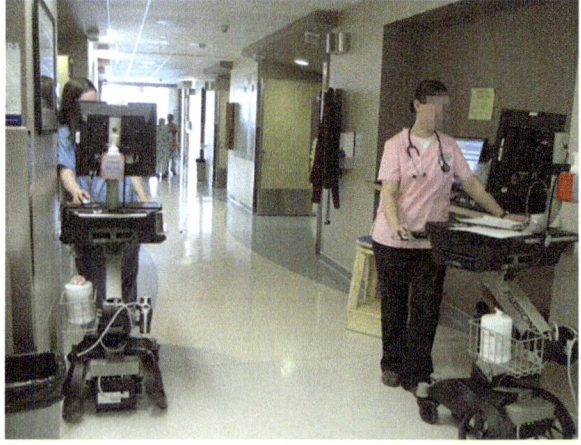

Fig. 11.1 The use of computer-on-wheels weakened interpersonal interaction. Source: Tang [142]

continue to use their familiar pen and paper to create their paper notes. The handwritten notes could be easily transformed into digital texts for documentation without navigating the hierarchical EHR system. The integrated paper-and-digital design was based on the findings that clinicians strongly preferred handwritten notes to the digital information in the EHR system. The feedback for this prototype gathered from six focus groups with nurses was generally encouraging and design guidelines were proposed for further development of the prototype to support both clinicians' preferred practices and the use of EHRs intended by the hospital. In a related study, a mobile digital pen meant to allow more flexible and mobile record keeping was viewed positively by nurses, but used little because of mechanical or physical limitations of the device [144]. If these issues are addressed, these novel designs can be useful in a variety of healthcare settings including hospitals, primary care clinics and community health centers.

Case Studies of Teamwork

As described above, communication and coordination of healthcare teams play a crucial role in achieving quality patient care. Therefore two case studies on different healthcare teams in different contexts are presented below. The first case study presents communication challenges encountered by healthcare teams dynamically and ephemerally formed in an ED, primarily for stabilizing the patients such that they can be quickly transferred out of the ED. The second case study describes the use of information artifacts and the communication processes during medical rounds that took place in a Pediatric Intensive Care Unit (PICU).

Communication Challenges for Loosely Formed Collaboration Teams
The following vignette was abstracted from our field study in an ED to show how mobile phones adopted in the ED failed to support the distributed teamwork.

> While Paul, a nurse in the ED, was at bedside drawing a blood sample from a patient, his mobile phone vibrated. Not knowing what the call was about, Paul decided to ignore it. This phone call turned out to be an emergency call to help with a critically ill patient in another room. Paul later commented why he didn't pick up the call "…when you are at the bedside with the patient, it [the mobile phone] rings; you pick it up to answer it. Sometimes they [the patients] may think it's rude. I don't think the patients know it's a work phone. I think they think it's a personal phone. Or it's ringing, ringing, ringing and you are in the middle of doing IV. The patients can go like 'okay it's ringing.' So that is a problem!"

Although mobile phones are highly appreciated in many other fields for the convenience it offers to distributed team members, clinicians in the ED actually often ignored mobile phone calls. Instead, they generally preferred to use overhead pagers to communicate work-related information inside the ED. This is because communication via mobile phones did not provide sufficient group awareness information for the patient care team members, which often led to unwanted interruptions at patients' bedside. More importantly, it failed to support role-based communication,

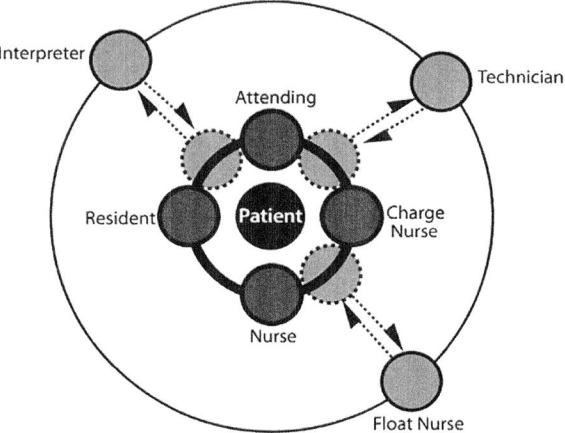

Fig. 11.2 The formation and disassembly of a loosely formed patient care team. Dark and light grey indicate core and peripheral members respectively. The dotted circles show that peripheral members join the care team temporarily. Source: Lee et al. [11]

which is important to the dynamic collaborative healthcare work that sometimes requires personnel of a specific role instead of a specific named person. The lack of role-based communication has caused considerable challenges in the ED teamwork communication since the team members are often formed dynamically and ephemerally in the ED (Fig. 11.2).

Our analysis of communication breakdowns in the ED revealed a unique characteristic of the collaborative teamwork that we regarded as *loosely formed* team collaboration. Specifically, patient care teams in the ED differ considerably from those in other medical wards, as ED care teams are often dynamically and quickly assembled upon patient arrival and the heterogeneous team members must immediately engage in interdependent and complex care activities. Since ED patients often require care from different providers including ED doctor, nurses, and various specialists. These team members come together dynamically and work with various collaborators for patients with different needs. Variations in shift cycles, temporal horizons, and collaborators' job nature further complicate the collaborative work. For example, ED nurses and residents have different shift cycles. ED nurses work on 12-h cycles and their bed assignment usually changes every 4 h, whereas ED residents work on 8–12 h shifts with different starting times. Thus, the residents may have to work with different nurses for a single patient during a shift, complicating the work collaboration. When individual care team members simultaneously work in multiple patient cases, the complexity in collaboration becomes highly intertwined and significantly more challenging. Finally, when an ED patient is stabilized, the responsible team dissolves right away. Thus the coordination required for achieving this kind of fluid work practices is highly challenging, and thus susceptible to breakdowns. In particular, the frequently changing collaborative teams require substantial spatial movement for collaboration, temporal coordination of the collaborative tasks, effective handling of unpredictable interruptions, and coordination across multiple healthcare teams comprising of team members of different roles and each team member may be concurrently involved in multiple patient cases.

The team members' spatial distribution explains why mobile phones were not preferred in the ED since each team member has to be reached separately. Moreover, sometimes when personnel of a particular role, such as a technician, instead of a specific person are needed, the current communication system did not support locating team members by their role. In addition, calls may interrupt patient care activities at the bedside as mobile phones used in the ED did not provide any caller information. In contrast, overhead pagers allowed ED-wide broadcasts alerting all team members at the same time. However, they might run the risk of disclosing private patient information over an open link. Hence the findings from this study pointed to the need for designing future communication technologies to meet the needs of loosely formed collaborative environments by providing team-based communication with lightweight feedback and point-to-point information transparency while preserving patient privacy.

Information Arena to Support Team Rounding in a Pediatric Intensive Care Unit

Hospital rounds are multi-disciplinary meetings convened at regular times (often daily), partly for purposes of coordinating care among workers. The complexity of hospital care [12] has made such rounds ever more essential for the safety and quality of care received by the patients. Hospital rounds are an example of teamwork for exchanging and updating critical information and responsibility under time constraints. Therefore, it is important for participants to select the most relevant details while providing an overall assessment. The following dialogue presents a typical segment from a "walking" round in a surgical Intensive Care Unit (ICU) during which the participants often ambulate. The information artifacts are underlined.

Resident: Mr. VVV is a 52-year old male with… His white cell count is continuing to increase. He is on antibiotics. Plan for him … [Resident provides a summary of the patient's current condition using her <u>summary sheet</u> while the attending looks at the <u>computer</u> for getting an update on patient's status]
Attending: Why don't we change his antibiotics to antibiotic x?
Pharmacist: Because he is allergic to Penicillin.
Attending: OK.
Resident: He has also developed a high fever last night.
[The charge nurse interrupts the conversation and asks]
Charge nurse: Excuse me Dr. B (the attending), how many empty beds will we have for today's admissions?
[Attending and the charge nurse walk together from the bedside to the <u>whiteboard</u> to check]

This case study highlights the findings of several studies on communication and coordination during rounds conducted in different settings (Fig. 11.3) including a pediatric intensive care unit [145] and a trauma specialty hospital [146]. A large number of physical artifacts (e.g. lists, bed boards, notes, charts) are used by round participants, both as memory aids for relevant patient information and as a record of goals and to-do lists (Fig. 11.3, left). Participants also spend considerable amount of

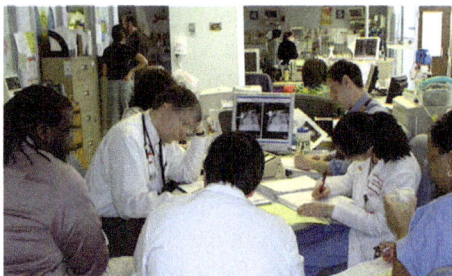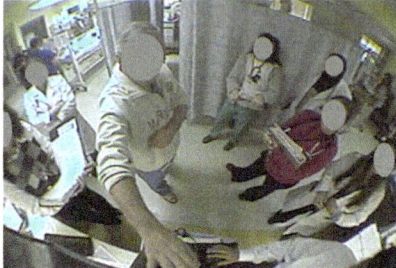

Fig. 11.3 (Left) Sit-down rounds in a pediatric intensive care unit: multi-disciplinary meetings convened for daily management of patient care. Note information artifacts scattered around the workplace and manipulated by participants (e.g., X-rays on computer screens, notes, papers on the wall, charts in binders); (right) A surgeon pointing at a chest X-ray on the computer

time in preparing for information exchanges during rounds so that they can quickly transfer information about status and tasks to another in order to sustain effective performance across task boundaries [68, 147].

The information processes took place during rounds were found to be multi-threaded and overlapping. Hence a "front-stage-back-stage" model was developed for capturing the choreographing of discourse and interaction with the information artifacts (Fig. 11.3). Information processes are considered front-stage when they were part of verbal exchanges or shared visual exchanges occupying the conversation "floor" whereas back-stage processes were those not occupying the floor, mostly non-verbal occasional side conversations or gestures, as well as private interactions between participants and their information sources and computer terminals. Below we illustrate the use of the front-stage-back-stage model in capturing the interactions between the multi-threaded information processes and discuss the model's implications on designing computing support for the information arena (Fig. 11.3).

1. *Front-stage activities driving front-stage activities* can be exemplified by a resident physician presenting data that the attending physician regards as a good teaching point and interrupts the presentation to launch into a didactic discussion.
2. *Front-stage activities driving back-stage activities* are most commonly represented by attending physicians filling in their personal notes (back-stage) as the presenting resident physician reads the data values out loud to the group (front-stage).
3. *Back-stage activities for supporting front-stage activities* include a resident on the computer listening to the presentation and locating relevant patient data on the computer while the resident later interjects to provide the latest values (e.g., laboratory results).
4. *Back-stage activities driving other back-stage activities* happen when a note-taking resident has difficulty keeping up with the presented data and conferring with another participant nearby. They would quietly exchange information as the round proceeds without interrupting the front-stage activities.

Based on the information arena just described, our field studies offer several implications for designing support for the interactions between activities in the front and the back stages. As the back-stage activity interacts with the front-stage both as an information contributor (e.g., during case presentation) as well as an information receiver (e.g., transcribing into personal notes), there is a potential to increase the "information density" of discourse. Newman and Smith [148] observed a similarly high requirement for ease of information access, beyond which people tended to disengage from the conversation. We thus speculate that the use of the front-stage may be improved with computing tools to support back-stage preparation and visual presentation in the front-stage so that communication of precise information (such as data value or medication dosages) may be more reliable. A major role of back-stage activities is to assist in developing a common information space by packaging and organizing relevant information ([149]; [150]) and to provide an annotated environment for fixing inadequacy in the physical space, artifacts, and technology [151] for facilitating front-stage information exchange. We believe that the front-stage-back-stage model provides useful guidance for both studies of critical discourse as well as the design of supporting tools.

Conclusion

Healthcare is a team activity, which entails intense coordination and collaboration among heterogeneous personnel who are typically distributed, both spatially and temporally. Healthcare teams exist in different types depending on individual teams' structural context and its functioning. An organization with a strong organizational shell, well-formulated team structures, and well-designed technology support is associated with lower coordination needs [5]. Yet, teamwork constantly faces a variety of challenges in the dynamic, information-rich, time-critical, and complex healthcare settings.

Recent developments in the use of health IT including the EHR systems and various mobile devices for enhancing real-time information access are discussed as new opportunities to enhance collaborative activities in healthcare. Given the complexity and diversity of healthcare settings, it is crucial to consider relevant sociotechnical issues when designing and deploying health IT for practical use in specific healthcare settings. These issues include design considerations to facilitate dynamic communication behaviors in healthcare settings and the use of medical records for enhancing collaborative healthcare teamwork through supporting relational coordination and social interactions, formal and informal work, and visible and invisible work. Recent technological development for supporting distributed healthcare teamwork is also described. Finally, two case studies on different healthcare teams in different contexts are presented to offer practical challenges in team communication in an ED and the complex information arena and processing involved in team-based medical rounds in an ICU. Both case studies concluded with design implications for supporting technologies.

Discussion Questions

1. What are the communication challenges facing healthcare providers using EHR systems?
2. What are the advantages and disadvantages of dashboard displays showing patient status in an emergency department?
3. How can EHR engage family members to be part of the care team for a patient in an intensive care unit?

References

1. Salas E, Dickinson TL, Converse S, Tannenbaum SI. Toward an understanding of team performance and training. In: Swezey RW, Salas E, editors. Teams: their training and performance. Norwood, NJ: Ablex; 1992. p. 3–29.
2. Dietz AS, Pronovost PJ, Mendez-Tellez PA, et al. A systematic review of teamwork in the intensive care unit: what do we know about teamwork, team tasks, and improvement strategies? J Crit Care. 2014;29(6):908–14. https://doi.org/10.1016/j.jcrc.2014.05.025.
3. Xiao Y, Jones A, Zhang BB, et al. Team consistency and occurrences of prolonged operative time, prolonged hospital stay, and hospital readmission: a retrospective analysis. World J Surg. 2015;39(4):890–6.
4. Xiao Y, Parker SH, Manser T. Teamwork and collaboration. Rev Hum Factors Ergon. 2013;8(1):55–102.
5. Ginnett R. Crews as groups: their formation and their leadership. In: Weiner E, Kanki B, Helmreich RL, editors. Cockpit resource management. London: Academic Press; 1993. p. 71–97.
6. MacMillan J, Paley MJ, Levchuk YN, Entin EE, Serfaty D, Freeman JT. Designing the best team for the task: optimal organizational structures for military missions. In: McNeese M, Salas E, Endsley M, editors. New trends in cooperative activities: system dynamics in complex settings. San Diego, CA: Human Factors and Ergonomics Society Press; 2002.
7. Xiao Y. Tools for distributed teamwork and rapid adaptation to change: COVID-19 and frontline learning. Jt Comm J Qual Patient Saf. 2021;47(5):273–4.
8. Abraham J, Reddy M. Moving patients around: a field study of coordination between clinical and non-clinical staff in hospitals. Paper presented at: Proceedings of the 2008 ACM Conference on Computer Supported Cooperative Work. 2008. p. 225–8.
9. Ash JS, Berg M, Coiera E. Some unintended consequences of information technology in health care: the nature of patient care information system-related errors. J Am Med Inform Assoc. 2004;11(2):104–12.
10. Henneman PL, Marquard JL, Fisher DL, et al. Bar-code verification: reducing but not eliminating medication errors. J Nurs Adm. 2012;42(12):562–6.
11. Lee S, Tang C, Park SY, Chen Y. Loosely formed patient care teams: communication challenges and technology design. Paper presented at: Proceedings of ACM Conference on Computer Supported Cooperative Work. 2012. p. 867–76.
12. Strauss A, Fagerhaugh S, Suczek B, Wiener C. Social organization of medical work. University of Chicago Press; 1985.
13. Aronsky D, Jones I, Lanaghan K, Slovis CM. Supporting patient care in the emergency department with a computerized whiteboard system. J Am Med Inform Assoc. 2007;15(2):184–94.
14. Benham-Hutchins MM, Effken JA. Multi-professional patterns and methods of communication during patient handoffs. Int J Med Inform. 2010;79(4):252–67.
15. Bardram JE, Bossen C. Mobility work: the spatial dimension of collaboration at a hospital. Comput Supported Coop Work. 2005;14(2):131–60.

16. Bardram JE, Bossen C. Moving to get ahead: local mobility and collaborative work. Paper presented at: Proceedings of the eighth conference on European Conference on Computer Supported Cooperative Work 2003. Kluwer Academic Publishers; 2003. p. 355–74.
17. Zerubavel E. Patterns of time in hospital life: a sociological perspective. University of Chicago Press; 1979.
18. Reddy M, Dourish P, Pratt W. Temporality in medical work: time also matters. Comput Supported Coop Work. 2006;15(1):29–53.
19. Reddy M, Pratt W, Dourish P, Shabot M. Asking questions: information needs in a surgical intensive care unit. Paper presented at: Proceedings of American Medical Informatics Association Fall Symposium (AMIA'02), San Antonio, TX. 2002. p. 647–51
20. Chen Y. Documenting transitional information in EMR. Paper presented at: Proceedings of the 2010 ACM Conference on Human Factors in Computing Systems. 2010. p. 1787–96.
21. Ebright PR, Urden L, Patterson E, Chalko B. Themes surrounding novice nurse near-miss and adverse-event situations. J Nurs Adm. 2004;34(11):531–8.
22. Gandhi TK. Fumbled handoffs: one dropped ball after another. Ann Intern Med. 2006;142(5):352–8.
23. Horwitz LI, Meredith T, Schuur JD, Shah NR, Kulkarni RG, Jenq GY. Dropping the baton: a qualitative analysis of failures during the transition from emergency department to inpatient care. Ann Emerg Med. 2009;53:701–10.
24. Patterson ES, Roth EM, Woods DD, Chow R, Gomes JO. Handoff strategies in settings with high consequences for failure: lessons for health care operations. Int J Qual Health Care. 2004;16(2):125–32.
25. Riesenberg LA, Leisch J, Cunningham JM. Nursing handoffs: a systematic review of the literature. Am J Nurs. 2010;110:24–34.
26. Bardram J. Temporal coordination: on time and coordination of collaborative activities at a surgical department. JCSCW. 2000;9(2):157–87.
27. Cabitza F, Sarini M, Simone C, Telaro M. When once is not enough: the role of redundancy in a hospital ward setting. Paper presented at: Proceedings of GROUP. 2005. p. 158–67.
28. Kovalainen M, Robinson M, Auramaki E. Diaries at work. Paper presented at: Proceedings of CSCW. 1998, p. 49–58.
29. Luff P, Heath C, Greatbatch D. Tasks-in-interaction: paper and screen based documentation in collaborative activity. Paper presented at: Proceedings of Computer Supported Cooperative Work. 1992. p. 163–70.
30. Randell R, Wilson S, Woodward P, Galliers J. Beyond handover: supporting awareness for continuous coverage. Cogn Technol Work. 2010;12(4):271–83.
31. Xiao Y, Lasome C, Moss J, Mackenzie C. Cognitive properties of a whiteboard: a case study in a trauma centre. Paper presented at: Proceedings of European Computer Supported Cooperative Work. 2001, p. 259–78.
32. Tang C, Carpendale S. An observational study on information flow during nurses' shift work. Paper presented at: Proceedings of the ACM Conference on Human Factors in Computing Systems. 2007, p. 219–28.
33. Tang C, Carpendale S. Evaluating the deployment of a mobile technology in a hospital ward. Paper presented at: Proceedings of the 2011 ACM Conference on Computer-supported Cooperative Work. ACM; 2008, p. 205–14.
34. Berg M. Practices of reading and writing: the constitutive role of the patient record in medical work. Sociol Health Illn. 1996;18(4):499–524.
35. Berg M, Bowker G. The multiple bodies of the medical record. Sociol Q. 1997;38(3):513–37.
36. Hackman JR. The design of work teams. In: Lorsch W, editor. Handbook of organizational behavior. Upper Saddle River, NJ: Prentice Hall; 1987. p. 315–42.
37. World Health Organization. Patient safety. 2019. Available from: https://www.who.int/patientsafety/en/
38. Marriage B, Kinnear J. Assessing team performance—markers and methods. Trends Anaesth Crit Care. 2016;7–8:11–6.

39. Ly O, Sibbald SL, Verma JY, Rocker GM. Exploring role clarity in interorganizational spread and scale-up initiatives: the 'INSPIRED' COPD collaborative. BMC Health Serv Res. 2018;18:680.
40. Ulrich B, Crider NM. Using teams to improve outcomes and performance. Nephrol Nurs J. 2017;44:141–51.
41. Agency for Healthcare Research and Quality. 2015 National Healthcare Quality and Disparities report and 5th anniversary update on the national quality strategy. Rockville, MD; 2016 Apr. AHRQ pub. no. 16–0015. Available from: https://www.ahrq.gov/sites/default/files/wysiwyg/research/findings/nhqrdr/nhqdr15/2015nhqdr.pdf
42. Fiscella K, Mauksch L, Bodenheimer T, Salas E. Improving care teams' functioning: recommendations from team science. Jt Comm J Qual Patient Saf. 2017;43:361–8. https://doi.org/10.1016/j.jcjq.2017.03.009.
43. Institute of Medicine. To err is human: Building a safer health system. Washington, DC: The National Academies Press; 2000. https://doi.org/10.17226/9728.
44. Baik D, Abu-Rish Blakeney E, Willgerodt M, Woodard N, Vogel M, Zierler B. Examining interprofessional team interventions designed to improve nursing and team outcomes in practice: a descriptive and methodological review. J Interprof Care. 2018;32:719–27.
45. Kilpatrick K, Paquette L, Jabbour M, et al. Systematic review of the characteristics of brief team interventions to clarify roles and improve functioning in healthcare teams. PLoS One. 2020;15(6):e0234416.
46. Patel RS, Bachu R, Adikey A, Malik M, Shah M. Factors related to physicians burnout and its consequences: a review. Behav Sci. 2018;8(11):98.
47. Maslach C, Jackson SE. The measurement of experienced burnout. J Organ Behav. 1981;2:99–113.
48. Gazelle G, Liebschutz JM, Riess H. Physician burnout: coaching a way out. J Gen Intern Med. 2015;30:508–13.
49. Shanafelt TD, Balch CM, Bechamps GJ, et al. Burnout and career satisfaction among American surgeons. Ann Surg. 2009;250:463–71.
50. Shanafelt TD, Gradishar WJ, Kosty M, et al. Burnout and career satisfaction among US oncologists. J Clin Oncol. 2014;32:678–86.
51. Shanafelt TD, Hasan O, Dyrbye LN, et al. Changes in burnout and satisfaction with work-life balance in physicians and the general US working population between 2011 and 2014. Mayo Clin Proc. 2015;90:1600–13.
52. Tawfik DS, Profit J, Morgenthaler TI, et al. Physician burnout, well-being, and work unit safety grades in relationship to reported medical errors. Mayo Clin Proc. 2018;93:1571–80.
53. Bianchi R, Schonfeld IS, Laurent E. Burnout-depression overlap: a review. Clin Psychol Rev. 2015;36:28–41.
54. Shanafelt TD, Sloan JA, Habermann TM. The well-being of physicians. Am J Med. 2003;114:513–9.
55. Miller C. What is the price of physician stress and burnout? 2016 [cited 2023 Mar 11]. Available from: http://www.medicaleconomics.com/medical-economics/news/what-price-physician-stress-and-burnout
56. Nantsupawat A, Nantsupawat R, Kunaviktikul W, Turale S, Poghosyan L. Nurse Burnout, Nurse-Reported Quality of care, and Patient Outcomes in Thai Hospitals. J Nursing Scholarship. 2016;48(1):83–90.
57. Galletta M, Portoghese I, D'Aloja E, Mereu A, Contu P, Coppola RC, Finco G. Campagna M. Relationship etween job burnout, psychosocial factors and health care-associated infections in critical care units. Intensive Crit Care Nurs. 2016;34:51–8.
58. Holmes EG, Connolly A, Putnam KT, et al. Taking care of our own: a multispecialty study of resident and program director perspectives on contributors to burnout and potential interventions. Acad Psychiatry. 2017;41:159–66.
59. IsHak W, Nikravesh R, Lederer S, Perry R, Ogunyemi D, Bernstein C. Burnout in medical students: a systematic review. Clin Teach. 2013;10:242–5.

60. Reith TP. Burnout in United States healthcare professionals: a narrative review. Cureus. 2018;10(12):e3681.
61. Chang KH, Lu F, Chyi T, Hsu YW, Chan SW, Wang E. Examining the stressburnout relationship: the mediating role of negative thoughts. Peer J. 2017;5:e4181.
62. Nayeri ND, Negarandeh R, Vaismoradi M, Ahmadi F, Faghihzadeh, S. Burnout and productivity among Iranian nurses. Nurs Health Sci. 2009;263–270.
63. Jun J, Ojemeni M, Kalamani R, Tong J, Crecelius M. Relationship between nurse burnout, patient and organizational outcomes: Systematic review. Int J Nurs Stud. 2021.
64. Pelissier C, Charbotel B, Fassier JB, Fort E, Fontana L. Nurses' occupational and medical risks factors of leaving the profession in nursing homes. Int J Environ Res Public Health. 2018;15:1850.
65. Morán E, Tentori M, González V, Favela J, Martinez-Garcia A. Mobility in hospital work: towards a pervasive computing hospital environment. Int J Electron Healthc. 2007;3(1):72–89.
66. Reddy M, Dourish P. A finger on the pulse: temporal rhythms and information seeking in medical work. Paper presented at: Proceedings of the 2002 ACM Conference on Computer-supported Cooperative Work. ACM; 2002. p. 344–53.
67. Coiera E, Tombs V. Communication behaviours in a hospital setting – an observational study. BMJ. 1998;316:673–7.
68. Gurses AP, Xiao Y, Gorman P, et al. A distributed cognition approach to understanding information transfer in mission critical domains. Proc Hum Factors Ergon Soc Annu Meet. 2006;50(10):924–8.
69. Baldwin L, McGinnis C. A computer-generated shift report. Nurs Manage. 1994;25(9):61–4.
70. Bates DW, Ebell M, Gotlieb E, Zapp J, Mullins HC. A proposal for electronic medical records in U.S. primary care. J Am Med Inform Assoc. 2003;10(1):1–10.
71. Currie J. Improving the efficiency of patient handover. Emerg Nurse. 2002;10(3):24–7.
72. Kerr M. A qualitative study of shift handover practice and function from a socio-technical perspective. J Adv Nurs. 2002;37(2):125–34.
73. Bossen C. The parameters of common information spaces: the heterogeneity of cooperative work at a hospital ward. Paper presented at: Proceedings of the Conference on Computer-supported Cooperative Work. ACM Press; 2002, p. 176–85.
74. Schmidt K, Bannon L. Taking CSCW seriously: supporting articulation work. Comput Supported Coop Work. 1992;1(1):7–40.
75. Hatten-Masterson SJ, Griffiths ML. SHARED maternity care: enhancing clinical communication in a private maternity hospital setting. Med J Aust. 2009;190(11 Suppl):S150–1.
76. Kraut R, Egido C, Galegher J. Patterns of contact and communication in scientific research collaboration. Paper presented at: Proceedings of Computer Supported Cooperative Work. 1988. p. 1–12.
77. Orlikowski WJ, Hofman JD. An improvisational model for change management: the case of groupware technologies. Sloan Manag Rev. 1997;38(2):11–21.
78. Vuckovic N, Lavelle M, Gorman PN. Eavesdropping as normative behavior in a cardiac intensive care unit. JHQ Online. 2004;W5:1–6.
79. Patterson ES, Watts-Perotti J, Woods DD. Voice loops as coordination aids in space shuttle mission control. Comput Supported Coop Work. 1999;8(4):353–71.
80. Wilson S, Galliers J, Fone J. Not all sharing is equal: the impact of a large display on small group collaborative work. Paper presented at: Proceedings of Computer Supported Cooperative Work. 2006, p. 25–8.
81. Staggers N, Jennings BM. The content and context of change of shift report on medical and surgical units. J Nurs Adm. 2009;39(9):393–8.
82. Collins S, Stein DM, Vawdrey DK, Stetson PD, Bakken S. Content overlap in nurse and physician handoff artifacts and the potential role of electronic health records: a systematic review. J Biomed Inform. 2011;44:704–12.
83. Strople B, Ottani P. Can technology improve intershift report? What the research reveals. J Prof Nurs. 2006;22(3):197–204.

84. Abraham J. Re-coordinating activities: an investigation of articulation work in patient transfers. Paper presented at: Proceedings of the 2013 ACM Conference on Computer Supported Cooperative Work. 2013. p. 67–78.
85. Berg M, Bowker G. The Multiple Bodies of the Medical Record. Sociological Quarterly 1997, 38(3):513–537.
86. Bates DW, Cohen M, Leape LL, Overhage JM, Shabot MM, Sheridan T. Reducing the frequency of errors in medicine using information technology. J Am Med Inform Assoc. 2001;8(4):299–308.
87. Paul S, Das A, Patel V. Specifying design criteria for electronic medical record interface using cognitive framework. AMIA Ann Symp Proc. 2003;2003:594–8.
88. Ackerman MS, Halverson CA, Erickson T, Kellogg WA, Reddy M, Dourish P. Representation, coordination, and information artifacts in medical work. In: Resources, co-evolution and artifacts. Springer London; 2008. p. 167–90.
89. Berg M, Pirnejad H, Stoop AP. Bridging information gaps between primary and secondary healthcare. Stud Health Technol Inform. 2006;124:1003–8.
90. Campbell EM, Sittig DF, Ash JS, Guappone KP, Dykstra RH. Types of unintended consequences related to computerized provider order entry. J Am Med Inform Assoc. 2006;13(5):547–56.
91. Edinger T, Cohen AM, Bedrick S, Ambert K, Hersh W. Barriers to retrieving patient information from electronic health record data: failure analysis from the TREC medical records track. AMIA Ann Symp Proc. 2012;2012:180–8.
92. Handel MJ, Poltrock S. Working around official applications: experiences from a large engineering project. Paper presented at: Proceedings of CSCW. 2011. p. 309–12.
93. Hardstone G, Hartswood M, Procter R, Slack R, Voss A, Rees G. Supporting informality: team working and integrated care records. Paper presented at: Proceedings of the 2004 ACM Conference on Computer-supported Cooperative Work. 2004. p. 142–51.
94. Gittel J. Coordinating mechanisms in care provider groups: relational coordination as a mediator and input uncertainty as a moderator of performance effects. Manag Sci. 2002;48(11):1408–26.
95. Havens DS, Vasey J, Gittell JH, Lin WT. Relational coordination among nurses and other providers: impact on the quality of patient care. J Nurs Manag. 2010;18:926–37.
96. Grudin J. Why CSCW applications fail: problems in the design and evaluation of organizational interfaces. Paper presented at: Proceedings of the 1988 ACM Conference on Computer-supported Cooperative Work. 1988. p. 85–93.
97. Nardi BA, Whittaker S, Bradner E. Interaction and outeraction: instant messaging in action. Paper presented at: Proceedings of the 2000 ACM Conference on Computer-supported Cooperative Work. 2000. p. 79–88.
98. Orlikowski WJ, Scott SV. Sociomateriality: challenging the separation of technology, work and organization. Acad Manag Ann. 2008;2(1):433–74.
99. Whittaker S, Frohlich D, Daly-Jones O. Informal workplace communication: what is it like and how might we support it? Paper presented at: Proceedings of the 1994 ACM Conference on Human Factors in Computing Systems. ACM; 1994. p. 131–7.
100. Bannon L, Schmidt K. Taking CSCW seriously: supporting articulation work. Comput Supported Coop Work. 1992;1:7–40.
101. Berg M. Accumulating and coordinating: occasions for information technologies in medical work. Comput Supported Coop Work. 1999;8(4):373–401.
102. Shipman FM, Marshall CC. Formality considered harmful: experiences, emerging themes, and directions on the use of formal representations in interactive systems. Comput Supported Coop Work. 1999;8(4):333–52.
103. Luff P, Heath C. Mobility in collaboration. Paper presented at: Proceedings of the 1998 ACM Conference on Computer Supported Cooperative Work. 1998. p. 305–14.

104. Poissant L, Pereira J, Tamblyn R, Kawasumi Y. The impact of electronic health records on time efficiency of physicians and nurses: a systematic review. J Am Med Inform Assoc. 2005;12(5):505–16.
105. Richardson J, Ash J. The effects of hands free communication devices on clinical communication: balancing communication access needs with user control. AMIA Ann Symp Proc. 2008;2008:621–5.
106. Bowers J, Button G, Sharrock W. Workflow from within and without: technology and cooperative work on the print industry shopfloor. Paper presented at: Proceedings of the First Conference of European Conference on Computer Supported Cooperative Work. Kluwer academic publishers; 1995. p. 51–66.
107. Dourish P. The appropriation of interactive technologies: some lessons from placeless documents. Comput Supported Coop Work. 2003;12(4):465–90.
108. Isaacs EA, Whittaker S, Frohlich D, O'Conaill B. Informal communication reexamined: new functions for video in supporting opportunistic encounters. In: Finn KE, Sellen AJ, Wilbur SB, editors. Video-mediated communication. Mahwah, NJ: Lawrence Erlbaum Associates; 1997. p. 459–85.
109. Kraut RE, Fish RS, Root RW, Chalfonte BL. Informal communication in organizations: form, function, and technology. In: People's reactions to technology in factories, offices, and aerospace. Sage Publications; 1990. p. 145–99.
110. Mejia DA, Morán AL, Favela J. Supporting informal co-located collaboration in hospital work. Paper presented at: Proceedings of the 13th International Conference on Groupware: Design Implementation, and Use. Springer-Verlag; 2007, p. 255–70.
111. Brown JB, Lewis L, Ellis K, Stewart M, Freeman TR, Kasperski MJ. Mechanisms for communicating within primary health care teams. Can Fam Physician. 2009;55(12):1216–22.
112. Ellingson LL. Interdisciplinary health care teamwork in the clinic backstage. J Appl Commun Res. 2003;31(2):93–117.
113. Koppel R, Wetterneck T, Telles JL, Karsh B. Workarounds to barcode medication administration systems: their occurrences, causes, and threats to patient safety. J Am Med Inform Assoc. 2008;15(4):408–23.
114. Novak LL, Holden RJ, Anders SH, Hong JY, Karsh BT. Using a sociotechnical framework to understand adaptations in health IT implementation. Int J Med Inform. 2013;82(12): e331–44.
115. Azad B, King N. Enacting computer workaround practices within a medication dispensing system. Eur J Inform Syst. 2008;17(3):264–78.
116. Zhou X, Ackerman Novak M, Zheng K. CPOE workarounds, boundary objects, and assemblages. Proc. Of the SIGCHI Conference on Human Factors in Computing Systems, 2011. 3353–62.
117. Park SY, Chen Y. Adaptation as design: learning from an EMR deployment study. Paper presented at: Proceedings of the 2012 ACM Conference on Human Factors in Computing Systems. ACM; 2012. p. 2097–106.
118. Fitzpatrick G. Integrated care and the working record. Health Inform J. 2004;10(4):291–302.
119. Hardey M, Payne S, Coleman P. 'Scraps': hidden nursing information and its influence on the delivery of care. J Adv Nurs. 2000;32(1):208–14.
120. Ames SA. Multiple spoken and written channels of communication: an ethnography of a medical unit in a general hospital. Ann Arbor, MI: UMI Dissertation Services; 1993.
121. Zhou X, Ackerman MS, Zheng K. I just don't know why it's gone: maintaining informal information use in inpatient care. Paper presented at: Proceedings of the 2009 ACM Conference on Human Factors in Computing Systems. ACM; 2009. p. 2061–70.
122. Gorman P, Ash J, Lavelle M, et al. Bundles in the wild: managing information to solve problems and maintain situation awareness. Libr Trends. 2000;49(2):266–89.
123. Sexton A, Chan C, Elliott M, Stuart J, Jayasuriya R, Crookes P. Nursing handovers: do we really need them? J Nurs Manag. 2004;12:37–42.

124. Mentis HM, Reddy M, Rosson MB. Invisible emotion: information and interaction in an emergency room. Paper presented at: Proceedings of the 2010 ACM Conference on Computer Supported Cooperative Work. 2010, 311–20.
125. Spence PR, Reddy MC. The "active" gatekeeper in collaborative information seeking activities. Paper presented at: Proceedings of the 2007 International ACM Conference on Supporting Group Work. ACM; 2007. p. 277–80.
126. Bossen C, Jensen L, Witt F. Medical secretaries' care of records: the cooperative work of a non-clinical group. Paper presented at: Proceedings of the 2012 ACM Conference on Computer Supported Cooperative Work. 2012. p. 921–30.
127. Holten Møller NL, Vikkelsø S. The clinical work of secretaries: exploring the intersection of administrative and clinical work in the diagnosing process. In: Dugdale J, Masclet C, Grasso MA, Boujut J-F, Hassanaly P, editors. From research to practice in the design of cooperative systems: results and open challenges. Springer London; 2012. p. 33–47.
128. Star SL, Strauss A. Layers of silence, arenas of voice: the ecology of visible and invisible work. Comput Supported Coop Work. 1999;8(1–2):9–30.
129. Nardi BA, Engestrom Y. A web on the wind: the structure of invisible work. Comput Supported Coop Work. 2001;8(1):1–8.
130. Suchman L. Making work visible. Commun ACM. 1995;38(9):56–64.
131. Hanada E, Fujiki T, Nakakuni H, Sullivan C. The effectiveness of the installation of a mobile voice communication system in a university hospital. J Med Syst. 2006;2006(30):101–6.
132. Tang C, Carpendale S. A mobile voice communication system in medical setting: love it or hate it? Paper presented at: Proceedings of the ACM Conference on Human Factors in Computing Systems. ACM; 2009, p. 2041–50.
133. Bardram J, Hansen T. The AWARE architecture: supporting context-mediated social awareness in mobile cooperation. Paper presented at: CSCW'04: Proceedings of the 2004 ACM Conference on Computer Supported Cooperative Work. New York: ACM Press; 2004. p. 192–201.
134. Bardram J, Hansen T, Søgaard M. AwareMedia: a shared interactive display supporting social, temporal, and spatial awareness in surgery. Paper presented at: Proceedings of the CSCW'06 Conference on Computer Supported Cooperative Work. New York: ACM Press; 2006. p. 109–18.
135. Thomas K. Wanted: a WhatsApp alternative for clinicians. BMJ. 2018;360:k622.
136. Karusala N, Wang D, O'Neill J. Making chat at home in the hospital: exploring chat use by nurses. Paper presented at: Proceedings of the 2020 ACM conference on Human Factors in Computing Systems. 2020. p. 1–15.
137. Bardram J, Hansen T. Why the plan doesn't hold: a study of situated planning, articulation and coordination work in a surgical ward. Paper presented at: CSCW'10: Proceedings of the 2010 ACM Conference on Computer Supported Cooperative Work. New York: ACM Press; 2010. p. 331–40.
138. France D, Levin S, Hemphill R, et al. Emergency physicians' behaviors and workload in the presence of an electronic whiteboard. Int J Med Inform. 2005;74(10):827–37.
139. Wong H, Caesar M, Bandali S, Agnew J, Abrams H. Electronic inpatient whiteboards: improving multidisciplinary communication and coordination of care. Int J Med Inform. 2009;78(4):239–47.
140. Silva J, Zamarripa M, Strayer P, Favela J, Gonzalez V. Empirical evaluation of a mobile application for assisting physicians in creating medical notes. Paper presented at: Proceedings of the 12th Americas Conference on Information Systems. 2006.
141. Zamarripa M, Gonzalez V, Favela J. The augmented patient charts: seamless integration of physical and digital artifacts for hospital work. In: Stephanidis C, editor. Universal access in HCI, part III, HCII 2007, LNCS, vol. 4556. Springer; 2007. p. 1006–15.
142. Tang C. Studying nurses' information flow to inform technology design [Ph.D. dissertation]. Department of Computer Science, University of Calgary, AB, Canada; 2009.

143. Tang C, Carpendale S. Supporting nurses' information flow by integrating paper and digital charting. Paper presented at: Proceedings of the European Conference on Computer Supported Cooperative Work. Springer; 2009. p. 43–62.
144. Yen PY, Gorman PN. Usability testing of a digital pen and paper system in nursing documentation. AMIA Annu Symp Proc. 2005;2005:844–8.
145. Cardarelli M, Vaidya V, Conway D, Jarin J, Xiao Y. Dissecting multidisciplinary cardiac surgery rounds: data, wisdom, time and money. Ann Thorac Surg. 2009;88(3):809–13.
146. Sen A, Xiao Y, Lee S, et al. Daily multi-disciplinary discharge rounds in a trauma center: a little time, well spent. J Trauma. 2009;66(3):880–7.
147. Gurses AP, Xiao Y, Hu P. User-designed information tools to support communication and care coordination in a trauma hospital. J Biomed Inform. 2009;42(4):667–77.
148. Newman W, Smith EL. Disruption of meetings by laptop use: is there a 10-second solution? Paper presented at: Extended Abstracts of the SIGCHI Conference on Human Factors in Computing Systems, CHI '06. New York, NY: ACM Press; 2006. p. 1145–50.
149. Bannon L, Bodker S. Constructing common information spaces. Paper presented at: Proceedings of the ECSCW, 1997, Kluwer. 1997. p. 81–96.
150. Fields B, Amaldi P, Tassi A. Representing collaborative work: the airport as common information space. Cogn Technol Work. 2005;7(2):119–33.
151. Coiera E. Communication spaces. J Am Med Inform Assoc. 2014;21(3):414–22. https://doi.org/10.1136/amiajnl-2012-001520.

Further Reading

Gorman P, Ash J, Lavelle M, et al. Bundles in the wild: managing information to solve problems and maintain situation awareness. Libr Trends. 2000;49(2):266–89.

Lee S, Tang C, Park SY, Chen Y. Loosely formed patient care teams: communication challenges and technology design. Paper presented at: Proceedings of the 2012 ACM Conference on Computer-supported Cooperative Work. ACM; 2012. p. 867–76.

Xiao Y, Schenkel S, Faraj S, Mackenzie CF, Moss JA. What whiteboards in a trauma center operating suite can teach us about emergency department communication. Ann Emerg Med. 2007;50(4):387–95.

Chapter 12
Designing and Deploying Mobile Health Interventions

Meghan Reading Turchioe, Albert M. Lai, and Katie A. Siek

Introduction

Early uses of mobile devices in healthcare were provider-focused which enabled physicians to communicate and access electronic health records whenever and wherever they were. Most healthcare providers are highly mobile and constantly moving throughout the healthcare environment—moving from patient to patient, making diagnoses, making treatment decisions, administering medications, and performing procedures—all of which need documentation.

As healthcare has moved from being acute care and physician-focused to a more patient- and wellness-centric model, applications of mobile devices in healthcare have shifted in focus as well. Many of the exciting innovations in the use of mobile devices have focused on targeting the healthcare consumer and enabling them to be better engaged in their own care and efforts to maintain their wellness. In this chapter, we introduce mobile technology, its use in healthcare, user interface aspects to consider when using mobile devices, and study design considerations.

We discuss a broad range of mobile devices—basic cellular (cell) phones, smartphones, tablets, and wearable devices. Strongly relevant to this chapter is the exciting and emerging field of *mHealth*. mHealth is defined broadly as the use of mobile

M. R. Turchioe (✉)
Columbia University School of Nursing, New York, NY, USA
e-mail: mr3554@cumc.columbia.edu

A. M. Lai
Department of Medicine, Washington University in St. Louis, St. Louis, MO, USA
e-mail: amlai@wustl.edu

K. A. Siek
Informatics, Indiana University, Bloomington, IN, USA
e-mail: ksiek@indiana.edu

© The Author(s), under exclusive license to Springer Nature Switzerland AG 2024
A. W. Kushniruk et al. (eds.), *Human Computer Interaction in Healthcare*, Cognitive Informatics in Biomedicine and Healthcare, https://doi.org/10.1007/978-3-031-69947-4_12

telecommunication devices for the delivery of healthcare services. The majority of the sections of this chapter are encompassed by the term mHealth, but we also cover mobile devices that are not telecommunication devices such as wearable devices, and are not traditionally included under mHealth.

This chapter is largely targeted at researchers, but we also discuss ideas that designers, software developers, and informaticians need to consider when designing and implementing mobile healthcare solutions. We place these mobile devices into their historical context and while this chapter does not provide a comprehensive systematic literature review, we cover important representative research that has been conducted using the variety of mobile devices covered in this chapter.

An Evolution of Mobile Devices

Since personal digital assistants and cell phones were introduced in the early 1990s, and later smartphones in the early 2000s, these mobile devices have rapidly become ubiquitous. In 2021, 97% of Americans own a cell phone of any kind, and 85% own a smartphone specifically (Fig. 12.1) [1]. Cell phone ownership is high (>92%)

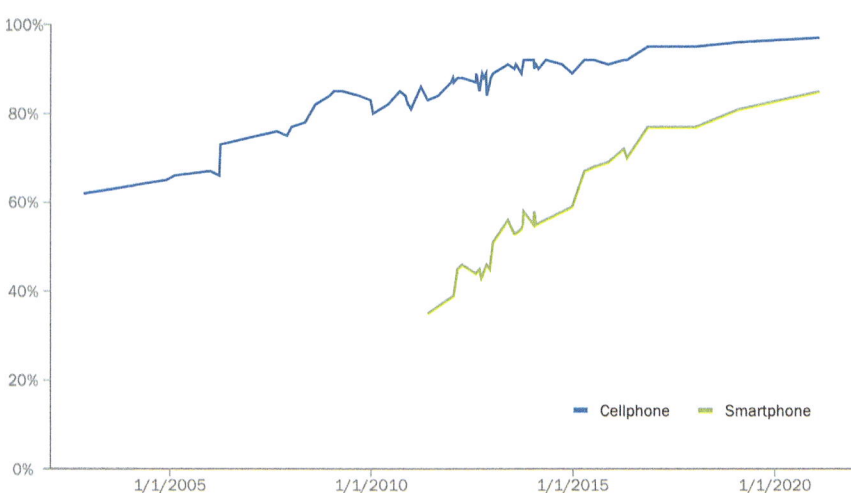

Fig. 12.1 Trends in mobile phone ownership among U.S. adults (Source: Pew Research Center [1])

regardless of age, gender, race, ethnicity, education, income, and urbanicity; smartphone ownership is also high but more variable across these groups (61–96%), with older age, low education levels, and low income having the lowest ownership rates [1]. This trend is mirrored globally as well. Although ownership is highest in upper-middle-income countries, even in lower-middle-income countries (LMIC), 83% of adults own a cell phone and 45% own a smartphone [2]. In LMIC, most smartphone owners are younger and have higher education. In the future, smartphone ownership may follow similar patterns as cellphone ownership so that as the technology becomes more affordable, demographic differences in ownership will decrease.

The widespread adoption of mobile devices has translated to a greater number and variety of mHealth interventions which rely upon such devices—either to deliver interventions directly (e.g., mobile applications or text messaging) or to transmit information to and from other health devices (e.g., wearables). Moreover, it has allowed us to move beyond prototyping and studying adoption, to pushing boundaries regarding the integrated smart solutions that are possible. It has also created space for researchers to consider patient engagement, inclusive design, implementation challenges, and the potential for mHealth to create intervention-generated inequities more thoughtfully [3]. However, a 2018 systematic review of mHealth interventions showed there is still limited evidence on the efficacy of these interventions [4]. Therefore, addressing these major challenges will be essential to improve patient outcomes with mHealth.

Mobile Health Devices

Smartphones

A smartphone is a mobile phone with advanced computing capabilities and Internet connectivity. Modern smartphones enable web browsing and installation of third-party applications (apps) and frequently include a relatively large color touchscreen display. The computational power, portability, and increased ownership of smartphones across multiple demographic segments have led to a surge in their use for healthcare purposes [5]. In the past decade, several customs and best practices for smartphone app interface design have been adopted to overcome issues related to the small size of the screen relative to a computer screen. The more that apps adopt the same customs and practices, the more users become familiar and experienced with them. For example, "hamburger" icons, consisting of three horizontal bars, provide a menu of options when they are clicked. They facilitate easier navigation on a small screen and are very commonly utilized in apps. Healthcare apps have successfully mimicked strategies used in apps used in other areas (e.g., personal finance, social media).

At the same time, even commonly used icons may not be recognized by inexperienced app users, which can cause confusion and frustration. Therefore, user testing and consideration of usability requirements are essential, as we discuss later in this chapter. In addition, smartphone interaction typically requires tapping, dragging, typing, and other gestures that may be challenging for individuals with limited dexterity and low vision. Large button sizes [6, 7], adequate spacing between targets [8], and utilizing tapping gestures as opposed to dragging or sliding [9] improve usability for these individuals. Voice-enabled input options also assist individuals who struggle to type or read written information. Guidelines for making interventions delivered via smartphone more accessible to individuals with challenges related to vision impairment, motor coordination, cognitive impairment, and other accessibility challenges are available to guide developers and researchers [10, 11].

Tablets

Compared to smartphones, modern tablets have larger displays, many are dependent on WiFi for internet connectivity (e.g., they do not possess the ability to connect to cellular service), and are generally not as widely adopted.

Tablets have been effectively deployed in healthcare settings to deliver interventions during inpatient hospitalizations or outpatient appointments (e.g., waiting rooms). For example, Epic Systems Corporation's MyChart Bedside enables an admitted patient the ability to gain access to more information about his or her stay in the hospital, such as treatment plans, the care team, and recent vital signs and laboratory tests. They have been adopted in many hospitals and have shown early success in improving patient outcomes. Researchers evaluating an inpatient portal available on tablets at Columbia University/New York Presbyterian Hospital conducted a randomized, controlled trial in which 426 English- and Spanish-speaking patients were randomized to usual care, tablet use with Internet connectivity but no portal, or tablet use with inpatient portal. They determined that participants with portal access had lower 30-day readmission rates and looked up health information online more often than patients in the other two groups [12].

Another application of inpatient clinical use of tablets is for clinicians to access the medical record. There have been two primary approaches to this: native apps and thin client access. Native apps provide a subset of functionality that is available in the desktop applications, such as reviewing patients' medications, lab results, and other data. Thin client access software (such as Citrix Workspace) enables devices such as tablets to access a remote virtual desktop hosted on a server where the full desktop application can be run. However, many full desktop EHR applications are not *responsive*, meaning pages do not automatically reformat to fit the size of the screen, which results in difficult interactions with the interface and a lot of scrolling. Desktop applications are rarely designed for a touch-first user interface, which can also result in difficult interactions from a tablet device. For these reasons, if the full functionality of the desktop app is not needed, native apps may be the ideal solution for such use cases.

There are several key issues to consider when considering using a tablet for a mHealth intervention. The cost of tablet ownership may create disparities in ownership, which is an important consideration when developing interventions. At the same time, the larger screen size may be preferable for individuals with lower levels of dexterity and vision. Many usability considerations are similar for smartphones and tablets despite their difference in screen size. For instance, as with smartphones, large touch targets and large spacing between targets are most appropriate in older adult populations. Some specific issues to consider when deploying tablets to patients in the inpatient domain are who will deploy the devices to the patients, how to keep them charged, how to secure the devices, who will reset the devices between patients, and, importantly after the COVID-19 pandemic, who will disinfect the devices before redeployment to the next patient.

Fundamentally, researchers should decide whether they want to use an existing app or build their own. Multiple operating systems could be used to develop a tablet-based intervention. Researchers should consider if they want their intervention to work on a device with a specific operating system or "cross-platform" where a developer creates an app that can work on devices with different operating systems. Specifically, researchers should consider if they want a "native" app, cross-platform app, or web app. A native app only works on a specific operating system but typically has access to more device functionality (e.g., accelerometers, cameras). A cross-platform app can work on multiple operating systems, but may not have access to the same functionality on the device. A web app typically is a website optimized for a mobile device, however, functionality could be limited based on internet connectivity and device functionality.

Wearable Systems

"Mobile technology," which is traditionally thought of in terms of cell phones, smartphones, and tablets, is quickly morphing into smaller, wearable systems. Many wearable systems are designed, built, and evaluated in the health and wellness domains to assist users assess specific metrics. Wearable devices are broadly defined to include any computational device that an individual wears—from pedometers to a computationally enhanced contact lens. Popular off-the-shelf wearable systems provide users with instant feedback on various metrics—the most popular metrics are step counts and sleep—and usually with the ability to connect their data to their social networks. On the horizon is industry research into more integrated systems that enhance everyday objects such as watches, glasses, rings, contact lenses, and even clothing.

Off-the-shelf wellness monitoring systems such as the Fitbit (fitbit.com), Apple Watch (apple.com/watch), and Oura Ring (ouraring.com) have become popular for many individuals who may wish to monitor their overall well-being, but may or may not have a specific health concern. The systems typically sense physical activity at a bare minimum but many also track sleep, heart rate and rhythm, and posture. All of the systems provide aggregate data via a mobile application or website. Oura Ring, for example, is a wearable ring containing small sensors that continuously measure physiologic signs, sleep, physical activity, and other metrics, and its accompanying app aggregates data to create personal health insights about one's health status. The aggregated data is done by proprietary algorithms, thus one's data accuracy is only as good as the proprietor's algorithm.

When researchers choose to use an off-the-shelf wearable sensing system, they must consider the accuracy of the system, if users can use the system, and how the system may interfere with users' lives [13]. Additionally, the ability to use the system may change depending on the user's health status. For example, the Oura Ring is worn on the finger, which may not fit individuals who experience swelling due to health conditions such as heart failure or pregnancy. Recently, a wearable evaluation framework was published to help researchers narrow their potential options in the ever-expanding world of medical wearables and determine appropriate options for a specific population and context [14]. The framework contains evaluation criteria relating to everyday use by users, device functionality, and infrastructure required to obtain the data.

Wearable textiles, which are articles of clothing that include smart sensors, are also a new area of development. For example, the Owlet smart sock is a small, wireless newborn monitoring device that wraps around the baby's foot like a sock. The Owlet uses embedded sensors to provide highly accurate, continuous monitoring of vital signs (oxygen saturation and heart rate) while babies are sleeping in home settings. The device connects to a base station using Bluetooth technology, which serves as the primary notification center, as well as to a smartphone app. This device has become extremely popular among parents who have specific concerns about their newborn's health, for example, newborns who spent time in the Neonatal Intensive Care Unit (NICU). In a large study of over 47,000 newborns using the Owlet sock, parents reported the top reason for owning it was "peace of mind" (75%) and nearly all (94%) reported a better quality of sleep for themselves because of it [15].

Some wearable systems now employ aspects of virtual reality (VR), immersive, three-dimension, simulated experiences, or augmented reality, in which information or enhanced/modified views are layered or integrated into the current view of the environment through eyewear. For example, There have also been applications of augmented reality to assist individuals with low vision in performing everyday functions, like distinguishing products of similar appearance and size on a shelf at a grocery store. Researchers at Cornell University created "ForeSee," a head-mounted system for individuals with low vision that enhances aspects of a visual field through magnification, contrast enhancement, edge enhancement, black and white reversal, and text extraction [16]. Whenever we use assistive technology, we must also consider possible privacy implications. For example, while a blind user was using the VizWiz app [17], an app where people can take pictures with a mobile phone and ask questions to crowd workers (e.g., Which hotel bottle is shampoo?), she learned from a crowd worker that there was a mirror in front of her, thus when she took the picture of the shampoo, she inadvertently shared a picture of herself without clothes on [18].

Wearable biosensors are small sensors that are worn on the body to provide continuous, automated measurement of physiologic data. As one example, continuous glucose monitors contain a smile wire inserted into the skin and adhere to the back of the arm. They have been available to individuals with diabetes for several years to support tight regulation of blood glucose levels, facilitate bolus dosing when needed, alert individuals about dangerous low or high levels, and even enable insights about personal trends. The NightScout Project (also called "CGM in the Cloud"; http://www.nightscout.info/) is a patient-driven platform enabling visualization and analysis of CGM data to facilitate personal health insights. Other wearable biosensors may be used to gather patient vital signs, step counts, and single-lead electrocardiograms to enable continuous vital sign monitoring both within and outside of healthcare settings [19, 20]. In the future, we may see more biosensors in smaller and more appealing devices, such as jewelry-like, on-skin temporary tattoos [21]. Biosensors may also be able to construct two- and three-dimension medical images. For instance, researchers at the Massachusetts Institute of Technology (MIT) created EIT-kit, a toolkit that allows users to design and fabricate health and motion sensing devices using Electrical Impedance Tomography (EIT), an imaging technique that measures conductivity, permittivity, and impedance of a subject [22].

Industry research continues to integrate intelligence into everyday artifacts to improve our physical, social, and emotional health. Most of the technology discussed here requires a smartphone, tablet, or computer to push or pull information to and from the enhanced artifact. Thus, researchers must be careful to consider the cost (material, developmental, and maintenance) and user burden (e.g., putting on sensors, charging them, and debugging the overall system) before deciding on a wearable system.

mHealth Interventions

Mobile Applications

Mobile applications (apps) are the most common methods of delivering mHealth interventions. The growth in tools and skilled personnel available to develop apps in recent years has led to a drastic rise in the number of apps available for any one condition. For example, in systematic reviews of apps in commercial marketplaces (Apple, Google Play, and Android stores), searches for apps related to heart failure [23], atrial fibrillation [24], cardiac rehabilitation [25], depression [26], and COVID-19 [27] have yielded between 1017 and 3636 apps each. The major benefit that apps provide is they leverage the ubiquity of smartphones and other devices in the population as an easy and cost-effective means of delivering health interventions and collecting data.

There are many considerations and potential drawbacks to apps that researchers must carefully consider, including Internet connectivity, consideration of whether a new app is needed or existing options meet the goals of the project and consideration of different platforms and devices. Apps may be stand-alone, meaning the app contains all data without requiring Internet access, or they may be Internet-connected. Some apps may offer the ability to toggle between the two options depending on the environment by enabling use in "offline mode" when users are in areas with poor Internet connectivity. This is useful when apps are being deployed in low-resource or rural settings with limited broadband access, especially in LMIC. For instance, researchers have developed and pilot-tested a mobile app for population health surveillance with 11,945 people across 33 villages in Western Myanmar, an extremely rural, mountainous region where cellular service (and often, electricity) is not routinely available and where population health monitoring does not exist [28]. The tool allowed nurses and community health workers to enter data into the app even if Internet connectivity is not available and upload the data to a centralized server when they were able to reconnect to the Internet. In interviews with stakeholders, researchers also learned that solar-powered charging packs and waterproof cases would also be helpful for future implementations to enable data collection when there was limited electricity and unpredictable weather.

Internet-connected applications require the following set of resources (that the designer, evaluator, and developer need to consider): (1) a mobile Internet-accessible area (which is still challenging in some rural communities); (2) a server or trusted cloud service that hosts data; (3) a mobile device that can easily access the Internet; (4) a data plan for each user to access the Internet; (5) and—especially relevant in health applications—a secure connection to share health information. If resources are restricted, then researchers may consider a mobile stand-alone application that hosts all of the data on the device. Researchers can download the data when they meet with the users, however, they also need to inform users of contingency plans and design software that alerts participants if they are not receiving accurate information because they are not transferring data in real-time. For these reasons, stand-alone mobile applications have been used in both rural, low-resource settings globally [29] and in the United States alike [30].

Another important consideration is determining whether building a new app is necessary for an intervention, or whether existing apps may be useful for a specific context or application. Given the sheer volume of health-focused apps that have been developed, researchers should consider reviewing what is presently available before embarking on the development of a new app. Additionally, patients may prefer to streamline their health self-management by using fewer apps, provided that the apps are high quality and meet their self-management needs. Evaluating the quality of existing apps is an important step in making this determination. Interaction designers can utilize an inspection method, such as specific types of heuristic evaluations, to evaluate quality. For instance, the Mobile Application Rating Scale (MARS) is a popular tool that has been used widely since it was first published in 2015, cited over 700 times as of this writing [31]. MARS evaluates apps along four objective quality scales (engagement, functionality, aesthetics, and information quality) and one subjective quality scale.

If existing apps are low quality but developers or researchers lack the time or funds to build their own high-quality apps, technical frameworks are available to facilitate more rapid development of custom apps. Apple's ResearchKit is an open-source framework for building mHealth apps that enables documentation of informed consent, subject enrollment, and data collection all in the app. ResearchKit includes multiple data collection options: self-reported data collection (e.g., completing surveys), "passive tasks" requiring no effort or input from the user (e.g., tracking step count), and "active tasks" in which the user completes a predefined task (e.g., a timed walk test). Several academic medical centers (including Harvard, NYU Langone, Mount Sinai Icahn, and the University of California San Francisco medical centers) have developed and deployed mHealth applications using ResearchKit.

Finally, those developing apps must consider the software platform and device on which the app will be deployed. The leading two platforms are Google's Android and Apple's iOS, with a total of over 90% of the worldwide market share. Android is vastly more popular worldwide, representing nearly three-quarters of the global market by some estimates [32]. However, there have been well-documented differences in the age, gender, and socioeconomic status of users of each platform; in the U.S., iPhone users tend to be in higher socioeconomic groups [33]. Therefore, the choice of software platform may have unintended consequences on the diversity of the patients that can use the app. For this reason, researchers are adopting platform-independent solutions, such as the open-source solution Apache Cordova (https://cordova.apache.org/), that allow developers to create the app using web technologies and deploy the apps on multiple platforms. Most of the app functionality can be used offline, however, researchers can benefit by being able to collect real-time data when the smartphone can access the Internet. Some researchers are also creating Android versions of native Apple apps, such as "Research Stack," an Android-enabled equivalent to Apple's ResearchKit from the Open mHealth group (https://www.openmhealth.org/).

The final consideration concerns which devices apps may be available on. Many apps can be downloaded on a smartphone, tablet, or wearable device, but function differently depending on the device. For example, Apple Watch versions of apps are limited to a few basic functionalities given the extremely small screen size but connect to an app with more complete functionality that can be viewed on a smartphone. Researchers must consider the device ownership rates, preferences, usability needs, and barriers to adoption and use (especially cost) of a target patient group when planning which devices the app will be available for.

Personal Health Records

Another area of significant interest has been the use of smartphones for Personal Health Records (PHRs). PHRs have been adopted by over one million patients in the U.S. alone since the federal *Meaningful Use* program began in 2014, which required organizations to allow patients to view, download, and transmit their health records [34]. There have been two main approaches to PHRs on smartphones: integrated and standalone. Within the category of integrated PHRs, they fall into two subcategories—those that integrate with EHRs and those that integrate with online PHR systems that contain data maintained by the patient. Integrated PHRs have been met with great interest and enable patients to access a subset of information that is stored in their health record that is maintained in their healthcare provider's EHR. They also frequently enable the patient to securely communicate with their provider. One such app is that of the MyChart for the iPhone from Epic Systems Corporation. Studies have demonstrated that integrated PHRs can facilitate shared decision-making, prevent medical errors, and improve certain health outcomes [35]. At the same time, numerous studies have documented disparities in the adoption of integrated PHRs. A systematic review demonstrated that technical training and assistance programs increase adoption and reduce disparities, but that more research evaluating barriers broadly, beyond individual-level factors, is needed [35].

There are a few PHR apps for smartphones that access information that is maintained by the patient themselves, but they have largely been unsuccessful due to the lack of adoption of these platforms, even on desktop computers [36]. For instance, many large technology companies have attempted but not succeeded with patient-maintained PHRs. One prominent example is HealthVault, launched by Microsoft in 2007 but closed in 2019 due to low user adoption [37]. Similarly, Google Health, the PHR created by Google, was launched in 2008 and closed just four years later, in 2012 [38].

Artificial Intelligence-Enabled Interventions

Within the last five years, there has been a sharp increase in the number of artificial intelligence (AI) models in healthcare. Most of these models focus on communicating results to researchers or clinicians, but patient-facing AI is currently in extremely nascent stages. The majority of patient-facing work has been in creating intelligent, patient-facing chatbots that facilitate psychotherapy [39], support symptom management [40], promote health behavior change [41], and provide other forms of health-related guidance. These have been explored in academic research as well as in industry. For instance, WoeBot is a commercially available personal mental health chatbot that provides routine check-ins and recommends evidence-based wellness interventions via chat functionality in a mobile app (Fig. 12.2). Although there is the promise for AI to assist in mental and digital health, more work must be

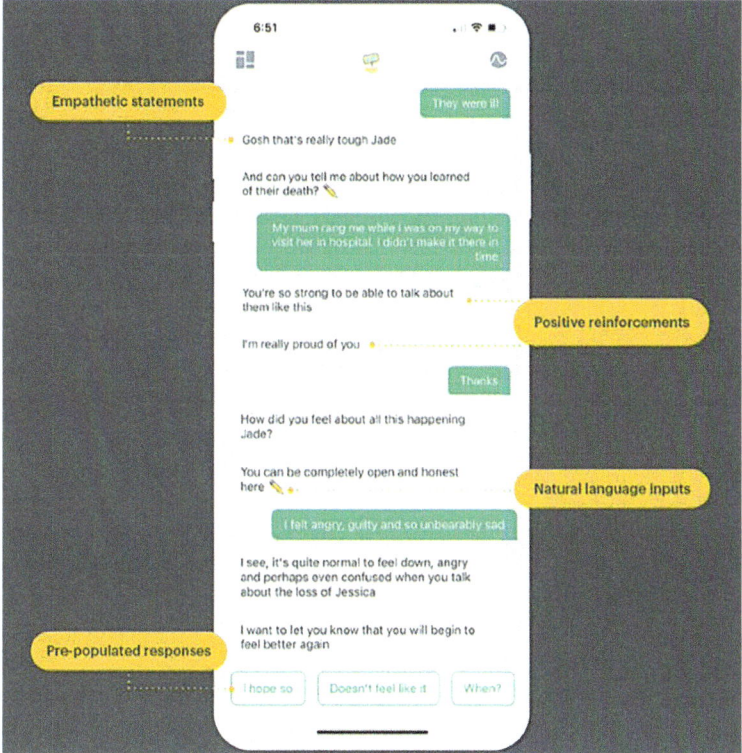

Fig. 12.2 Example interaction with the Woebot chatbot (Source: Darcy et al. [42])

done to ensure validated interventions are deployed while maintaining people's privacy and regularly reviewing apps for efficacy [43].

The large amounts of data that can be captured using wearable devices and smartphones have created opportunities to integrate predictive or diagnostic AI models into mHealth. The incorporation of AI into mHealth raises important questions about strategies for communicating model output to lay audiences who may have limited statistical and medical knowledge. Nonetheless, to date, there have been early successful applications of AI in mobile interventions. For example, in 2018 Apple released a single-lead electrocardiogram (ECG) recording feature in the Apple Watch along with a machine-learning algorithm that identifies atrial fibrillation from the ECG tracing with high accuracy [44]. In the Apple Heart study, researchers at Stanford University recruited over 419,000 participants in 8 months to wear the Apple Watch to monitor for atrial fibrillation. They reported that 2161 participants received abnormal heart rhythm notifications, and 34% of participants who completed follow-up testing were ultimately diagnosed with atrial fibrillation [45].

Text Messaging Interventions

Text messaging interventions involve sending short text messages (Short Message Service or SMS) or pictures, videos, or other multimedia (Multimedia Messaging Service or MMS) to provide information—textual or multimedia—to individuals. Text messaging interventions are a low-cost, quick way to send data to and receive data from consumers and health professionals. Currently, there are two main text messaging programs—*push programs* that deliver information to people and *two-way programs* that can deliver and receive information from users. Current mass consumption text messaging programs are *"push"* systems in that they *push* information to the public to inform them about specific health-related issues but do not expect user responses. Push systems are fairly straightforward to implement—researchers could choose to manually send text messages from a phone or text message app (e.g., iMessage). Alternatively, researchers could create a more robust and automatic system by maintaining an SMS gateway or using an SMS gateway service (e.g., Twilio) to automatically send text messages at specific times. Some health text messaging programs provide *two-way* communication so that users can communicate with other users or healthcare professionals. Two-way communication is slightly more complex to implement than *push* programs because the researcher needs to use an SMS gateway service and program some logic into the system to accommodate the various inputs a user may send to the system.

Although smartphones have amazing capabilities, effort needs to be spent on making sure that interventions are designed appropriately and that the new capabilities of smartphones add substantive improvement in healthcare interventions over what is available in phones of lesser capabilities. For example, Buller, Borland [46] performed a randomized trial comparing the effectiveness of a smartphone mobile application to text messaging to support smoking cessation. They found that text messaging can be as effective—if not more effective—interventions than those that require smartphones while enabling a wider audience to participate and lowering the costs of the intervention. Thus, although text messaging interventions may seem outdated compared to those that use more novel mHealth technologies, they are still highly effective in reaching specific populations who do not own, or prefer, smartphones. Text4baby is an excellent example of an effective and enduring text messaging intervention. In 2012, the U.S. Centers for Disease Control (CDC) launched Text4baby as a free text messaging intervention providing health information and reminders to pregnant women or women with children under age one. It has remained a popular intervention in underserved communities, such as urban women of color in New York City [47], and has inspired similar interventions for breast-feeding support [48].

Text messaging is also an effective strategy for sending reminders about data collection and upcoming appointments to older adults. In a large randomized, controlled trial evaluating a Mobile Integrated Health intervention that leverages community paramedics and telehealth to deliver urgent care in patient homes, researchers used Twilio to send text message reminders to patients about completing patient-reported outcomes surveys at regular intervals [49]. Twilio integrates with survey databases such as REDCap to deliver automated text messages to patients' cell phones at predetermined times (e.g., 30, 60, and 90 days after recruitment). Text messages include links to the surveys and the text can be customized and translated into other languages to allow for more personalized outreach.

Text messaging interventions may increase accessibility to mHealth interventions for populations without smartphones but should be considered thoughtfully to avoid exacerbating disparities. For example, individuals need to be able to read and, in the case of two-way communication interventions, type a text message, which may be challenging for individuals with language, literacy, vision, or dexterity barriers. "Talk-to-text" features available on cell phones transcribe users' spoken language into typed messages and may be a helpful additive feature in such cases. Individuals with certain phone plans may need to pay for each text message sent and received, which may create financial barriers to participation. A final consideration is that text messaging interventions are ideal for short messages and interactions, but may not work well when large amounts of information need to be communicated.

A Summary of Mobile Technology

When selecting a mobile technology, researchers should consider mobility, input, output, uses, connectivity, and cost. We summarize these key points, as shown in Table 12.1, in relation to the technologies covered in this chapter. By mobility, we mean how often the technology will be available for participants to use—either all of the time ⊘ or when an event occurs ①. Tablets are the only mobile devices that we would argue are mostly event-driven because of their larger size—thus participants would be less likely to carry them around all of the time. Digital pens are sometimes used all of the time, thus the dotted line around the 24/7 icon, however, they have mostly been used in event-driven studies (e.g., in an emergency room

Table 12.1 An overview of mobile technology based on functionality. Grey icons mean that the functionality is typically not available. Dashed icons mean that the functionality is sometimes available

Technology	Mobility	Input	Output	Uses	Connectivity	Cost
Stand alone	⊘①	⋮⋮⋮ ✓	▯ ⇔ ⊚	8	IR 📶 ✳ ⇄ ⏵⏵	1×
Text messaging	⊘①	⋮⋮⋮	▯ ⊚	🕸	📶 💬 ✳ ⏵⏵	1× 1st
Feature phones	⊘①	⋮⋮⋮	▯ ⇔	8 🕸	IR 📶 💬 ✳ ⏵⏵	1× 1st
Smartphones	⊘①	⋮⋮⋮ ✓ 🎤	▯ ⇔ ⊚	8 🕸	📶 💬 ✳ ⇄ ⏵⏵	1× 1st
Tablets	①	⋮⋮⋮ ✓ 🎤	▯ ⇔ ⊚	8 🕸	IR 📶 ✳ ⇄	1× 1st
Wearable systems	⊘①	⋮⋮⋮	▯ ⇔ ⇧	8	IR 📶 ✳ ⇄	1× 1st
Digital pens	⊘①	🎤 ▯ ⇔		8	IR 📶 ✳ ⇄ ⏵⏵	1×

during a trauma incident). Although we note that most mobile technology is available 24/7 to participants, most users want breaks from continuously being monitored or burdened with inputting something into a device. Thus, researchers should consider how much a sociotechnical intervention will burden the user and what implications could occur from having continuous monitoring. For example, are there repercussions for a user not being compliant? In addition, if continuous monitoring/input is part of the study, the researchers must seriously consider the robustness of the technology. Mobile devices with glass screens easily crack when dropped—thus a case may be needed (and a budget for fixing the device). Wearable technology must be comfortable and not get in the way of users' everyday activities. If a target population already has a preferred mobile or wearable device (e.g., Fitbit), they may be less inclined to use a device chosen by the study (e.g., a Garmin watch). In addition, battery power is always a significant challenge when doing continuous monitoring because monitoring requires computation and computation requires power—thus, researchers must conduct small, beta tests to ensure the device can handle the continuous monitoring without burdening users to change batteries or recharge in the middle of the day.

Input mechanisms include buttons, touchscreen interaction, voice, photos or videos, handwriting recognition via a stylus, touchscreen, or pen, and sensor input. All of the technologies discussed here can accept some sort of button input—whether it is a physical device button, touch screen button, or touch-sensitive button on a wearable item. Only standalone devices, smartphones, and tablets have specific touchscreen inputs. For voice input, we specifically meant that the voice can be recorded and acted on, thus only smartphones, tablets, and digital pens can use voice input in this way. Most higher-end phones and tablets can take photos and videos for input. Handwriting recognition requires either a touch-sensitive screen or a camera embedded in the writing instrument, as is the case with digital pens. Only smartphones, tablets, and wearable systems have sensors for input.

Since we are working with mobile devices, the major output concern is how much screen space there is— a small, medium, or large screen. Mobile devices can also provide vibrotactile or audio, lights/LEDs, and multimedia outputs. Most mobile devices can accommodate designs for small displays where information must be abstracted or divided into small, readable chunks. Some newer mobile devices, such as smartphones and tablets, have medium to large size displays, thus these technologies have more real estate to work with to design an interface with more information. All of the technologies except for text messaging provide vibrotactile or audio feedback to the user. Stand-alone, feature phones with screens, smartphones, and tablets can provide researchers with the ability to present multimedia information. Finally, wearable systems are currently the only systems that regularly use lights/LEDs to communicate information to users.

In terms of uses, we looked at what each technology performed best at—individual usage, one-to-one, one-to-many, and many-to-one. The standalone, wearable, and digital pen technologies are best when used individually, however, we do note that the latter two could connect one-to-many and many-to-one depending on connectivity (e.g., sharing over the Internet). Feature phones are good at individual or one-to-one communication since the device has limited inputs and connectivity. Finally, text messaging, smartphones, and tablets excel at one-to-many, one-to-one, and many-to-one communication because it is easy to communicate with multiple people using multiple connectivity mechanisms (e.g., text messages, emails, and social networking). Researchers should consider the possible privacy issues that users may encounter when sharing information between various people—just because technology provides users with the ability to easily *share* information does not necessarily mean that it is in the user's best interest to share information—especially information related to one's health.

We briefly note the type of connectivity each device has—infrared IR, wireless Internet 🛜, text messaging 💬, short-range wireless (e.g., Bluetooth ✱), docking the technology to another device to connect the technology to a network ⇌, and voice 🔊. The connectivity is tightly tied to the cost of the technology—either a one-time cost 1× or a reoccurring cost 🗓 which can take the form of a monthly plan or a pay-as-you-go plan. All of the technologies except text messaging have a one-time cost to purchase the device. Although it can be argued that text messaging requires a phone or computer to text message, we were looking at the costs of the specific technologies. If a researcher would like to automate text messaging, then in addition to the recurring text messaging costs, the researcher would have to pay for a text messaging gateway service—another reoccurring cost. Any technology that supports text messaging or voice connectivity has a reoccurring cost associated with it. We noted that tablets sometimes have a reoccurring cost because some tablets have data plans to receive Internet connectivity. We also identified that wearable systems sometimes have reoccurring costs because some systems are paired with a device, such as a smartphone, to connect to the Internet. Thus, in these wearable systems, researchers should be prepared for two one-time costs—the wearable cost and device cost—in addition to the reoccurring cost. Digital pens do not have a monthly or pay-as-you-go cost, but some may require special paper that has to be purchased or printed. Researchers should carefully consider the privacy and security of information when sharing information digitally—since mobile devices are small and computation drains batteries faster, information is typically not encrypted.

Based on the examples and overview provided in this section, researchers should be able to find a mobile technology that can meet their needs *if* their intervention truly needs to be relatively small, easy to carry, and available most of the time.

Methodological Considerations for mHealth Design

Much has been written about the optimal design of mHealth interfaces; indeed, entire textbooks and book chapters have been devoted to this subject and some are provided here as references [50–52]. Rather, we have highlighted three areas that are particularly important to consider: visualizing personal health data, designing for sustained engagement, and contextual inquiry, particularly in underserved communities.

As massive amounts of personal health data are being collected and stored about one's health, individuals increasingly expect to be able to view and engage with their health data. Examples include viewing data collected from wearables through the accompanying smartphone app or viewing information collected during clinical care in one's patient portal. This has raised questions about the optimal strategies for displaying personal health data given issues of limited health literacy (as high as 88% of U.S. adults [53]), inadequate graph literacy (40% of U.S. adults [54]), and the potential for unnecessary anxiety or even harm from misunderstanding one's data. Many studies have created novel visualizations for displaying personal health data but few have been designed in user-centered ways or evaluated rigorously [55]. If researchers or developers are planning to return data to users, they should be sure to include visualizations that have been rigorously tested with end users and meet their specific goals for showing data to the patient, such as appropriate risk perception. For example, researchers at the University of Michigan compared several visualizations and demonstrated that number lines with "anchors" and color-coding indicating normal ranges helped lay audiences distinguish between normal, abnormal but non-urgent, and urgent laboratory values [56]. Similarly, when displaying changes in patient-reported outcomes, visual analogies such as gas gauges representing different levels of physical function may be better comprehended among all adults, including older adults with cognitive impairment, compared to line graphs or text alone [57]. As AI-generated predictive models are increasingly integrated into these interventions, questions regarding the ideal strategy for communicating properties of the model (fairness, explainability, accuracy), as well as the output itself (one's personal risk and risk factors, recommended actions, confidence ranges) will need to be determined.

Many participants will abandon a mHealth intervention within weeks or months of initiating use. In most cases, sustained use of the intervention is required to receive its full benefit. Therefore, researchers should think critically about sustained engagement at the *beginning* of the design process—this includes defining the goal for engagement at the outset. For example, researchers created a protocol for one randomized, controlled trial in which atrial fibrillation patients were randomized to a mHealth intervention involving recording a mobile electrocardiogram using the AliveCor Kardia device twice daily for 6 months [58]. However, in follow-up interviews, patients and clinicians pointed out that this was not only burdensome but also unnecessary—if patients do not experience atrial fibrillation for several months, titrating usage to once per day or a few times per week may be more appropriate [59].

When designing technologies, it is important to engage with patients and other stakeholders to optimize the chances of sustained engagement. The literature can provide examples of features that may promote adoption and sustained engagement, including ease of use, summary graphs or statistics, and data sharing with friends and clinicians [60]. However, much of this research has been conducted with individuals who may already be predisposed to use mHealth, such as higher education levels, non-minoritized racial and ethnic groups, and younger adults. Individuals who do not fall into these categories, but who nonetheless could benefit from mHealth, may need unique design approaches. For example, researchers at Columbia University conducted qualitative interviews and focus groups with low-income, Latino adults with Type 2 Diabetes living in an urban environment to co-develop a mHealth app for diabetes self-management. They found that these individuals needed support and guidance to collect, make sense of, and act on their personal health data (such as meal information and blood glucose levels), and that clinician involvement and/or recommender systems may be needed to promote sustained engagement [61, 62].

Researchers can use contextual inquiry methods [63] to learn about current processes and information resources so that the researcher can integrate these processes and artifacts earlier into their design and analysis cycle. Contextual inquiry methods typically include researchers interviewing (*the inquiry*) target users where they conduct the targeted activity (*the context*) and asking users to walk through typical activities to gain a better understanding of what is done when and how the process works. Researchers can gain rich data on users' processes—specifically understanding *if* technology is appropriate and *how* technology could enhance these processes. Contextual inquiry in underserved communities converges community-based participatory research and informatics to apply basic concepts of contextual inquiry to the unique and specific social determinants of health faced by many underserved communities. For example, researchers creating a dietary intake monitoring application (DIMA) app spent 2 years meeting with health professionals and patients in an iterative user-centered design process to design the application. The mobile application used icons, barcode scanning, and voice recording to provide users with an easy way to input what they ate and receive real-time feedback. In a pilot study, participants were able to successfully use DIMA and some noted that it helped them change their diet by becoming more compliant with their dietary restrictions [64]. Since the application needed to provide real-time feedback, the researchers had to ensure that the database was primed with everything users could possibly input into the system. In addition, the researchers had to iteratively design the interface because they were working with a low literacy population—a population often overlooked in the human-computer interaction community. The research team had to consider everything from how to present dietary limits and organize food items [30], to the application's navigation structure [65].

There are a number of unique challenges with conducting evaluation studies with mobile devices. Many of the challenges are because (1) users are mobile and (2) capturing real-world usage is challenging. Unlike capturing interactions on desktop computers, screen capture software generally cannot be used to conduct usability studies on phones and tablets. Problems with the screen capture approach include, generally, the lack of good software for the variety of mobile devices available in the ecosystem and that screen capture software cannot effectively capture the interactions of the user with the screen. When users interact with mobile devices, they frequently interact with touch screens. Without the ability to visually capture the user's finger taps on the screen, it can be difficult to determine whether or not some of the usability challenges are related to a failure of the hardware device to pick up the user's taps or related to the design of the user interface.

To solve this issue, researchers have designed "sleds" to capture a user's interaction with the devices. These sleds usually have a camera focused on the mobile device and occasionally have an additional camera focused on the user (Fig. 12.3). They attach to the mobile device to maintain a consistent view of the device, even when the user picks up the device to use it.

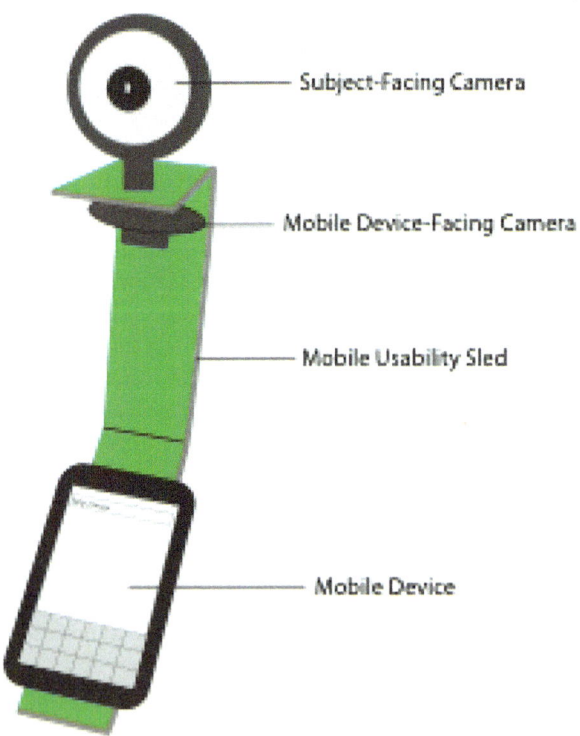

Fig. 12.3 Illustration of a low-cost mobile usability sled. These sleds are frequently made from a sheet of acrylic and bent into shape

Methodological Considerations for mHealth Implementation

When designing a user study to evaluate mobile systems in health informatics, researchers should carefully consider the goal of the mobile system and how it may impact the study. For example, if a dietary monitoring application was designed to help users be more compliant with specific dietary restrictions, then researchers must account for how the research team and users think about compliance. Contextual factors influencing the outcomes of interest should also be considered, such as the time of year for the study. If a study is to investigate a group's everyday diet, then the study should not be planned around holidays when people may eat more than normal. If an intervention is aimed to increase physical activity, then the time of year, the weather during that year, and the safety of where people live should be considered. If a study is being conducted in a clinical environment, then the unit and time of year should be considered. For example, conducting a study in pediatrics in August when children need physicals before school starts in comparison to the summertime when families are away or busy with summer activities.

We always encourage researchers to report on users' mobile system usage to provide the research community with an idea of how users appropriated the system into their daily lives. Usage statistics can take many forms—when the user opened the application; what screens they used most; how many items were input at one time; where they navigated to (a normal navigation segment or are they getting "stuck" somewhere?). Another issue related to usage is to report on when participants used the system to help create a rich picture of the participant's interactions with the system. For example, if a participant was instructed to use a mobile system throughout the day, but only used the system once during a certain time period, then the research team has to acknowledge the possibility of recall bias. If participants only used the system when the research team contacted them—either to remind them of an upcoming meeting or right before a meeting—then the researchers have to acknowledge that usage spiked when the research team contacted the participants and the accuracy of the data may have been compromised. For example, Stone et al. coined the term "parking lot compliance" for when participants do their study participation in the parking lot of the building where they will meet the research team [66]. Qualitative research can be a very useful tool in providing a richer picture of how and why participants used or didn't use a particular system.

It will also be important for researchers to document how certain mHealth interventions translate across different disease contexts, patient populations, and geographical areas. This is particularly important in LMICs. The focus of mHealth interventions in many UMICs has been on chronic disease prevention and management, reflecting this as a top cause of morbidity and mortality in these nations, and most interventions leverage the popularity of smartphones. By contrast, mHealth interventions in LMIC countries in Africa, Asia, and Latin America focus predominantly on infectious disease and maternal health and leverage text messaging interventions more often. Additionally, mHealth interventions in these areas face unique barriers including funding and infrastructure, lack of equipment, and technology disparities [67]. To adapt mHealth interventions to other settings, ways that individuals represent and interpret knowledge and make decisions will need to be formally studied to guide adaptations and implementation. For example, researchers who created a culturally adapted app for community health nurses to conduct suicide risk and depression assessments in Fiji Islands conducted "think aloud" methods and other cognitive tasks to determine whether the app supported information processing and decision-making compared to paper-based assessments (Fig. 12.4). They found that the app support faster information processing, more accurate decision-making, and different reasoning patterns, compared to paper-based assessments [68].

Since we use mobile systems to manage some health metrics, we need to investigate ways to measure the metric through baseline data, validated instruments, physiological data, and self-report. This may be conducted through the mHealth tools themselves, which streamline data collection for the participant but depend upon sustained use of the tool—which, as we noted above, can be variable. Researchers may instead opt to collect important endpoints through other means, such as telephone outreach, automated electronic survey invitations to email addresses, or secondary data collection through sources such as electronic health records and insurance claims data.

If a research team decides to use a fairly new mobile system, we would strongly recommend that they start the study with a small participant pool and a short duration—similar to some of the studies discussed in this chapter. Although the results may not be generalizable and behavior will not change, researchers will have the opportunity to understand how and why people use the system and what changes are needed to provide easier interactions with the system. After the research team has assured that users want and can use the mobile system, they can decide to increase the study size and duration.

mHealth devices are becoming more ubiquitous and pervasive, and as a result, the amount and type of data that may be collected by researchers has increased dramatically. Some of these data may be identifiable, personal, and/or sensitive. For

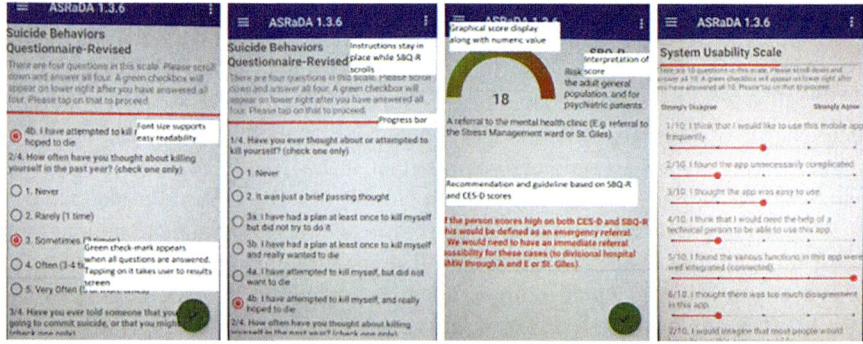

Fig. 12.4 Screens from a culturally adapted app for community health nurses to conduct suicide risk and depression screening in Fiji Islands

example, geolocations, infectious disease status, menstrual cycles, pregnancy status, and mental health symptoms may be captured. This raises questions about how these data can and should be used by researchers in ethically sound ways. For example, funders and publishers frequently require data transparency and open-access repositories. Researchers may collaborate and share data for secondary analyses or future applications, such as artificial intelligence. Security and privacy standards also vary dramatically across consumer-grade devices and may be susceptible to hacking and other malicious activities. While the European Union has implemented the General Data Protection Regulations to regulate data sharing and protect data privacy (https://gdpr-info.eu/), standards in the U.S. and other countries are not as strict. Therefore, researchers should consider how and where their data is collected and stored, which parties can access it, and how informed patients are about sharing and reuse of their personal health data.

Finally, as mHealth interventions move from novel prototypes and proof-of-concept testing to large trials and evaluations, and eventually become embedded in individuals' lives and clinical care, implementation science frameworks may guide researchers and developers who wish to describe and disseminate successful implementation strategies. Some general-purpose frameworks may be suitable for adaptation and use in these contexts, while in other cases frameworks specifically addressing technology implementation may be a better fit. For example, the Consolidated Framework for Implementation Research (CFIR) is a general framework that specifies characteristics of interventions, inner and outer settings, processes, and individuals, and can be useful in planning an implementation [69]. The Reach Effectiveness Adoption Implementation Maintenance (RE-AIM) framework is a widely used framework for evaluating implementation efforts after initial trials or pilot tests and identifies strategies for sustained integration of technologies (https://re-aim.org/). The general RE-AIM questions are useful when applied to mHealth, but additional questions evaluating predisposing, enabling, and reinforcing factors to technology implementation have also been proposed to better adapt the framework to informatics interventions [70]. Finally, the Non-adoption, Abandonment, Scale-up, Spread, Sustainability (NASSS) framework describes the adoption, non-adoption, and abandonment and the challenges to scale-up, spread, and sustainability of technologies in health systems [71]. All of these frameworks have freely available training, as well as sample survey questions and interview guides which may be tailored for use in a particular mHealth project. For example, RE-AIM has been used to study the implementation of a mobile app for heart failure self-monitoring in a heart failure clinic primarily consisting of older adults in New York City [72]. The RE-AIM framework was useful in identifying aspects of the app that were effective, and those that required continued refinement, to meet patients' needs.

Conclusion

In this chapter, we provided a brief overview of how mobile technology has evolved from novelty to ubiquity, with now the majority of adults globally owning a cell phone and many owning a smartphone. We presented research, industry, and government examples for each technology to show best practices in design, implementation, and dissemination. We also closely examined the various functionalities available in each type of technology to assist researchers in understanding what types of mobile technologies they should consider for their own work. Finally, we concluded with some considerations one should make when designing and conducting studies related to healthcare with mobile technology. With the information in this chapter, researchers can make an informed decision about whether mobile technology is right for their system design, what technology they could use, and key considerations they must make when conducting their study.

Discussion Questions
1. Compare and contrast the similarities and differences in designing a system and study for a text messaging, smartphone, and wearable system intervention.
2. What are our responsibilities as researchers to consider:
   (a) How do people want to use a mobile intervention in their everyday lives versus how the research team envisions the participants using the application?
   (b) What happens to the application after the study and funding are completed, but participants still want to use it?
   (c) How we use AI in mHealth interventions to provide feedback and interventions to people?

References

1. Pew Research Center. Mobile fact sheet 2021. Available from: https://www.pewresearch.org/internet/fact-sheet/mobile/
2. Silver L. Smartphone ownership is growing rapidly around the world, but not always equally 2019. Available from: https://www.pewresearch.org/global/2019/02/05/smartphone-ownership-is-growing-rapidly-around-the-world-but-not-always-equally/
3. Veinot TC, Mitchell H, Ancker JS. Good intentions are not enough: how informatics interventions can worsen inequality. J Am Med Inform Assoc. 2018;25(8):1080–8.
4. Marcolino MS, Oliveira JAQ, D'Agostino M, Ribeiro AL, Alkmim MBM, Novillo-Ortiz D. The impact of mHealth interventions: systematic review of systematic reviews. JMIR Mhealth Uhealth. 2018;6(1):e23.
5. McKay FH, Cheng C, Wright A, Shill J, Stephens H, Uccellini M. Evaluating mobile phone applications for health behaviour change: a systematic review. J Telemed Telecare. 2018;24(1):22–30.
6. Motti LG, Vigouroux N, Gorce P. Interaction techniques for older adults using touchscreen devices: a literature review. Paper presented at: 25ème conférence francophone sur l'Interaction Homme-Machine (IHM 2013), AFIHM: Association Francophone de

l'Interaction Homme-Machine, Nov 2013, Bordeaux, France. 2013. p. 125–34. https://doi.org/10.1145/2534903.2534920
7. Kobayashi M, Hiyama A, Miura T, Asakawa C, Hirose M, Ifukube T. Elderly user evaluation of mobile touchscreen interactions. Paper presented at: Proceedings of the 13th IFIP TC 13 International Conference on Human-Computer Interaction - Volume Part I; Lisbon, Portugal: Springer-Verlag; 2011. p. 83–99.
8. Jin ZX, Plocher T, Kiff L. Touch screen user interfaces for older adults: button size and spacing. Paper presented at: Proceedings of the 4th International Conference on Universal Access in Human Computer Interaction: Coping with Diversity; Beijing, China. Springer-Verlag; 2007. p. 933–41.
9. Nischelwitzer A, Pintoffl K, Loss C, Holzinger A. Design and development of a mobile medical application for the management of chronic diseases: methods of improved data input for older people. Paper presented at: Proceedings of the 3rd Human-Computer Interaction and Usability Engineering of the Austrian Computer Society Conference on HCI and Usability for Medicine and Health Care; Graz, Austria. Springer-Verlag; 2007. p. 119–32.
10. Liu N, Yin J, Tan SS, Ngiam KY, Teo HH. Mobile health applications for older adults: a systematic review of interface and persuasive feature design. J Am Med Inform Assoc. 2021;28(11):2483–501.
11. Valdez RS, Lyon SE, Wellbeloved-Stone C, et al. Engaging the disability community in informatics research: rationales and practical steps. J Am Med Inform Assoc. 2022;29(11):1989–95.
12. Masterson Creber RM, Grossman LV, Ryan B, et al. Engaging hospitalized patients with personalized health information: a randomized trial of an inpatient portal. J Am Med Inform Assoc. 2019;26(2):115–23.
13. Chen Z, Lin M, Chen F, et al. Unobtrusive sleep monitoring using smartphones. Paper presented at: 2013 7th International Conference on Pervasive Computing Technologies for Healthcare (PervasiveHealth); Venice, Italy. 2013. p. 145–52.
14. Connelly K, Molchan H, Bidanta R, et al. Evaluation framework for selecting wearable activity monitors for research. Mhealth. 2021;7:6.
15. Dangerfield MI, Ward K, Davidson L, Adamian M. Initial experience and usage patterns with the owlet smart sock monitor in 47,495 newborns. Glob Pediatr Health. 2017;4:2333794x17742751.
16. Zhao Y, Szpiro S, Azenkot S. ForeSee: a customizable head-mounted vision enhancement system for people with low vision. Paper presented at: Proceedings of the 17th International ACM SIGACCESS Conference on Computers & Accessibility; Lisbon, Portugal: Association for Computing Machinery; 2015. p. 239–49.
17. Bigham JP, Jayant C, Ji H, et al. VizWiz: nearly real-time answers to visual questions. Paper presented at: Proceedings of the 23nd Annual ACM Symposium on User Interface Software and Technology; New York: Association for Computing Machinery; 2010. p. 333–42.
18. Ahmed T, Shaffer P, Connelly K, Crandall D, Kapadia A. Addressing physical safety, security, and privacy for people with visual impairments. Paper presented at: Proceedings of the Twelfth USENIX Conference on Usable Privacy and Security; Denver, CO: USENIX Association; 2016. p. 341–54.
19. Miller K, Baugh CW, Chai PR, et al. Deployment of a wearable biosensor system in the emergency department: a technical feasibility study. Proc Annu Hawaii Int Conf Syst Sci 2021;2021:3567–72.
20. Li T, Divatia S, McKittrick J, Moss J, Hijnen NM, Becker LB. A pilot study of respiratory rate derived from a wearable biosensor compared with capnography in emergency department patients. Open Access Emerg Med. 2019;11:103–8.
21. Kao H-L, Holz C, Roseway A, Calvo A, Schmandt C. DuoSkin: rapidly prototyping on-skin user interfaces using skin-friendly materials. Paper presented at: Proceedings of the 2016 ACM International Symposium on Wearable Computers; Heidelberg, Germany: Association for Computing Machinery; 2016. p. 16–23.

22. Zhu J, Snowden JC, Verdejo J, et al. EIT-kit: an electrical impedance tomography toolkit for health and motion sensing. Paper presented at: The 34th Annual ACM Symposium on User interface Software and Technology; Virtual Event, USA: Association for Computing Machinery; 2021. p. 400–13.
23. Masterson Creber RM, Maurer MS, Reading M, Hiraldo G, Hickey KT, Iribarren S. Review and analysis of existing mobile phone apps to support heart failure symptom monitoring and self-care management using the mobile application rating scale (MARS). JMIR Mhealth Uhealth. 2016;4(2):e74.
24. Turchioe MR, Jimenez V, Isaac S, Alshalabi M, Slotwiner D, Creber RM. Review of mobile applications for the detection and management of atrial fibrillation. Heart Rhythm O2. 2020;1(1):35–43.
25. Meddar JM, Ponnapalli A, Azhar R, Turchioe MR, Duran AT, Creber RM. A structured review of commercially available cardiac rehabilitation mHealth applications using the mobile application rating scale. J Cardiopulm Rehabil Prev. 2022;42(3):141–7.
26. Myers A, Chesebrough L, Hu R, Turchioe MR, Pathak J, Creber RM. Evaluating commercially available mobile apps for depression self-management. AMIA Annu Symp Proc. 2020;2020:906–14.
27. Schmeelk S, Davis A, Li Q, et al. Monitoring symptoms of COVID-19: review of mobile apps. JMIR Mhealth Uhealth. 2022;10(6):e36065.
28. Benda NC, Zawtha S, Anderson K, et al. Developing population health surveillance using mHealth in low-resource settings: qualitative assessment and pilot evaluation. JMIR Form Res. 2022;6(10):e36260.
29. Grisedale S, Graves M, Grünsteidl A. Designing a graphical user interface for healthcare workers in rural India. Paper presented at: Proceedings of the ACM SIGCHI Conference on Human Factors in Computing Systems; Atlanta, Georgia: ACM; 1997. p. 471–8.
30. Siek KA, Connelly KH, Rogers Y. Pride and prejudice: learning how chronically ill people think about food. Paper presented at: Proceedings of the SIGCHI Conference on Human Factors in Computing Systems; Montréal, QC: ACM; 2006.
31. Stoyanov SR, Hides L, Kavanagh DJ, Zelenko O, Tjondronegoro D, Mani M. Mobile app rating scale: a new tool for assessing the quality of health mobile apps. JMIR Mhealth Uhealth. 2015;3(1):e27.
32. GlobalStats. Mobile operating system market share worldwide. 2021. Available from: https://gs.statcounter.com/os-market-share/mobile/worldwide/2021
33. Shaw H, Ellis DA, Kendrick LR, Ziegler F, Wiseman R. Predicting smartphone operating system from personality and individual differences. Cyberpsychol Behav Soc Netw. 2016;19(12):727–32.
34. HealthIT.gov. 2014 Edition Ehr certification criteria grid mapped to meaningful use stage 2.
35. Grossman LV, Masterson Creber RM, Benda NC, Wright D, Vawdrey DK, Ancker JS. Interventions to increase patient portal use in vulnerable populations: a systematic review. J Am Med Inform Assoc. 2019;26(8–9):855–70.
36. Kharrazi H, Chisholm R, VanNasdale D, Thompson B. Mobile personal health records: an evaluation of features and functionality. Int J Med Inform. 2012;81(9):579–93.
37. Muoio D. Microsoft will officially shut down HealthVault later this year. 2019. Available from: https://www.mobihealthnews.com/content/microsoft-will-officially-shut-down-healthvault-later-year
38. Mearian L. Why Google Health failed: too little, too soon. 2011. Available from: https://www.computerworld.com/article/2509515/why-google-health-failed%2D%2Dtoo-little%2D%2Dtoo-soon.html
39. Lim SM, Shiau CWC, Cheng LJ, Lau Y. Chatbot-delivered psychotherapy for adults with depressive and anxiety symptoms: a systematic review and meta-regression. Behav Ther. 2022;53(2):334–47.
40. Geoghegan L, Scarborough A, Wormald JCR, et al. Automated conversational agents for post-intervention follow-up: a systematic review. BJS Open. 2021;5(4):zrab070.

41. Aggarwal A, Tam CC, Wu D, Li X, Qiao S. Artificial intelligence-based Chatbots for promoting health behavioral changes: systematic review. J Med Internet Res. 2023;25:e40789.
42. Darcy A, Daniels J, Salinger D, Wicks P, Robinson A. Evidence of human-level bonds established with a digital conversational agent: cross-sectional, retrospective observational study. JMIR Form Res. 2021;5:e27868.
43. Kahane K, François J, Torous J. PERSPECTIVE: the digital health app policy landscape: regulatory gaps and choices through the lens of mental health. J Ment Health Policy Econ. 2021;24(3):101–8.
44. Pepplinkhuizen S, Hoeksema WF, van der Stuijt W, et al. Accuracy and clinical relevance of the single-lead Apple Watch electrocardiogram to identify atrial fibrillation. Cardiovasc Digit Health J. 2022;3(6 Suppl):S17–s22.
45. Perez MV, Mahaffey KW, Hedlin H, et al. Large-scale assessment of a smartwatch to identify atrial fibrillation. N Engl J Med. 2019;381(20):1909–17.
46. Buller DB, Borland R, Bettinghaus EP, Shane JH, Zimmerman DE. Randomized trial of a smartphone mobile application compared to text messaging to support smoking cessation. Telemed J E Health. 2014;20(3):206–14.
47. Blackwell TM, Dill LJ, Hoepner LA, Geer LA. Using text messaging to improve access to prenatal health information in urban African American and Afro-Caribbean immigrant pregnant women: mixed methods analysis of Text4baby usage. JMIR Mhealth Uhealth. 2020;8(2):e14737.
48. Demirci JR, Suffoletto B, Doman J, et al. The development and evaluation of a text message program to prevent perceived insufficient milk among first-time mothers: retrospective analysis of a randomized controlled trial. JMIR Mhealth Uhealth. 2020;8(4):e17328.
49. Masterson Creber RM, Daniels B, Munjal K, et al. Using mobile integrated health and telehealth to support transitions of care among patients with heart failure (MIGHTy-Heart): protocol for a pragmatic randomised controlled trial. BMJ Open. 2022;12(3):e054956.
50. Sethumadhavan A, Sasangohar F. Design for health: applications of human factors. Elsevier Science; 2020.
51. Turchioe MR, Creber RM. User-centered development and evaluation of patient-facing visualizations of health information. In: Hsueh P-YS, Wetter T, Zhu X, editors. Personal health informatics: patient participation in precision health. Cham: Springer; 2022. p. 371–96.
52. Sharp H, Preece J, Rogers Y. Interaction design: beyond human-computer interaction. Wiley; 2019.
53. Lopez C, Kim B, Sacks K. Health literacy in the United States: enhancing assessments and reducing disparities. Milken Institute; 2022.
54. Galesic M, Garcia-Retamero R. Graph literacy: a cross-cultural comparison. Med Decis Mak. 2011;31(3):444–57.
55. Turchioe MR, Myers A, Isaac S, et al. A systematic review of patient-facing visualizations of personal health data. Appl Clin Inform. 2019;10(4):751–70.
56. Zikmund-Fisher BJ, Scherer AM, Witteman HO, et al. Graphics help patients distinguish between urgent and non-urgent deviations in laboratory test results. J Am Med Inform Assoc. 2017;24(3):520–8.
57. Reading Turchioe M, Grossman LV, Myers AC, Baik D, Goyal P, Masterson Creber RM. Visual analogies, not graphs, increase patients' comprehension of changes in their health status. J Am Med Inform Assoc. 2020;27(5):677–89.
58. Hickey KT, Hauser NR, Valente LE, et al. A single-center randomized, controlled trial investigating the efficacy of a mHealth ECG technology intervention to improve the detection of atrial fibrillation: the iHEART study protocol. BMC Cardiovasc Disord. 2016;16:152.
59. Reading M, Baik D, Beauchemin M, Hickey KT, Merrill JA. Factors influencing sustained engagement with ECG self-monitoring: perspectives from patients and health care providers. Appl Clin Inform. 2018;9(4):772–81.

60. Lazard AJ, Babwah Brennen JS, Belina SP. App designs and interactive features to increase mHealth adoption: user expectation survey and experiment. JMIR Mhealth Uhealth. 2021;9(11):e29815.
61. Reading Turchioe M, Burgermaster M, Mitchell EG, Desai PM, Mamykina L. Adapting the stage-based model of personal informatics for low-resource communities in the context of type 2 diabetes. J Biomed Inform. 2020;110:103572.
62. Turchioe MR, Heitkemper EM, Lor M, Burgermaster M, Mamykina L. Designing for engagement with self-monitoring: a user-centered approach with low-income, Latino adults with type 2 diabetes. Int J Med Inform. 2019;130:103941.
63. Holtzblatt K, Wendell J, Wood S. Rapid contextual design: a how-to guide to key techniques for user-centered design (interactive technologies). Morgan Kaufmann; 2004.
64. Connelly K, Siek KA, Chaudry B, Jones J, Astroth K, Welch JL. An offline mobile nutrition monitoring intervention for varying-literacy patients receiving hemodialysis: a pilot study examining usage and usability. J Am Med Inform Assoc. 2012;19(5):705–12.
65. Chaudry BM, Connelly KH, Siek KA, Welch JL. Mobile interface design for low-literacy populations. Paper presented at: Proceedings of the 2nd ACM SIGHIT International Health Informatics Symposium; Miami, FL: ACM; 2012.
66. Stone A, Shiffman S, Schwartz J, Broderick J, Hufford M. Patient compliance with paper and electronic diaries. Control Clin Trials. 2003;24(2):182–99.
67. Kruse C, Betancourt J, Ortiz S, Valdes Luna SM, Bamrah IK, Segovia N. Barriers to the use of mobile health in improving health outcomes in developing countries: systematic review. J Med Internet Res. 2019;21(10):e13263.
68. Patel VL, Halpern M, Nagaraj V, Chang O, Iyengar S, May W. Information processing by community health nurses using mobile health (mHealth) tools for early identification of suicide and depression risks in Fiji Islands. BMJ Health Care Inform. 2021;28(1):e100342.
69. Damschroder LJ, Reardon CM, Widerquist MAO, Lowery J. The updated consolidated framework for implementation research based on user feedback. Implement Sci. 2022;17(1):75.
70. Bakken S, Ruland CM. Translating clinical informatics interventions into routine clinical care: how can the RE-AIM framework help? J Am Med Inform Assoc. 2009;16(6):889–97.
71. Greenhalgh T, Wherton J, Papoutsi C, et al. Beyond adoption: a new framework for theorizing and evaluating nonadoption, abandonment, and challenges to the scale-up, spread, and sustainability of health and care technologies. J Med Internet Res. 2017;19(11):e367.
72. Reading Turchioe M, Mangal S, Goyal P, et al. Special section on patient engagement in informatics: a RE-AIM evaluation of a visualization-based electronic patient-reported outcomes system. Appl Clin Inform. 2023;14(2):227–37.

Further Reading

Klasjna P, Pratt W. Healthcare in the pocket: mapping the space of mobile-phone health interventions. J Biomed Inform. 2012;45(1):184–98. https://doi.org/10.1016/j.jbi.2011.08.017.

Motti LG, Vigouroux N, Gorce P. Interaction techniques for older adults using touchscreen devices: a literature review. Paper presented at: 25ème conférence francophone sur l'Interaction Homme-Machine (IHM 2013), AFIHM: Association Francophone de l'Interaction Homme-Machine, Nov 2013, Bordeaux, France. 2013. p. 125–34. https://doi.org/10.1145/2534903.2534920

Siek KA, Hayes GR, Newman MW, Tang JC. Field deployments: knowing from using in context. In: Olson JS, Kellogg WA, editors. Ways of knowing in HCI. New York, NY: Springer; 2014. p. 119–42. https://doi.org/10.1007/978-1-4939-0378-8_6.

Part IV
Applications

Chapter 13
Human-Computer Interaction in Medical Devices

Todd R. Johnson, Harold Thimbleby, Peter Killoran, and Franck Diaz-Garelli

Introduction

Intuitively, we might think of a medical device as any tool specifically designed for health or promoting health. Although this intuitive notion is sufficient for everyday purposes, it is not sufficient for medical device designers. What counts as a medical device, and the requirements for testing, using, and selling a device, are defined through regulations and standards that are designed to protect the safety of patients and caregivers. These regulations are one of several factors that affect the user interface design (how to use devices) and evaluation of medical devices (how effective they are). Other factors include the safety-critical nature of medical devices, the diversity of users, extreme and noisy use environments, the lack of user interface standards for medical devices, and the small physical space often available for the user interface.

This chapter provides an introduction to medical device HCI (Human Computer Interaction—the scientific field that includes user interface design) regulations, and the challenges that result from the regulatory requirements and the complexity and variation within healthcare. We demonstrate these challenges using specific examples along with two case studies: one showing how HCI and broader human factors

---

T. R. Johnson (✉) · P. Killoran
University of Texas Health Science Center, McWilliams School of Biomedical Informatics, Houston, TX, USA
e mail: Todd.R.Johnson@uth.tmc.edu

H. Thimbleby
Swansea University, Swansea, Wales, UK

F. Diaz-Garelli
Biomedical Engineering Department, Wake Forest School of Medicine, Winston-Salem, NC, USA

Data Science R&D, Medtronic Diabetes, Northridge, CA, USA

© The Author(s), under exclusive license to Springer Nature Switzerland AG 2024
A. W. Kushniruk et al. (eds.), *Human Computer Interaction in Healthcare*, Cognitive Informatics in Biomedicine and Healthcare,
https://doi.org/10.1007/978-3-031-69947-4_13

engineering played a major role in reducing deaths related to the use of anesthesia machines, and another showing how critical changes to number entry interfaces can decrease the chance of serious medical errors.

Changes Since the First Edition

Since the first edition of this chapter was published, the biggest change affecting HCI for medical devices has been the development of regulatory guidance for software as a medical device (SaMD). Under SaMD regulations, once software meets the definition of a medical device, it is subject to the same regulatory oversight and requirements as traditional medical devices. SaMD may be designed for or run on a range of devices and software thus producing a set of HCI challenges. Another recent development is the emerging recommendations for SaMD with embedded artificial intelligence (AI). In this revised chapter we include updates on the regulations affecting medical devices, including SaMD, AI as part of medical devices, and the additional HCI challenges that result from these developments.

Human Computer Interaction and Related Fields

The field of human computer interaction is intimately concerned with medical devices because medical devices are used by humans (usually caregivers, but increasingly patients) and they often include computers. HCI is not concerned so much with whether a device performs within technical specifications, but with other important matters like whether it is usable, helps reduce error, and is enjoyable to use [1]. HCI helps make informed trade-offs, for example, how to make a device smaller without making it too small for people to use (for instance because the screen is illegible), or how to make a system secure, but not so secure that nobody can use it or so secure that everybody reverts to sticking password reminders up, and thus circumventing the security features. HCI thus covers a very broad range of important topics that help improve the safety, ease of use and user satisfaction of medical devices. Different emphases on analytic foci and different types of methods emerge from different but interrelated areas of inquiry concerned with devices:

- **HF**, Human Factors (sometimes called **ergonomics**)—the study of how humans perform and behave, particularly while operating complex systems or working in complex environments, often with tough working conditions such as interruptions, fatigue, vibration and so forth. HF includes less obvious factors, such as back strain and eye strain, that impact the user.
- **HFE**, Human Factors Engineering—human factors specifically used to help engineer or design improved working environments and systems.

- **HCI**, Human Computer Interaction (sometimes CHI, which is more pronounceable)—many complex systems involve computers; hence, HCI is HF and HFE in the context of complex, computer-based systems. HCI is not concerned with exactly what a "computer" is, so it includes mobile phones, infusion pumps, beds, and many devices where the computer is embedded and not visible like a desk-top computer.
- **UCD**, User Centered Design—a key slogan of HCI and HFE. UCD means to design a system for human use, one must focus, or center, design efforts on the user and their actual tasks.
- **UX**, User Experience—originally, HFE focused on work environments and performance of work-related goals; in contrast, UX emphasizes the experience of the user rather than the organization. Do they enjoy their work? Of course, if users have a good experience, their work will improve too!

What Is a Medical Device?

The U.S. Federal Food, Drug, and Cosmetic Act [2] defines a medical device as "an instrument, apparatus, implement, machine, contrivance, implant, *in vitro* reagent, or other similar or related article, including a component part, or accessory that is:

- Recognized in the official National Formulary, or the US Pharmacopoeia, or any supplement to them,
- Intended for use in the diagnosis of disease or other conditions, or in the cure, mitigation, treatment, or prevention of disease, in man or other animals, or
- Intended to affect the structure or any function of the body of man or other animals, and which does not achieve any of its primary intended purposes through chemical action within or on the body of man or other animals and which is not dependent upon being metabolized for the achievement of any of its primary intended purposes."

This definition offers an initial starting point for device manufacturers. In practice, whether a device is considered a "medical device" and the legal requirements to market a medical device are complex. In addition, in 2013 the FDA began to issue guidance on regulating software functions that meet the definition of medical devices [3]. The latest, nonbinding policy recommendations, published in 2022, distinguish between "Software as a Medical Device (SaMD)" and "Software in a Medical Device (SiMD)" [4]. If a software function meets the definition of a medical device, the medical device regulatory policies apply, independent of the platform that the software runs on. The distinction between SaMD and SiMD, along with their definitions mirrors that of the 2013 International Medical Device Regulators Forum [5]. By extending the definition of a medical device from a physical product to software functions, these changes increase the number and variety of products that may require regulatory approval. The European Union (EU) uses a similar, but not identical, definition of medical devices [6]. Specific details and differences of the definitions and regulations around the world are beyond the scope of this chapter. In the rest of this chapter, we will use the FDA framework as an example of how regulations affect HCI. Since regulations vary by region and change over time, HCI designers must be aware of current regulations for their target market early in the design process. When a medical device is marketed in different countries, HCI expertise is also needed to balance international issues, cultural differences, and so on to ensure devices are usable where they are needed.

Regulatory History and Human Factors Engineering Requirements

The Federal Food, Drug, and Cosmetic Act (FFDCA) of 1938 contributed to the formal definition of a medical device and its status in law. The Food and Drug Administration's (FDA) mission was to determine whether a device was safe and effective as opposed to defective, unsafe, filthy, or produced in unsanitary conditions (contaminated), or against statements, designs, or labeling that was false or misleading (misbranded). Enforcement was predominantly based on post-market inspection and complaints until the 1960s when the FDA shifted to more proactive oversight of life-saving devices and medical equipment as opposed to screening for fraudulent and dangerous products.

In 1976, new legislation defined devices and divided them into three classes based on potential risks, with varying regulatory control for each class [7]. Class I devices are those that have minimal potential for harm, such as dental floss and elastic bandages. Many Class I devices are exempt from the regulatory process. Class II devices have greater potential for harm, such as powered wheelchairs. Class III devices are those with the highest potential risks, such as replacement heart valves, breast implants, and implantable pacemakers.

The Medical Device Amendments Act of 1976 also established the provisions for pre-market notifications (the so-called 510k) [8], and inspection and enforcement of good manufacturing practices [9].

In 1995, the Association for the Advancement of Medical Instrumentation (AAMI) and the FDA held a joint conference in Washington D.C. to discuss human factors and medical devices [10]. This was the first large scale attempt to include human factors in FDA regulations. Two publications were key to the evolution of manufacturing standards and made human factors an active part of the design process for the first time. *Quality System—Design Controls Regulations* were published under 21 CFR part 820 in 1996 (61 FR 52602) and went into effect in 1997, harmonizing requirements to international standards, primarily, the International Organization for Standards (ISO) 9001:1994 series of quality standards [11]. From an HCI perspective, the most important clause in the Design Controls Regulations states "Design validation shall ensure that devices conform to defined user needs and intended uses and shall include testing of production units under actual or simulated use conditions." The second important publication, *Do it by design: An introduction to human factors in medical devices,* was issued in 1996 as guidance to help medical device manufacturers take human factors into account during product design phases [12].

In 2000, the FDA's Center for Devices and Radiological Health (CDRH) released human factors guidance including that "human error" should be considered in risk analysis [13]. In 2001, the American National Standards Institutes (ANSI) and the AAMI released standard HE74 *Human Factors Design Process for Medical Devices* [14]. In 2006, the International Electrical Commission (IEC) released standard 60601-1-6 on medical electrical equipment, which included human factors of alarm systems (Part 1–6: *General requirements for basic safety and essential performance—Collateral standard: Usability*) [15]. In 2007, the IEC released standard 62,366, *Application of usability engineering to medical devices* [16], and ANSI/AAMI/ISO released 14971:2007, detailing how human factors engineering can be used as part of risk analysis [17]. In 2009, the ANSI and the AAMI released standard HE75:2009 *Human Factors Engineering—Design of Medical Devices* [18].

As noted in the prior section, beginning in 2013, the FDA issued regulatory guidance on software as (or in) a medical device (SaMD and SiMD). More recently, the FDA has begun to consider how to regulate medical devices that use artificial intelligence or machine learning (AI/ML) [19, 20]. This is a challenging new area of device regulation, because a device using AI/ML may continue to learn and adapt once on the market, or may be fixed at market time, but include regular software updates based on new training data or algorithm improvements. All SaMD and SiMD, with or without AI/ML, is subject to the human factors engineering requirements that apply to all medical devices; however, SaMD, SiMD, and AI/ML bring new challenges to human factors engineering that require additional research to address [21, 22].

In addition to pre-market requirements, regulations also cover post-market surveillance of medical devices. Manufacturers, importers, and device user facilities are required to report all device-related adverse events and product problems, including "use errors": outcomes that are different than intended due to how a device was used, but not caused by malfunctions. In addition, the FDA encourages healthcare professionals, patients, caregivers, and consumers to submit reports voluntarily. Reports going back to 1991 are publicly available online through a web-based search engine called MAUDE (Manufacturer and User Facility Device Experience) [23]. MAUDE can be used for downloading data for importing into databases. These reports are an important source of information regarding possible human factors issues with medical devices; however, they must be used with caution because there is often insufficient data to determine whether a use error was due to a design problem or to a user problem. In addition, the data cannot be used to evaluate rates of adverse events or compare rates across devices, due to the incomplete nature of the reports and lack of availability of the number of devices in use at the time of the report.

At present, the regulatory environment continues to evolve. For example, the Institute of Medicine issued a report, at the FDA's request, of the 510(k) clearance process [24]. This refers to Section 510(k) of the FFDCA, which outlines a streamlined pre-market approval process for medical devices that are "substantially equivalent" to an existing device that was cleared through the same process. The IOM report found that the 510(k) process is flawed because many existing devices were never assessed for safety and effectiveness. As a result, 510(k) clearance is not a determination that a device is safe and effective. They recommend that the FDA develop a new integrated pre-market and post-market regulatory system, instead of continuing to modify the existing system.

Taken together, the regulations, guidance documents and recognized standards offer both general and specific guidelines and recommendations for applying human factors engineering to medical device design including documentation requirements for devices that require FDA approval. Many of the standards include extensive background material and references for further reading. Before beginning any medical device interface design project, it is essential for HCI designers to have a thorough understanding of these documents.

Impact of Medical Device Design on Patient Safety

Many studies have examined the role and extent of human factors issues on errors involving medical devices. Overall, these reports indicate that more problems are caused by device-use errors than device failures. An early study showed that 82% of all preventable medical errors involving anesthesia devices were due to human error [25]. Another suggested that patients may be 3–10 times more at risk due to user error than to device failure [26]. A study of errors involving infusion pumps found that the most frequent cause of patient harm was user error and inadequate device education [27]. It is important to note that use error does not mean the user is at fault; many use errors have multiple causes, including poor training, poor device design, overwork, fatigue and interruptions, poor operating procedures and even poor handwriting. In fact, FDA data collected between 1985 and 1989 demonstrated that 45–50% of device recalls stemmed from poor product design [28]. Studies suggest that, despite efforts to improve device user interfaces and safety, device use errors continue to be a substantial source of adverse events. For example, studies of "smart" infusion pumps (which contain dose error reduction systems sensitive to drugs and safe dosing ranges) have found that they have had only limited effects on patient safety [29–32]. A recent analysis of medical device error reports from 2010 to 2018 found that 28.1% of reports labeled with a device problem code, were device use errors [33]. Of those device use errors, 15.3% resulted in patient injury and 0.432% in death. A review of medical device recall data from the U.S. for the years 2012 to 2015 found that 423 device recalls were due to user interface software issues [34].

The limited impact of efforts to improve device safety mirrors the generally limited results of more than a decade of effort to improve patient safety in the US, despite demonstrated success in controlled studies of specific interventions [35]. More recently, a review of 11 hospitals during 2018 found that patients experienced an adverse event in nearly one in four admissions and that one in four of those events were preventable [36].

Unique Challenges of Medical Device Design

Usability is ultimately a product of the interplay of a device (including its user interface), its use environment, its user(s), the characteristics of the patients who are being treated, and the tasks being performed with the device. Although device manufacturers must consider all of these elements, the diversity, complexity, and ever-changing nature of healthcare poses design problems that common methods of user-centered design do not adequately address. Below we review each of these areas in the context of medical device design.

Medical Device Users

Users of medical devices range from healthcare professionals to patients and their family members. Professionals are more likely to understand the medical role of devices, have experience using the devices, and may be familiar with similar devices. However, professionals often must use a number of similar devices of different models by the same or multiple manufacturers. For example, the same hospital may use different models of infusion pumps, each with user interfaces that may be very or just slightly different. This diversity in design may be for historical reasons (older and newer devices in the same setting), clinical reasons (some models are better for certain areas of care or tasks), or because the user works in multiple healthcare settings. Although familiarity with a family of devices can have positive transfer of skill effects, it can also lead to negative transfer where the user's knowledge of one device leads to use errors on a different device [37]. Healthcare professionals also tend to be extremely busy, which can result in limited time for formal training on new devices. This increases their need to rely on their mental models and operating knowledge of previous devices—knowledge that may not correctly transfer to the new device. For example, we have found that users of infusion pumps use undocumented and unintended device-specific methods to speed reprogramming. Those methods will not transfer to other devices and may not work on the same device with different firmware or configuration settings.

An increasing number of devices are being used outside traditional healthcare settings by patients or lay-caregivers. In some cases, these devices are specifically designed for non-professional users and settings. One common example are glucose meters, which had significant problems in early designs [38]. In other cases, patients and lay caregivers must use devices that were designed for healthcare professionals operating in a clinical setting.

Designing medical devices for non-professional users is challenging because these users exhibit much more variation in abilities and knowledge than healthcare professionals. They may have a wide range of physical, cognitive or perceptual disabilities, and their educational background and understanding of the clinical context can vary greatly. Although non-professional users may need to undergo training before device use, their actual use is much harder to monitor than in more controlled, professional settings.

In April 2010, the FDA issued the Medical Device Home Use Initiative guidance document [39]. It lists caregiver knowledge, device usability, and environmental unpredictability as three unique challenges. A companion draft guidance document, issued in 2012, provides design considerations for medical devices intended for home use [40]. Many of the recommendations address the differences between professional and non-professional users. For instance, the guidance recommends that designers consider literacy level and emotional issues, and design the interface so that it is "inherently apparent to users how to use the device."

There is considerable need for additional research on designing medical devices to accommodate a wide variety of user characteristics. More accessible medical devices could benefit both non-professional and professional users, because as the workforce ages, professional users will face some of the same challenges as non-professional users. Existing medical devices designed for professionals rarely consider even common disabilities, making it difficult for caregivers with disabilities to use, or even access, the devices [41].

Variability in Patients

Even when a patient is not a direct user of a device, characteristics of the patient being treated, tested, or monitored can still affect device use, and thus must be considered during device design. For example, adults, young children, and neonates (premature and newborn infants) have very different dosing limits for medications. As a result, vendors have designed infusion pumps that the user can place in different operating modes, depending on the patient being treated. This has caused mode confusion errors when a pump is inadvertently placed in the wrong mode, but operated as if it is in the correct mode [42]. Patients with several comorbidities increase task complexity and often the number of devices involved in their care. Device designers must also consider patient disabilities. For instance, patients who cannot stand on their own, such as those who use wheelchairs, may have difficulty getting a mammogram because most mammography equipment requires that the patient stand and remain still [43].

Use Environments

The diversity and complexity of medical device use environments present several design challenges. There are roughly four different environments: inpatient facilities (such as hospitals and nursing homes), pre-hospital emergency settings, outpatient clinics, and homes. Although variation is more extreme across these settings, there is also considerable variation within each. Here we highlight some of the major differences among these environments.

The hospital setting is the most controlled of all healthcare settings. Equipment, staffing, room and unit layout, and room assignments may all be managed to optimize care. However, patients in hospitals tend to be those who require immediate medical monitoring and intervention, ranging from nearly constant monitoring and therapy (such as in an intensive care unit) to relatively infrequent observation. Multiple devices are often in use for a single patient, which can lead to connector and alarm confusion, as well as equipment placement that is less than ideal for optimal use. For instance, many medical devices have digital displays that are inset in a bezel, such that if viewed from an angle above the device, the bezel will obscure the top or sides of the numbers, perhaps making a 7 appear as a 1 [44].

In this and other healthcare environments, many safety-critical devices are in constant operation even when a trained provider is not present. Although medical devices include visual and audible alerts, these may not be heard outside a patient's room. Some devices also have high rates of false alarms, so the alarms tend to be ignored, or patients ask providers to lower the alarm volume so that they are not woken at night. There is considerable body of research on medical device alarm design; for a review see [45].

The inpatient environment is also subject to numerous interruptions, and it may be noisy, have non-optimal lighting and limited space for equipment placement. Multiple devices are often mounted on a single wheeled pole, which can become unstable and pose a hazard to patients and providers. Providers are typically time-constrained due either to workload or emergent clinical situations. This has design implications for speed and ease of use that we explore below.

Pre-hospital emergency settings include injury scenes and ground or air ambulances. Ambulances present unique design challenges due to the available space and vehicle motion, vibration, and noise. A user interface that works well at the hospital bedside may not be suited for use in ambulances. For example, during an observational session of paramedics who were operating in an ambulance equipped with an early telemedicine system, one of the authors (TRJ) observed that the paramedics used a raised bezel around a wall-mounted computer touchscreen to anchor their fingers so they could successfully use the telemedicine interface: the bezel allowed the user's hand to rise and fall with the movement of the vehicle and the touchscreen. To access menus on the top half of the screen, the paramedics hooked their fingers on top of the bezel and used their thumb to touch the screen. To access menus on the lower half, the paramedics hooked their thumb on the bezel at the bottom of the screen and used a finger to touch the screen. The bezel was not intentionally designed for this purpose—it was simply an artifact of method used to mount the screen. Without the bezel, the paramedics would have had trouble using the touchscreen interface while the ambulance was moving.

Outpatient clinics are perhaps the simplest environment with respect to medical devices; however, efforts to reduce the number of emergency department visits and inpatient stays are increasing the complexity of care in outpatient clinics. With increased complexity of care comes an increase in the number and complexity of medical devices. Similar economic pressures are demanding faster and faster visits, meaning that common outpatient medical devices that are easier and faster to use can play a role in assisting the shift to "better care for less." For example, medical devices that directly send patient vital signs to the electronic medical records can offer significant efficiency gains, but also pose design challenges in terms of patient identification and preventing errors that result from removing the user from overseeing the data entry process.

The home care environment, which may also include work and recreational sites, is a growing but challenging environment for medical device design. An aging population, patient preference, and economic pressures, along with constantly wired mobile technology, are leading to new ways to monitor and care for patients who would normally require care in a traditional healthcare setting. However, the home setting is one of the most diverse and uncontrolled environments. The FDA's draft guidance on home-use medical devices lists a number of environmental considerations, including contaminants, childproofing, resistance to tampering, and possible implications of security screenings while traveling with medical devices [40].

Tasks

The safety-critical nature and complexity of tasks in which medical devices play a role, greatly affect device usability and safety. In HCI the notion of task is broadly defined. It may be used to refer to something very general that a person wants or needs to do, such as diagnosing or monitoring a patient, or to something very specific, such as turning off an infusion pump. When designing and evaluating a medical device interface, it is important for designers to consider both device-specific tasks and broader tasks in which the device plays a role. For example, clinicians sometimes manage a patient's pain by using a patient-controlled analgesia pump. This is a type of infusion pump that is loaded with pain control medication, then programmed to allow the patient to deliver the medication as needed—up to a programmed dose and rate limit. Device-specific tasks include programming the pump (typically done by a nurse) and signaling the need for more pain medication (typically done by the patient). However, these tasks are just subtasks of the broader pain management task. Likewise, pain management is just one subtask of treating a patient. While a single device-specific task might seem relatively simple when analyzed in isolation, designers need to consider that that task is being done in the context of a complex suite of tasks involving multiple agents and multiple devices, often over extended periods of time.

As medicine has progressed, the complexity of clinical tasks has increased. As with other areas of technology, the introduction of computer-controlled medical devices has supported and enabled more and more complex interventions, further raising task complexity. To support more complex interventions, designers have added additional functionality to medical devices, in much the same way that mobile phones have continued to gain functionality. For example, some infusion pumps can deliver several medications, each with their own rate and total doses. Infusions may also be programmed to change over time. Medical devices are increasingly connected to other devices and clinical information systems. They may be operated or reconfigured remotely or even automatically. Many can be customized at the institutional level to provide default values and modes designed to ensure efficiency of care and safe dose limits.

When devices are designed to perform more and more functions, their user interfaces necessarily increase in complexity. At the same time, designers are pressured to keep device size as small as possible to maximize space utilization and the ability to transport the device (and to reduce manufacturing and storage costs). The pressure to keep devices as small as possible can lead to serious compromises in display and control design. For example, multi-channel infusion pumps may only display the program for a single channel, requiring user interaction to view other channels. Physical controls may be placed too close together with each control serving multiple functions. On some devices controls are placed at the back of the device where they are hard to see and may be inadvertently changed when moving or holding the device. Small screen and font sizes may also make it difficult for users to accurately read the display, particularly when not standing directly in front of the screen, such as when a provider is on the opposite side of a patient's bed. A user may not realize a screen is difficult to use; they may just misread it and not know they have misread the display.

Infection control is a major concern in nearly all healthcare settings. It is an overarching task in which almost all device tasks are embedded. To prevent infection, providers often use medical devices while gloved, so traditional consumer-oriented interaction technology and user interfaces may not work or work reliably. Devices must also be easy to disinfect, and must work under extreme conditions, such as when splashed with fluids.

Because users are often time-constrained, they must be able to quickly and accurately assess and change the state of the device, or use the device to get an accurate assessment of the patient's clinical state. Small displays, confusing icons and information displays, and the need to change modes to access critical information, all raise the probability of adverse events. When used in the context of multiple medical devices, the time element increases the chance of alarm, connector, and device confusion. For instance, nurses have correctly programmed the wrong infusion channel, because they had difficulty tracking down which tube was connected to which pump and which channel on the pump.

Many devices must continue to operate when removed from a main power source, such as during a power outage or during patient transport. Devices typically have built-in batteries in addition to a power cord. The design of power source and battery status displays is critical for the safe operation of these devices. Since the devices continue to operate while unplugged, and since operators are not always present, patients have been harmed when devices have run out of battery power because they were either inadvertently unplugged or were not plugged in after transportation or setup. In some cases, these errors were the result of poorly designed power status displays.

Devices

Unlike consumer applications that have user interfaces based on mature operating systems with standardized user interface elements and interaction guidelines, medical devices are often completely custom-designed user interface projects involving blends of custom hardware, software, displays, and interaction devices. Although this gives designers tremendous flexibility to develop innovative devices, it also means that designers do not benefit from the years of user interface development and research experience embedded in modern consumer products. In particular, users familiar with everyday devices may be caught up by medical device idiosyncrasies. The small form-factor of many medical devices adds additional challenges to user interface design, both in terms of the amount of information that can be displayed at once and the design of physical controls.

With the advent of mobile technology, such as smartphones and tablets, the number and importance of mobile medical applications continues to increase. As noted above, the FDA regulation of mobile medical applications is part of its broader regulation of software in (or as) a medical device (SiMD or SaMD). Mobile medical applications can offer additional HCI challenges [21, 46]. Unlike dedicated medical devices, they share the device with several other applications that could affect the functioning of the mobile health application. For example, a mobile health alert may be lost among a number of other, non-health related application alerts. Mobile app developers and users vary more than for traditional medical devices. Because users typically have their mobile devices on or near them at all times, the same user may use the mobile health app under a wide range of environmental and social conditions. In addition to standard usability factors, such as the design of visual and audible feedback, designers must also address battery issues, Internet connectivity, security, and privacy. There is also a need to integrate information from a number of health-related devices and display it in a way that permits a user to understand relationships. For example, a person might want to view weight, blood pressure, sleep, and exercise in an integrated display by date, despite the fact that each is collected by different devices and applications.

Methods for Medical Device Interface Design and Evaluation

The FDA provides comprehensive draft guidance on the human factors engineering process for medical device design along with recommended methods [45]. The main goal of the process is to understand and mitigate use-related hazards so that device use is safe and effective. The process has four main steps: identifying and investigating anticipated and unanticipated use-related hazards, prioritizing risks associated with use-related hazards, developing and implementing risk mitigation and control strategies, and validation testing. The steps must be carried out in the context of an analysis of the intended users, tasks, use environments, and (once designed or prototyped) the device user interface.

It is never possible to design a good device without doing user testing. How users will use a device is unknown until they try it in a realistic environment; even in the lab, user behavior can be misleading. Crucially, if designers modify a design to improve user performance, it becomes necessary to do more user testing in case new problems have been accidentally introduced. Hence all devices should be tested *iteratively* until they meet the design criteria appropriate for their intended use. International standards such as ISO 9241 [47] and 14971 [17] should be referred to for more details on design processes.

Since medical devices are used in safety-critical settings where even infrequent errors can result in major harm, user tests are not sufficient for ensuring safety. Testing with humans gets harder and harder as user interface design improves. For example, if only 1% of user actions are errors, user tests have to be performed 100 times longer to get reliable results. As a result, user tests must be supplemented by two further approaches. The first is to use computer models of users to "stress test" devices. These simulated users try to get the device to do everything it is intended to do, while making key-press slips. Using this approach, it is easy to perform billions of tests, and to cover all of a device's features [44].

Secondly, devices should be designed using formal methods—modern software engineering—so that it can be proved they satisfy their design requirements [48]. Programming medical devices without proof today is irresponsible, but as we have emphasized it is always essential to perform user tests—a device might be "correct" but correctly implementing a poorly-conceived design!

Our own experiments, discussed in Case Study 2 [49], show that user interfaces can be made from 2 times to 20 times safer, and that the improvements to the user interface do not need to disadvantage error free behavior, so users need no retraining to benefit from the improved safety.

Since medical device user interface design challenges stem from the interplay of a number of factors as we described in the previous section, it is also important to use a human factors framework that takes a systems-based approach to design. Contextual Design offers a systematic set of methods and tools to help designers analyze the context in which devices are used and then to use this information to inform user interface design [50]. Universal Design [51] and Inclusive Design [52] are two design frameworks that provide design guidelines and methods for producing devices and applications for a broader range of user abilities and disabilities.

The moral of the story is that Human Factors and HCI can help make better and safer medical devices, and that current devices unfortunately leave much to be desired in terms of their quality, but this is primarily because manufacturers are not using HCI well enough given the complexity of healthcare.

Case Study 1: Human Factors in the Evolution of Anesthesia Machines

The progressive improvement in anesthesia machine safety over the last century is a striking example of how risks associated with increased complexity have been mitigated through improvements in design. More than 50 years after the first public demonstration of ether in 1846 [53], anesthesia machines at the start of the twentieth century looked more like industrial equipment than a medical device [54]. Early development had focused on increasing the efficiency of drug delivery and to control cost, so that the benefits of anesthesia during dental and surgical procedures could reach as many patients as possible. Techniques for accurately measuring gas flow rates were still decades away and patient monitoring was limited to "keeping a finger on the pulse". Interaction with the device was limited to adjusting valves that regulated the flow of anesthetic gasses and oxygen to the patient without the assistance of safety features that might prevent overdose or alert the anesthetist to an interruption in gas delivery.

Over the subsequent decades, advances in technology led to gradual design enhancements. For example, as the ability to accurately measure flow rates and drug concentration became available, these components were incorporated into the design. Engineering approaches to improving machine safety were also developed in this period. In response to patient deaths involving delivery of hypoxic gas mixtures due to incorrect attachment of gas supply tanks to the machine, the pin-index safety system was introduced in 1948, making it virtually impossible to connect a nitrous oxygen cylinder to an oxygen intake valve. While the introduction of this technology undoubtedly reduced errors and saved lives, deaths associated with incorrect gas connections continued for decades. In short, although technological solutions to specific safety issues improved anesthesia practice and mitigated the potential for errors, a paradigmatic shift in perspective by considering the "human factor" was ostensibly missing.

By the 1950s, anesthesia machines began to resemble contemporary designs. One of the most striking changes in appearance during this period was driven by the desire to integrate the device into the clinical workflow. Early machines, which appeared like collections of tubes, valves, and tanks assembled on a wheeled platform, had evolved into a workstation with a flat surface where documentation could be completed or drugs and procedural equipment placed for immediate access. In addition, storage drawers were also integrated into the design where additional emergency equipment could be available in easy reach. The appearance of these enhancements signaled a shift in design priorities away from purely technological enhancements to a design that addressed the global needs of the anesthetist using the machine in a clinical setting, where regulating gas flow is only one of the many tasks to be completed.

By modern standards, anesthesia was still a hazardous business in the 1950s, with one study of nearly 600,000 patients reporting anesthetic related mortality in 1 in 1560 patients [55]. However, the pace of innovation in machine design continued to advance utilizing both engineering and human factors approaches. Innovations in engineering included development of fail-safe components to detect and alert clinicians to the presence of hypoxic gas mixtures, enhancing safety beyond what the pin-index system had been able to achieve. Human factors approaches included efforts to standardize equipment and machine design across manufacturers. For example, the variation between manufacturers in tubing diameter used to connect patient endotracheal tubes to the anesthesia circuit was widely recognized as a hazard, because incompatibility could have disastrous implications. Standardization of equipment to ensure compatibility regardless of manufacturer would improve safety by reducing the number of variables a clinician needed to consider while preparing for a case or in response to an unexpected circumstance.

Broad design issues were addressed by the American National Standards Association Committee z79, which further advocated for safety standards in anesthesia machine design that would reduce the potential for human error [56]. For example, the relative ordering of gas flow control knobs was specified, so that the oxygen control valve would be located in the same relative position on every machine regardless of manufacturer. Similarly, the texture of the oxygen control valve was specified so that it would always have a ridged feel, while nitrous oxide and air would be smooth, giving the anesthetist a tactile cue for the valve being adjusted. While earlier approaches to improving safety had emphasized enhanced mechanical engineering, these enhancements were more directed at improving cognitive performance. Standard positioning of gas control valves could eliminate the clinician's need to remember the specific model of the machine in use during a crisis, while the standard "feel" of the oxygen control knob could enhance cognitive performance by engaging other senses.

By the 1970s, enhanced designs had started to make their way into clinical use as older equipment was retired. However, adverse events due to poor equipment design continued to be reported. In a 1976 report Dr. Rendell-Baker expressed his concerns about the role of poor design and inadequate consideration of human factors in anesthetic gas delivery systems [57]. He noted numerous examples where safe operation of the machine required strict compliance with specific operating instructions by the anesthetist that were not necessarily explicit. In one instance, he described a design where oxygen delivery could be entirely routed through the vaporizer. If the breathing circuit needed to be flushed with fresh oxygen, as might be required after induction of anesthesia, all gas flow (including oxygen) would be vented to the atmosphere rather than to the patient. If the clinician then neglected to re-open the vaporizer, no gas would flow to the patient. The only acknowledgement of this risk from the manufacturer was in an informational brochure that stated:

> "should the anesthesiologist turn the Shunt Valve to the OFF position, he will automatically isolate the vaporizer, and the O_2, previously passing through the vaporizer will be vented to atmosphere. It will then be necessary to maintain a flow of metabolic O_2, from a direct O_2 flowmeter to the patient circuit. By thus acknowledging the performance characteristics of the apparatus, the operator can fully appreciate its efficiency with complete safety." This final sentence must rate as a masterpiece of Orwellian "1984" logic! ([57], p. 28)

As a result of this design, the patient's well-being under anesthesia was critically dependent on the cognitive performance of the anesthetist to compensate for the design flaws of the equipment. Dr. Rendell-Baker went on to advocate for a fail-safe gas delivery system that incorporated continuous delivery of oxygen to the patient, an approach that would allow the anesthetist to recover from an operational error with much less risk of harm to the patient. While acknowledging the role of human error in anesthesia mishaps, there clearly were many areas where safety could be improved with engineering approaches that limited the potential for human error. Dr. Rendell-Baker recommended that "The aim of the design engineer should be to eliminate as many mechanical hazards as possible. Safety should not depend upon the user's memory and ability to carry out the correct procedure."

At the same time, rigorous analysis of anesthetic mishaps using formal human factors techniques was also underway. Cooper et al. [58] used a modified critical-incident analysis technique to examine the characteristics of human error and equipment failure in anesthetic practice. In most cases, they found that preventable incidents were related to human error (82%), rather than overt equipment failure (14%), but poor design was often contributory in cases of human error and inadequate experience in cases of equipment failure. The complexity of both gaining an initial understanding of machine safety and then designing a mitigation strategy is illustrated by one of their findings. At some point prior to the start of the study, the hospital had changed the shape of the oxygen control valve to a large, protruding, square knob, presumably in response to recommendations previously discussed. This change in equipment design was intended to improve the cognitive performance of the anesthetist, but as an unintended consequence, the impact of an object on the work surface could cause unintentional rotation of the knob and result in decreased oxygen flow. Clearly, improved safety would depend on deep understanding of the clinical environment, engineering requirements, and human factors.

Recognizing that improvements in machine design had largely progressed in an ad hoc manner for nearly 50 years, Cooper et al. [59] later noted "Improvements and developments have been individual and narrow, arising in response to each specific safety problem as discovered and designed". In response to the existing machine design where "new concepts, as they have emerged, have been added to the system in the form of new and separate boxes and gadgets that further complicate the maze of wires, cords, and objects which currently clutters the operating room and the anesthetist's visual field", he proposed a complete redesign. His proposed machine would explicitly "eliminate human-factors problems… and lay a suitable technological foundation for the development of new techniques in anesthesia management". The importance of man-machine communication links that operated with a minimum of attention and effort was emphasized, and the anesthetist was conceived of as a controller, processing both patient physiologic sensors and machine effectors that would support decision-making and action-taking by the anesthetist.

The innovations advocated by Cooper et al. would take years to reach routine clinical practice. So, despite these technological innovations and awareness of human factors, anesthesia in the early 1980s was still considered risky. Anesthetic related mortality had improved, but was still estimated to be 1–2 per 10,000 anesthetics [60, 61]. Malpractice insurance was very expensive for anesthesiologists, and a disproportionate amount of payments were related to anesthesia [62].

The issue of patient safety was brought to public attention in 1982 when a documentary entitled "The Deep Sleep" aired on television. The program asserted that more than 6000 patients would die or suffer brain damage from preventable causes associated with anesthesia that year. Its broadcast was followed by an immediate public outcry [63]. The American Society of Anesthesiologists (ASA) responded, and by dedicating significant resources to making anesthesia safer, was able to make a big difference in a short period of time.

The ASA started by gathering consensus and studying technological and human issues. In 1985, the Anesthesia Patient Safety Foundation (APSF) was created with a mission that "no patient shall be harmed by anesthesia," [64] and a year later the Anesthesia Closed Claims project was launched as a collaborative effort between anesthesiologists, hospitals, lawyers, and insurance carriers to develop a standardized method of analyzing and learning from anesthesia related mishaps [65].

Closed claims data have been used extensively to analyze anesthesia related risks and improve outcomes. While incidents related to equipment have been analyzed repeatedly since its inception, claims related to gas delivery systems have decreased to 1% since 1990, with a similar decline in the severity of harm [66].

Anesthesia today is safer than it has ever been. Some estimates of mortality are now as low as 1–2 per 250,000 [67] and malpractice premiums and payouts are now similar to other specialties. Such rapid, dramatic declines in mortality are rare in medicine, and have been achieved in part by improved fail-safe engineering, but also by addressing human factors that inherently pose error risks. As we celebrate the decline of equipment related injury in the Closed Claims Database, it is important to remember that the majority of the claims involving gas delivery (85%) are still related to human error without equipment failure [66]. Clearly, Human Factors will play a central role in future advancements in anesthesia machines related patient safety.

Case Study 2: User Interface Details—Illustrating the Value of HCI

HCI encompasses a wide range of subjects, yet its influence becomes evident even in minute details. Take numbers. You press buttons and a number appears in the medical device, perhaps the infusion rate in mL/h. On the Baxter Colleague 3 infusion pump, you can type 1.5 and that's what you will get, but if you type 100.5 the Baxter ignores the decimal point and you will get 1005, which is ten times larger. The designers obviously decided that large numbers do not need decimal points; no number needs to be given to four digits of precision. So the Baxter ignores decimals, which sort of makes sense, but a rule of HCI is to provide useful feedback to the user. On the Baxter, when you press keys, they click, confirming that you pressed them hard enough. This is good feedback. Unfortunately, when you press a decimal point you get a click whether or not the Baxter ignores it. This is a design defect. In fact, the whole idea is an HCI defect: we know from eye tracking experiments [68] that users do not look at displays as much as they look at keyboards, so a user will not notice the display shows 1005 instead of 100.5, which is what they expect. We know this and HCI dictates we should design to accommodate what users expect.

The BBraun Infusomat infusion pump handles numbers differently; instead of a numeric keypad there are four arrow keys and a cursor. The user can move the cursor left or right by using the left and right arrow keys, and can increase or decrease the digit the cursor is over by using the up and down arrow keys (see Fig. 13.1). The behavior of the Infusomat depends on its mode. In VTBI (Volume To Be Infused) if the display shows 0.0 with the cursor on the tenths position and the user presses the right arrow key (to move the cursor to the right from the tenths to the hundredths position) and then presses 'up' to increase the 0 to a 1, the display will change to 0.1, not to 0.01. The designers have made a decision to change what the users do to

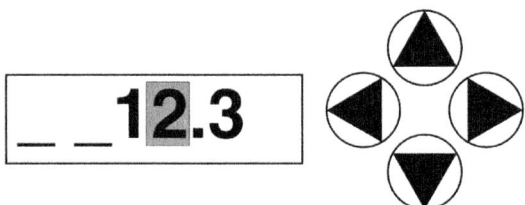

Fig. 13.1 A 4-key number entry design. The left/right "arrows" move the cursor left and right, and the up/down arrows increase or decrease the digit the cursor is over. The cursor is shown here as a gray box, but on many designs it will flash, and perhaps invert video as well. Some defective designs allow left/right arrows to wraparound the cursor position: e.g., pressing too many rights will bring the cursor round to the far left, so a user trying to enter a fractional digit could accidentally enter a 1000s digit. Some designs adjust digits independently, and others have "carry" so incrementing a digit goes –8–9–10, rather than –8–9–0. The four-key design has a low user error rate but it is complex to ensure it handles boundary cases correctly and in the best way for the user. For example, an easy way of changing 10 to 100 goes via 0, which may be a prohibited value and automatically set a minimum value like 1, which the user will find counter-productive!

mean something else, and (worse) the keystroke feedback (click sounds) seem to confirm the device is obeying the keystrokes. The design is likely to cause problems. The solution would be to make an alarm sound so as to draw the user's attention to the divergence of what the pump is doing and what it was told to do. Moreover, the alarm should stay activated until the user acknowledges it, for instance by pressing [CLEAR].

Many devices keep a log, which may be used as legal evidence after an incident. If the log says the infusion pump delivered 15 mL, then it is tempting to think the user told it to deliver 15 mL, and if this is the cause of the incident, then it would seem the user is to blame. But it is not so simple. On some devices, the delete key does not work as expected. For example, keying 1.. [DEL] 5 may result in 5 rather than the intended 1.5, an error that is 3.33 times out yet the log will say the user keyed 5, not 1.5 (or even 1.. [DEL] 5). Thus the log in this case probably correctly describes what the infusion pump did, but not what the user asked it to do. Logs are also susceptible to key bounce errors, where the user presses a key once but the device treats it as two or more presses; again the log will say what the device does, but is a misleading account of what the user did.

Reducing the number of keys to enter numbers makes using a device easier and reduces the time a user needs to look at the keyboard. Some devices use up/down arrows to increase and decrease numbers (see Fig. 13.2). Not only are there fewer keys, but the user model is that the displayed number has to be changed to be correct; like the 4-key style mentioned above, therefore, 2-key number entry has lower error rates. Instead of the design being "the user keys a number" the design is "the

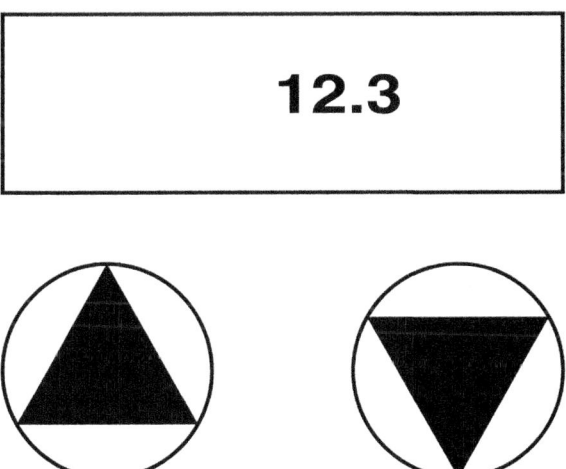

Fig. 13.2 2-key number entry. Pressing the "up" triangle (on the left) increases the number and pressing the "down" triangle decreases the number. Typically, holding a button down repeatedly increments or decrements the number, and holding it down for several seconds speeds up the rate of change. Some devices swap the up/down keys, and some additionally have "fast" keys (e.g., which increment and decrement in 10s or 100s rather than 1s)

number displayed is wrong; the user corrects it" and therefore they are forced to look at the display and to expect errors they will correct. Such interfaces are much more reliable, yet they are slower and therefore some might claim they are "less usable." However, to say they are less usable is to confuse speed with ease of use; but in a healthcare environment, ease of use is not as important as whether a device can be used reliably. Obviously it is an advantage that people like a design, but it should not be the top criterion. A better way to understand the trade-off is that speed limits slow vehicles down, making trips longer, but with the goal of making those trips safer for all. Likewise, slowing down a user may improve their performance overall.

Feedback is important—users cannot always pay full attention to a device (they have distracting jobs) so devices must make clear whether user actions "work" or not. In all the designs discussed, keys normally change the display, but in boundary cases (e.g., when too many digits have been pressed) the display cannot change or possibly changes in a non-standard way (e.g., not going above a preset maximum value). Hence buttons should make two sorts of noise: that they have been pressed successfully, and possibly that they have been pressed but nothing can happen. Many designs beep once for success and twice for failure, as of course a double beep for a single key press is an error in any case. Some buttons (such as [cancel] or buttons that cause confirmatory displays to appear) should make distinctive sounds.

Conclusions

The HCI of medical devices is an important but complex topic due to their safety-critical nature, regulatory requirements, and the complexity and heterogeneity of their users and use environments. This chapter provided only a brief overview of HCI for medical devices. The key messages are:

1. Humans make errors sooner or later and designers should design for error. The key point in medical device design is that use error should be managed and so far as possible not lead to patient harm. For example, correctly implemented UNDO or DELETE keys allows users to make errors and to correct them.
2. Designers, too, are human and can never know enough about the context of use of a device. Medical devices help highly trained professionals in complex, stressful environments, and they do not understand complex issues of engineering design. It is *inevitable* that design requirements are going to have oversights. Devices have to be user-tested in realistic environments and improved in light of experimental results, in a repeating process called *iterative design*.
3. To fully assess device usability, designers should augment user tests with simulation and formal software engineering approaches. Simulated users that make keystroke errors can exercise the full range of device operations. Formal methods, such as model checking, can prove that the device works as intended.

4. There are numerous relevant international standards, and these are both a regulatory framework of minimum standards as well as an excellent resource of authoritative literature.

There is considerable need for research that addresses common issues across medical devices; more so, there is considerable need for the research to be applied! Research on medical device alarms and data entry interfaces are good examples of such work, but additional work is needed in other areas, such as improving situational awareness when using one or more devices. Recent developments with respect to the variety of devices and software that are considered medical devices, along with the growing use of AI, have created additional challenges that require extensive empirical and theoretical work on the HCI of medical devices.

This chapter gives only a basic introduction to the challenges of designing interfaces for medical devices. A comprehensive review can be found in the *Handbook of Human Factors in Medical Device Design* [69] and in the FDA guidance documents and regulatory standards.

Acknowledgments This work was partly funded by EPSRC grant [EP/L019272/1].

Discussion Questions

1. What are the similarities and differences between HCI for medical devices vs. non-medical devices?
2. Pick a type of medical device, such as an insulin pump, and then search MAUDE for related reports. Can you separate use-related errors from other types of problems, such as malfunctions or unrelated issues? Are they consistent kinds of use errors? Do they vary based on the model? What kinds of data would you like to gather to further clarify possible use-related errors?
3. Discuss the definition of a medical device with respect to sample mobile apps or other device software functions. Can you find examples of apps or software functions that meet and do not meet the definition?
4. Pick a simple mobile device, such as a blood pressure monitor, and consider how well it meets the needs of a diverse set of users and use environments.
5. Pick an AI/ML-based medical device, such as a skin cancer detection app, and analyze it with respect to human factors considerations for a typical end user. See, for example, Felmingham, et al. on incorporating human factors into AI-based skin cancer diagnostic tools [70].
6. Based on the definition of a medical device, do you think electronic health record systems (EHRs) are medical devices? If EHRs were regulated as medical devices, how might this affect the stakeholders, including EHR vendors, doctors, and patients?

References

1. Carroll JM. HCI models, theories, and frameworks: toward a multidisciplinary science. 1st ed. Morgan Kaufmann; 2003.
2. FDA. Federal Food, Drug, and Cosmetic Act FD&C Act 21 CFR 201(H) [21 U.S.C. 321], § 21 CFR 201(h). 2002. Available from: http://www.fda.gov/regulatoryinformation/legislation/federalfooddrugandcosmeticactfdcact/fdcactchaptersiandiishorttitleanddefinitions/ucm086297.htm
3. U.S. Department of Health and Human Services, Food and Drug Administration. Mobile medical applications: guidance for industry and food and drug administration staff. 2013. Available from: http://www.fda.gov/downloads/MedicalDevices/DeviceRegulationandGuidance/GuidanceDocuments/UCM263366.pdf
4. U.S. Department of Health and Human Services, Food and Drug Administration. Policy for device software functions and mobile medical applications: guidance for industry and food and drug administration staff. 2022. Available from: https://www.fda.gov/media/80958/download
5. IMDRF SaMD Working Group. Software as a medical device (SaMD): key definitions. International Medical Device Regulators Forum; 2013. Available from: https://www.imdrf.org/sites/default/files/docs/imdrf/final/technical/imdrf-tech-131209-samd-key-definitions-140901.pdf
6. The Council of the European Communities. EU medical devices directive—MDD 93/42/EEC and 2007/47/EC. 2007. Available from: http://www.emergogroup.com/resources/regulations-europe/regulations-EU-MDD93-42-EEC#1
7. Medical Device Amendments of 1976. Pub. L. No. 94–295. 1976.
8. U.S. Food and Drug Administration, Center for Devices and Radiological Health. Premarket notification (510k). 2014. Available from: http://www.fda.gov/medicaldevices/deviceregulationandguidance/howtomarketyourdevice/premarketsubmissions/premarketnotification510k/default.htm
9. U.S. Food and Drug Administration. Good manufacturing practice (GMP) guidelines/inspection checklist. 2008. Available from: http://www.fda.gov/cosmetics/guidanceregulation/guidancedocuments/ucm2005190.htm
10. Association for the Advancement of Medical Instrumentation. Human factors in medical devices: design, regulation, and patient safety (conference report). 1996. Available from: http://www.fda.gov/MedicalDevices/DeviceRegulationandGuidance/HumanFactors/ucm126018.htm
11. International Organization for Standardization. ISO 9001:1994—quality systems—model for quality assurance in design, development, production, installation and servicing. 1994. Available from: http://www.iso.org/iso/iso_catalogue/catalogue_tc/catalogue_detail.htm?csnumber=38193
12. Sawyer D. Do it by design—an introduction to human factors in medical devices. U.S. Food and Drug Administration, Center for Devices and Radiological Health; 1996. Available from: http://www.fda.gov/medicaldevices/deviceregulationandguidance/guidancedocuments/ucm094957.htm
13. Kaye R, Crowley J. Medical device use-safety: incorporating human factors engineering into risk management. U.S. Food and Drug Administration, Center for Devices and Radiological Health; 2000. Available from: http://www.fda.gov/downloads/MedicalDevices/DeviceRegulationandGuidance/GuidanceDocuments/UCM094461.pdf
14. Association for the Advancement of Medical Instrumentation. Human factors design process for medical devices. 2001.
15. International Electrochemical Commission. IEC 60601-1-6: medical electrical equipment—part 1–6 general requirements for basic safety and essential performance—colateral standard: usability. Author; 2006.
16. International Electrochemical Commission. IEC 62366—medical devices—application of usability engineering to medical devices. Author; 2007.

17. International Organization for Standardization. ISO 14971:2007—medical devices—application of risk management to medical devices. 2007. Available from: http://www.iso.org/iso/iso_catalogue/catalogue_tc/catalogue_detail.htm?csnumber=38193
18. Association for the Advancement of Medical Instrumentation. Human factors engineering—design of medical devices. 2009.
19. U.S. Food and Drug Administration. Artificial intelligence/machine learning (AI/ML)-based software as a medical device (SaMD) action plan. 2021a. Available from: http://www.fda.gov/media/145022/download
20. U.S. Food and Drug Administration. Proposed regulatory framework for modifications to artificial intelligence/machine learning (AI/ML)-based software as a medical device (SaMD). 2021b. Available from: https://www.fda.gov/files/medical%20devices/published/US-FDA-Artificial-Intelligence-and-Machine-Learning-Discussion-Paper.pdf
21. Groenborg T. In the face of new challenges; effective human factors engineering for software as medical device products. Proc Int Symp Hum Factors Ergon Health Care. 2022;11(1):13–7. https://doi.org/10.1177/2327857922111002.
22. Sujan M, Furniss D, Grundy K, et al. Human factors challenges for the safe use of artificial intelligence in patient care. BMJ Health Care Inform. 2019;26(1):e100081. https://doi.org/10.1136/bmjhci-2019-100081.
23. MAUDE - Manufacturer and User Facility Device Experience. n.d. [cited 2014 May 30]. Available from: http://www.accessdata.fda.gov/scripts/cdrh/cfdocs/cfMAUDE/search.CFM
24. Woltz DJ, Gardner MK, Bell BG. Negative transfer errors in sequential cognitive skills: strong-but-wrong sequence application. J Exp Psychol Learn Mem Cogn. 2000;26(3):601–25. https://doi.org/10.1037/0278-7393.26.3.601.
25. Cooper JB, Newbower RS, Kitz RJ. An analysis of major errors and equipment failures in anesthesia management: considerations for prevention and detection. Anesthesiology. 1984;60(1):34–42.
26. Grant L. Medical equipment. Devices and desires. Health Serv J. 1998;108(5603):34–5.
27. McConnell EA, Cattonar M, Manning J. Australian registered nurse medical device education: a comparison of simple vs. complex devices. J Adv Nurs. 1996;23(2):322–8.
28. O'Connel GW. Human factors in the GMP inspection process. n.d. [cited 2014 May 30]. Available from: http://www.fda.gov/MedicalDevices/DeviceRegulationandGuidance/HumanFactors/ucm128186.htm
29. Brannon TS. Ad hoc versus standardized admixtures for continuous infusion drugs in neonatal intensive care: cognitive task analysis of safety at the bedside. AMIA Ann Symp Proc. 2006;2006:862.
30. Cummings K, McGowan R. "Smart" infusion pumps are selectively intelligent: nursing 2013. Nursing. 2011;41(3):58–9.
31. Rothschild JM, Keohane CA, Cook EF, et al. A controlled trial of smart infusion pumps to improve medication safety in critically ill patients. Crit Care Med. 2005;33(3):533–40.
32. Trbovich PL, Pinkney S, Cafazzo JA, Easty AC. The impact of traditional and smart pump infusion technology on nurse medication administration performance in a simulated inpatient unit. Qual Saf Health Care. 2010;19(5):430–4. https://doi.org/10.1136/qshc.2009.032839.
33. Knisely BM, Levine C, Kharod KC, Vaughn-Cooke M. An analysis of FDA adverse event reporting data for trends in medical device use error. Proc Int Symp Hum Factors Ergon Health Care. 2020;9(1):130–4. https://doi.org/10.1177/2327857920091024.
34. Zhang Y, Masci P, Jones P, Thimbleby H. Research: user interface software errors in medical devices: study of U.S. recall data. Biomed Instrum Technol. 2019;53(3):182–94. https://doi.org/10.2345/0899-8205-53.3.182.
35. Wachter RM, Pronovost P, Shekelle P. Strategies to improve patient safety: the evidence base matures. Ann Intern Med. 2013;158(5_Part_1):350–2. https://doi.org/10.7326/0003-4819-158-5-201303050-00010.
36. Bates DW, Levine DM, Salmasian H, et al. The safety of inpatient health care. N Engl J Med. 2023;388(2):142–53. https://doi.org/10.1056/NEJMsa2206117.

37. Gosbee J. Human factors engineering and patient safety. Qual Saf Health Care. 2002;11(4):352–4. https://doi.org/10.1136/qhc.11.4.352.
38. Rogers WA, Mykityshyn AL, Campbell RH, Fisk AD. Analysis of a "simple" medical device. Ergon Des. 2001;9(1):6–14.
39. U.S. Food and Drug Administration Center for Devices and Radiological Health. Medical device home use initiative. 2010. Available from: http://www.fda.gov/downloads/medicaldevices/productsandmedicalprocedures/homehealthandconsumer/homeusedevices/ucm209056.pdf
40. U.S. Food and Drug Administration, Center for Devices and Radiological Health. Draft guidance for industry and FDA staff—design considerations for devices intended for home use. 2012. Available from: http://www.fda.gov/medicaldevices/deviceregulationandguidance/guidancedocuments/ucm331675.htm
41. Winters JM, Story MF. Medical instrumentation: accessibility and usability considerations. CRC Press; 2007.
42. Obradovich JH, Woods DD. SPECIAL SECTION: users as designers: how people cope with poor HCI design in computer-based medical devices. Hum Factors. 1996;38(4):574–92. https://doi.org/10.1518/001872096778827251.
43. Todd A, Stuifbergen A. Barriers and facilitators related to breast cancer screening. Int J MS Care. 2011;13(2):49–56. https://doi.org/10.7224/1537-2073-13.2.49.
44. Thimbleby H. Press on: principles of interaction programming. The MIT Press; 2007.
45. U.S. Food and Drug Administration Center for Devices and Radiological Health, Center for Devices and Radiological Health. Draft guidance: applying human factors and usability engineering to optimize medical device design. 2011. Available from: http://www.fda.gov/medicaldevices/deviceregulationandguidance/guidancedocuments/ucm259748.htm
46. Poole ES. HCI and mobile health interventions. Transl Behav Med. 2013;3(4):402–5. https://doi.org/10.1007/s13142-013-0214-3.
47. International Organization for Standardization. ISO 9241—ergonomics of human-system interaction. 2006. Available from: http://www.iso.org/iso/iso_catalogue/catalogue_tc/catalogue_detail.htm?csnumber=38193
48. Dix AJ. Formal methods. In: Soegaard M, Dam RF, editors. The encyclopedia of human-computer interaction. 2nd ed. The Interaction Design Foundation; 2013. Available from: http://www.interaction-design.org/encyclopedia/formal_methods.html
49. Cauchi A, Gimblett A, Thimbleby H, Curzon P, Masci P. Safer "5-key" number entry user interfaces using differential formal analysis. Paper presented at: Proceedings of the 26th Annual BCS Interaction Specialist Group Conference on People and Computers. 2012. p. 29–38. Available from: http://dl.acm.org/citation.cfm?id=2377916.2377921
50. Holtzblatt K, Beyer HR. Contextual design. In: The encyclopedia of human-computer interaction. 2nd ed. Interaction Design Foundation; 2013. Available from: http://www.interaction-design.org/encyclopedia/contextual_design.html
51. Story MF, Mueller JL, Mace RL. The universal design file: designing for people of all ages and abilities. Revised edition. 1998. Available from: http://eric.ed.gov/?id=ED460554
52. Clarkson J. Inclusive design: design for the whole population. Springer Science & Business Media; 2003.
53. Viets HR. The earliest printed references in newspapers and journals to the first public demonstration of ether anesthesia in 1846. J Hist Med Allied Sci. 1949;IV(2):149–69. https://doi.org/10.1093/jhmas/IV.2.149.
54. Drägerwerk AG. The history of anaesthesia at Dräger 1898–1966. 2nd revision. 2012. Available from: http://www.draeger.com/sites/assets/PublishingImages/Generic/UK/Booklets/4212-Br-History-of-Anaesthesia_A5_en_191212-LR.pdf
55. Beecher HK, Todd DP. A study of the deaths associated with anesthesia and surgery: based on a study of 599, 548 anesthesias in ten institutions 1948-1952, inclusive. Ann Surg. 1954;140(1):2–35.
56. Betcher AM. Historical development of the American Society of Anesthesiologists, Inc. In: Volpitto P, Vandam L, editors. The genesis of contemporary American anesthesiology, vol.

134. Charles C. Thomas; 1982. p. 185–211. Available from: http://www.woodlibrarymuseum.org/Finding_Aid/ASA/ASA/Betcher%20Historical%20Development%20of%20The%20American%20Society%20of%20Anesthesiologists,%20Inc..pdf
57. Rendell-Baker L. Some gas machine hazards and their elimination. Anesth Analg. 1976;55(1):26–33. Available from: http://journals.lww.com/anesthesia-analgesia/Fulltext/1976/01000/Some_Gas_Machine_Hazards_and_Their_Elimination_.6.aspx
58. Cooper JB, Newbower RS, Long CD, McPeek B. Preventable anesthesia mishaps: a study of human factors. Anesthesiology. 1978a;49(6):399–406.
59. Cooper JB, Newbower RS, Moore JW, Trautman ED. A new anesthesia delivery system. Anesthesiology. 1978b;49(5):310–8.
60. Keenan RL, Boyan CP. Cardiac arrest due to anesthesia: a study of incidence and causes. JAMA. 1985;253(16):2373–7.
61. Lunn JN, Mushin WW. Mortality associated with anaesthesia. Anaesthesia. 1982;37(8):856.
62. Pierce EC. The 34th Rovenstine lecture: 40 years behind the mask: safety revisited. Anesthesiology. 1996;84(4):965–75.
63. Pierce EC Jr. Looking back: doctor pierce reflects. Anesth Patient Saf Found Newsl. 2007;22(1):1–24. Available from: http://www.apsf.org/newsletters/html/2007/spring/02_looking_back.htm
64. Cooper JB, Pierce EC. Safety foundation organized. Anesth Patient Saf Found Newsl. 1986;1(1):1–8.
65. Cheney FW. The American Society of Anesthesiologists Closed Claims Project: what have we learned, how has it affected practice, and how will it affect practice in the future? Anesthesiology. 1999;91(2):552–6.
66. Mehta SP, Eisenkraft JB, Posner KL, Domino KB. Patient injuries from anesthesia gas delivery equipment: a closed claims update. Anesthesiology. 2013;119(4):788–95.
67. Haller G, Laroche T, Clergue F. Morbidity in anaesthesia: today and tomorrow. Best Pract Res Clin Anaesthesiol. 2011;25(2):123–32.
68. Oladimeji P, Thimbleby H, Cox A. Number entry interfaces and their effects on errors and number perception. Paper presented at: Proceedings IFIP Conference on Human-Computer Interaction, Interact 2011, Volume IV. 2011. p. 178–85.
69. Weinger MB, Wiklund ME, Gardner-Bonneau DJ. Handbook of human factors in medical device design. CRC Press; 2011.
70. Felmingham CM, Adler NR, Ge Z, Morton RL, Janda M, Mar VJ. The importance of incorporating human factors in the design and implementation of artificial intelligence for skin cancer diagnosis in the real world. Am J Clin Dermatol. 2021;22(2):233–42. https://doi.org/10.1007/s40257-020-00574-4.

Further Reading

Kaye R, Crowley J. Medical device use-safety: incorporating human factors engineering into risk management. Silver Spring, MD: U.S. Food and Drug Administration, Center for Devices and Radiological Health; 2000. Available from: http://www.fda.gov/downloads/MedicalDevices/DeviceRegulationandGuidance/GuidanceDocuments/UCM094461.pdf

Sawyer D. Do it by design - an introduction to human factors in medical devices. Rockville, MD: U.S. Food and Drug Administration, Center for Devices and Radiological Health; 1996. Available from: http://www.fda.gov/medicaldevices/deviceregulationandguidance/guidancedocuments/ucm094957.htm

Weinger MB, Wiklund ME, Gardner-Bonneau DJ. Handbook of human factors in medical device design. CRC Press; 2011.

Chapter 14
Applying HCI Principles in Designing Usable Systems for Dentistry

Elsbeth Kalenderian and Muhammad F. Walji

Introduction

Currently over 201,000 active dental practitioners provide care to at least 150 million dental patients in dental offices throughout the United States [1, 2]. Dentists, like physicians, routinely perform highly technical procedures in complex environments, work in teams [3], and have rapidly begun to adopt electronic health records (EHRs). Unfortunately, there is another parallel to medical practice: the usability of dental EHRs is a growing concern. Data stored in dental EHRs are not only used to coordinate care for an individual patient, but also can be aggregated and mined to determine the efficacy of treatments or adherence to standards of care. One of the biggest limitations of data stored in dental EHRs has been the lack of adoption of a standardized terminology to document dental diagnoses. As a structured diagnosis code is still not required as part of dental billing, there continues to be little to no emphasis on the importance of accurately documenting a diagnosis as part of a patient's health record. In this chapter, we review our previously published research (in context with other research in this area), in developing and disseminating the Dental Diagnostic System (DDS) Dental Diagnostic Terminology (formerly called the EZCodes) amongst dental school clinics. In order to bring DDS into the clinic,

---

E. Kalenderian (✉)
University of Pretoria, School of Dentistry, Pretoria, South Africa
e-mail: elsbeth.kalenderian@marquette.edu

M. F. Walji
UTHealth Houston McWilliams School of Biomedical Informatics, Houston, TX, USA

© The Author(s), under exclusive license to Springer Nature Switzerland AG 2024
A. W. Kushniruk et al. (eds.), *Human Computer Interaction in Healthcare*, Cognitive Informatics in Biomedicine and Healthcare,
https://doi.org/10.1007/978-3-031-69947-4_14

we applied human computer interaction (HCI) principles to re-designing a treatment-planning module in a widely used dental EHR called axiUm (Exan Corp., Vancouver, Canada) [4] in close collaboration with the vendor. American academic dentistry is well positioned to leverage on the promise of the EHR to advance scientific knowledge and improve health care quality, as the majority of the 65 U.S. dental schools use axiUm as their EHR. To contextualize this undertaking, we begin by describing the dental profession and practice, with a major focus on the United States. We then describe our human-computer interaction studies, highlighting the relevance of the work to usability studies, secondary use of data, and inter-professional practice.

In order to ensure effectiveness in practice we assessed the utilization and correct use of the diagnostic terminology over a four-year period in the academic setting as well as a large private dental group practice [5]. The utilization and validity proportions of the DDS statistically significant increased from 2013 to 2016 ($P < 0.0001$). Academic dental sites were more likely to document diagnoses associated with orthodontic and restorative procedures, while the private dental site was equally likely to document diagnoses associated with all procedures. Although the results show an ongoing improvement in the utilization and validity of the dental terminology, ensuring that providers use standardized methods for documenting a diagnosis remains a challenge within the dental arena. A positive development has been the harmonization of the DDS terminology with the American Dental Association's SNODENT terminology in 2016 (and renamed SNODDS) and its subsequent approval as an ANSI standard in 2017, allowing for integration into SNOMED [6].

Characteristics of the Dental Team

The dental practitioner will rarely perform care without a dental assistant present chair-side as "fourhanded" dentistry significantly improves productivity [7], efficiency [8], as well as ergonomics [9]. Hygienists and sometimes a nurse further round out the clinical dental team. Front- and back-office personnel are responsible for patient scheduling, billing and other administrative duties.

The majority of the 201,000 dentists in the U.S. work in small practices, although ownership declined from 91% to 73% between 1991 and 2021 [10, 11]. During the same period, solo practitioners declined from 67% to 46% [10, 12], and as one might imagine, group practices increased in number: between 2008 and 2010, the number of dentists joining a company-owned practice grew from 5.4% to 6.4% [10], although opinions vary to what extent large managed group practices will become the predominant setting for oral health care [13]. By contrast, in the medical profession physicians started to integrate in large group practices as early as the 1990s, associated with the rise of managed care in medicine [14]. This is in contrast to our Canadian colleagues where 98.3% of the 19,563 [15] Canadian licensed dentists work in private practice, of whom 79% are owners [16].

In the teaching practices within dental schools, the workflow is different than in private practices. Students provide care under the supervision of full-time or adjunct faculty members. In most dental schools, students frequently practice without a dedicated dental assistant or are assisted by a fellow dental student. Thus, the students themselves are responsible for data entry into the EHR and might also schedule appointments for their patients.

Workflow in the Dental Operatory

Even before the introduction of computers, a lot was happening in a small space within the modern dental operatory, the space in which the dental team performs its clinical work. Dentists may have two to three operatories occupied at the same time; on average, the operatory turnover occurs every 30 min.

The EHR-endowed dental operatory is typically set up in one of two ways: either with the EHR at the 12 o'clock position, essentially behind the dentist, or attached to the dental chair. The latter more readily allows the patient to be included in treatment planning and education as documents, instructional videos and digital radiographs can easily be displayed by swiveling the EHR within eyesight of the patient. Most often, the dental assistant enters data into the EHR via a wireless keyboard chair-side. The most intensive data entry occurs during the intra-oral exam, when the dentist calls out findings that the dental assistant documents in the EHR. Figure 14.1.

Dentistry has a unique clinical workflow [17], yet only a few studies have been conducted on workflow and the role of technology in the dental clinic [17, 18]. Nevertheless, previous studies have demonstrated that limited consideration of HCI related issues often interferes with the dental clinic workflow. For example, Irwin et al. showed that over 60% of the 27 "breakdowns" during initial examination and treatment planning using EHRs in general dentist practices were associated with technology [19]. Usability issues and unfamiliarity with chair-side use of clinically relevant electronic data were major barriers to EHR adoption for dental practitioners [20–24], not unlike the barriers associated with medical provider encounters [25–27]. In the U.S., the axiUm EHR has achieved near ubiquity in dental academic

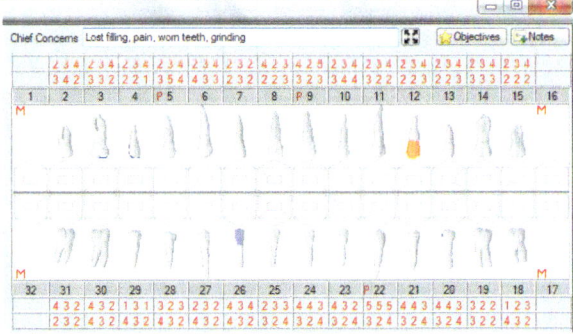

Fig. 14.1 Recording of pocket depth (numbers in mm in red), bleeding points (P), missing teeth (M) and existing restorations (colored areas on teeth) in the EHR

settings. This is not to say that the axiUm EHR has surmounted the usability challenges of the private practice dental EHRs; indeed, a survey and interview study conducted during the implementation of axiUm at the University of Texas Health Science Center at Houston Dental Branch identified usability as a major concern [28].

Development of a Standardized Dental Diagnostic Terminology

A complete list of patient problems and diagnoses is a cornerstone of the medicolegal document that is the patient record. It serves as a valuable tool for providers assessing a patient's clinical status, succinctly communicates this information between providers and to front desk and administrative personnel and serves as a fulcrum around which research and quality improvement levers pivot.

Early efforts to standardize dental diagnostic terms have fallen short with respect to comprehensiveness and availability [29, 30]. Subsequently, the ICD-DA (application of the International Classification of Diseases to Dentistry and Stomatology) was added to ICD-8 in 1965 [29]. However, the oral health coverage of the ICD terminology continues to call for improvement [30]. Over the years, some groups independently generated dental diagnostic terminologies [31–33]. Of these, the Toronto Codes [34] have been systematically evaluated [35], while we do not know to what extent the other terminologies have met dental teams' diagnostic documentation needs [36]. In the early 1990s, the American Dental Association (ADA) started the development of SNODENT, a Systematized Nomenclature for Dentistry. In 1998, the ADA entered into an agreement to incorporate SNODENT Version I into SNOMED [37]. SNODENT is composed of diagnoses, signs, symptoms and complaints, and currently includes over 7700 terms [38, 39]. In 2012, SNODENT Version II was incorporated into the SNOMED CT. Until its recent inclusion into SNOMED CT, SNODENT was only available by license and was maintained by the ADA. As a result, SNODENT was not widely implemented. In 2007, our research team developed the EZCodes [40], renamed Dental Diagnostic System or DDS for short, to enhance the proper and consistent registration of diagnostic findings. The DDS has been mapped to SNOMED, ICD 9, ICD 10, ICD 9-CM and ICD 10-CM (CM is the American version of ICD 9 and 10). With 1518 terms, the DDS is developed as an interface terminology (a set of terms designed to be compatible with the natural language of the user, used to mediate between a user's colloquial conceptualizations of concept descriptions and an underlying reference terminology [41]) to be used in the dental clinic with SNOMED CT as its back-end reference terminology (a terminology where each term has a codable, computer-usable definition to support retrieval and data aggregation [42]). The few DDS terms that did not have adequate coverage with SNOMED terms were submitted for integration with SNOMED, of which the majority has been accepted. Through this process the team started working with the ADA which resulted in the harmonization of the DDS with SNODENT into a renamed SNODDS terminology. As such, SNOMED truly functions as the reference terminology first for the DDS and now for the SNODDS terminology. Similarly, we have submitted terms to ICD in an effort to enhance the ICD oral health classification and improve the mapping between DDS and ICD oral health terms. The DDS terminology also became a norm in The Netherlands, meaning that it is the standardized diagnostic terminology that all Dutch dentists are expected to use [43].

However, prior analyses of the EZCodes (DDS) terminology in use in an EHR demonstrated both low utilization and frequent errors [40]. Between July 2010 and June 2011, the EZCodes were utilized 12% of the time in three dental schools. More than 1000 terms of the available 1321 terms were never chosen. Caries and periodontics were the most frequently used categories. 60.5% of the EZCodes entries were found to be valid [44]. The low utilization rate reiterated findings from an earlier study [45], but also suggested the need to conduct more training, improve the EHR interface, and add descriptions and synonyms to the terms.

In section "Applying Theory to Practice: Redesigning A Treatment Planning Module in a Dental EHR" we describe our approach in using HCI principles to systematically identify usability problems, and to drive the re-design of an existing EHR to enhance the effective and efficient entry of dental diagnostic terms.

To put this work in context, we first review some of the recent and relevant literature regarding usability, dental EHRs and interface terminologies. A number of researchers have established that dental EHRs have some distance to go to be usable. Reynolds and colleagues provide a brief overview of dental informatics, reiterating that usability challenges represent a primary hurdle to the adoption of dental EHRs [46]. In 2008, Hill, Stewart, and Ash explored the impact of EHRs on dental faculty and students in the dental academic setting. Newly developed clinical processes were considered more time consuming than previous paper processes. The end users' needs appeared to be intense, immediate and significant. Here too, the authors reported significant usability problems standing in the way of smooth implementation. Additionally, changes in workflow were significant and often cumbersome [47]. Juvé-Udina reported on the evaluation of the usability of the diagnosis axis in a nursing interface terminology. Utilization of the diagnostic terms was high at 92.3% where some of the concepts were used rarely and others as often as 51.4% [48]. Thyvalikakath et al. similarly concluded that using a combination of heuristic evaluation and user tests methods showed that the four major commercial dental EHRs had significant usability problems [49]. Despite the fact that dental EHR usability is an established problem, little has been published on the use of cognitive engineering approaches, like think-aloud protocols, workflow observations and semi-structured interviews, to remedy the issues [50].

Challenges of Dental EHR Use and Usability

Although healthcare providers, including dental providers, increasingly adopt EHRs, in part driven by current significant governmental incentives [51] and the hope for increased efficiency and quality [44, 52], usability issues remain a major barrier to adoption [53–55]. As with medical EHRs, a user-centered designed dental

EHR facilitates good usability, assuring that the user can efficiently and effectively complete work tasks satisfactorily and successfully [56]. It is also understood that, on the contrary, a poorly designed EHR with poor usability can lead to potential patient safety issues [57–59].

There is a plethora of challenges of dental EHR use and usability concerns. Usability challenges include visual as well as functional interface design problems [49]. Illogical button placement, unanticipated button functionality, difficulty switching between the odontogram and periodontal chart, inability to easily delete a mistaken entry on the odontogram, the need for better visual representation of dental findings and the fact that many icons resemble each other in shape and color are just some specific examples of interface design problems detected in the dental EHR [46, 49, 60, 61].

Low chair-side adoption rate of dental EHRs is also thought to be, in part, due to the unsuitability of the conventional EHR set-up in the dental operatory [46]. Keyboards and mice are potential sources of infection and need protective covers [62]. Electronic clinical data entry is often believed to take longer than entering this information in the paper chart or is thought to be impractical because the dental assistant is needed to perform other duties [46]. Additionally, the inability to effectively use clinical decision support within the dental EHR to positively influence dental patient care outcomes [63] and the lack of integration of evidence based guidelines [61] into the EHR have limited adoption by dental practitioners.

Applying Theory to Practice: Redesigning a Treatment Planning Module in a Dental EHR

Design Challenge

Because the axiUm EHR is widely used amongst dental school clinics to document patient care, it was possible to work in close collaboration with the vendor to redevelop one of its existing modules, using a participatory, work-centered design approach with an aim to better support the diagnostic-centric treatment planning process for dental students. Specifically, the existing treatment planning module within the EHR was deemed too complicated and difficult to use. Several dental institutions had also recently adopted the then called DDS Dental Diagnostic Terminology, which drove the diagnostic entry functionality of the Treatment Planning module.

The work of treatment planning in dentistry is the process of using information obtained from the patient history, clinical examination and diagnostic tests to formulate a sequence of treatment steps designed to eliminate disease and restore efficient, comfortable aesthetic and masticatory function to a patient. When developing a treatment plan, the provider should follow a general phasing and sequencing format designed to solve the patient's dental problems in a way that first manages the patient's emergent concerns (e.g., pain and infection). The next step is disease (e.g., caries) removal and tooth restoration; then, tooth replacement and reconstruction. Once these priorities have been met, aesthetic and cosmetic concerns are addressed, and lastly, preventive and maintenance measures are ensured. Any given phase may contain several individual procedures, some of which may be sequenced in a specific order [64].

The Treatment Planning module in the axiUm EHR was originally developed with input from dental educators and thought leaders, and follows the treatment planning philosophy of Stefanac [64]. In order to develop a treatment plan within axiUm, a user (1) enters the patient's problems/complaints; (2) selects the appropriate diagnoses from a comprehensive list; (3) enters the treatment objectives, which represent the intent or rationale for the final treatment plan, usually expressed as short statements and clear goals from both the student's and patient's perspectives; and (4) enters a detailed plan for treating each of the selected diagnoses (Fig. 14.2). Following treatment planning, the student obtains instructor approval and patient consent before beginning treatment.

Design Approach

A participatory design process to systematically identify challenges in the use of the existing Treatment Planning Module was used to inform an improved user interface that effectively supports the underlying needs of the end users. As summarized in Fig. 14.3, usability challenges were first identified and prioritized. New mockups were then developed, tested, refined and implemented in the EHR by the vendor. After further usability assessments, the new module was released to customers. Post-implementation usability assessments were conducted to determine the impact of the re-design in comparison to the original version.

Usability Assessment to Identify Challenges in Existing Treatment Planning Module

In general, a terminology is evaluated in terms of its ability to represent relevant concepts, and user interfaces are evaluated in terms of their usability. As Patel and Cimino noted, a combined approach towards evaluating both the terminology and the user interface offers a more holistic perspective on how the task is carried out and where it can be improved [66]. Consider when a user would like to enter a diagnosis into the Treatment Planning module but faces significant hurdles or fails. The reason for the failure might be any one or a combination of the following: inadequate completeness of the terminology (e.g., the terminology does not represent the diagnosis), poor usability (e.g., the interface does not provide adequate access to the diagnostic terminology), or insufficient representation within the terminology (e.g., poor organization of the terminology). The same problems could underpin the

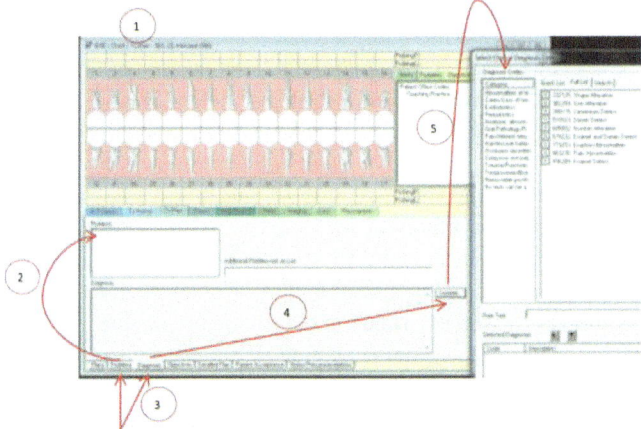

In the (1) 'treatment planning' module, the student (2) enters the problems and (3) moves to the 'Diagnosis' tab. Here, the appropriate diagnoses may be selected by (4) clicking on the 'update' button and working through (5) the list of the 'Clinical Diagnosis Codes'.

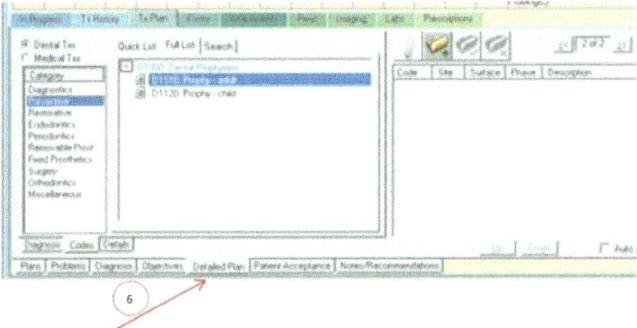

Treatment is added for each diagnosis by clicking on the (6) 'Detailed Plan' tab, selecting the appropriate treatment category and subsequently, the suitable treatment from the full list.

Fig. 14.2 Original treatment planning process in axiUm. Reproduced with permission from Tokede et al. [65]

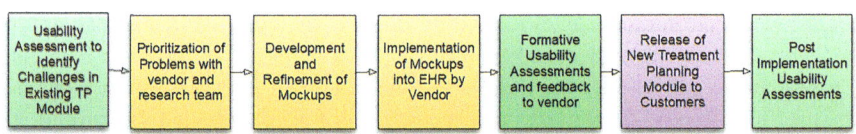

Fig. 14.3 Overall process for assessing, improving and implementing the Treatment Planning (TP) Module in axiUm

selection of a term that does not capture the intended meaning. By attending to both the terminology and the user interface, we can begin to characterize the breadth of the causes of failure. Thus, we analyzed the following when considering this human computer interaction challenge: (1) use of the DDS terminology itself, (2) use of the existing Treatment Planning interface and (3) use of the DDS terminology as part of clinic workflow.

We conducted usability assessments of EHRs at two dental schools: Harvard School of Dental Medicine (HSDM) and University of California, San Francisco (UCSF). Both institutions have university-owned clinics to train dental students as well as residents (post graduate students). Both dental schools also have a private faculty practice, use the axiUm EHR system, and were early adopters of the DDS dental diagnostic terminology. Study participants included a sample of third- and fourth-year dental students (who were actively involved with delivering patient care), residents, and faculty. These groups represent the primary users of the DDS dental diagnostic terminology. As mentioned previously, dental students are responsible for updating the dental patient record under the supervision of attending faculty. Because one does not get many opportunities to overhaul a major module within the EHR, we conducted three complementary usability assessments in order to maximize our ability to capture challenges. We will summarize that work here; we have published full details in the International Journal of Medical Informatics [56, 60].

Think-Aloud User Testing We created two pre-defined scenarios to assess users' interactions with DDS in the axiUm Treatment Planning module: a simple task of entering one diagnosis and a more complex treatment-planning task. Participants were asked to think aloud [67] and verbalize their thoughts as they worked through each scenario. As part of user testing, quantitative data was captured to assess if tasks were completed successfully (a measure of effectiveness) and the amount of time spent in accomplishing the task (a measure of efficiency). To evaluate whether a user successfully completed the tasks, we had to define the correct path to complete the tasks. We did this using Hierarchical Task Analysis (HTA) [68] after gathering input from expert dentists at each site. After determining the appropriate path to complete the tasks, we calculated the expert performance time, which is the time it would take an expert (who makes no errors) to complete the tasks. We did this using CogTool [69], an open source software that predicts performance time on the basis of application screenshots and the specification of a path to complete a specific task. After completing the exercises, participants were asked to provide additional feedback on the use of the module, and complete a user satisfaction survey using the validated and widely used System Usability Scale [70].

Observations Using Ethnography Observational data were collected over a three-day period by a trained researcher in order to provide insight into the clinical workflow, information gathering and diagnostic decision-making process in the clinical environment where the dentists and dental students worked. To minimize any impact on patient care, a non-participatory observational technique was used. The researcher engaged with the dental team members only if there was a need for any clarification or during downtime such as when a patient did not show for an appointment. Observational data were captured using paper-based field notes. Each set of observations occurred for approximately 4 h, in two separate shifts (morning and afternoon). The primary purpose of the observations was to capture overall clinical workflow and to identify how diagnoses were made and captured in the EHR using the DDS dental diagnostic terminology, and to identify any associated challenges. Actual clinical work was not part of the observation.

Semi-Structured Interviews The third approach we took for evaluating the terminology and interface was to conduct semi-structured interviews with open-ended questions. The semi-structured format ensured uniformity of questions asked, while the open-ended format allowed the interviewees to express themselves. New questions were allowed to arise as a result of the discussion. The prepared questions focused on two broad themes: (1) the perception and internal representation of the clinic, patient care and role of dentists/students within the clinic; and (2) the nature of the workflow and environment of care within this dental clinic with the use of EHR. The questions were influenced by the knowledge gained from the observations. Interviews lasted approximately 30 min each. The interview data were collected in order to assess information on the role, situational awareness and general work philosophy of the subjects in the dental clinic. The sample was representative of those who are usually present in the clinical environment and as such included dental third- and fourth-year students, residents and faculty.

Findings User testing revealed that only 22% of users were able to successfully complete all of the steps in the simple task of entering one diagnosis, while no user was able to complete the more complex treatment-planning task. Table 14.1 provides an overview of the 24 high-level usability problems that were found through the use of the three methods. The methods together identified a total of 187 usability violations: 54% via user testing, 28% via the semi-structured interview and 18% from the survey method, with modest overlap [56]. Interface-related problems included unexpected approaches for displaying diagnosis, lack of visibility, and inconsistent use of user interface widgets. User interface widgets are elements of the interface with which a user interacts. Terminology related issues included missing and mis-categorized concepts. Work domain issues involved both absent and superfluous functions. In collaboration with the vendor, each usability problem was prioritized, and a timeline set to resolve the concerns.

Participatory Prioritization of Problems with the Vendor and Broad-Based Research Team

Based on the findings from the usability studies, a diverse group comprising of clinicians, secondary data users, usability experts, terminology developers/researchers, and the vendor design team assessed each of the 24 findings and prioritized each issue, and how it may be addressed in future versions of the EHR. Involvement of the vendor was critical at this stage. Several problems had solutions or workarounds that could be implemented immediately by re-configuration or customization in the

Table 14.1 Summary of usability problems, priorities and timeframe to address and implement solutions. Reproduced with permission from Walji et al. [60]

	Usability problem(PRIORITY) Description/example	Timeframe to implement solutions
Interface	1. Illogical ordering of terms (HIGH) Terms are ordered based on numeric code rather than alphabetically	Immediate: Reorder alphabetically <1 year: Users to customize ordering
	2. Term names not fully visible(HIGH) Users select incorrect diagnosis as they are unable to read the full name	<6 months
	3. Time consuming to enter a diagnosis(HIGH) User must navigate several screens and scroll through a long list to find and select a diagnosis	<1 year
	4. Inconsistent naming and placement of user interface widgets(HIGH) To add a new diagnosis, a user must click a button labeled "Update"	<6 months
	5. Ineffective feedback to confirm diagnosis entry(HIGH) User only sees the numeric code for the diagnosis and not the name of the term.	<1 year
	6. Search results do not match users expectations(MEDIUM) A search for "pericornitis" retrieves three concepts with the same name but a different numerical code	<1 year
	7. Users unaware of important functions to help find a diagnosis(MEDIUM) System defaults to "quick list", so some users do not navigate the "full list" or discover the use of the search feature	<1 year
	8. Limited flexibility in user interface(MEDIUM) User unable to modify an entered diagnosis on the "details" page and must go back to previous screens to edit diagnosis	<1 year
	9. Distinction between category name and concept unclear(MEDIUM) Users attempt to select a category name.	Immediate

Table 14.1 (continued)

	Usability problem(PRIORITY) Description/example	Timeframe to implement solutions
Terminology	10. Inappropriate granularity/specificity of concepts(MEDIUM) Some sub-categories have a large number of concepts making it very difficult for users to find an appropriate term	<1 year
	11. Some concepts appear missing/not included(HIGH) Examples of missing concepts according to users include: Missing tooth, arrested caries, and attritional teeth	<6 months
	12. Some concepts not classified in appropriate categories/sub categories(HIGH) Example: Aesthetic concerns	<6 months
	13. Abbreviations not recognized by users(HIGH) Example: F/U, NOS, VDO	<6 months
	14. Visibility of the numeric code for a diagnostic term(HIGH) Although the numeric code is a meaningless identifier, users had an expectation that the identifier should provide some meaning	Immediate: Use Quicklist to hide code <1 year: Remove numeric code in UI
	15. Users not clear about the meaning of some concepts(MEDIUM) Novice users (students) had difficulty distinguishing between similar terms, and definitions and synonyms were not provided	<1 year
Work domain	16. Free text option can be used circumvent structured data entry(HIGH) Instead of selecting a structured term, some users free text the name of the diagnosis	Immediate: Disable option <1 year: Remove option altogether
	17. Synonyms not displayed(HIGH) Users must search by preferred term name	<1 year
	18. Knowledge level of diagnostic term concepts and how to enter in EHR limited(HIGH) Users appear to have had little concerted education and training either by institution or vendor	<1 year
	19. Only one diagnosis can be entered for each treatment(HIGH) Endodontic discipline require that treatments are justified using both a pulpal and periapical diagnosis	<1 year
	20. Diagnosis cannot be charted using the Odontogram or Periogram(HIGH) Users chart findings using	<2 year
	21. No historical view of when a diagnosis has been added or modified(HIGH)	<1 year
	22. No decision support to help suggest appropriate diagnoses, or alert if inappropriate ones are selected(MEDIUM)	<2 year
	23. No way to indicate state of diagnosis (i.e., differential, working or definitive)(MEDIUM)	<1 year
	24. Users forced to enter a diagnosis for treatments that may not require them(MEDIUM)	<1 year

existing version of the Treatment Planning module. For example, the ability to enter free text could be disabled for end users. The research team also gained greater appreciation of the vendor's development schedule and rationale for some of their earlier design decisions. The vendor's development team, for the first time, had empirical evidence of specific usability problems faced by users. The prioritization process, which occurred during a face-to-face meeting with the CEO as well as several follow-up phone calls, provided a common understanding of the major usability problems and a process by which they could be addressed.

Development and Refinement of Mockups

Over 2–3 months, the usability team developed low fidelity mockups and made presentations of this work to the larger, broad-based team in weekly conference calls. After several iterations, a consensus design was developed. As shown in Fig. 14.4, key design features included (1) one screen for entering problems, diagnoses and treatments to provide situational awareness to users, (2) autocomplete functionality to enter problems, diagnoses and treatments, and (3) ability to explicitly link problems, diagnoses and treatments.

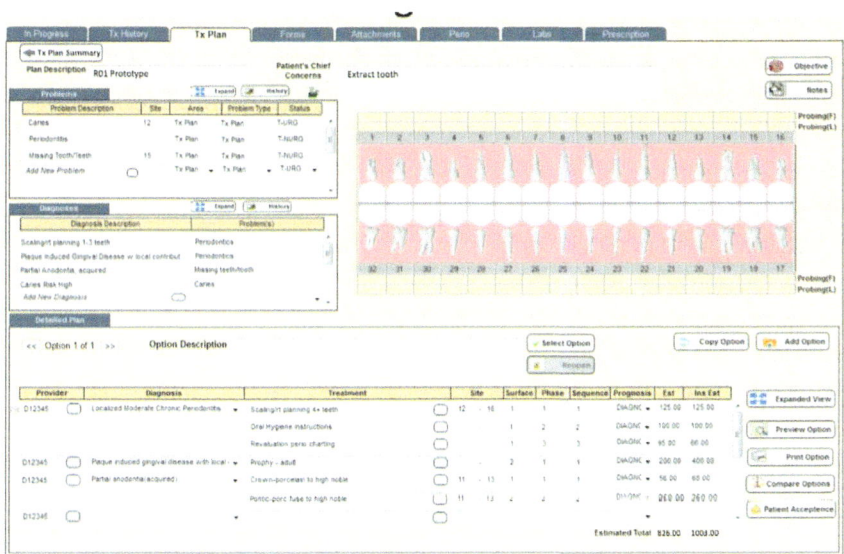

Fig. 14.4 Example of a mature mockup of a new Treatment Planning interface

Implementation of Mockups into EHR

The vendor's design team was then responsible for determining how to implement the mockups within its EHR using their existing development tools (Microsoft Visual C++ .Net). Some of the desired functionality, such as drag and drop to reorder concepts, was not possible due to the underlying design architecture. In each case, the vendor would provide alternative solutions to meet the intent of the enhancement. Figure 14.5 shows a screenshot of the newly developed Treatment Planning module in the axiUm EHR. The approximate development time from receiving the mockups to full implementation was 6 months.

Next Steps: Assessing Impact of the New Treatment Planning Module

This design case demonstrates how a participatory, work-centered design process can be used to re-design an EHR module to support the treatment planning process in dentistry. The vendor released the new Treatment Planning module in February 2014. In ongoing work, the research team is conducting comprehensive assessments to determine the impact of the new interface on efficiency, effectiveness, and satisfaction.

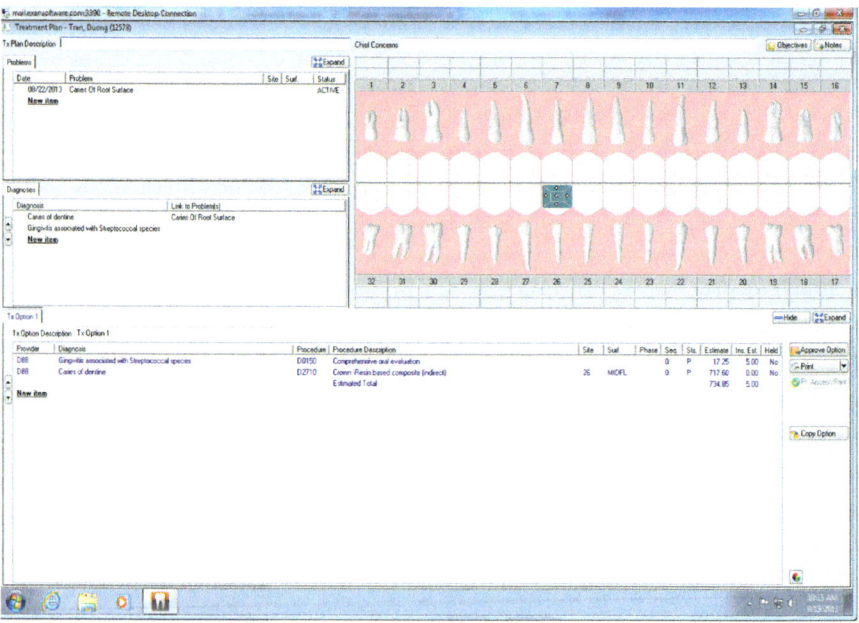

Fig. 14.5 Treatment Planning interface in axiUm after implementation by vendor

Implications for Practice

Importance of Collaborative Teams for the Design of Usable Systems

"It takes work, and new ways of thinking, and new kinds and methods of openness, to bring substantively new voices into a conversation. Similarly, to bring users' knowledges and perspectives directly into computer specification and design, it is necessary to do more than "just add users and stir" [71].

Human-computer interaction has, as a field, undergone an evolution from technological solutions to complex problems of human interaction with computers, to user-centered design [72], to participatory design [73]. This evolution represents shifts from designing without users to designing with users in mind to designing with users. This last approach, called participatory design, is a set of theories and practices engaging end-users as full participants in design. Rather than replacing user-centered design, participatory design has subsumed user-centered approaches, like the work-centered design approach we used, into its rich and diverse toolbox, which draws upon fields such as graphic design, architecture, psychology, anthropology, software engineering, and communications studies. Participatory design has likewise been applied to a diverse set of applications, as wide ranging as land use in Africa [74] to designing technology for children with special needs [75].

In a strict user-centered design process, the researcher serves as the interface between the user and designer. The researcher collects primary data or uses secondary sources to learn about the user's needs, which are translated by the researcher into design criteria. The designer interprets these criteria, typically through mockups. The researcher and user reappear in the process for usability testing. In user-centered design, the researcher, designer, and user have distinct roles: the user is not integral to the design team but is instead spoken for by the researcher. A key participatory design principle is to blur and bridge the distinctions among these roles through mutual learning, often through face-to-face interaction and prototyping.

The way that we have operationalized participatory design principles in the context of standardized dental diagnostic term entry into the EHR has been to bring together a broad range of stakeholders in a series of virtual and face-to-face working sessions. The breadth of the stakeholders at each meeting reflected the wide-ranging impact of building and implementing the terms and the interface to the terms. Each team member brought a different, relevant perspective; they included the CEO of the dental EHR company, the lead architect of the dental EHR company, practicing dentists, usability experts, epidemiologists, data warehouse experts, and dental clinic administrators. Through close interaction and real-time problem solving, we were able to learn from each other and to find solutions that would meet each stakeholder's needs while respecting the limitations other stakeholders faced.

Participatory design was a good fit with our goal of enhancing standardized dental diagnostic term entry in the context of an EHR. We had a committed, and funded, set of core participants who were willing to devote scores of hours to the project; we had sufficient technical latitude to accommodate end-user feedback given the close partnership with the EHR vendor; and as the developers of the diagnostic terminology, we had the ability to make necessary changes to the terms as required. In addition, as has been the case in many participatory design applications, our scope was tightly focused [76]. Were we to have considered the totality of the user experience when interacting with the EHR, the type of participatory approach we took would have been infeasible given our timeline and budget. As has been noted elsewhere, participatory design is costly [76]. A much leaner approach to usability analysis is the use of heuristics evaluation, i.e., assessing how well a given system adheres to best practices for interaction design, which is well-suited to eliminating initial design decisions that would violate a heuristic. As design progresses to implementation, though, more user engagement is needed to identify usability challenges. In a 2009 study of four dental EHRs, heuristic evaluation was found to anticipate half of the usability problems identified through empirical testing with end users [49]. User testing is not, of course, the only way to incorporate user participation. Other approaches include interviews and surveys. Though we found the survey approach to be comparatively less effective in our own work, surveys have the advantage of being inexpensive and quick to yield results, which may be the best option in some circumstances [56]. We have used surveys and interviews to further assess the impact of the implementation of the SNODDS terminology and found it to be an effective option, yielding excellent results [77].

Impact on Secondary Use of Data

Although the discussion of whether the use of EHRs will lower costs and improve care is still open, there are fewer questions about the significance of the data generated through clinical care. Given the monetary and time expense of clinical trials, it is only sensible to use the informational and biological by-products of health care delivery to expand our knowledge and improve practice [78]. Before being the object of a researcher's analysis, these data were entered in a variety of systems, which in turn, sit in a variety of contexts, both of which may have usability implications. Here, it is useful to draw out what is meant by the term usability, as it covers a large swath of concepts. Over the decades, the literature has surfaced a wide range of both narrow and broad definitions of usability. A frequently-referenced definition is that framed within the ISO 9241 standard, in which usability is defined as the "[e]xtent to which a product can be used by specified users to achieve specified goals with effectiveness, efficiency, and satisfaction." [79] In turn, satisfaction is defined as "freedom from discomfort, and positive attitudes towards the user of the product"; efficiency is defined as the "resources expended in relation to the accuracy and completeness with which users achieve goals"; and effectiveness is defined as the "accuracy and completeness with which users achieve specified goals."

It would be tempting to surmise that effectiveness, efficiency, and satisfaction depend on one another, but alas, the field has an under-developed understanding of the relationships among usability measures [80]. Indeed, some have posited that any relationships among them depend on other factors, such as application domain, use context, user experience, and task complexity [81]. What this means is that distinct aspects of usability need to be measured separately, that we cannot rely upon efficiency to tell us about effectiveness, for example.

In the setting of secondary use of data, effectiveness is key: in the context of dental diagnostic terms, for instance, secondary users of data rely upon the primary users to have effectively entered valid diagnostic terms, even if such entry entailed discomfort and expenditure of resources on the part of the individual who entered the data. Indeed, part of the challenge of promoting the valid documentation of standardized diagnostic terms is that it has not been a professional norm in dentistry and thus inherently involves additional effort than does failing to enter the diagnosis. Thus, the assessments we conducted captured utilization, the proportion of times that any diagnostic term was entered when a diagnosis was appropriate, as well as valid use, the proportion of diagnostic terms entered that were an appropriate match for the treatment provided. Institutions that have adopted standardized dental diagnoses are reaping the rewards. For example, BigMouth [82, 83] is a dental data repository that has aggregated data from 11 dental institutions, many of which use SNODDS. Researchers have used BigMouth to investigate a wide variety of clinical questions relating to periodontal diseases [84, 85], endodontics [86], social determinants of health [87], and head and neck cancers [88]. Standardized diagnoses have also allowed dental clinics to measure the quality of care [89] using data from the EHR for process [90] and outcome measures [91].

Impact on Inter-Professional Practice

It is an artifact of the history of dentistry in the United States [92, 93], rather than anatomy or physiology, that oral health is perceived as separable from general health, as if there were an impenetrable firewall between the two. Unfortunately, in the case of bridging medical and dental data, there most often is such a technical and policy-based firewall, with no broadly adopted ways to communicate efficiently across the divide. In 2013, the Advisory Committee on Training in Primacy Care Medicine and Dentistry wrote, "the separation between oral health and systemic health does not serve the needs of patients. There must be a mutual interaction between oral health and systemic health using efficient inter-professional communication." Inter-professional practice is being promoted as a way to achieve the so-called Triple Aim of (1) enhanced population health, (2) reduced costs of care, and (3) optimal patient care experience [94, 95]. Informatics infrastructure can pose both barriers to and opportunities for collaborative practice between medicine and dentistry; the Advisory Committee recommended that dental practices should interact and integrate more effectively with medicine and other health professions in terms of quality measure and health information systems [94].

A survey of medical and dental providers at academic centers in the USA and Germany "found that 77% of dentist respondents and 57% of physician respondents believed that the connection between oral and systemic health impacted their patients and that access to medical and dental information through their HER would improve care." [96] The need for linking a patient's complete health profile was further elucidated in a study analyzing data recorded in a patients dental record compared with their medical record. Alarming discrepancies were discovered; 15.1% misreported their diabetes condition to their dental clinicians, while 29.0% of patients failed to report their hypertension [97].

Under the right conditions, EHRs in the dental clinic setting could serve to bridge the inter-professional information gap in a way that is not possible in a paper-based world. In the most straightforward scenario, the medical and dental records would be integrated into a single system. EHR systems with oral health modules are deployed through the Indian Health Service, the Department of Veteran's Affairs, as well as the Cattails medical and dental EHRs developed and used at the Marshfield Clinic in Marshfield, WI [94, 98]. More recently, large healthcare systems that have both medical and dental practices are adopting a common EHR platform Epic, that has recently developed a dental module called Wisdom. Unfortunately, these cases are the rare exception rather than the rule. As noted by Powell and Din, "the essential core improvement to bring medicine and dentistry closer together is the integration of medical and dental care and data. Currently, many medical records and data exist separate and distinct from dental records and data for the same patient." [99] Even in the context of clinical care, there are no routine channels through which to exchange data between medical and dental EHRs. In practice, thus, the little information that is exchanged between the medical and dental settings is typically done through letters or telephone calls. Information exchanged in this way can make its way into the record only as a PDF or image or as free-text notes entered by a clinician. In 2009, the ADA announced an agreement with HL7 (Health Level 7) to enhance the coordination of patient care between medical and dental practices using a dental extension to the Continuity of Care Document (CCD) [100, 101], though the routine exchange of such documents still has not yet come to pass. More recently, the HL7 Fast Health Interoperability Resource (FHIR) that defines the format and structure is an "emerging communication standard for health data being widely adopted by the health care industry" [102]. However, the use of FHIR in dentistry is still in its infancy.

In addition to the technical details of how clinical information is exchanged across the professional divide, we should consider the communicative value of the information. One of the primary goals of standardizing dental diagnostic terms is to enhance communication between providers, with patients, and with third parties like payors [40]. Thus, ensuring that both the terminology itself as well as the EHR design, deployment, and use support effective and efficient documentation of standardized dental diagnostic terms serves inter-professional practice at its most basic level [103]. Taking a step back, it is also worth noting that poor usability and a steep learning curve have been reported as barriers to adoption of EHRs in dentistry, as was mentioned in section "Development of a Standardized Dental Diagnostic

Terminology" of this chapter. Even in the dental academic setting, in which EHRs are widespread, users have expressed doubt that the systems improve efficiency and effectiveness [50].

Improving EHR usability could not only enhance inter-professional practice but also could heal the fractured perceptions of EHRs within larger dental practices in which administrative and clinical duties are divided. In a study in a large dental teaching practice at an academic center, administrators articulated the most and broadest benefits of an EHR: in fact, the technology had so enhanced the quantity and quality of accessible information to the point that it was described as indispensable. By contrast, the faculty and student dentists saw the EHR as a mixed blessing with a not entirely positive impact on their clinical practice or teaching [104]. This gap again underscores the importance of broad-based collaborative teams participating in the design of usable systems that maximize efficiency, effectiveness, and satisfaction across user groups. We have seen similar success with a large dental practice, in part due to a relentless pursuit for perfection during implementation of the terminology and a culture of strictly adhering to evidence-based guidelines for using treatments that tie logically to diagnoses [77, 105].

Future Directions

Utilization and validity of the DDS terminology improves over time. In a study with four academic sites and one large dental practice we noted a 1.5-fold increase in the number of unique diagnoses documented during the four-year study period (2013–2016). The utilization and validity proportions of the DDS had statistically significant increases from 2013 to 2016 ($P < 0.0001$). We believe that utilization and validity are influenced by the professional and clinic-led cultural direction and the level and quality of the implementation efforts. It also raises the need for more focused training of the dental students and residents. Our data suggest that the longer a terminology is used, the higher the chances that it will be understood and better utilized by end users [5].

The debate on the routine use of standardized diagnostic terminologies (DxTMs) in dentistry is slowly moving towards how to do it, instead of if or why. Through unstructured interviews a group of dental stakeholders at a 2016 National Conference provided input on how to enhance the uptake of DxTMs. Key strategies suggested to further enhance the adoption of DxTMs in dentistry included the use of mandates, a value proposition for providers, communication and education, and integration with EHRs and existing systems. Clearly, all groups across the dental healthcare delivery spectrum will need to work together for the success of the widespread and consistent use of DxTMs. Understanding the provider perspective is however the most critical step in achieving this goal, as they are the group who will ultimately be saddled with the critical task of ensuring DxTM use at the point of care [106]. Medical cognition has been defined as the study "of cognitive processes, such as perception, comprehension, reasoning, decision making, and problem solving in medical practice itself" [107], and a better understanding of these mental processes can be used to design and develop technologies for supporting the diagnostic process in dentistry. For instance, applying the principles of human-centered design can help to develop systems that support the work and mental models of dental practitioners. New technology should also minimize and not increase the cognitive load of users. Decision support systems should help dentists make faster and more accurate diagnoses, reduce errors, and ultimately help improve patient outcomes.

Summary

Policy and socio-cultural factors have brought dental EHR adoption to a tipping point [108]. This adoption is occurring in the context of high expectations for software that can "help improve [your] patient care and communication, streamline [your] clinical workflow, improve [your] referral process, and reduce overall practice liability…" [109] In light of these hopes, it should not come as a surprise that dental practices are advised to consider the usability of and ease of navigation within the EHR software when making their purchasing decisions [109]. If the research base matched the enthusiasm of end-users for usable systems, the literature would be replete with HCI work in the unique dental setting. As it stands, literature review demonstrates that there remains a knowledge gap in dental informatics, particularly with respect to HCI research that directly engages end-user stakeholders.

A more robust dental HCI ecosystem can help to close the gap between end-user goals and the status quo of dental EHRs, which have been found to have "significant usability problems." [49] Within this chapter, we have illustrated a practical example of how this iterative improvement can occur, by describing how we undertook a multi-modal participatory design process to redesign the treatment planning module in a dental EHR to better support the documentation of standardized dental diagnostic terms. The enhanced usability resulting from this and similarly directed efforts holds the promise to enhance clinical care, empower secondary data analysis, and lower the barriers to inter-professional care of our patients, who are the ultimate beneficiaries of usable systems.

The dental profession has slowly started to acknowledge that routine use of standardized diagnostic terminologies is imperative as part of providing comprehensive care. Understanding and supporting the providers' perspective and cognitive processes will be the most critical step in achieving implementation, as they are the group who will ultimately be saddled with the critical task of ensuring use at the point of care.

Discussion Questions
1. Identify the challenges for the average general dentist and primary care physician to collaboratively manage and thus be able to exchange electronically patient information, specifically regarding diagnoses and chronic care management.

2. Discuss the strengths and limitations of user testing, interviews and observations in detecting usability problems.
3. Identify the unique challenges in dentistry, e.g., the slow adoption of meaningful use, workflow issues and various practice structures, and specifically how lessons learned in medicine can help advance the field.

References

1. Munson B, Vujicic M. Projected supply of dentists in the United States, 2020–2040. Chicago, IL: American Dental Association; 2021 [cited 2022 Jun 2]. Available from: https://www.ada.org/-/media/project/ada-organization/ada/ada-org/files/resources/research/hpi/hpi-brief_0521_1.pdf?rev=b5f3e8a7c15f4fd5a238314d0f58945c&hash=1688579EF176F8C6B240A4BBC5477E30
2. Manski R, Rohde F, Ricks T, Chalmers NI. Statistical brief #544. Number and percentage of the population with any dental or medical visits by insurance coverage and geographic area, 2019. Rockville, MD: AHRQ, MEP Survey; 2022.
3. Taichman R, Pinsky H, Sarment D. Pilot safety protocol could help dentists reduce errors. Ann Arbor, MI: University of Michigan; 2010 [cited 2011 Apr 25]. Available from: http://ns.umich.edu/htdocs/releases/story.php?id=7906
4. Exan Vancouver, Canada. [cited 2014 Jul 29]. Available from: http://www.axiumdental.com
5. Yansane A, Tokede O, White J, et al. Utilization and validity of the dental diagnostic system over time in academic and private practice. JDR Clin Trans Res. 2019;4(2):143–50.
6. Kalenderian E, Ramoni RB, Walji MF. Standardized dental diagnostic terminology. Ann Dent Oral Health. 2018;1:1002.
7. Finkbeiner BL. Four-handed dentistry revisited. J Contemp Dent Pract. 2000;1(4):74–86.
8. University of Alabama at Birmingham. Four-handed dentistry. Birmingham, AL: UAB; 2011 [cited 2014 May 2]. Available from: https://www.uab.edu/uabmagazine/breakthroughs/healthcare/four-handed-dentistry
9. Finkbeiner BL. Selecting equipment for the ergonomic four-handed dental practice. J Contemp Dent Pract. 2001;2(4):44–52.
10. Guay AH, Wall TP, Petersen BC, Lazar VF. Evolving trends in size and structure of group dental practices in the United States. J Dent Educ. 2012;76(8):1036–44.
11. Health Policy Institute. Practice ownership among dentists continues to decline. Chicago, IL: American Dental Association; 2022 Mar.
12. Health Policy Institute. Solo practice continues to decrease. Chicago, IL: American Dental Association; 2022 Mar.
13. Cole JR, Dodge WW, Findley JS, et al. Will large DSO-Managed Group practices be the predominant setting for oral health care by 2025? Two viewpoints: viewpoint 1: large DSO-Managed Group practices will be the setting in which the majority of oral health care is delivered by 2025 and viewpoint 2: increases in DSO-Managed Group practices will be offset by models allowing dentists to retain the independence and freedom of a traditional practice. J Dent Educ. 2015;79(5):465–71.
14. Anderson GD, Grey EB. The MSO's prognosis after the ACA: a viable integration tool? Phoenix, AZ: Physicians and Physician Organizations Law Institute; 2013 [cited 2014 May 2]. Available from: http://www.healthlawyers.org/Events/Programs/Materials/Documents/PHY13/B_anderson_grey.pdf
15. Canadian Dental Association Dental Health Services in Canada. Fact and Fifures 2010. 2010 [cited 2014 Jul 6]. Available from: http://www.med.uottawa.ca/sim/data/Dental/Dental_Health_Services_in_Canada_June_2010.pdf

16. Service Canada Dentists. Government of Canada. 2014 [cited 2014 Jul 6]. Available from: http://www.servicecanada.gc.ca/eng/qc/job_futures/statistics/3113.shtml
17. Button PS, Doyle K, Karitis JW, Selhorst C. Automating clinical documentation in dentistry: case study of a clinical integration model. J Healthc Inf Manag. 1999;13(3):31–40.
18. Wotman S, Lalumandier J, Nelson S, Stange K. Implications for dental education of a dental school-initiated practice research network. J Dent Educ. 2001;65(8):751–9.
19. Irwin JY, Torres-Urquidy MH, Schleyer T, Monaco V. A preliminary model of work during initial examination and treatment planning appointments. Br Dent J. 2009;206(1):E1; discussion 24–5.
20. Schleyer TK, Thyvalikakath TP, Spallek H, et al. Clinical computing in general dentistry. J Am Med Inform Assoc. 2006;13(3):344–52.
21. John JH, Thomas D, Richards D. Questionnaire survey on the use of computerisation in dental practices across the Thames Valley region. Br Dent J. 2003;195(10):585–90; discussion 579.
22. Schleyer T, Spallek H, Hernandez P. A qualitative investigation of the content of dental paper-based and computer-based patient record formats. J Am Med Inform Assoc. 2007;14(4):515–26.
23. Thyvalikakath TP, Schleyer TK, Monaco V. Heuristic evaluation of clinical functions in four practice management systems: a pilot study. J Am Dent Assoc. 2007;138(2):209–10, 212–8.
24. Thyvalikakath TP, Monaco V, Thambuganipalle HB, Schleyer T. A usability evaluation of four commercial dental computer-based patient record systems. J Am Dent Assoc. 2008;139(12):1632–42.
25. Miller RH, Sim I. Physicians' use of electronic medical records: barriers and solutions. Health Aff (Millwood). 2004;23(2):116–26.
26. Fitzpatrick J, Koh JS. If you build it (right), they will come: the physician-friendly CPOE. Not everything works as planned right out of the box. A Mississippi hospital customizes its electronic order entry system for maximum use by physicians. Health Manag Technol. 2005;26(1):52–3.
27. Simon SR, Kaushal R, Cleary PD, et al. Correlates of electronic health record adoption in office practices: a statewide survey. J Am Med Inform Assoc. 2007;14(1):110–7.
28. Walji MF, Taylor D, Langabeer JR 2nd, Valenza JA. Factors influencing implementation and outcomes of a dental electronic patient record system. J Dent Educ. 2009;73(5):589–600.
29. World Health Organization. Application of the international classification of diseases to dentistry and stomatology. 1st ed. Geneva: WHO; 1973.
30. Ettelbrick KL, Webb MD, Seale NS. Hospital charges for dental caries related emergency admissions. Pediatr Dent. 2000;22(1):21–5.
31. Orlowsky WJ, Glusman M. Recovery of aversive thresholds following midbrain lesions in the cat. J Comp Physiol Psychol. 1969;67(2):245–51.
32. Gregg TA, Boyd DH. A computer software package to facilitate clinical audit of outpatient paediatric dentistry. Int J Paediatr Dent. 1996;6(1):45–51.
33. Bader JD, Shugars DA, White BA, Rindal DB. Development of effectiveness of care and use of services measures for dental care plans. J Public Health Dent. 1999;59(3):142–9.
34. Leake JL, Main PA, Sabbah W. A system of diagnostic codes for dental health care. J Public Health Dent. 1999;59(3):162–70.
35. Leake JL. Diagnostic codes in dentistry--definition, utility and developments to date. J Can Dent Assoc. 2002;68(7):403–6.
36. Sabbah W. Assessing the validity of North York dental diagnostic codes. Faculty of Dentistry, University of Toronto; 1999.
37. SNODENT update. National Committee on Vital and Health Statistics (NCVHS); Subcommittee on Standards and Security. Chicago, Ill: American Dental Association; 2004.
38. Goldberg LJ, Ceusters W, Eisner J, Smith B. The significance of SNODENT. Stud Health Technol Inform. 2005;116:737–42.

39. Torres-Urquidy MH, Schleyer T. Evaluation of the systematized nomenclature of dentistry using case reports: preliminary results. AMIA Annu Symp Proc. 2006;2006:1124.
40. Kalenderian E, Ramoni RL, White JM, et al. The development of a dental diagnostic terminology. J Dent Educ. 2011;75(1):68–76.
41. Clinical Information Modeling Initiative (CIMI). Category:interface terminology. 2012 [cited 2014 Jul 14]. Available from: http://informatics.mayo.edu/CIMI/index.php/Category:Interface_Terminology
42. Clinical Information Modeling Initiative (CIMI). Category:reference terminology. [cited 2013 Apr 1]. Available from: http://informatics.mayo.edu/CIMI/index.php/Category:Reference_Terminology
43. Nederlands Tandartsenblad Nederlandse Norm voor diagnostische termen. Nieuwegein, Nederland: Nederlandse Maatschappij van Tandartsen; 2014 [cited 2014 Jul 14]. Available from: http://www.ntblad.nl
44. Blumenthal D, Glaser JP. Information technology comes to medicine. N Engl J Med. 2007;356(24):2527–34.
45. White JM, Kalenderian E, Stark PC, et al. Evaluating a dental diagnostic terminology in an electronic health record. J Dent Educ. 2011;75(5):605–15.
46. Reynolds PA, Harper J, Dunne S. Better informed in clinical practice - a brief overview of dental informatics. Br Dent J. 2008;204(6):313–7.
47. Hill HK, Stewart DC, Ash JS. The training and support needs of faculty and students using a health information technology system were significant: a case study in a dental school. AMIA Annu Symp Proc. 2010;2010:301–5.
48. Juve-Udina ME. What patients' problems do nurses e-chart? Longitudinal study to evaluate the usability of an interface terminology. Int J Nurs Stud. 2013;50(12):1698–710.
49. Thyvalikakath TP, Monaco V, Thambuganipalle H, Schleyer T. Comparative study of heuristic evaluation and usability testing methods. Stud Health Technol Inform. 2009;143:322–7.
50. Thyvalikakath TP, Dziabiak MP, Johnson R, et al. Advancing cognitive engineering methods to support user interface design for electronic health records. Int J Med Inform. 2014;83(4):292–302.
51. Marcotte L, Seidman J, Trudel K, et al. Achieving meaningful use of health information technology: a guide for physicians to the EHR incentive programs. Arch Intern Med. 2012;172(9):731–6.
52. Chaudhry B, Wang J, Wu S, et al. Systematic review: impact of health information technology on quality, efficiency, and costs of medical care. Ann Intern Med. 2006;144(10):742–52.
53. Patel VL, Zhang J, Yoskowitz NA, Green R, Sayan OR. Translational cognition for decision support in critical care environments: a review. J Biomed Inform. 2008;41(3):413–31.
54. Zhang J. Human-centered computing in health information systems part 2: evaluation. J Biomed Inform. 2005;38(3):173–5.
55. Zhang J. Human-centered computing in health information systems. Part 1: analysis and design. J Biomed Inform. 2005;38(1):1–3.
56. Walji MF, Kalenderian E, Piotrowski M, et al. Are three methods better than one? A comparative assessment of usability evaluation methods in an EHR. Int J Med Inform. 2014;83(5):361–7.
57. Horsky J, Kuperman GJ, Patel VL. Comprehensive analysis of a medication dosing error related to CPOE. J Am Med Inform Assoc. 2005;12(4):377–82.
58. Horsky J, Zhang J, Patel VL. To err is not entirely human: complex technology and user cognition. J Biomed Inform. 2005;38(4):264–6.
59. Ash JS, Berg M, Coiera E. Some unintended consequences of information technology in health care: the nature of patient care information system-related errors. J Am Med Inform Assoc. 2004;11(2):104–12.
60. Walji MF, Kalenderian E, Tran D, et al. Detection and characterization of usability problems in structured data entry interfaces in dentistry. Int J Med Inform. 2013;82(2):128–38.

61. Song M, Spallek H, Polk D, Schleyer T, Wali T. How information systems should support the information needs of general dentists in clinical settings: suggestions from a qualitative study. BMC Med Inform Decis Mak. 2010;10:7.
62. D'Antonio NN, Rihs JD, Stout JE, Yu VL. Computer keyboard covers impregnated with a novel antimicrobial polymer significantly reduce microbial contamination. Am J Infect Control. 2013;41(4):337–9.
63. Schleyer T, Thyvalikakath TP. Alert fatigue. J Am Dent Assoc. 2012;143(4):332–3; author reply 333–4.
64. Stefanac SJ, Nesbit SP. Treatment planning in dentistry. 2nd ed. St. Louis, MO: Mosby; 2007.
65. Tokede O, Walji MF, Ramoni RL, et al. Treatment planning in dentistry using an electronic health record: implications for undergraduate education. Eur J Dent Educ. 2013;17(1):e34–43.
66. Cimino JJ, Patel VL, Kushniruk AW. Studying the human-computer-terminology interface. J Am Med Inform Assoc. 2001;8(2):163–73.
67. Ericsson KA, Simon HA. Protocol analysis: verbal reports as data. Rev. ed. Cambridge, MA: MIT Press; 1993.
68. Diaper D, Stanton NA. The handbook of task analysis for human-computer interaction. Mahwah, NJ: Lawrence Erlbaum; 2004.
69. John B, Prevas K, Salvucci D, Koedinger K. Predictive human performance modeling made easy. Paper presented at: Proceedings of CHI, 2004; Vienna, Austria.
70. Brooke J. A "quick and dirty" usability scale. London: Taylor and Francis; 1996.
71. Muller M, Druin A. Participatory design: the third space in HCI. The human-computer interaction handbook. Hillside, NJ: L. Erlbaum Associates Inc.; 2003.
72. Thursky KA, Mahemoff M. User-centered design techniques for a computerised antibiotic decision support system in an intensive care unit. Int J Med Inform. 2007;76(10):760–8.
73. Teixeira L, Saavedra V, Ferreira C, Santos BS. Using participatory design in a health information system. Conf Proc IEEE Eng Med Biol Soc. 2011;2011:5339–42.
74. d'Aquino P, Bah A. Multi-level participatory design of land use policies in African drylands: a method to embed adaptability skills of drylands societies in a policy framework. J Environ Manag. 2014;132:207–19.
75. Frauenberger C, Good J, Keay-Bright W. Designing technology for children with special needs: bridging perspectives through participatory design. CoDesign. 2011;7(1):1–28.
76. Pilemalm S, Timpka T. Third generation participatory design in health informatics--making user participation applicable to large-scale information system projects. J Biomed Inform. 2008;41(2):327–39.
77. Ramoni RB, Walji MF, Kim S, et al. Attitudes toward and beliefs about the use of a dental diagnostic terminology: a survey of dental care providers in a dental practice. J Am Dent Assoc. 2015;146(6):390–7.
78. Kohane IS. Secondary use of health information: are we asking the right question? JAMA Intern Med. 2013;173(19):1806–7.
79. International Organization for Standardization. Ergonomic requirements for office work with visual display terminals. Part 11: guidance on usability. Geneva: International Organization for Standardization; 1998.
80. Hornbaeck K. Current practice in measuring usability: challenges to usability studies and research. Int J Hum-Comput Stud. 2006;64:79–102.
81. Association for Computing Machinery CHI. Measuring usability: are effectiveness, efficiency, and satisfaction really correlated? Paper presented at: Conference on Human Factors in Computing Systems, 2000; The Hague, The Netherlands.
82. Walji MF, Kalenderian E, Stark PC, et al. BigMouth: a multi-institutional dental data repository. J Am Med Inform Assoc. 2014;21(6):1136–40.
83. Walji MF, Spallek H, Kookal KK, et al. BigMouth: development and maintenance of a successful dental data repository. J Am Med Inform Assoc. 2022;29(4):701–6.
84. Saleh MH, Decker A, Wang HL. Using the BigMouth repository for periodontal medicine. Breaking the chains? J Periodontol. 2023;94(3):311–2.

85. Tokede B, Yansane A, White J, et al. Translating periodontal data to knowledge in a learning health system. J Am Dent Assoc. 2022;153(10):996–1004.
86. Messing M, de Souza LC, Cavalla F, et al. Investigating potential correlations between endodontic pathology and cardiovascular diseases using epidemiological and genetic approaches. J Endod. 2019;45(2):104–10.
87. Rodriguez JL, Thakkar-Samtani M, Heaton LJ, Tranby EP, Tiwari T. Caries risk and social determinants of health: a big data report. J Am Dent Assoc. 2023;154(2):113–21.
88. Saenthaveesuk P, Kiat-Amnuay S, Walji MF. Using electronic dental records to assess osteoradionecrosis risk in irradiated head and neck cancer. JDR Clin Trans Res. 2023;8(3):244–56.
89. Kalenderian E, Tokede B, Ramoni R, et al. Dental clinical research: an illustration of the value of standardized diagnostic terms. J Public Health Dent. 2016;76(2):152–6.
90. Kumar SV, Yansane A, Neumann A, et al. Measuring sealant placement in children at the dental practice level. J Am Dent Assoc. 2020;151(10):745–54.
91. Brandon RG, Bangar S, Yansane A, et al. Development of quality measures to assess tooth decay outcomes from electronic health record data. J Public Health Dent. 2023;83(1):33–42.
92. Centers for Medicare & Medicaid Services. Medicare dental coverage. Baltimore, MD: Centers for Medicare & Medicaid Services; 2013. Available from: http://cms.hhs.gov/Medicare/Coverage/MedicareDentalCoverage/index.html
93. Bebinger M. Put back the teeth? Why we separate dental and medical care. WBUR's CommonHealth Reform and Reality; 2014.
94. Advisory Committee on Training in Primary Care Medicine and Dentistry. Interprofessional education. Rockville, MD: Health Resources and Services Administration; 2013.
95. Berwick DM, Nolan TW, Whittington J. The triple aim: care, health, and cost. Health Aff (Millwood). 2008;27(3):759–69.
96. Simon L, Obadan-Udoh E, Yansane AI, et al. Improving oral-systemic healthcare through the interoperability of electronic medical and dental records: an exploratory study. Appl Clin Inform. 2019;10(3):367–76.
97. Adibi S, Li M, Salazar N, et al. Medical and dental electronic health record reporting discrepancies in integrated patient care. JDR Clin Trans Res. 2020;5(3):278–83.
98. Schleyer T, Eisner J. The computer-based oral health record: an essential tool for cross-provider quality management. J Calif Dent Assoc. 1994;22(11):57–8; 60–1;63–4.
99. Powell VJH, Din FM. Rational and need to articulate medical and dental data. New York: Springer; 2011.
100. Health Level 7 International. HL7/ASTM implementation guide for CDA® R2 -continuity of care document (CCD®) release 1. Ann Arbor, MI: Health Level 7 International. [cited 2014 May 4]. Available from: http://www.hl7.org/implement/standards/product_brief.cfm?product_id=6
101. Health Level 7 International. Health Level Seven and the American Dental Association sign agreement to develop joint healthcare IT standard initiatives. Ann Arbor, MI: Health Level 7 International; 2009.
102. Rajkumar N, Muzoora M, Thun S. Dentistry and interoperability. J Dent Res. 2022;101(11):1258–62.
103. Kalenderian E, Halamka JD, Spallek H. An EHR with teeth. Appl Clin Inform. 2016;7(2):425–9.
104. Hill HK, Stewart DC, Ash JS. Health information technology systems profoundly impact users: a case study in a dental school. J Dent Educ. 2010;74(4):434–45.
105. Ramoni RB, Etolue J, Tokede O, et al. Adoption of dental innovations: the case of a standardized dental diagnostic terminology. J Am Dent Assoc. 2017;148(5):319–27.
106. Obadan-Udoh E, Simon L, Etolue J, et al. Dental providers' perspectives on diagnosis-driven dentistry: strategies to enhance adoption of dental diagnostic terminology. Int J Environ Res Public Health. 2017;14(7):767.
107. Patel VL, Kaufman DR. Medical informatics and the science of cognition. J Am Med Inform Assoc. 1998;5(6):493–502.

108. Uretz M. 10 reasons why your dental practice will soon be using Electronic Health Records (EHRs). 2014 [cited 2014 Jul 14]. Available from: http://practicemanagement.dentalproductsreport.com/technology-ehr/10-reasons-why-your-dental-practice-will-soon-be-using-electronic-health-records-ehrs
109. Uretz M. ADA professional product review. 2014;9(2). Available from: http://www.dentalsoftwareadvisor.com/wp-content/uploads/2014/05/PPR_Vol_9_Iss_2_April_2014_PDF.25-29.pdf

Further Reading

Benoit B, Frédéric B, Jean-Charles D. Current state of dental informatics in the field of health information systems: a scoping review. BMC Oral Health. 2022;22(1):1–17.

Kalenderian E, Ramoni RL, White JM, et al. The development of a dental diagnostic terminology. J Dent Educ. 2011;75(1):68–76.

Muller M, Druin A. Participatory design: the third space in HCI. The human-computer interaction handbook. Hillside, NJ: L. Erlbaum Associates Inc.; 2003.

Norman DA. Human-centered design considered harmful. Interactions. 2005;12(4):14–9.

Obadan-Udoh E, Simon L, Etolue J, et al. Dental providers' perspectives on diagnosis-driven dentistry: strategies to enhance adoption of dental diagnostic terminology. Int J Environ Res Public Health. 2017;14:767. https://doi.org/10.3390/ijerph14070767.

Yansane A, Tokede B, Etolue J, Walji M, Obadan-Udoh E, Kalenderian E. Utilization and validity of the dental diagnostic system over time in academic and private practice. JDR Clin Trans Res. 2019;4(2):143–50. https://doi.org/10.1177/2380084418815150.

Chapter 15
The Unintended Consequences of the Technology in Clinical Settings

Amy Franklin and Jeritt Thayer

Introduction

Unintended consequences (UCs) are direct and indirect outcomes that are outside of expectation. In the context of healthcare, this includes the unanticipated impact of health information technology (HIT) on clinical practice. For example, although electronic health record (EHR) systems may improve access to information through the use of standardized fields, the increased documentation demands may cause busy doctors to enter data into free text fields rather than attempt to search for the "right" location in a structured field. Downstream effects of this extra documentation burden include additional effort required for subsequent users of that data by other stakeholders. This is because other users must either assume that the information is unavailable or search for it outside its expected location.

The recent surge in HIT, particularly EHR systems, has spurred discussion and research into its potential consequences, including unanticipated outcomes. From physician complaints and praise of EHRs to patients' reports regarding the impact on visits, interaction with HIT has altered healthcare processes. Headlines in the

---

A. Franklin
D. Bradley McWilliams School of Biomedical Informatics at UTHealth Houston, Houston, TX, USA
e-mail: Amy.Franklin@uth.tmc.edu

J. Thayer
D. Bradley McWilliams School of Biomedical Informatics at UTHealth Houston, Houston, TX, USA

Department of Pediatrics, Perelman School of Medicine at the University of Pennsylvania, Philadelphia, PA, USA

popular media have pointed out the changes to how medicine is practiced in the digital age [1–3]. One often-cited example of unintended consequences in HIT is the changing dynamics of the doctor-patient interaction when using an EHR system. It is no longer just the doctor and the patient in the room: EHRs add a "third party", the computer, to the patient visit. This results in changes to workflow, including alteration of the patient's narrative [4] as well as changes in communication behaviors such as eye contact [5]. All of these may adversely impact patient care quality and patient satisfaction. These are **unintended consequences** of technology that is not intended in its design. As healthcare delivery evolves, for example in the use of telemedicine during the Covid pandemic, we must remain mindful of the unanticipated outcomes of technology use.

Although HIT systems, including EHRs, have great potential for improving healthcare quality and safety, it is necessary to elucidate and manage the outcomes that were not foreseen or intended in the design and implementation of the system. Unintended consequences, though commonly thought of as being unexpected *problems* created by a system, are not always negative. Technology may provide benefits beyond its intended design. Serendipitous benefits may include repurposing of tools beyond their original purpose. For example, Kuziemsky et al. [6] provide examples in which physicians found a new use for their data entry and process monitoring system developed for palliative care. By leveraging the features that helped physicians visualize data for developing care plans, doctors found that sharing the visual depictions of patient's disease progression (e.g., medication needs, pain reports) aided difficult conversations with family members regarding end of life decision-making. Similarly, the Covid pandemic spurred the use of virtual clinical rounds to limit contact and the need for protective equipment. Although some results indicate challenges with this shift in format [7], there are positive unintended consequences seen by some in which virtual rounds demonstrated improvements in patients' length of stay along with positive changes to standardize round content [8].

This chapter discusses the unintended consequences (UC) of HIT in clinical practice. We begin with examples of how computerized physician order entry (CPOE) created unforeseen outcomes in clinical care. Additionally, we consider how the architecture of organizational systems of HIT can impact clinical practices as well as the consequences of increased access to clinical information on doctor-patient relationships. We also consider how changes in care delivery and policies, such as telemedicine use from Covid demands, have led to ongoing consequences to patient care. Following a literature review, we use these instances to discuss the dimensions of different frameworks for classifying UCs. Next, we consider potential mechanisms underlying UCs and touch on issues regarding the constraints of human cognition, usability of devices, and work processes described in other chapters of this volume. Finally, we look at reported issues on common UCs in HIT and outline proposed solutions. Through a better understanding of UCs, particularly those generated through human-computer interaction (HCI), we can build systems that mitigate negative UCs and reap the benefits of serendipity in unanticipated positive outcomes.

Defining Unintended Consequences

The idea of unexpected outcomes is not unique to healthcare, nor is it always mediated by technology. The disciplines of philosophy, sociology, and even economics have discussed unintended consequences over the course of the past few centuries (see for example Adam Smith's The Theory of Moral Sentiments [9]). An analogous phenomenon is commonly observed in biological systems. For example, introducing new sources of food such as rabbits or new crops can solve a short-term food supply problem, while leading to long-term issues including the disruption of the ecosystem (e.g., lack of predation leads to overpopulation of rabbits that decimate other food sources such as crops). The first modern definition of UCs as direct and indirect outcomes not intended by purposeful action was popularized in the 1930s by the sociologist Robert Merton [10]. Through his research, Merton attempted to explain why human actors were unable to anticipate outcomes in complex systems. Although Merton's argument was a philosophical discussion regarding the limitations of human reasoning, his ideas have been applied in other domains for understanding outcomes that are outside of expectation.

Merton's treatise centered on understanding UCs via potential sources of causation. UCs could be understood as leading from errors in assumptions, (un)-informed tradeoffs in short versus long term gain, and the impact of culture/policy. This theme of classifying UCs by causation re-emerges in later frameworks. However, Merton's ideas on UCs continued to evolve over time to include other components. For example, rather than focusing solely on causation, other frameworks have separated UCs along dimensions of outcome (e.g., negative or positive results, expected or unanticipated from design).

Research by Ash and colleagues [11] provides the seminal framework for unintended consequences in HIT. In their hierarchy, the singular notion of unintended consequences has been broadened. First, consequences are split into anticipated or unanticipated outcomes, i.e., not predicted. Next, the dimension of the **desirability** of the outcome is considered. This allows for the traditional negative/undesirable, unanticipated and thus unintended consequence as well as unexpected and yet desirable outcomes of serendipity. The inclusion of desirability shifts the focus from prediction (i.e., anticipation) of the outcome to a new examination of the actual outcomes (i.e., positive or negative results). In this framework, expected negative outcomes can be considered **risks or tradeoffs** (*undesired but anticipated results*), which differ substantively from the negative surprises of UCs.

Figure 15.1 depicts the hierarchy created by Ash et al. [11] expressing both benefits and negative consequences through direct process measures as well as indirect outcomes. In this framework, only unanticipated and undesired consequences are deemed unintended. Although this hierarchy focused on CPOE use, the attributes of anticipation, desirability and direct/indirect outcomes can be generalized to classifying consequences in other domains (including those outside HIT). The above hierarchy highlights both the positive and negative consequences; however, much of the literature (and the popular press) has focused on *unintended adverse consequences*.

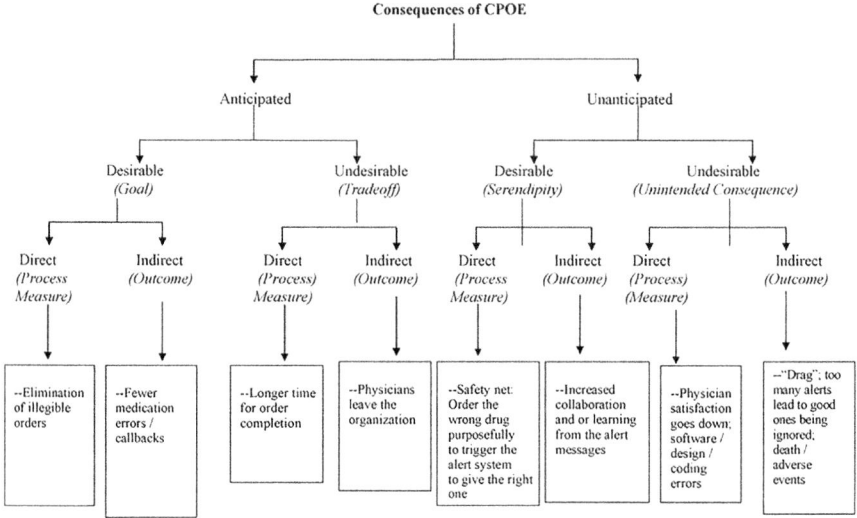

Fig. 15.1 Ash et al.'s [11] hierarchy (Reprinted with permission from Ash et al. [11])

Campbell et al. [12] provide a typology for looking just at these negative outcomes, again with a CPOE focus.[1] Campbell and her team interviewed and observed clinicians (including physicians, nurses, pharmacists, and allied healthcare providers) at five hospital sites. Using a grounded theory approach and card sorting techniques, they first distilled shared themes from across observations and interviews. Next, in the card sort, with clinician assistance, they grouped the ideas presented into nine classes of negative unanticipated outcomes. These categories, organized as a typology, add a finer classification grade to the discussion of UCs.

Campbell's typology included categories for generalizing across problems and mapped UCs to their underlying outcomes. For example, the additional work generated by technologies can vary from transformed work practices and workflow to additional required effort (e.g., documentation, and handling new decision support alerts). Respondents noted that there is simply more work to be done compared to the paper-based clinical practice at sites within their study. Other classes of UCs include a poor fit between the human-computer interface and the context of use, unintended overload of individual cognitive and collective work processes, and changes to coordination and communication practices. Of course, at this point in time, some of those consequences can be construed as anticipated. As with Ash et al.'s hierarchy, several instances within this typology are extensible to other forms of healthcare products beyond CPOE, including medical devices, communication tools and other technology.

While the above typologies focus on an expectation of outcomes, sociotechnical models reevaluate UCs through a systems' lens. Rather than focusing only on the

---

[1]CPOE is often the HIT component under study given its rich and tangible connection between design and potential safety events such as medication errors.

technology, these models were developed with foundations in systems research. They were based on the idea that the impact of HIT can only be understood while considering its social, organizational and technical context of use [13, 14]. They depict complex and interdependent components of the health care system, including users' characteristics, workflow, organizations, policy, and the health information technology itself.

In Harrison et al.'s Interactive Sociotechnical Analysis (ISTA) [15], UCs were not seen as created by the HIT system (e.g., failure to fully understand the impact of design); instead the consequences were understood as resulting from different types of interactions. ISTA depicts the emergent relationships between HIT, clinicians, and workflows. Technology is viewed as part of the complex system that is shaped by the technical and physical infrastructure within which it resides. The system as a whole is understood as the interaction and interdependence among its components. UCs in this framework are not solely classified by *anticipation* of their design (e.g., anticipated use/unanticipated outcomes), rather ISTA considers how HIT is actually *used* within a given context. Thus, interaction type is used to define UCs rather than the intent or outcome. The five interaction types include: (1) new HIT changes existing social system, (2) technical and physical infrastructure mediates HIT use, (3) social system mediates HIT use, (4) HIT-in-use changes social systems, and (5) HIT-social system interactions engender HIT redesign. Instances of new HIT changing the existing social system include UCs such as new/more work on tasks such as documentation, changes to informal interactions yielding communication changes, or alterations in workflow such as shifts in roles and responsibilities. As illustrated in Table 15.1, Harrison et al. incorporate both Campbell's typology [14] as well as the work on communication and information transfer by Ash et al. [11, 18] into their interaction types. Importantly, ISTA shifts the focus from causation or outcome of UCs to pointing out the impact and differences of *systems in use* from the ways in which the *systems were*

Table 15.1 Unintended consequences by ISTA type (Reprinted with permission from Harrison et al. [15])

ISTA type	Unintended consequences[a]
1. New HIT changes social system	***More/new work for clinicians*** [12] • Physicians spend more time on documentation and justification. ***Changes in communication patterns and practices*** • Introduction of IT leads to decline of vital interactions among care providers, ancillary services and units.[b] • IT system eliminates informal interactions and redundant checks that help catch errors. ***Workflow*** • CPOE undermines informal gatekeeping by clerk who decided whether patients really needed daily X-rays.
2. Technical and physical infrastructure mediate HIT use	***Paper persistence*** [12] • Paper used to solve problems of lack of integration of CPOE and other clinical information systems.

(continued)

Table 15.1 (continued)

ISTA type	Unintended consequences[a]
3. Social system mediates HIT use	***New types of errors*** [12] • Busy physicians enter CPOE data in miscellaneous section rather than scrolling for optimal location. Improper placement can impede use by other physicians and by CPOE systems. • Causing cognitive overload by overemphasizing structured and "complete" information entry or retrieval [16] ***Fragmentation*** • Distribution of information over several screens sometimes leads busy physicians to miss key parts of record, such as interpretations or reports by other types of physicians. ***Structure, overcompleteness*** • Extensive reporting requirements lead physicians to cut and paste whole reports, rather than extracting pertinent facts. ***Paper persistence*** [12] • Counter to hospital directives and recommended IT practice, MDs who prefer paper records annotate CPOE printouts and place these in patient charts as formal documentation. ***Misrepresenting collective, interactive work as linear, clear cut, predictable workflow*** [16] • *Inflexibility*: *Transfers*: Inflexible EHR reporting requirements generate failures to record clinically appropriate drug administration and cause difficulties in managing patient transfers. • *Urgency*: Nurses and Physicians refuse to follow data-entry rules requiring physician pre-authorization for urgent care. • *Workarounds*: Physicians and nurses provide urgent care by working around cumbersome procedures. ***Misrepresenting communication as information transfer*** [16] • *Decision support overload*: Alert fatigue: Physicians ignore warnings and reminders. • *Loss of communication*: Urgent requests and some test results from accident and emergency, admissions are never viewed on ward terminal. • *Loss of feedback*: Nurses initial orders on receipt, rather than administration, so physicians cannot tell if orders have been carried out. ***Human-computer interface unsuitable for highly interruptive context*** [16] • Juxtaposition errors • Entry of orders for or on behalf of the wrong person
4. HIT-in-use changes social system	***Changes in the power structure*** [12] • Narrow, role-based authorizations redistribute work—Requiring physicians to enter orders directly. • Remote monitoring by the organizations undermines physicians' autonomy. • IT, quality assurance departments, administration gain power by requiring physician to comply with CPOE-based directives. • In decentralized systems, internal variations in CPOE uses and configurations increase interdepartmental conflicts and competition.
5. HIT-social system interactions engender HIT redesign	***Never-ending system demands*** [12] • As implemented CPOE systems evolve, users rely more on the software, demand more sophisticated functionality, & customize software (e.g., physicians create their own order sets). New features must be added to original software. Interactions among multiple variations of the software in use make CPOE system unmanageable & require replacement with newer versions.

Table 15.1 (continued)

[a]The headings for the types of unintended, negative consequences cited by Campbell and colleagues [12] are the short forms that appear in the Discussion section of their paper. A subsequent paper [17] uses the same headings with minor variations

[b]Also treated in Ash and colleagues [16] (misrepresenting communication as information transfer—loss of communication). The italicized and bold type headings from the paper by Ash and colleagues are abbreviated versions of headings appearing in italics in the body of their paper. Their subtypes appear in [15] in italics but without bold and are shown as modifiers to the main headings

[c]Also treated in Ash and colleagues [16] under misrepresenting communication as information transfer—loss of communication catching errors

designed. Harrison's framework offers a richer and more nuanced analysis and provides significant potential for remediation through redesign.

The 2009 American Medical Informatics Association (AMIA) Annual Health Policy meeting focused on outlining "outcomes of actions that are not originally intended in a particular situation (e.g., HIT implementation)." The resulting publication [19] from a panel of experts considered another perspective on sociotechnical systems and consequences. In their article, Bloomrosen et al. put forth a model with inputs and outputs that span domains including:

- *Technology*: hardware and software systems that are implemented and the constraints they impose.
- *Human factors and cognition*: thought processes, habits of behavior, and mental capabilities that humans bring to the use of HIT tools and processes.
- *Organization*: embedding of technology in the complex environment of healthcare organizations.
- *Fiscal/policy and regulation*: the legislative and regulatory environment governing the design, implementation, and use of HIT such as HIPPA requirements, indicators of meaningful use and standards for health information exchange.

In this input-output model, interactions define the model as they did in ISTA. The domains of technology, organization and human factors, along with the addition of policy and regulations converge into a sociotechnical system with an even broader scope. Complicated interactions yield outcomes that can be understood in terms of types of consequences and the affected stakeholders. Like the ISTA framework, Bloomrosen's efforts frame UCs as a study of interactions. The input-output model specifies stakeholders (i.e., inputs) as well as results or outcomes as components within the sociotechnical system. The complexity of the system underscores the need to understand points of input to the unintended consequences. For example, poor usability of an interface can increase the cognitive burden on the clinicians by requiring searching for a returned laboratory value in a sea of electronic, scanned, and paper data. Cognitive factors such as limited memory and attention coupled with a poorly designed or cluttered interface may engender potential UCs. These inputs can lead to output (i.e., consequences) that may impact both cognitive (e.g., diagnostic reasoning) and clinical processes for patients and providers. At another level of analysis, organization

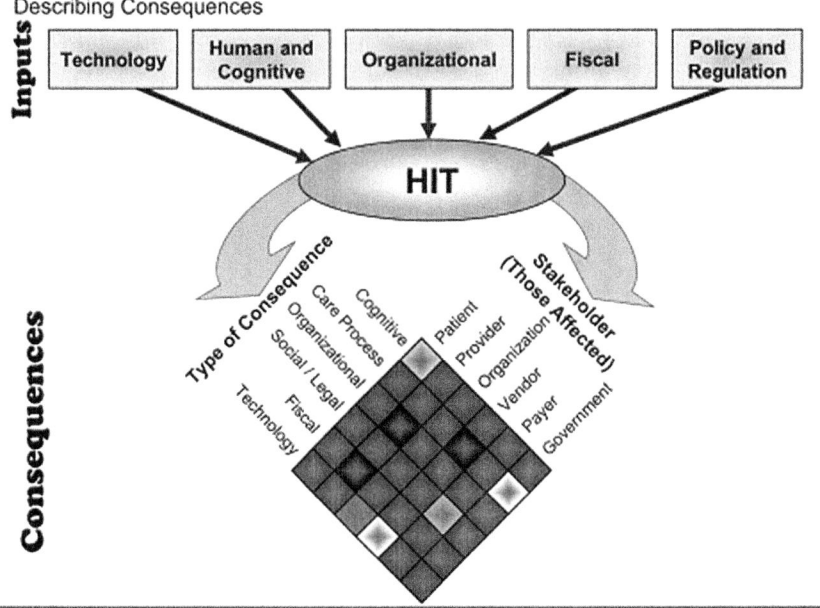

Fig. 15.2 Input-output model (Reprinted with permission from Harrison et al. [15])

policy may serve to mitigate or exacerbate these consequences. In this example, documentation requirements could lead to workflow changes generating further unanticipated outcomes.

This multi-faceted model depicted in Fig. 15.2 underscores the shifting view of UCs as an individual problem to a perspective in which UCs is considered as complex and situated in system-wide issues. Embedding HIT into sociotechnical frameworks highlights the need to consider all the interactions of inputs and products of work in design.

Exploring Unanticipated Consequences

The potential unintended impacts of HIT in clinical settings are wide-ranging, including the risk of harm to patients, inefficiencies in work practices, and unnecessary costs [20]. Just as UCs can occur with technology [21], introducing new devices, or new processes, have the potential for both beneficial and harmful effects beyond the expectation of the product developers. CPOE-based problems are well documented issues related to unintended consequences of the use of healthcare technology [11, 12, 16, 18–24].

Some of the technology-induced errors are derived from the user interface. Reckman and colleagues [25] review identified problems created by poor usability including incorrect drug selection induced by lengthy drop-down menus [26], and duplicate orders or failures to discontinue medications [27]. Subsequent problems also arose when unexpected consequences led to downstream issues. For example, Computers on Wheels (CoW) were used to move computers to the patient's bedside seamlessly. Having a computer at the point of care can potentially prevent errors in identification, reduce interruptions, and improve the completeness of procedures such as documentation. Combined with bar code technology, CoW can improve medication administration by reducing medication errors (i.e., scan the patient, scan the medication to prevent errors). However, Koppel et al. identified 15 kinds of modified workflows in use while using the barcode medication administration technology [23]. For example, the authors identified an instance where the potential benefits of bar code/CoW systems were thwarted when these units were too large to fit into the patients' rooms. Rather than scanning patient wrist identification at the *bedside*, nurses would print out extra bar codes *outside* the room. Such alterations to clinical practice can have downstream effects and, in fact, can lead to identification errors this technology was originally intended to prevent.

Similarly, the introduction of order sets into emergency medicine was intended to safeguard patients and moderate physician burden by prompting ordering tests and procedures. However, a recent study found these generalized order sets lead to potentially unnecessary costs and resource consumption [20].

HIT may not function as expected in the real world implementation. For example, alerts for drug-drug or drug-allergy problems triggered during the prescribing process. If too many alerts are delivered, clinicians may fail to acknowledge the appropriate and relevant alerts. Additionally, the high rate of potential notifications can lead to *alert fatigue* [28], and subsequently introduce technology-induced errors. Often drug-drug and drug-allergy alerts were simply overridden. Payne et al. [29] found an 88% override rate for drug interaction alerts, and a 69% override rate for drug-allergy alerts. Similarly, Weingart et al. [30] found ambulatory physicians overrode 91% of drug-allergy alerts, and 89% of high-severity drug-drug interaction alerts. A percentage of these alerts may have provided limited detail (e.g., notifying the physician that no drug information was available in system) and perceived to be uninformative, presented information with unknown clinical significance (e.g., lacking indicators of the severity of an interaction), or may have repeated the content of previous messages.

Carspecken et al. [31], in a case study, described an instance where a two-year-old child was admitted to a pediatric intensive care unit (PICU) with a documented antibiotic allergy. Over a 1-month, more than 100 alerts related to a drug-allergy cross-reactivity were overridden, as the treatment was deemed a requirement for the patient's condition (i.e., ignoring what was considered an inappropriate alert). Over time, it was determined that the child had an allergic hypersensitivity, and his medical record was eventually amended. However, even after this change, the now appropriate alert (i.e., acknowledging that the child does have an allergy) was *still* overridden. Due to the routine rejection of the alert, clinical staff had become desensitized to drug-allergy alerts in this child's case.[2]

---

[2]This case has additional complications regarding the appropriateness of sulfonamide allergies. Please see the original publication for details.

There are multiple issues at the heart of this example. First, the unintended consequence of new/additional work led to an increased burden on the physicians. Subsequently, the repeated alerts decreased clinicians' sensitivity to the message resulting in inappropriate persistence of behavior (i.e., continued override of the alert.) Additionally, the EHR did not make the addition/change to the allergy list salient to the users of the system. Finally, the unintended changes to the workflow, particularly around communication practices regarding medications, may have led to less feedback and decreased opportunities to prevent this error.

We can break the case down into its component parts to situate it within the previously described UC frameworks. Within Campbell's CPOE typology and Ash's work on communication, this case study includes communication failures (e.g., misrepresenting communication as information transfer [21]), demonstrates new types of errors not found in paper-based systems, and shows how changes to communication practices can lead to unanticipated outcomes. Sociotechnical system models could also include discussion regarding how the social system mediated HIT use including changes in assignment of roles (i.e., who maintains the allergy list and notifies others) as well as workflows. To prevent these types of errors in the future, changes to the work system would be necessary to provide more nuanced and context-sensitive decision support. This would include having appropriate content, including severity of interactions, visible changes for new alerts, and appropriate timing of alerts in the decision process.

Ongoing research shows potential improvement in adherence to alerts (rather than overriding them) by improving the relevance of alert messages [32]. Shah et al. [33] found that with appropriate design, it is possible to generate high rates of alert acceptance by clinicians. In their study of 18,115 drug alerts generated during a 6-month study period, 67% of *interruptive* but informative alerts were accepted in spite of its impact on workflow.

Modifying a system to prevent or fix an existing problem can also introduce other unintended consequences. For example, Strom et al. [34] identified the complexities surrounding the unintended consequences of trying to prevent errors in a CPOE system that in turn created new problems. In this study, a hard stop, or a required step in the ordering process by which no further action can occur until a response is produced, was added to the ordering process. It was intended to promote adherence to decision support by preventing concomitant orders for a known hazardous sulfa drug interaction (i.e., warfarin and trimethoprim-sulfamethoxazol). Their clinical trial exploring the effectiveness of this hard stop was halted when it was determined that four patients received delayed treatment as a consequence of changes to the medication-ordering process. In those cases, concurrent prescribing was in fact appropriate and the hard stop should have been overridden. Like the pediatric study, this case provides an example of the complicated process for determining system rules, workflows, and challenges to anticipating all potential outcomes for decision support choices. Other ways in which unintended consequences emerge are through workarounds or additional unplanned innovations [35]. When systems fail to support workflow in an acceptable fashion, users may innovate and introduce new paths for completing their tasks and goals.

Just as with consequences, workarounds can have positive or negative impacts. For example, Vogelsmeier et al. [36] studied five nursing homes to uncover workaround practices related to electronic medication administration records. They found two types of workarounds: those associated with the system interface, and those related to organizational processes. For example, when the CDS alerted that medication was "excessive" in dose, nurses entered multiple within-range doses in order to measure up to the requested dose (rather than directly speaking with a physician or pharmacist). Other system requirements were managed by a "flouting" policy. For example, in these nursing homes, there was a requirement for separate documentation, one for preparation of medication and another one subsequent to the administration of the medication. Nurses would often only note the process prior to administration of medication, and ignore the post-administration records. If delays occurred, or if the medication was not actually administered, it would not be accurately reflected on the patient record. Similarly, when voluminous printouts of medication orders were required to complete the policy-driven fax for prescription, nurses often elected to follow a speedier (but not supported) process of calling-in medication orders.

Some workaround cases are complex events for which it may be difficult to define a singular unintended outcome, potential cause, or solution. As Bloomrosen's input-output model suggests, to understand the triggers of these events, and to work towards managing such outcomes, the inputs (clinicians, technology, organizational policy and the social structure), interactions, and outputs must all be considered in the system in which the work occurs. In these circumstances, triggers to the event include the changes to the interactions of the nurses and physicians, the adaption of clinicians to technology, workers negotiating organizational policy and the social structure that guides their actions. All of these contribute to the "excessive" dose workaround. The way in which a nurse enters drug information is only one of the many problems. Solutions to these kinds of cases are not as straightforward as changing specific algorithms in decision support systems. Rather, consideration should be given to the communication practices and policies that lead to these events, as well as the HIT demands.

Workarounds arising from a gap between the system intended workflow and actual practice are so prolific that a framework for understanding them has been created. The Sociotechnical EHR Workaround Analysis (SEWA) defines the work system and the sociotechnical components in which EHR workarounds emerge along with explicating the rationales for their creation as well as defining workaround attributes, and their impact on clinical processes and outcomes [37]. Ongoing iterative assessments are needed to help redesign systems that accomplish their needed function without creating negative unintended outcomes.

In addition, here are basic computer functions that lead to significant frustration. For example, the onerous demands of documentation are an often-touted (perhaps, even shouted) unintended consequence of EHR implementation. All of that new work could be supported by judicious copy and paste within clinical notes. Seventy-four to ninety percent of physicians use the copy-paste function in their EHRs, and between 20 and 78 percent of physician notes are copied text [38]. However, many are concerned that this function is not being used appropriately [39, 40]. Issues with copied text include the potential for lost information as reviewing notes becomes a hunt for new or different information. In addition, other clinicians caring for the same patient may elect not to read the patient notes which contain copious amounts of redundant or uninformative text. There is also a concern that copying and pasting could lead to inappropriate billing [41]. The American Health Information Management Association (AHIMA) provides a stakeholder perspective on the issues of copy and paste. As the association for health information management (as compared to clinicians using the health record system), this organization has a broad interest in the use of these basic computer functions. In their position paper [41], AHIMA proposes that copy and paste (i.e. cloning, identical documentation) should be used only under technical and administrative control and with well-trained users, potentially limiting the adverse outcomes of this function. This example also demonstrates how multiple sources (i.e., stakeholders) must be considered as input to the event and the solution. While copy and paste may be an individual activity, organizational policy, technological constraints and socio-cultural practice can define (or even regulate) how this activity is completed. Copy and paste could well be an issue within the EHR systems that may someday be constrained by Federal regulation.

Paper persistence, similar to copy and paste, offer short-term solutions to HIT problems that may have an impact on long-term consequences. The inability to satisfy the demand of having access to an EHR system, as well as simple preference for physical documents can lead to the persistence of paper in the presence of electronic solutions. Some people like that napkin as a note tucked in their pocket, while others are forced to create paper-based workarounds due to the constraints of their HIT systems. In a study on consultation practices at a Veterans Affairs Medical Center, Saleem et al. [42] explored how paper persisted as a means of communicating and coordinating between physicians, even in the presence of electronic consultation tools. They found that the use of paper documents and informal notes persisted for a 5-year period when electronic processes were already in place. Coordination workarounds were a common response to limitations in the EHR system, for example, delays in notifying primary care physicians that a consult report was available. Preferences for homegrown solutions such as compact spreadsheets listing multiple patients and individual checklists, were also common workarounds.

Concerns for these behaviors include maintenance of dual paper and electronic records: paper persistence engenders the potential consequence that handwritten information may not become part of the electronic record, and gaps in information retrieval may occur as individuals may not be exhaustive in their search for information. When evaluating the differences across paper and electronic sources, Kannampallil et al. [43] found that a local optimization process drove information-seeking across paper and electronic documents. Physicians gathered information from sources that maximized their information gain even though it required significantly more cognitive effort. Unintended consequences are often the product of poorly supported cognitive processes. We may mitigate these consequences if we are able to better support processes like information search.

Following the rapid adoption of EHRs within the United States, unintended outcomes of EHR have been seen from the health-system level through failed expectations and the challenges at the bedside [44]. As EHR systems have been implemented and even replaced by new systems, we continue to the proliferation of new forms of unintended consequences [45]. For example, as systems have changed from monolithic structures to newer distributed architectures the data used as part of the HIT may no longer reside on the same physical infrastructure where the computation of that data may occur. In these situations, data must be transferred across an information network, which is subject to "unbounded delays", meaning the data may be transfered immediately (e.g. within a few milliseconds) or take an indeterminate amount of time [46]. This is especially problematic in a clinical environment, where delays can directly impact patient care, and violates widely held beliefs about the importance of the speed of health information systems [47]. Rubins et al. [48] recently highlighted the potential clinical impact of delayed CDS on providers while placing imaging orders with some requests taking up to 60 s to return. Stemming in part from the challenge of delays in information transfer are problems of concurrency (or race conditions), where two separate processes (can be from the same or different systems) attempt to access and/or update a piece of data simultaneously. Documented examples of race conditions are rare within the health literature, but two examples include near-simultaneous order entry silencing duplicate alert CDS [49] and the rapid opening and closing of an externally embedded CDS [50]. Race conditions are particularly concerning given their ability to create discordant views of the data in question, which can lead to clinical decisions based on inaccurate data. Additional administrative and legal factors must be considered beyond the technical consequences of transitioning to distributed systems. For example, a common model within the distributed system community is the service-oriented architecture, where several software services (known as components) are connected to create a single application. This has several advantages including scalability and reusability, but it can also create a reliance on several external vendors who may have different service level agreements and data use agreements.

Human Factors Models

The sociotechnical frameworks for understanding UCs focus on the systems in which technology is used. Macroergonomic models that emerged from a human factors engineering approach to patient safety (including UCs) similarly embrace a systems-centered perspective [51]. Karsh et al.'s Human Factors (HF) Paradigm [52] is exemplified by a principle that the goal should be to *"design work systems that support and enhance work process performance"* and that safety, risk, and all other outcomes then flow from the accommodation of the system to this work. Well-designed systems would support typical efforts and should be robust and resilient enough to reinforce work under *challenging conditions*, such as high patient load. Although the HF paradigm focuses on error and harm (the worrisome potential outcomes of UCs), Holden [53] suggests that HIT improves or worsens outcomes depends on how that system impacts cognitive performance. In his extension of this paradigm to EHRs, Holden proposes that cognitive performance processes are the mediating mechanism between a work system and outcomes. Rather than saying failures in design lead to error, harm or unintended consequences, Holden outlines how the work system either positively or negatively affects cognitive performance.[3] The resulting themes from Holden's interviews of clinicians surface many of the same unintended consequences previously outlined in the UC literature such as the burden of extra cognitive effort generated from poor displays, impacts on workflow including extra steps, and communication changes including simply less face-to-face time. Likewise, the SEIPS (Systems Engineering Initiative for Patient Safety) models [54–56] echo many of the components of Bloomrosen's Input-Output model in that they both share the idea of interacting components encompassing clinicians, technology, human interaction, and external factors such as policy. Importantly, the SEIPS model includes feedback loops between the work system and care processes, and between the work system and outcomes that provide support for redesign. These human factors engineering models provide a means for discussing potential interventions to systems to safeguard patient safety. Federal programs have recently provided more direct and immediate methods for assessing the risk of UCs as briefly discussed in the next section.

Solutions

Finding productive means to manage unintended consequences can take many forms. As Holden [53] suggests, redesigning work systems to support cognitive processes is necessary. We view that this redesign would include not only features of the technology but also the social and organizational structures. As Bloomrosen et al. [19] suggest, regulation and policy may also play a role. Funding through the Office of the National Coordinator (ONC) and the Agency for Healthcare Research and Quality (AHRQ) has spawned research programs along the development of guidelines to understand and mitigate UCs. Examples of the output from these efforts are the AHRQ *Guide to Reducing Unintended Consequences of Electronic Health Records* [45] and the *Safety Assurance Factors for EHR Resilience (SAFER) Guides* [57]. The AHRQ Guide provides detailed support in understanding and identifying unintended consequences in EHR systems as well as suggestions for remediation. Through a series of case studies, this guide highlights areas of concern and references research in each area. For example, the guide describes a case in which the implementation of a nursing documentation system unintentionally duplicated efforts (both paper and electronic forms were completed) as part of a policy requirement for a specific type of documentation (here, patient social function). Process assessment and redesign are provided as suggested solutions.

---

[3] In line with Hollnagel and Woods, all performance, or work, in healthcare is considered cognitive, from procedures to decision-making, including the cognitive processes of mental, physical, social, and behavioral activities.

As Jones et al. suggests in this guide [58], corrective actions may fall into one or more broad categories: (a) software change, (b) training for local IT staff, (c) configuration change, (d) custom programming, (d) care process change and (e) policy change. As these corrective actions may be costly both in terms of time and effort, remediation plans detailing the problem, its impact, the scope of the request, stakeholder involvement as well as benefits from change may all be necessary to justify the price of change. Such plans may therefore vary in their ranking of importance for patient safety, user satisfaction and desirability for corrective action.

The *SAFER* guidelines [59]), also put out by ONC and AHRQ, are designed to help care delivery organizations conduct self-assessments of recommended practices in those areas important to the safe use of health information technology. These efforts are part of the Health IT Patient Safety Action and Surveillance Plan. Some of the guides such as those targeting CPOE and Lab results detail unintended consequences in these systems and provide assessments of system function.

Other federal efforts include ONC initiatives for EHR certification requirements for usability testing with public reporting. These requirements have increased the dialogue regarding user and system performance. Summative testing is one way of uncovering unintended consequences in ready-to-deploy or implemented products. The potential inclusion of formative testing requirements as part of the 2015 rule may prevent some UCs from reaching end users through discovery and recovery during development. Regional Extension Centers (RECs) and Health Information Technology Research Centers (HITRC) are other programs funded by ONC which may help in supporting UC capture and remediation by providing support directly to providers.

Professional organizations such as the American Medical Informatics Association (AMIA), Healthcare Information and Management Systems Society (HIMSS) and American Health Information Management Association (AHIMA) have also sponsored efforts supporting HIT implementation and the identification of unintended consequences.

Serendipity and Struggle: Unintended Consequences of HIT and the Covid Pandemic

The impact of the recent pandemic echoes in all aspects of modern life from work practices to supply chain struggles. Throughout this public health event we saw the interdependence of our sociotechnical systems. Policies regarding vaccines, social distancing, and masking changed how we interacted and drove the adoption of different means of achieving our healthcare needs. As we shift into post-pandemic times, we see the continued use of some of the need driven solutions.

Telemedicine is one such aspect [59–61]. The need to provide ongoing care for patients while preserving safety practices led to increased use of technology to support care at a distance. As with other forms of HIT, the benefits of continued care and drivers of innovation within telemedicine are offset by the challenges incurred by shifting a previously physically based interaction to a new virtual medium. Changes to the physical assessment and documentation of the physical state were one such loss [62]. Additionally, disparities occur in groups with difficult access to the necessary technology [63] or virtual conferencing systems [64]. Persistence of telemedicine following policy changes has continued to reap the benefits of improvements in triage processes, reach of services, and meeting new desires in patient preferences [65–67]. As with EHR systems, federal agencies and academic organizations are developing guidance to support telehealth practices including the AHRQ 2023 Safety Program for Telemedicine.

Conclusions

To understand and support HIT in clinical practice, we must recognize the impact of the complex sociotechnical system of healthcare in both contributing to unintended consequences as well as discovering solutions to managing these emerging issues. Through a better understanding of UCs, particularly those generated through human-computer interaction, we can build systems that mitigate negative UCs and reap the benefits of serendipity in unanticipated outcomes.

Discussion Questions
1. Sociotechnical models highlight the interwoven factors of individual, organizational, and technical components surrounding unintended consequences (UCs). Do solutions for UCs necessarily have to bridge domains? For example, can solutions occur at only one level such as the technical component, or does the management of UCs require responses from multiple inputs? As an example, consider the impacts of Covid policies on HIT use.
2. How can we capture the unintended consequences of HIT experienced by clinical users (i.e. patients and communities)? How should healthcare systems weigh the benefits and burdens across the full system?

References

1. Campbell KR. Embrace the age of digital medicine. KevinMD.com; 2014.
2. Meisel ZF. The health IT paradox: why more data doesn't always mean better care. 2011 Jan 12 [cited 2014 Aug 29]. Available from: http://content.time.com/time/health/article/0,8599,2041900,00.html
3. Campbell KR. Practicing medicine in the digital age: challenges & opportunities of the virtual encounter. 2014 [cited 2014 Aug 29]. Available from: http://www.eplabdigest.com/blog/Practicing-Medicine-Digital-Age-Challenges-Opportunities-Virtual-Encounter
4. Lown B, Rodriguez D. Lost in translation? How electronic health records structure communication, relationships and meaning. Acad Med. 2012;87(4):3.
5. Al-Jafar E. Exploring patient satisfaction before and after electronic health record implementation: the Kuwait experience. Perspect Health Inf Manag. 2013;10(Spring):1c.

6. Kuziemsky CE, Borycki E, Nøhr C, Cummings E. The nature of unintended benefits in health information systems. Stud Health Technol Inform. 2012;180:896–900.
7. Bavare AC, Goldman JR, Musick MA, et al. Virtual communication embedded bedside ICU rounds: a hybrid rounds practice adapted to the coronavirus pandemic. Pediatr Crit Care Med. 2021;22(8):e427–36. https://doi.org/10.1097/PCC.0000000000002704.
8. Nimmagadda K, Pancrazi S, Martino A, et al. Virtual multidisciplinary rounds to reduce length of stay, decrease variation, and promote accountability. Jt Comm J Qual Patient Saf. 2023;49(9):450–7.
9. Smith A. The theory of moral sentiments (Soares SM, editor). MetaLibri; 2005.
10. Merton RK. The unanticipated consequences of purposive social action. Am Sociol Rev. 1936;1(6):894–904.
11. Ash JS, Sittig DF, Dykstra RH, et al. Categorizing the unintended sociotechnical consequences of computerized provider order entry. Int J Med Inform. 2007;76(Suppl 1):S21–7.
12. Campbell EM, et al. Types of unintended consequences related to computerized provider order entry. J Am Med Inform Assoc. 2006;13(5):547–56.
13. Fox W. Sociotechnical system principles and guidelines: past and present. J Appl Behav Sci. 1995;31(1):91–105.
14. Cummins TS, Srivastva S. Management of work: a sociotechnical systems approach. San Diego: University Associates; 1977.
15. Harrison MI, Koppel R, Bar-Lev S. Unintended consequences of information technologies in health careDOUBLEHYPHENan interactive sociotechnical analysis. J Am Med Infom Assoc. 2007;14(5):542–9.
16. Ash JS, Berg M, Coiera E. Some unintended consequences of information technology in health care: the nature of patient care information system-related errors. J Am Med Inform Assoc. 2004;11(2):104–12.
17. Ash JS, Sittig DF, Poon EG, Guappone K, Campbell E, Dykstra RH. The extent and importance of unintended consequences related to computerized provider order entry. J Am Med Inform Assoc. 2007;14(4):415–23. https://doi.org/10.1197/jamia.M2373.
18. Ash JS, Sittig DF, Dykstra RH, Campbell EM, Guappone KP. The unintended consequences of computerized provider order entry: findings from a mixed methods exploration. Int J Med Inform. 2009;78(Suppl 1):S69–76.
19. Bloomrosen M, Starren J, Lorenzi NM, et al. Anticipating and addressing the unintended consequences of health IT and policy: a report from the AMIA 2009 Health Policy Meeting. J Am Med Inform Assoc. 2011;18(1):9.
20. Frutos EL, Muñoz AM, Rovegno L, et al. Can CPOE based on electronic order sets cause unintended consequences (expensive and unnecessary tests) at the emergency department? Stud Health Technol Inform. 2022;290:192–6. https://doi.org/10.3233/SHTI220059.
21. Tenner R. Why things bite back: technology and the revenge of unintended consequences. New York: Randon House; 1997.
22. Campbell EM, Sittig DF, Guappone KP, Dykstra RH, Ash JS. Overdependence on technology: an unintended adverse consequence of computerized provider order entry. AMIA Annu Symp Proc. 2007;2007:94–8.
23. Koppel R, Metlay JP, Cohen A, et al. Role of computerized physician order entry systems in facilitating medication errors. JAMA. 2005;293(10):1197–203.
24. Weiner JP, Kfuri T, Chan K, Fowles JB. "e-Iatrogenesis": the most critical unintended consequence of CPOE and other HIT. J Am Med Inform Assoc. 2007;14(3):387–8; discussion 389.
25. Reckmann MH, Westbrook JI, Koh Y, Lo C, Day RO. Does computerized provider order entry reduce prescribing errors for hospital inpatients? A systematic review. J Am Med Inform Assoc. 2009;16(5):613–23.
26. Shulman R, Singer M, Goldstone J, Bellingan G. Medication errors: a prospective cohort study of hand-written and computerised physician order entry in the intensive care unit. Crit Care. 2005;9(5):R516–21.

27. Koppel R, Leonard CE, Localio AR, et al. Identifying and quantifying medication errors: evaluation of rapidly discontinued medication orders submitted to a computerized physician order entry system. J Am Med Inform Assoc. 2008;15(4):461–5.
28. Steele AM, DeBrow M. Efficiency gains with computerized provider order entry. In: Henriksen K, Battles JB, Keyes MA, Grady ML, editors. Advances in patient safety: new directions and alternative approaches (Vol. 4: Technology and medication safety). Rockville, MD: AHRQ; 2008.
29. Payne TH, Nichol WP, Hoey P, Savarino J. Characteristics and override rates of order checks in a practitioner order entry system. Proc AMIA Symp. 2002;2002:602–6.
30. Weingart S, Toth M, Sands DZ, et al. Physicians' decisions to override computerized drug alerts in primary care. Arch Intern Med. 2003;163(21):2625–31.
31. Carspecken CW, Sharek PJ, Longhurst C, Pageler NM. A clinical case of electronic health record drug alert fatigue: consequences for patient outcome. Pediatrics. 2013;131(6):e1970–3.
32. Weingart SN, Seger AC, Feola N, Heffernan J, Schiff G, Isaac T. Electronic drug interaction alerts in ambulatory care: the value and acceptance of high-value alerts in US medical practices as assessed by an expert clinical panel. Drug Saf. 2011;34(7):587–93.
33. Shah NR, Seger AC, Seger DL, et al. Improving acceptance of computerized prescribing alerts in ambulatory care. J Am Med Inform Assoc. 2006;13(1):5–11.
34. Strom BL, Schinnar R, Aberra F, et al. Unintended effects of a computerized physician order entry nearly hard-stop alert to prevent a drug interaction: a randomized controlled trial. Arch Intern Med. 2010;170(17):1578–83.
35. Strauss A, Fagerhaugh S, Suczek B, Wiener C. Social organization of medical work. Transaction Publishers; 1997.
36. Vogelsmeier AA, Halbesleben JR, Scott-Cawiezell JR. Technology implementation and workarounds in the nursing home. J Am Med Inform Assoc. 2008;15(1):114–9.
37. Blijleven V, Koelemeijer K, Jaspers M. SEWA: a framework for sociotechnical analysis of electronic health record system workarounds. Int J Med Inform. 2019;125:71–8.
38. Bowman S. Impact of electronic health record systems on information integrity: quality and safety implications. Perspect Health Inf Manag. 2013;10:1c.
39. Hripcsak G, Vawdrey DK, Fred MR, Bostwick SB. Use of electronic clinical documentation: time spent and team interactions. J Am Med Inform Assoc. 2011;18(2):112–7.
40. Hirschtick RE. A piece of my mind. Copy-and-paste. JAMA. 2006;295(20):2335–6.
41. McCann E. EHR copy and paste? Better think twice. Healthcare IT NEWS; 2013.
42. Saleem JJ, Russ AL, Neddo A, et al. Paper persistence, workarounds, and communication breakdowns in computerized consultation management. Int J Med Inform. 2011;80(7):466–79.
43. Kannampallil TG, Franklin A, Mishra R, Almoosa KF, Cohen T, Patel VL. Understanding the nature of information seeking behavior in critical care: implications for the design of health information technology. Artif Intell Med. 2013;57(1):21–9.
44. Colicchio T, Cimino J, Del Fiol G. Unintended consequences of nationwide electronic health record adoption: challenges and opportunities in the post-meaningful use era. J Med Internet Res. 2019;21(6):e13313. https://doi.org/10.2196/13313.
45. Huang C, Koppel R, McGreevey JD 3rd, Craven CK, Schreiber R. Transitions from one electronic health record to another: challenges, pitfalls, and recommendations. Appl Clin Inform. 2020;11(5):742–54. https://doi.org/10.1055/s-0040-1718535.
46. Kleppmann M. Designing data-intensive applications: the big ideas behind reliable, scalable, and maintainable systems. 1st ed. O'Reilly Media; 2017.
47. Bates DW, Kuperman GJ, Wang S, et al. Ten commandments for effective clinical decision support: making the practice of evidence-based medicine a reality. J Am Med Inform Assoc. 2003;10(6):523–30. https://doi.org/10.1197/jamia.M1370.
48. Rubins D, Wright A, Alkasab T, et al. Importance of clinical decision support system response time monitoring: a case report. J Am Med Inform Assoc. 2019;26(11):1375–8.
49. Schreiber R, Sittig DF, Ash J, Wright A. Orders on file but no labs drawn: investigation of machine and human errors caused by an interface idiosyncrasy. J Am Med Inform Assoc. 2017;24(5):958–63.

50. Thayer JG, Miller JM, Fiks AG, Tague L, Grundmeier RW. Assessing the safety of custom web-based clinical decision support systems in electronic health records: a case study. Appl Clin Inform. 2019;10(2):237–46. https://doi.org/10.1055/s-0039-1683985.
51. Carayon P, Xie A, Kianfar S. Human factors and ergonomics as a patient safety practice. BMJ Qual Saf. 2014;23(3):196–205.
52. Karsh BT, Holden RJ, Alper SJ, Or CKL. A human factors engineering paradigm for patient safety: designing to support the performance of the healthcare professional. Qual Saf Health Care. 2006;15(Suppl 1):i59–65.
53. Holden RJ. Cognitive performance-altering effects of electronic medical records: an application of the human factors paradigm for patient safety. Cogn Tech Work. 2011;13(1):11–29.
54. Carayon P, Hundt AS, Karsh BT, et al. Work system design for patient safety: the SEIPS model. Qual Saf Health Care. 2006;15(Suppl 1):i50–8.
55. Carayon P, Smith M. Work organization and ergonomics. Appl Ergon. 2000;31(6):649–62.
56. Carayon P, Wooldridge A, Hoonakker P, Hundt AS, Kelly MM. SEIPS 3.0: Human-centered design of the patient journey for patient safety. Appl Ergon. 2020;84:103033. https://doi.org/10.1016/j.apergo.2019.103033.
57. SAFER guides. Washington, DC: Office of National Coordinator for Health Information; 2017.
58. Jones SS, Koppel R, Ridgely MS, et al. Guide to reducing unintended consequences of electronic health records. Rockville, MD: Agency for Healthcare Research and Quality (AHRQ); 2011.
59. Smith AC, Thomas E, Snoswell CL, et al. Telehealth for global emergencies: implications for coronavirus disease 2019 (COVID-19). J Telemed Telecare. 2020;26(5):309–13.
60. Monaghesh E, Hajizadeh A. The role of telehealth during COVID-19 outbreak: a systematic review based on current evidence. BMC Public Health. 2020;20(1):1193.
61. Zhou X, Snoswell CL, Harding LE, et al. The role of telehealth in reducing the mental health burden from COVID-19. Telemed J E Health. 2020;26(4):377–9.
62. Hiremath RN, Sinha P, Ghodke S, Manjunath SR, Vishwanath K. Telemedicine: basics, utilization and challenges during covid pandemic. Res Highlights Dis Health Res. 2023;4:39–46. https://doi.org/10.9734/bpi/rhdhr/v4/5591A.
63. Crawford A, Serhal E. Digital health equity and COVID-19: the innovation curve cannot reinforce the social gradient of health. J Med Internet Res. 2020;22(6):e19361. https://doi.org/10.2196/19361.
64. Alsabeeha NHM, Atieh MA, Balakrishnan MS. Older adults' satisfaction with telemedicine during the COVID-19 pandemic: a systematic review. Telemed J E Health. 2023;29(1):38–49. https://doi.org/10.1089/tmj.2022.0045.
65. Gupta VS, Popp EC, Garcia EI, et al. Telemedicine as a component of forward triage in a pandemic. Healthc (Amst). 2021;9(3):100567. https://doi.org/10.1016/j.hjdsi.2021.100567.
66. Hincapié MA, Gallego JC, Gempeler A, Piñeros JA, Nasner D, Escobar MF. Implementation and usefulness of telemedicine during the COVID-19 pandemic: a scoping review. J Prim Care Community Health. 2020;11:2150132720980612. https://doi.org/10.1177/2150132720980612.
67. Tenforde AS, Borgstrom H, Polich G, et al. Outpatient physical, occupational, and speech therapy synchronous telemedicine: a survey study of patient satisfaction with virtual visits during the COVID-19 pandemic. Am J Phys Med Rehabil. 2020;99(11):977–81. https://doi.org/10.1097/PHM.0000000000001571.

Further Reading

Bloomrosen M, Starren J, Lorenzi N, Ash JS, Patel VL, Shortliffe E. Anticipating and addressing the unintended consequences of health IT and policy: a report from the AMIA 2009 Health Policy Meeting. J Am Med Inform Assoc. 2011;18(1):9.

Colicchio TK, Cimino JJ, Del Fiol G. Unintended consequences of nationwide electronic health record adoption: challenges and opportunities in the post-meaningful use era. J Med Internet Res. 2019;21(6):e13313.

Sittig DF, Salimi M, Aiyagari R, Banas C, et al. Adherence to recommended electronic health record safety practices across eight health care organizations. J Am Med Inform Assoc. 2018;25(7):913–8. https://doi.org/10.1093/jamia/ocy033.

Turner P, Kushniruk A, Nohr C. Are we there yet? Human factors knowledge and health information technology–the challenges of implementation and impact. Yearb Med Inform. 2017;26(01):84–91.

Chapter 16
The Role of Human Computer Interaction in Consumer Health Applications: Current State, Challenges and Future

Holly B. Jimison and Misha Pavel

Introduction

Health technologies for use by consumers and patients run the gamut from Web pages for browsing health information to disease management systems involving real-time measurement and tailored feedback on mobile phones, watches and ubiquitous devices throughout the home. In this chapter, we will consider consumer health applications to be the set of technologies used by consumers to promote their health and wellbeing. One of the distinctions of this chapter, from the rest of the medical informatics applications described in this book, is that the primary user of the technology is the consumer or patient. Interactive consumer health technologies offer a scalable and potentially cost-effective mechanism for engaging individuals in their own care, certainly an important component of healthcare reform, as healthcare becomes more proactive and takes place outside the hospital and clinic.

In contrast to medical technologies designed for specific clinicians with common training and levels of education, with consumer health applications we find additional challenges in designing for a broad base of consumers with varying educational, cultural, language and literacy levels. The need to communicate medical and health information in lay language with meaningful graphics adds an additional level of complexity. The following sections will provide an overview of the field, as well as background and guidance on addressing the needs of specific populations of consumers of healthcare.

H. B. Jimison (✉) · M. Pavel
Khoury College of Computer Information Sciences, Northeastern University, Silicon Valley Campus, San Jose, CA, USA
e-mail: h.jimison@northeastern.edu; m.pavel@northeastern.edu

© The Author(s), under exclusive license to Springer Nature Switzerland AG 2024
A. W. Kushniruk et al. (eds.), *Human Computer Interaction in Healthcare*, Cognitive Informatics in Biomedicine and Healthcare,
https://doi.org/10.1007/978-3-031-69947-4_16

Overview of Consumer Health Informatics

Interactive consumer health technology applications are increasingly recognized as an important component of healthcare services. The Institute of Medicine's (IOM) report on Crossing the Quality Chasm [2] discussed fostering self-management support by encouraging providers to use education and other supportive interventions in order to systematically increase patients' skills and confidence in managing their health problems. Two of their recommended initiatives refer to patient-centered care and informatics. Patient-centered care is aligned with consumer health informatics in that it aims to inform and involve patients and their families in their decision-making and self-management, apply principles of disease prevention and behavioral change appropriate for diverse populations, and understand patients' concepts regarding their illness and their cultural beliefs. They additionally recommended informatics approaches to communicate, manage knowledge, and support decision-making using information technology [1]. Examples of basic consumer-facing technologies for health include searchable Web portals for health information (e.g., WebMD.com or MayoClinic.com) and Web access to curated patient education content, such as the Healthwise Knowledgebase [2]. These are currently perhaps the most commonly used consumer health applications. Although they include some degree of tailoring information for the user (e.g., body mass index calculators), real-time monitoring systems that adapt to individual users' inputs and provide tailored responses or advice can be much more powerful [3, 4]. For example, such interactive health technologies may include home monitoring sensors with interactive disease-management or self-management technology, educational or decision-aid software that is interactively tailored to a patient's needs, online patient support groups, tailored interactive health reminder systems where interactions are linked with electronic medical records, and patient-physician electronic messaging [3].

Johnson et al. used a framework of modes of engagement to categorize basic types of consumer health informatics applications, with categories of communication, data storage, behavior management, and decision support. Table 16.1, adapted from their chapter in Shortliffe and Cimino's book on Biomedical Informatics Computer Applications in Health Care and Biomedicine [5], provides definitions and examples of such systems. This framework and classification scheme shows that consumer health applications range from simple browsing for health information to interactive systems that provide tailored advice and interventions. In the category of Communication, we include online support groups and social networking sites that deal with health issues.

For example, a person interested in learning about multiple sclerosis (MS) could find structured background information at a Web site like Johns Hopkins Medicine's Health Site [6] or the Cleveland Clinic's Site on MS. [7] The first steps would be viewing the sections on learning the basics, which would cover symptoms, vocabulary, causes, risk factors, tests and diagnoses, and complications of the disease. The use of video, graphics, simple language and a clear organization can help users successfully navigate these sites and help them obtain the information they need.

Table 16.1 Categorization of types of consumer health informatics applications (adapted from Johnson et al. [5])

Mode of engagement	Definition	Examples
Communication	Support for patient-to-patient, computer-to-patient and patient-to-provider communication or information dissemination	Patient portals Patient-physician secure email Online support groups Social networking sites
Data storage	A patient-centered and managed repository for patient-entered data	Personal health records Data portals for home monitoring devices
Behavior management	Tools to support personal health goals, often by combining data storage, care protocols, information dissemination, and communication	Weight management tools Physical activity tools Medication reminder systems
Decision support	Tools to prepare patients to participate in 'close call' decisions that involve weighing benefits, harms, and uncertainty	Interactive tools for treatment decisions for breast ca, prostate ca, back pain, end of life, heart disease

Further sections on treatment options, finding a doctor, advice on managing the condition, and links to ongoing clinical trials become important for those diagnosed with MS. Many health websites with disease specific information also offer online support groups. There are several ways in which patients can reach out to one another online. Some sites offer a service where patients can rate their therapies and share results, load and share video testimonials, share tips for living with a particular disease, and have ongoing remote text discussions as a group. Many support groups link through Reddit or Facebook. Some organizations offer online support groups with expert moderators, such as myHealthteam.com's set of community support groups [8]. Both types of services serve important functions. Much of the care for chronic conditions, such as MS, occurs at home and has to do with managing symptoms and adhering to treatment goals. Oftentimes, other patients who have long-term experience with a condition can be most helpful. Additionally, the health benefits of social support from patients in the same situation can be very powerful [9, 10]. Researchers have found improved quality-of-life outcomes not only for patients enrolled in face-to-face support groups for diagnoses like breast cancer [11], but also for online patient support groups [12]. The social support provided by patients with similar issues can serve to provide empathy and encouragement in a way that is difficult for clinicians or even family members. Additionally, patients who have already learned to cope with self-management challenges can offer just-in-time information to patients struggling to cope. The website PatientsLikeMe.com addresses these issues and includes the feature of crowd-source answers to patients' questions [13]. An online venue makes these connections more accessible and convenient. Additionally, the anonymity encourages a more honest and open dialogue [12]. It is important that the computer interface design of the online systems facilitate these important features for patients. Representative interface design issues include clearly communicating the level of privacy and security of the data being shared, and helping the consumer in distinguishing advertising and misinformation from legitimate health information.

Other examples of consumer health applications include personal health records, decision support tools, and health behavior change systems. Personal health records offer users a mechanism to store and retrieve their health information. Those that are linked to specific health systems often additionally offer secure patient-physician email, appointment setting, and medication renewals. Decision support tools for patients have run the gamut from early interactive video systems designed to integrate patient preferences on potential health outcomes into medical treatment decisions such as prostate or breast cancer treatments to Web-based systems that lead patients through background material and assessments for tailored feedback on their health care decisions [14]. Finally, systems that offer monitoring and performance feedback (i.e., the Fitbit or Apple Watch devices) can be clustered in Table 16.1 under Health Behavior Change systems. User feedback from the monitoring itself has been shown to influence behavior change [15], but for many chronic conditions such as diabetes, asthma and heart failure, it is important to have sophisticated behavior change protocols in consumer systems that can be facilitated by a coach or nurse care manager [16]. Changing health behaviors is challenging, and user interface design for the necessary prompts and reminders becomes critical to the success of these systems.

Consumer health applications may be implemented on a variety of platforms using Web/Internet technology, desktop computer applications, touch screen kiosks or tablets, cell phones, smart watches, or combinations of the above. The human computer interaction implications of deploying these types of health interventions on varying display devices with varying types of consumers generates many challenges for designers. The subsequent sections further elucidate these challenges and offer potential design guidance.

Needs Assessment as Part of Interface Design for Consumers

Interface design for a new health information technology must originate with a careful needs assessment and understanding of goals and tasks to be performed. In the case of designing a system for consumers, it is important to anticipate the characteristics of the intended users. A first step is to define the varying age ranges, different cultures, and different education levels. It is important to determine whether there will be separate systems for use by specific groups or whether the interface and content need to be adapted to the type of user. Needs assessment techniques such as focus groups and interviews with stakeholders can provide feedback to inform these design choices. An example of an iterative needs assessment is described in Jimison's study on multimedia tools for informed consent [17]. The initial challenge in this example was to address the needs of patients with varying forms of cognitive impairment as they went through the informed consent process for a medical intervention or research trial. Standard consent materials were often written at above the college level when considering trials with complex protocols. The study addressed how best to tailor materials to address both literacy (addressed in more detail in a following section) and cognitive complexity of the consent process. To explore these challenges, the researchers selected consent procedures associated with trials for patients with schizophrenia, depression, and newly diagnosed patients with breast cancer. Design specifications for a tool to help patients decide whether or not to volunteer for a trial were developed with input from a series of focus groups with representative patients with experience in these types of trials. The resulting prototype was then tested again as stimulus material with similar focus groups, followed by usability testing of a following iteration and then a trial comparing paper consents to the multimedia decision aid. Interestingly patients newly diagnosed with breast cancer patients were found to be the most decisionally impaired, wanting almost uniformly to defer to their doctor. Patients with schizophrenia were better able to focus with a tool that kept the amount of material on any one screen minimal, let patients browse for further information, and then bring them back to the main points. A needs assessment with users, encouraging participatory design, is helpful, especially for rapidly changing technologies.

How Culture Influences Design Choices

Culture is an umbrella term used to refer to a multi-layered construct influenced by language, education, societal rules and religion [18, 19]. Designing user interfaces for people with different cultural and health beliefs requires adapting and incorporating a variety of factors. People from different countries/cultures use interfaces in different ways, prefer different graphical layouts and have different expectations in how the health technology interacts [16]. Therefore, user interfaces should be designed to accommodate the cultural differences of the target end users to provide an optimal user experience [19]. If you have ever tried to assemble furniture produced in another country using instructions roughly translated to your language, you probably have a sense of the frustration or confusion non-native consumers have when using health information systems that have been crudely adapted to their language using word-by-word translations instead of looking for the cultural meaning to convey. The success of a consumer health intervention in a new culture critically depends on careful and meaningful message adaptation. Additionally, visuals containing graphics with colors may seem to have an agreed upon interpretation for many people in the United States with common experiences, but quite different when shown to immigrant populations or subgroups with a nonstandard exposure to the media.

As an example of the benefits of user testing of health content, the Los Angeles Cancer Education Project conducted a learner verification of a number of national and local publications with potential users from their Hispanic community [20]. The materials were found to be unsuitable "because they dealt with facts rather than with people and their concerns," meaning that the patients' emotional responses were felt to be more salient and of concern than finding out medical facts about cancer. The feedback from this resulted in a new publication based on one extended family's experiences with cancer: Hablaremos Sobre Cancer de la Familia (Let's Talk About Cancer Among the Family) [20]. This became the centerpiece for a comprehensive community effort to detect early cancer. Family participation for cancer detection was more culturally appropriate than individual participation. Culture involves common beliefs, values, traditions, lifestyle, communication, region, and the way you look at the world. Another interesting location requiring multiple styles of communication and influencing interface design occurs in the Hawaiian Islands. There are several ethnic subcultures there, including Hawaiian, Portuguese, Chinese, Japanese, Korean, Caucasian, Filipino, Vietnamese, Samoan, and other Pacific Island ethnic groups, often identified as native Hawaiian. Each group, on average, has different cultural expectations for communication styles and this influences how best to use (or not use) technology to communicate health messages (e.g., screening for cancer or appointments) [21, 22]. Chinese and Caucasian cultures tend to prefer a more direct style, Japanese a more formal style, and native Hawaiians a more indirect approach that first addresses social needs. It is important for designers of health technology tools to consider communication styles as part of the human computer interaction design process.

Designing for Populations with Health Disparities

There are several subpopulations in the United States who are predisposed to worse health outcomes than other groups. For example, African Americans when compared to non-Hispanic white Americans, have higher rates of obesity, hypertension, cardiovascular disease and higher infant mortality [23]. Similarly, Hispanic populations also have worse health outcomes when compared to whites. Latino and Hispanic populations have higher incidences of diabetes, hypertension and obesity in addition to double the amount of cervical cancer among Latino/Hispanic women [23]. Perhaps most strikingly, Native Americans are twice as likely to have diabetes as compared with whites [24]. However, in addition to race and ethnicity, health disparities occur across a broad range of factors, such as age, gender, income, geography, language, educational level, and sexual orientation [25]. It is critical for new health technologies to address the needs of underserved and disadvantaged populations.

When designing user interfaces for these groups, there are several key considerations to address [26]. Disparities in education and income levels are intertwined with health disparities. Approximately 16% of African Americans and Hispanics live below the federal poverty line. 37.7% of Hispanics and 16.1% of African Americans aged 25 and older did not complete high school [27]. It is important that the design of health technology interfaces facilitate bridging the digital divide and embrace disenfranchised populations or those who are medically underserved.

Several studies have demonstrated creative designs targeted to the needs and preferences of a variety of populations. These studies have shown that interfaces that contain culturally appropriate content are more effective than purely language translations [27, 28].

Access Issues and the Digital Divide

The access to technology for consumer health information and patient-facing interventions has presented a challenge to researchers, policy makers and clinicians with an interest in the equitable delivery of care. Populations who most need health information often lack the means, knowledge, and skills necessary to benefit from Internet health resources. The adoption of internet connectivity in households initially became a large factor in the digital divide with regard to health care and health access in the United States. Many demographic groups, including African Americans, Latinos, non-English speaking Asians, rural and elderly were slow to adopt the new technologies. Over the years, the Pew Research Foundation has continued to track internet and technology use. They have found that adoption challenges included (1) no service available in their area, (2) lack of affordability, (3) not understanding how to use it, (4) lack of trust, and (5) not perceiving the usefulness [29, 30]. These factors drove disparities for communities of color [31], low-income households [30], and rural populations [32]. Government and industry groups have subsequently made progress in closing the gaps, primarily with wireless connectivity. By 2011, wireless internet use was nearly equal for African Americans, Latinos and whites, with usage rates between 62% and 63% [32]. Remarkably, one of the Pew Reports found that 15% of African Americans and 11% of Hispanics had downloaded a mobile app to track or manage their health, as compared to only 7% of whites [29]. Internet usage has been changing rapidly over the years. As of 2021, 91% of adults in the U.S. are connected to wired or wireless broadband and 85% own a smartphone [33]. About 15% of adults solely use their smartphones for internet access, with an increase to 25% for Latino and 17% for African Americans [33]. It is important to track and understand these trends when addressing health issues for minority populations with health disparities with new technologies and interfaces for health interventions.

The design choices that developers of consumer health informatics systems make with regard to media and format have a direct impact on the degree of use by populations of interest. Access by definition affects degree of use. Even though conventional access to health information through more traditional Web interfaces on desktop computers may have less use in minority populations, a design choice to use mobile phones to communicate may actually increase use above the norm in targeted populations.

Design Considerations According to Age

The population of older adults in the U.S. is increasing dramatically. In 2018, there were 52 million people age 65 and older, accounting for 16% of the total U.S. population. The Older Americans report of 2020 projects an increase to 73 million people in this segment by the year 2030 (20% of total U.S. population) [34]. In parallel to this trend is the projected increase in healthcare expenditures for older adults. According to the Centers for Disease Control, Medicare spending has grown in the past 25 years, increasing from $37 billion to $336 billion, a trend that is expected to continue due to the increases in aging populations [35].

Empowering patients will apply to all ages, but age must be taken into account in addition to all other user characteristics in order to optimize the user experience with consumer health technologies. There are age-related declines in several cognitive and sensory-motor skills. For example, psychomotor skills such as dexterity and hand–eye coordination decline with age and these limitations can make it more challenging for older users to learn to use a keyboard or control a mouse device [36]. Age-related declines in working memory and divided attention have very direct implications for interface design [37]. Interface content must be much simpler and less cluttered to allow older users to attend to pertinent material. Rogers and Fisk have found that older adults are limited in their ability to develop automated responses [38], which also has implications for needing to keep interface designs simple and easy to learn. Further, it is important to minimize tasks that might maintain a high cognitive load over time without the development of an automated response. Although there are several types of age-related declines, and many are quite severe with the onset of various pathologies, such as dementia, healthy older adults are quite adaptive in compensating and can continue to perform interactive tasks with technology quite successfully.

An equally important aspect of the design is matching the communication style of the interface to that of the users, as vocabulary changes over time. The communication styles vary significantly across generations and ages, but are very important in creating trust and acceptance on the part of the users. The rapid evolution of communication styles is greatly influenced by the advances in communication technology including email, short message service (SMS) and various social media. Even adults in their 30s and 40s have a hard time keeping up with the rapidly changing tech lingo of the next generation. Language is dynamic and technology content must match the vocabulary of the targeted audience.

The matching of communication styles is not limited to textual information, but rather generalizes to all modalities. In particular, audio and pictorial representation as well as icon-based systems must be adjusted in accordance with the expected age and style of the users. Figure 16.1 shows a simple example of various choices of icons to represent a phone call. The icon on the left is recognizable to older adults, however, most young people will never have seen a dial phone, or perhaps even a land line. Additionally, with the advent of smartphones, physical keypads on a cell phone may not look familiar to some.

Fig. 16.1 Examples of phone icons, showing how the choice of a visual icon may be different for different age groups (Courtesy dreamstime.com)

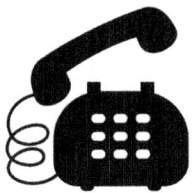
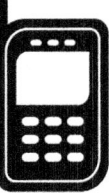
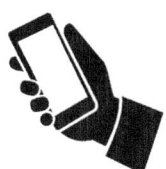

Given the effectiveness of video-based communication as demonstrated by YouTube and similar sites, it is expected that this style of information communication will find increasing applicability in the domain of consumer health informatics. Much like text-based communication, these video-based approaches are likely to comprise a wide range of styles, ranging from cartoon animation, to interactive avatars and human actors.

To summarize this section, the dynamics of the cognitive and sensory-motor skills combined with the heterogeneity in users' knowledge present significant challenges to the developers of interactive systems. Although consumer health information technology has the potential to empower patients to become more active in the care process, the elderly may be disadvantaged unless the designers of both software and hardware technology consider their needs explicitly [37]. The mitigation of these challenges in designing for consumer health technologies across ages and skill levels will be addressed in the section on the Future of Human Computer Interaction for Consumer Health. Despite the concerns addressed in this section, there is evidence suggesting older adults are connecting with technology more than ever before. According to Pew Research again [33], more than 75% of older adults use the Internet or email, however, a majority of older adults preferred simpler technology with fewer features [39, 40].

Additional Design Considerations Based on Chronic Conditions

If designed appropriately, health technology interventions for older adults could contain the costs burden on the healthcare system while simultaneously improving health outcomes for this population. Older populations also experience higher incidences of chronic conditions, and many of these conditions affect a user's ability to interact successfully with health information technology unless specific adaptations are in place. For example, approximately a third of adults between ages 65 and 74 have hearing loss, and most people notice visual problems around the age of 40 [35]. Having adaptable visual and auditory interfaces as options for technology addresses much of the problem. For example, varying font size and contrast options can often address the needs of individuals with mild to medium vision impairment. Common tools with many computers include auditory feedback and screen magnifying software. There are also several software packages for screen reading, converting text to speech. The American Foundation for the Blind provides a review of

18 such systems [41]. An additional visual factor related to designing consumer health systems is that about 8% of the population (mostly males) has a form of color blindness, and confuse either red and green and/or blue and green. The implication here is that interfaces should not rely on just color to convey information.

Arthritis is another common condition that affects users' ability to interact with keyboards, mouse devices and small phone interfaces. Arthritis is a leading cause of work disability, and those with the disease may have difficulty performing physically demanding jobs, and may select jobs that appear less strenuous but require intensive computer use. In 2010–2012, arthritis was the most frequently occurring chronic condition among older persons. 50% of people over 65 were diagnosed with arthritis [35]. A study of 315 arthritis patients found that 84% percent of respondents reported a problem with computer use attributed to their underlying disorder and 77% reported some discomfort related to computer use, mainly reporting problems with finding a comfortable position while using the computer and in manipulating the keyboard and mouse [42, 43]. Newer speech interfaces may serve to alleviate these issues. For example, voice browsers for the Web usually adhere to the World Wide Web Consortium guidelines [34] and use Voice Dialog Extensible Markup Language (VoiceXML) to interpret and encode the Hypertext Markup Language (HTML) of a Web page. Voice browsers serve to both interpret human speech with speech recognition software and generate text-to-speech while interacting with a given Web page. Speech recognition and text-to-speech technology has improved remarkably in recent years, allowing users to interact seamlessly with many devices in the home and workplace. It is important that interface designers take advantage of the opportunities voice technologies allow in improving access and convenience for users.

Health Literacy

Health literacy of the target population is a key concern for the design of both the content and interface of consumer health informatics systems. The lack of understanding of the material will hinder both the use and usefulness of a system. Health Literacy, defined by an IOM report as "the degree to which individuals have the capacity to obtain, process, and understand basic health information and services needed to make appropriate health decisions," is measured across the following domains: (1) cultural and conceptual knowledge, (2) oral literacy, including speaking and listening skills, (3) print literacy, including writing and reading skills, and (4) numeracy [44, 45]. Individual health literacy is most commonly assessed by using the Rapid Estimate of Adult Literacy in Medicine (REALM) and Test of Functional Health Literacy in Adults (TOFHLA) tests. Both these instruments measure reading skills, word recognition, vocabulary, reading fluency and to some extent numeracy [44]. The impact of low health literacy, while a general concern, is particularly important to address when designing for groups with known literacy problems. For example, low health literacy is common among racial and ethnic minorities, older adults, and patients with chronic conditions [3, 46]. Nearly nine of ten adults have trouble using the everyday health information that is routinely available in our healthcare facilities, retail outlets, media, and communities [29]. Among adult age groups, those aged 65 and older have the smallest percentage of people with proficient health literacy skills and the largest percentage with "below basic" health literacy skills [3].

There are several tools for helping designers of consumer health applications to provide appropriate text content. For example, Web sites like the Readability Test Tool [47] and ReadabilityScore.Com [48] provide measures of the reading grade level of any English language text submitted. These tools typically include several standard measures, such as

- Flesch Kincaid Reading Ease [49]
- Flesch Kincaid Grade Level [49]
- Gunning Fog Score [50]
- Coleman Liau Index [51]
- SMOG Index [52]
- Automated Readability Index [53]

The guidelines for developing patient education materials call for maintaining a reading level of grade 5 or below [54]. This can sometimes be quite challenging for designers not trained in writing at this level. FirstClinical.com has a Web tool that assists in this process by providing a glossary of simple health terms [55] and a document analysis tool [56] to ensure readability by a majority of the population.

When considering human computer interaction design in consumer health applications, it is also important to consider what has been termed "eHealth" literacy. The term eHealth refers to health interventions or information using Internet, wireless services, and related technologies [51]. These types of consumer-oriented applications are used to engage consumers in managing their own health care, communicating with clinicians, making health decisions, and adhering to their health behavior change goals [3]. Several researchers have proposed methods for measuring eHealth literacy. For example, vander Vaart et al. use eHEALs, an 8-item scale that measures perceived skills in finding, evaluating and applying electronic health information to health problems [57]. Chan and Kaufman created a theoretical framework for evaluating eHealth literacy [58]. They first considered the dimensions proposed by Norman and Skinner [59] consisting of computer literacy, information literacy, media literacy, traditional literacy and numeracy, science literacy and health literacy. They then integrated a second model to include variation in task performance along a continuum of cognitive demands (e.g., remembering, understanding, applying, analyzing, evaluating, and creating). The goal of this new framework was to elucidate the barriers to effective user performance on intended health management tasks. Given that self-management and consumer engagement are critical to the success of our new models of care, it is now well recognized that we must address the barriers of health literacy and eHealth literacy more specifically as part of healthcare services. This is increasingly recognized as a problem that impacts healthcare quality and costs. However, again, given the recent advances in speech recognition and language translation software that is widely used, the opportunities are great for adapting interfaces to rely much less on text communication or an understanding of the English language. Many of the technology advances can be used to reduce health disparities and make health technologies easier to use.

The Future of Human Computer Interaction for Consumer Health

One important, but often ignored, aspect of interface design involves the consequences of rapid advances in technologies that affect design approaches. We see several important trends in the development of systems used to communicate health information to consumers. First, the interfaces and user designs will be tailored to target populations and potentially to individuals as well. More importantly, these interfaces will continuously adapt to changing user needs, for example, as a consequence of the aging process. Secondly, we will be conducting real-time remote usability testing using video-conferencing techniques for protocol analysis and ecological momentary assessment using just-in-time feedback from mobile phones. Thirdly, many of new health interventions will be delivered via robots, virtual reality headsets, and new immersive technologies [60]. In general, new artificial intelligence approaches (e.g., ChatGPT) will have major impacts on health technologies and how we design user interfaces. It is clear that the move toward pervasive and ubiquitous computing will impact the design of consumer health systems, especially our notion of user interface design and usability testing. The following sections describe the newer approaches to health technology development and user interface design.

New Horizons: Approaches to Developing Adaptive User Interfaces

Throughout this chapter, we noted that interfaces for consumer health informatics systems need to be user specific. In particular, the effectiveness of interactions depends on how closely the interface style is matched to that of the users. In addition, the state, ability and functionality of the user are not constant over time. Some of these changes are predictable; others are highly variable. For example, it is well documented that an individual's perceptual, cognitive and physical functionality declines with aging [3, 36–38]. In contrast, users' health literacy is likely to improve with exposure to information. Less well documented is the short-term variability, for example, as function of the daily variability in the quality of sleep [36]. Given the dynamics of users' characteristics, an important question faced by the designer is how to optimize interfaces with respect to these characteristics. There are many options, but two approaches stand out. The first is based on a prior, population-based characterization of the users, perhaps by clustering them with respect to their age, functionality, communication styles, demographics, socio-economic status, etc. The interface design would then be tailored to the cluster and its characteristics. Individual users would be categorized and assigned to the most appropriate interface. Recent advances in commercial systems (e.g., Amazon.com) have demonstrated the potential of adaptation strategies. For example, a number of Internet-based marketing strategies use history of users' visits to various sites and the targets of their prior clicks. Much like these commercial approaches, using algorithms for collaborative filtering, one could develop interfaces that adapt their style, knowledge level and information content to the specific user. Collaborative filtering methods [61] are based on using large amounts of information on users' quantifiable characteristics, behaviors, activities or preferences and determining similarity among users that is then used to infer their preferences and aspects of interactions. Some early work in this area is described by Yue et al. [62], where researchers used collaborative clustering to anticipate users' intended tasks. We note that this type of implementation would require more basic research concerning the types of data and their implication on the interactions before it can be used as a standard interface design practice.

In an alternate approach, interfaces would be designed to adapt to the communication styles and task-specific information processing capabilities, e.g., domain-specific health literacy of the individual users. A user may be relatively naïve about health issues in general, but in short time acquires significant information about a specific health issue. For example, following a diagnosis of diabetes, an individual may acquire a sophisticated diabetes-related vocabulary. The recent advances in sensor technology, networking and inference algorithms open the opportunity to monitor users' interactions and make inferences about the individuals' states. These inferences can then be used to adapt aspects of the interfaces. Examples of such adaptive actions can be found in the commercial settings where advertisements are geared to the search activities of the users. Emotional responses, as assessed by physiological measurements, can be used to modify consumer information delivery and presentation. In the field of education, interfaces have been adapted in real time through signals of pressure-sensitive mouse devices and wrist sensors for heart rate variability and galvanic skin response. Research versions have been used to categorize level of understanding for users of interactive educational materials (tentative movements and pressure correspond to low levels of understanding, and firm clicks and movements to higher levels of understanding) [63]. There is also indication that in the more distant horizon it is likely that brain-computer interfaces will enable even finer adaptation and thus track the changing functionality of elderly users. This fits within the field of Neuroergonomics—the study of the human brain in relation to performance in everyday settings, including interactions with devices and systems [64, 65]. One of the objectives of this nascent discipline is to enhance our understanding of how humans interact with technology and thereby improve the scientific underpinning of user interface design.

New Horizons: Remote Usability Testing of Consumer Health Systems

Given that most consumer health systems are used in the home or workplace, it is important that future usability testing occur in these naturalistic settings and occur in real-time. Traditional usability testing takes place in a controlled laboratory setting where a sample of users are asked to perform representative tasks with the technology being tested, typically while talking aloud as in protocol analysis or task analysis. The advantages to this approach have been that video recordings of the user's face, speech, and interactions with the technology can be carefully recorded and later analyzed. However, the set of interactions tested can be quite limited and typically do not have normal background distractions or a normal context. Early attempts at remote usability testing of naturally occurring interactions with Web sites used sequences and timings of user clicks to infer intent and to look for potential misunderstandings. The advantages were that the data collection was inexpensive and it was possible to test all users of a site. The downside was not truly knowing what users were thinking or whether they were successful. For mobile phone health interventions it is possible to use the newer techniques of Ecological Momentary Assessment (EMA) [66, 67] for testing some aspects of usability. EMA is used more generally for health assessments, where questions are sent to a user's phone based on time, location, and/or context. These questions can be adapted to verify a system's inference on context, intended task, and other aspects that influence the content and interface. This was an important aspect to the participatory design of Goodman et al.'s work on technology for older adults in the home [68].

Kaufman et al. used a more thorough approach to field testing their diabetes technology in the homes of older adults [69]. The researcher participated in the usability testing in the home environment with cameras recording the user, the researcher and the screen interactions. The usability testing was coupled with cognitive walkthrough analysis of the telemedicine system. Jimison et al. developed a novel approach to usability testing of health technologies. They developed and evaluated remote usability testing on an ongoing basis (without researchers in the home) for participatory design. An initial implementation of the approach involved a cohort of older adult participants in their "Living Lab" (a group of approximately 50 cognitively healthy adults over 70 years of age living independently in their homes) [70]. As part of a study of health coaching technology, as well as sensors for monitoring of movement, sleep, socialization, medication management, physical exercise and cognitive exercise, these seniors were used to using Web cameras and video conferencing as part of their coaching and socialization interventions with family members. Usability researchers in a central academic setting used the seniors' Web cameras with video conferencing software and screen capture software to conduct low-cost iterative usability tests of new software while users remained in their homes using their own computers, as shown in the diagram in Fig. 16.2.

Testers were able to remotely control the computer in the home and obtain video (face and computer screen) and audio recordings of talk-aloud task analyses as

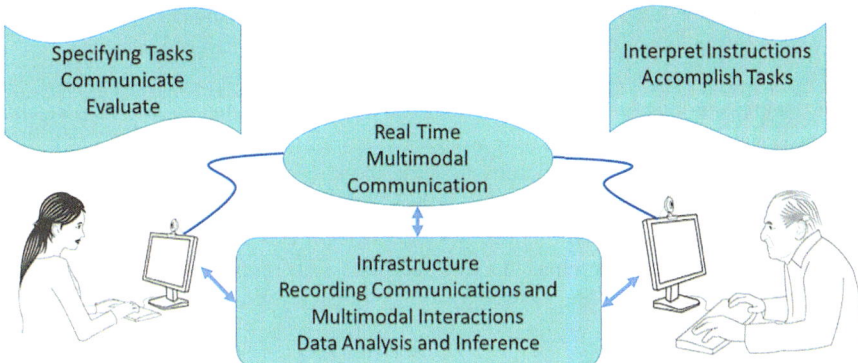

Fig. 16.2 Schematic of the video conferencing set-up for remote usability testing from the research lab to the home; figure rendered by Jesse Pavel of Electrika Inc.

subjects used the technology in their familiar setting [71]. Recordings of the computer screen during the test were synced with the Web camera recording of the participant's facial expressions and audio for later analysis. This form of user testing could be performed quickly and conveniently, allowing for frequent iterations of software design with user participation and immediate feedback. It also allows the user to feel more comfortable in their own environment with a familiar computer. The convenience on the part of the developers and usability testers, being able to conduct the tests from their office or home, is also important in encouraging frequent iterations to optimize the interface. These remote usability approaches allow researchers and developers to perform frequent low-cost remote usability tests of new screen designs and content as part of a participatory iterative design process. An additional advantage of this approach is that rapid usability testing can easily include participants from any remote location and not be bound by the demographics close to the lab setting. Being inclusive in obtaining feedback in the early stages of design will lead to better products and equitable health outcomes.

New Horizons: Human Computer Interaction with Distributed Computing

The advances in technology, computation and engineering alluded to in the section on adaptive interfaces have much farther-reaching implications than those discussed thus far. Perhaps for the first time in history, we have access to technology that is capable of monitoring, inference and interpretation of behaviors, ranging from physical activity to emotional responses. We are in the midst of a rapid expansion in the availability of sensors to measure motion, acceleration, location, sleep quality and many physiological quantities. These sensors are now smaller and cheaper than ever before. There have been advances in energy harvesting, and enhancing battery life will continue to make these more convenient to use in wearable versions.

These sensors add to our ability to collect routine physiological measures in the home, such as blood glucose for diabetes, peak flows for asthma, and blood pressure for cardiovascular disease. The new wearable sensors now allow us continuous and unobtrusive monitoring, and thereby provide more effective tailored interventions in a variety of areas ranging from cardiovascular monitoring to physical exercise and weight management. Among the consequences of this technological revolution is the rise of movements such as "Quantified Self" [72] on the monitoring side and "PatientsLikeMe" [73] on the networking side. Both of these directions are suggestive of future trends in consumer health informatics that incorporate behavioral inferences, social connectivity and data analytics, but will require appropriate human computer interfaces and data visualization. The raw data from monitoring converted to information will be increasingly useful in matching consumer needs with available sources of information and knowledge.

The concurrent rising ubiquity of smartphones will also play a large role in the future of interface design. In fact, for many, smartphones are the main method of interfacing with the Internet. The user interface issues in attempting to convey complex information on a small screen will remain a challenge. However, more importantly, users will likely be interacting with displays of varying sizes throughout their environment, much as the newer displays on cars now can show applications from the driver's mobile phone. Linking to displays in varying locations and of varying dimensions will offer a potentially much improved user experience and certainly convenience. The sophistication of user interface algorithms will necessarily grow, making this a fertile area for discovery and innovation.

New Horizons: Emergence of Artificial Intelligence and Machine Learning

Recent advances in Machine Learning (ML), Artificial Intelligence (AI), and Data Science enable revolutionary developments in interactive environments closer to human-human interactions. The recently implemented large language models such as ChatGPT use generative pretrained transformer models fitted to very large data sets capable of producing texts indistinguishable from those generated by humans. The huge training data sets, large amounts of parameters, and attention-based sequential processing techniques enable the AI systems to produce grammatical and semantically appropriate texts. Unsurprisingly, GPT applications are leading to the development of advanced, interactive systems. Applications for consumer health technologies include the automated generation of answers to frequently asked questions by patients, recommendations for when to see a doctor, and for possible treatments. A key issue for these applications is to limit the database of web sites used for the generation of the models to vetted sites with legitimate information. Using speech interfaces, context recognition, and sophisticated individual identification is likely to reduce or eliminate many barriers for individuals with cognitive impairments to using technology.

Merging the interface-related benefits of the large language models with equally powerful computational models and assessment techniques will enable the estimation and prediction of the health and mental individuals' states. Researchers have been investigating approaches to assessing individuals' stated and improving health behaviors over the last two decades using these emerging computer science-based, engineering approaches. The general idea is that the ability to assess the individuals' states enable the systems to interact more effectively with the participants [74].

Conclusion

Overall, user interfaces and user-centered design more generally will play a large role in the success of health interventions in the future, as more healthcare is provided in the home and environments outside a hospital or clinic. The challenges in designing systems for a highly variable set of consumers are great, but the opportunities provided by new monitoring and communications technologies, along with advances in AI and machine learning, are also great. This will certainly be a dynamic field for both research and development of successful systems for consumers of healthcare.

Discussion Questions
1. Imagine that you are working for a clinic that provides consumer technology for diabetes care in the home, consisting of blood glucose meters, a Web site with educational material, and automated reminders by cell phone. You have been asked to develop design specifications to adapt it for a low-income Spanish-speaking immigrant population living in an urban setting. Describe your process in adapting this set of technology for this new population.
2. For a new era of pervasive computing, where sensors and communication displays are distributed throughout the home, workplace, and general environment, describe the challenges and potential solutions to usability testing of a new device or tailored health communications tool.

References

1. Committee on Quality Health Care in America. Crossing the quality chasm: a new health system for the 21st century. Washington D.C.: Institute of Medicine; 2001.
2. Healthwise Knowledgebase. Available from: https://www.healthwise.org/solution/articulate/kbdemo/index.html#/

3. Jimison H, Gorman P, Woods S, et al. Barriers and drivers of health information technology use for the elderly, chronically ill, and underserved. Evid Rep Technol Assess (Full Rep). 2008;175:1–1422.
4. Demeris G, Eysenbach G. Internet use in disease management for home care patients: a call for papers. J Med Internet Res. 2002;4(2):E6.
5. Johnson K, Jimison H, Mandl K. Consumer health informatics, Ch 17. In: Shortliffe EH, Cimino JJ, editors. Biomedical informatics: computer applications in health care and biomedicine. 4th ed. Springer; 2014.
6. Johns Hopkins Medicine Health – Multiple sclerosis. Available from: https://www.hopkinsmedicine.org/health/conditions-and-diseases/multiple-sclerosis-ms
7. Cleveland Clinic. Multiple sclerosis (MS). Available from: https://my.clevelandclinic.org/health/diseases/17248-multiple-sclerosis?view=print
8. myHealthteam. Expert support groups. Available from: myhealthteam.com/experts/
9. Umberson D, Montez JK. Social relationships and health: a flashpoint for health policy. J Health Soc Behav. 2010;51:S54.
10. Würtzen H, Dalton SO, Elsass P, et al. Mindfulness significantly reduces self-reported levels of anxiety and depression: results of a randomised controlled trial among 336 Danish women treated for stage I-III breast cancer. Eur J Cancer. 2013;49(6):1365–73.
11. Klemm P, Bunnell D, Cullen M, Soneji R, Gibbons P, Holecek A. Online cancer support groups: a review of the research literature. Comput Inform Nurs. 2003;21(3):136–42.
12. Hsuing RC. The best of both worlds: an online self-help group hosted by a mental health professional. CyberPsychol Behav. 2000;3(6):935–50.
13. PatientsLikeMe. 2023 [cited 2023 Jun 21]. Available from: https://www.patientslikeme.com
14. O'Connor AM, Rostom A, Fiset V, et al. Decision aids for patients facing health treatment or screening decisions: systematic review. BMJ. 1999;319:731.
15. Bravata DM, Smith-Spangler C, Sundaram V, et al. Using pedometers to increase physical activity and improve health: a systematic review. JAMA. 2007;298(19):2296–304.
16. Demiris G, Afrin LB, Speedie S, et al. Patient-centered applications: use of information technology to promote disease management and wellness. J Am Med Inform Assoc. 2008;15(1):8–13.
17. Jimison HB, Sher PP, Appleyard R, LeVernois YM. The use of multimedia in the informed consent process. J Am Med Inform Assoc. 1998;5(3):245–56.
18. The provider's guide to quality and culture. Available from: http://erc.msh.org/mainpage.cfm?file=5.2.0h.htm&module=provider&language=English
19. McCrickard S, Doswell F, Barksdale J, Piggot D. Understanding cool and computing for African-American youth. Paper presented at: CHI 2012 May 5–10 2012, Austin, Texas, USA.
20. Briceno C, Killam B. Designing an effective web presence for the Hispanic audience. Available from: http://www.upa-dc-metro.org/Resources/Documents/conference/2011/Presentations/UsabilityofHispanicWebsites_09_16_2011(2)-1.pdf
21. Evercare, developing cultural proficiency: understanding and serving the people of Hawai'i. Available from: https://www.uhccommunityplan.com/content/dam/communityplan/plandocuments/culturalcompetency/en/HI-Evercare-QExA-Cultural-Competency.pdf
22. Goebert D, Morland L, Frattarelli L, Onoye J, Matsu C. Mental health during pregnancy: a study comparing Asian, Caucasian and Native Hawaiian women. Matern Child Health. 2007;11:244–55. https://doi.org/10.1007/s10995-006-0165-0.
23. Braveman PA, Cubbin C, Egerter S, et al. Socioeconomic status in health research: one size does not fit all. JAMA. 2005;294(22):2879–88.
24. Ndugga N, Artiga S. Disparities in health and health care: 5 key questions and answers. Kaiser Family Foundation report on racial equity and health policy. Available from: https://www.kff.org/racial-equity-and-health-policy/issue-brief/disparities-in-health-and-health-care-5-key-question-and-answers/
25. National Academies of Sciences, Engineering, and Medicine, Health and Medicine Division, Board on Population Health and Public Health Practice, et al., editors. Communities in action: pathways to health equity: 2. The state of health disparities in the United States. Washington

(DC): National Academies Press (US); 2017. Available from: https://www.ncbi.nlm.nih.gov/books/NBK425844/
26. Reinecke K, Gajos KZ. One size fits many westerners - how cultural abilities challenge UI design. Available from: http://reinecke.people.si.umich.edu/Publications_files/CulturalAbilities.pdf
27. Chang CL, Su Y. Cross-cultural interface design and the classroom learning environment in Taiwan. Available from: http://www.tojet.net/articles/v11i3/1139.pdf
28. Kreuter M, McClure S. The role of culture in health communication. Annu Rev Public Health. 2004;25:439–55.
29. Branson R, Davis D, Gadson M. Wireless in communities of color: bridging the digital divide, Multicultural Media, Telecom & Internet Council report. 2002. Available from: https://www.mmtconline.org/wp-content/uploads/2022/07/Wireless-in-Communities-of-Color-July-2022-B.pdf
30. Smith A. Home broadband adoption 2010. Pew Research Center; 2010 Aug 11. Available from: www.pewresearch.org/internet/2010/08/11/trends-in-broadband-adoption/
31. Atske S, Perrin A. Home broadband adoption, computer ownership vary by race, ethnicity in the U.S. Pew Research Center; 2021 Jul 16. Available from: www.pewresearch.org/fact-tank/2021/07/16/home-broadband-adoptioncomputer-ownership-vary-by-race-ethnicity-in-the-u-s/
32. Vogels EA. Digital divide persists even as Americans with lower incomes make gains in tech adoption. Pew Research Center; 2021 Jun 22. Available from: https://www.pewresearch.org/fact-tank/2021/06/22/digital-divide-persists-even-asamericans-with-lower-incomes-make-gains-in-tech-adoption/
33. Perrin A. Mobile technology and home broadband, 2021. Pew Research Center; 2021 Jun 3. Available from: https://www.pewresearch.org/internet/2021/06/03/mobile-technology-and-home-broadband-2021/
34. Federal Interagency Forum on Aging-Related Statistics. Older Americans 2020: key indicators of Well-being. Washington, DC: U.S. Government Printing Office; 2020. This report is available from: https://agingstats.gov
35. Promoting health for older adults. 2022 Sep 8. National Center for Chronic Disease Prevention and Health Promotion. Centers for Disease Control and Prevention. Available from: www.cdc.gov/chronicdisease/resources/publications/factsheets/promoting-health-for-older-adults.htm#:~:text=By%202040%2C%20the%20number%20of,diabetes%2C%20arthritis%2C%20and%20cancer
36. Hedden T, Gabrieli JDE. Insights into the ageing mind: a view from cognitive neuroscience. Nat Rev Neurosci. 2004;5(2):87–96.
37. Fisk AD, Rogers WA, Charness N, Czaja SJ, Sharit J. Designing for older adults: principles and creative human factors approaches. 2nd ed. Boca Raton, FL: CRC Press; 2009.
38. Rogers WA, Fisk AD. Age-related differences in the maintenance and modification of automatic processes: arithmetic stroop interference. Hum Factors. 1991;33:45–56.
39. Gell NM, Rosenberg DE, Demiris G, LaCroix AZ, Patel KV. Patterns of technology use among older adults with and without disabilities. Gerontologiest. 2015;55(3):412–21.
40. Anderson M, Perrin A. Tech adoption climbs among older adults. Pew Research Center: internet, science & technology. 2017. Available from: www.pewinternet.org/2017/05/17/tech-adoption-climbs-among-older-adults/
41. American Foundation for the Blind. Review of screen readers. [cited 2023 Jun 21]. Available from: https://www.afb.org/aw/full-issue?id=14060
42. Baker NA, Rogers JC, Rubinstein EN, Allaire SH, Wasko MC. Problems experienced by people with arthritis when using a computer. Arthritis Rheum. 2009;61(5):614–22.
43. World Wide Web Consortium. 2023 Jun 15. Available from: www.w3.org
44. Baker D. The meaning and the measure of health literacy. J Gen Intern Med. 2006;21(8):878–83.
45. Schillinger D, Grumbach K, Piette J, et al. Association of Health Literacy with diabetes outcomes. J Am Med Assoc. 2002;288(4):475–82.

46. Eysenbach G. What is e-health? J Med Internet Res. 2001;3(2):E20. Available from: http://www.jmir.org/2001/2/e20/
47. The readability test tool. [cited 2014 Sep 25]. Available from: http://read-able.com/
48. ReadabilityScore.Com. [cited 2014 Sep 25]. Available from: https://readability-score.com/
49. Kincaid JP, Braby R, Mears J. Electronic authoring and delivery of technical information. J Instr Dev. 1988;11:8–13.
50. The Gunning's fog index (or FOG) readability formula. Readabilty Formulas. [cited 2014 Sep 10]. Available from: https://readabilityformulas.com/the-gunnings-fog-index-or-fog-readability-formula/
51. Coleman M, Liau TL. A computer readability formula designed for machine scoring. J Appl Psychol. 1975;60:283–4.
52. Hedman AS. Using the SMOG formula to revise a health-related document. Am J Health Educ. 2008;39(1):61–4.
53. Senter RJ, Smith EA. Automated readability index. Wright-Patterson Air Force Base; 1967 Nov. p. 3. AMRL-TR-6620. [cited 2014 Sep 25]. Available from: http://en.wikipedia.org/wiki/Automated_Readability_Index
54. Ochsner Health System. Development guidelines for patient education materials. Available from: http://academics.ochsner.org/editingdyn.aspx?id=51327
55. First Clinical research glossary. [cited 2014 Sep 25]. Available from: http://firstclinical.com/icfglossary/
56. First Clinical research document analysis. [cited 2014 Sep 25]. Available from: http://www.firstclinical.com/words/
57. van der Vaart R, van Deursen A, Drossaert C, Taal E, van Dijk J, van de Laar M. Does the eHealth literacy scale (eHEALS) measure what it intends to measure? Validation of a Dutch version of the eHEALS in two adult populations. J Med Internet Res. 2011;13(4):e86.
58. Kaufman DR, Starren J, Patel VL, et al. A cognitive framework for understanding barriers to the productive use of a diabetes home telemedicine system. AMIA Annu Symp Proc. 2003;2003:356–60.
59. Norman CD, Skinner HA. eHealth literacy: essential skills for consumer health in a networked world. J Med Internet Res. 2006;8(2):e9.
60. Mesko B. Guide to the future of medicine: technology & human touch. The Medical Futurist. Available from: https://medicalfuturist.com/ten-ways-technology-changing-healthcare/#
61. Su X, Khoshgoftaar TM. A survey of collaborative filtering techniques. Adv Artif Intell. 2009;2009:421425.
62. Yue Y, Wang C, El-Arini K, Guestrin C. Personalized collaborative clustering. Available from: http://www.cs.princeton.edu/~chongw/papers/YueWangEl-AriniCuestrin.pdf
63. Viadero D. Scholars test emotion-sensitive tutoring software. Educ Week. 2010;29(16):6.
64. Parasuraman R, Rizzo M. Neuroergonomics: the brain at work. Oxford University Press; 2008.
65. Parasuraman R. Neuroergonomics: brain, cognition, and performance at work. Curr Dir Psychol Sci. 2011;20(3):181–6.
66. Dunton GF, Liao Y, Kawabata K, Intille S. Momentary assessment of adults' physical activity and sedentary behavior: feasibility and validity. Front Psychol. 2012;3:260.
67. Heron KE, Smyth JM. Ecological momentary interventions: incorporating mobile technology into psychosocial and health behaviour treatments. Br J Health Psychol. 2010;15(Pt 1):1–39.
68. Goodman CA, Jimison HB, Pavel M. Participatory design for home care technology. Paper presented at: Proceedings of the 24th Annual Engineering in Medicine and Biology Conference, vol. 3. 2002.
69. Kaufman DR, Patel VL, Hilliman C, et al. Usability in the real world: assessing medical information technologies in patients' homes. J Biomed Inform. 2003;36(1–2):45–60.
70. Jimison HB, Pavel M. Integrating computer-based health coaching into elder home care, technology and aging. In: Mihailidis A, Boger J, Kautz H, Normie L, editors. Technology and aging. Amsterdam: IOS Press; 2008.

71. Yu CH. Evaluation of remote usability techniques in an elderly cohort. Available from: http://digitalcommons.ohsu.edu/.
72. Adventures in self-surveillance, aka the quantified self, aka extreme navel-gazing. Forbes. 2011 Apr 7.
73. Wicks P, Massagli M, Frost J, et al. Sharing health data for better outcomes on PatientsLikeMe. J Med Internet Res. 2010;12(2):e19.
74. Spruijt-Metz D, Hekler E, Saranummic N, et al. Building new computational models to support health behavior change and maintenance: new opportunities in behavioral research. Transl Behav Med. 2015;5(3):335–46.

Further Reading

Agency for Healthcare Quality and Research. Designing consumer health IT: a guide for developers and systems designers. Available from: https://digital.ahrq.gov/sites/default/files/docs/page/designing-consumer-health-it-a-guide-for-developers-and-systems-designers.pdf

Cronin RM, Jimison HB, Johnson KB. Personal health informatics, Ch 11. In: Shortliffe EH, Cimino JJ, Chiang MF, editors. Biomedical informatics: computer applications in health care and biomedicine. 5th ed. Springer; 2021.

Reinecke K, Gajos KZ. One size fits many westerners: how cultural abilities challenge UI design. Paper presented at: Proceedings of the Workshop on Dynamic Accessibility: Detecting and Accommodating Differences in Ability and Situation at CHI'11, 2011.

Chapter 17
Intelligent Decision Support in Personal Health: Personalized Health Coaching in Type 2 Diabetes

Lena Mamykina, Elliot Mitchell, Pooja Desai, and David Albers

Introduction

Chronic conditions like type 2 diabetes (T2D) continue to present a considerable challenge to the affected individuals and to the society at large [1]. Chronic conditions are particularly burdensome because they require that individuals engage in proactive self-management and make numerous adjustments to their lifestyles, including their diet, levels of physical activity, sleep routines, and many others [2]. However, identifying changes that can lead to improved health requires literacy, and sustaining these changes requires motivation. Self-management is further complicated by high individual differences in pathophysiology of diseases and in the way individuals respond to lifestyle modifications [3–5]. These challenges contribute to growing health disparities; low income and minority communities have higher prevalence and worse outcomes from chronic diseases and lower access to resources like diabetes education [6–8].

In response to these trends, *personal informatics* emerged as a field that examines ways individuals use personal data for reflection and increased self-knowledge [9]. While personal informatics is not limited to health, most publications in this

---

L. Mamykina (✉) · P. Desai
Department of Biomedical Informatics, Columbia University, New York, NY, USA
e-mail: lena.mamykina@columbia.edu; pmd2137@cumc.columbia.edu

E. Mitchell
Steele Institute for Health Innovation, New York, NY, USA
e-mail: emitchell3@geisinger.edu

D. Albers
Department of Biomedical Informatics, University of Colorado School of Medicine, Aurora, CO, USA
e-mail: david.albers@cuanschutz.edu

© The Author(s), under exclusive license to Springer Nature Switzerland AG 2024
A. W. Kushniruk et al. (eds.), *Human Computer Interaction in Healthcare*, Cognitive Informatics in Biomedicine and Healthcare, https://doi.org/10.1007/978-3-031-69947-4_17

field focused on health and wellness [10]. Li et al. proposed a stage-based model of personal informatics that outlines several stages of individuals' engagement with personal data, from deciding what data to collect, to the actual data collection, to integration of data from multiple sources, to reflection and analysis, and, finally, to action [9, 11]. Many personal informatics tools use visual representation of data captured with self-monitoring to help individuals to identify patterns in their records, which could lead to increased self-awareness and enable more informed future choices (e.g. [11–16]. However, many data-driven health interventions place the burden on individuals to derive insights from their data and determine how to change their behavior [17, 18], and, as a result, suffer from high user burden and low adoption [9, 19, 20]. As a consequence, individuals with low technology and health literacy, who are most impacted by chronic diseases, are least equipped to reap the benefits [21, 22].

Advances in *machine learning* (ML) create new opportunities to reduce the burden of data analysis and to rely on computational techniques instead or in addition to analysis by humans. Typical ML techniques learn patterns and associations in large datasets and use these learned patterns to make inferences and predict future states. Recent research initiatives have demonstrated high accuracy of ML models in many health-related tasks [23, 24]. In the context of personal health, ML methods can be applied to personal health data to find patterns of association between multiple streams of self-tracking data [25] or forecast changes in relevant biomarkers, such as blood glucose (BG) levels [26]. However, incorporating ML into personal health applications can present new challenges. First, traditional ML techniques require vast amounts of data and typically learn patterns for cohorts, rather than trends unique to each individual. Even more importantly, while both inferences and predictions can be informative and lead to increased self-knowledge, they may suffer from the same limitations as many personal informatics solutions in that they focus on pointing out patterns in the past, rather than making suggestions for future choices.

Generating suggestions that inform individual action is the heart of the field of *recommender systems* (RecSys) [27, 28]. Past research explored applicability of RecSys techniques for providing nutritional recommendations [29–31]. However, most health-related RecSys developed thus far focused primarily on tailoring suggestions to individuals' preferences inferred from their past choices, rather than on helping individuals meet their goals or improve their health. Thus, there a need for new approaches to translating inferences achieved with ML into recommendations that can guide individuals' action.

To address these research gaps, we developed an approach to generating recommendations for self-management goals using a combination of ML with individuals' self-monitoring data, an expert system for translating ML inferences into action-oriented goals, and an interactive mHealth application (app), GlucoGoalie, that helps individuals choose personal self-management goals and provides in-the-moment decision support for attaining these goals in daily lives. We evaluated GlucoGoalie's computational engine on its accuracy of inferences and GlucoGoalie's interactive mHealth app on its' ability to generate easy to understand and actionable self-management goals. In this chapter, we describe each of these components and the results of the evaluation study.

Related work

Diabetes Self-Management and Personalization

In chronic conditions like T2D, daily lifestyle behaviors, including food choices and physical activity, impact short- and long-term health status. A key goal in T2D self-management is keeping blood glucose (BG) levels within target ranges. Dietary decisions have a direct impact on BG after each meal, but there is a high degree of variability between and within individuals. The same meal can have wildly different glycemic impacts across individuals [4], and the American Diabetes Association (ADA) recommends 1-on-1 counseling with diabetes educators to determine personalized nutrition goals and macronutrient targets [3]. Notably, it can be difficult for individuals to anticipate the impact of a particular meal on BG, even for experts [17].

Personal Informatics

The increasing availability of data related to individuals' personal histories inspired a new wave of research in Human-Computer Interaction with the focus on facilitating individuals' engagement with personal data. Li et al. proposed a stage-based model of personal informatics that outlines a number of stages of individuals' engagement with personal data [9, 11]. To promote reflection and identification of trends, many personal informatics tools rely on visualizations of data captured with self-monitoring (e.g. [11–16]. For example, Medynskiy and Mynatt's system Salud! allowed its users to specify activities with suspected impact on wellbeing and related biomarkers (for example time spent in the office and mood) and visually examine possible dependencies in these data using interactive visualizations [14]. Epstein et al. developed visualizations of variables related to specific questions posed by individual users based on their self-tracking goals [15]. Similarly, SleepExplorer by Liang et al. visualized patterns of sleep in conjunction with other data tracked by participants [16]. However, many of these previous works focused on technologically-savvy individuals who were already engaged in active self-monitoring. Somewhat in contrast to these visual approaches, Bentley et al. used simple statistical inferences to computationally identify correlations in the captured data and present their users with discoveries [25]. Self-experimentation framework proposed by Karkar et al. helped individuals to evaluate hypotheses in regards to the associations between specific behaviors and health outcomes [32]. However, similarly to other personal informatics solutions, both of these approaches focus on recognizing trends, and leave it up to the users to identify mitigating strategies.

In the context of diabetes self-management, previous research examined the feasibility of using dense datasets of blood glucose levels captured with CGM to personalize self-management. Most notably, Zeevi et al. used CGM data of 800 individuals combined with their nutritional records as a foundation for development of computational models of postprandial glycemic response (PPGR) [4]. These models were then used to devise personally tailored nutritional therapy for individuals with T2DM shown to help individuals achieve better glycemic control (lower postprandial BG levels). However, this approach requires dense data streams captured with CGM; attempts to utilize machine learning to model glycemic function using sparse data were not successful [33].

Recommender Systems

Recommender systems take a different approach to providing individuals with personalized support for making daily decisions [27]. Instead of focusing on reflection and self-knowledge, RecSys provide more direct support for action in the form of recommendations. RecSys are especially common in the consumer space, for example recommending items for purchase on an e-commerce site, or videos on a streaming platform. Previous research has explored RecSys in health, and, in particular, in nutrition management [29–31]. Past nutritional recommender systems often delivered recommendations in the form of recipes and focused on tailoring recommendations to individuals' preferences for different foods expressed in the past. However, applying RecSys approach to health management introduces new challenges. The focus on preferences, typical for RecSys, may lead to recommendations that are at odds with individuals' health goals. While there is emerging research on incorporating health constraints as part of nutritional recommendations, these constrains are often derived from population-level guidelines, rather than learned from or informed by individuals' personal data [31, 34–36].

GlucoGoalie

GlucoGoalie was designed following a user-centered design process with individuals with T2D from a predominantly Black and Latino economically disadvantaged community [37]. Figure 17.1 presents an overview of the different components of GlucGoalie from collection of self-monitoring data to generation of personalized nutritional goals. GlucoGoalie's goal-generating engine includes two main components that combine a data-driven and a knowledge-drive approaches. First, in a data-driven approach, a machine learning algorithm uses self-management data to identify patterns of association between nutrition in meals and changes in BG

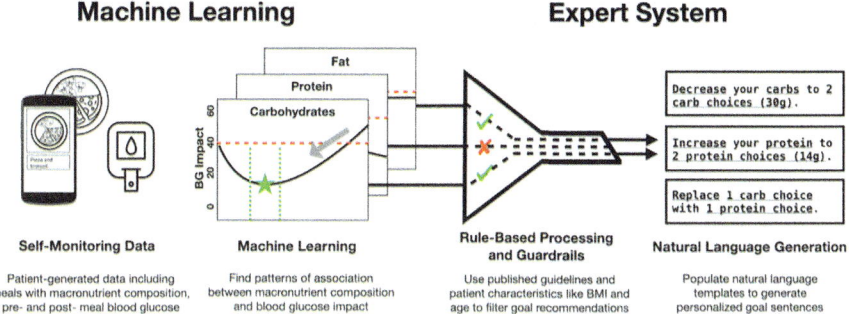

Fig. 17.1 An overview of the pipeline for generating personalized goal recommendations in GlucoGoalie

levels, thus learning which nutritional patterns are associated with mild impact on BG levels and which patterns systematically lead to an undesired increase in BG levels. Second, an expert system incorporates knowledge of expert dietitians to generate recommendations for changes in diet based on patterns learned with ML. We describe these in more detail below.

Approach to Goal Setting

One of the main challenges in designing nutrition recommendation systems is to develop an actionable and easy to understand and follow approach for displaying recommendations. A typical approach used by many nutritional RecSys is to provide recommendations in the form of recipes. However, individuals in economically disadvantaged communities may have many barriers to following recipes as they may lack access to ingredients and time and equipment for cooking. Furthermore, focusing recommendations on specific foods greatly increases the space for ML as there are many foods and food combinations. Furthermore, individuals may only eat these foods infrequently and learning associations between events that occur with low frequency may be difficult. To overcome these challenges, GlucoGoalie nutritional goals focus on amounts of different macronutrients in meals, such as carbohydrate, protein, and fat, rather than the specific foods and ingredients used to prepare these meals. This approach has several important advantages. First, the macronutrient composition of a meal is directly related to its impact on BG, but the specifics of the relationship vary between individuals [38]. Second, nutrition education in diabetes emphasizes macronutrients to help individuals think flexibly about the nutritional composition of similar foods [39]. Third, using macronutrients as features has advantages for machine learning, offering a denser, low-dimensional feature representation compared to other representations like the specific food items in a meal. We worked with a group of Certified Diabetes Educators (CDEs, $n = 3$) to formulate goals that are consistent with the ones used in typical diabetes self-management education and that focus on changes to macronutrient composition of meals and to create templates for goals that could be populated by an ML algorithm. We identified three types of changes to meal composition that could impact post-meal BG: increase the amount of a particular macronutrient, decrease the amount of a macronutrient, or replace one macronutrient with another. Goals are formulated at a level of a single meal, rather than as a daily target because the balance of each meal has its own impact on BG, making day-level goals (e.g., daily calories) less appropriate. See Table 17.1 for a selection of goals.

Machine Learning

The first step in generating personalized nutritional goals is in identifying what nutritional patterns are associated with systematic increase in post-meal blood glucose levels. To accomplish this, we used a machine learning method called Attributable Component Analysis (ACA), a non-parametric method for estimating the conditional expectation of a quantity of interest based on a set of covariates [40]. This method uses amounts (grams) of macronutrients in individuals' logged meals as its input. The outcome of interest—change in BG after a meal—is the difference between self-reported BG before the meal, compared with 2 h after. Expert RDs suggested 40 mg/dL as a minimal clinically-meaningful post-meal increase in BG

Table 17.1 A selection of nutritional goals available in GlucoGoalie. Generic goals are available for all users from when they first use the app. Personalized goals are recommended for an individual based on ML-based analysis of recorded meals and blood glucose readings. Underlined words are personalized for each user based on their data

Type	Title	Description
Personalized	Decrease your carbs to 2½ carb choices	For high carb lunches, decrease your carbs to be about 2½ carb choices (38 g). An example of 1 carb choice is 1 slice of whole wheat toast, $\frac{1}{3}$ cup of plantains, or $\frac{1}{3}$ cup of brown rice.
Personalized	Increase your protein to 3 protein choices	For low protein dinners, increase your protein to be about 3 lean protein choices (21 g). An example of 1 lean protein choice is 1 ounce of lean ground beef, $\frac{1}{2}$ cup of tofu, or 1 ounce of chicken breast.
Personalized	Replace 2 carb choices with 2 protein choices	For high carb dinners, replace 2 carb choices with 2 lean protein choices. For example, replace $\frac{2}{3}$ cup of rice with 2 ounces of ground turkey or 2 ounces of tilapia.
Generic	Choose whole fruits	Choose whole fruits instead of fruit juices. For example, have a whole orange, an apple, or a cup of berries with your meals.
Generic	Choose plant proteins	Include proteins that come from plants, such as beans, nuts and seeds, and legumes. For example, choose a cup of beans, a handful of peanuts, or a cup of lentils to add protein to your meal.

Note: A food "choice" is a unit similar to a serving size that identifies servings of different foods with similar macronutrient compositions

and ACA learns nutritional composition of meals that are associated with this or greater increase in BG [41]. Because self-monitoring data are manually entered by users, there are often a small number of data points that are prone to include errors and outliers. These characteristics pose challenges for ML, and ACA has advantages over other methods like linear regression because it is able to capture non-linear relationships, is less sensitive to erroneous data points, and more effectively estimates uncertainty [42]. As its output, ACA identifies ranges of different macronutrients that are systematically associated with an increase in BG levels of 40 mg/dL or greater.

Expert System Interpretation and Guardrails

While ML can identify ranges of macronutrients associated with undesired changes in BG levels, these ranges alone may not be sufficient to inform future choices. In a series of ten sessions, we worked with CDEs to establish rules for interpreting the ML output and translating it into goal recommendations described above. In addition, we took several steps to make goals easier to understand and more actionable for individuals with mixed levels of nutritional literacy. First, each goal included examples of specific foods rich in the targeted macronutrient drawn from an ADA resource [39]. Second, we explored different approaches to communicating amounts of macronutrients mentioned within each goal. Here, we used the ADA-endorsed language of food "choices," a system meant to simplify nutrition education [39]. A food "choice" is a unit similar to a serving size; it identifies servings of different foods with similar macronutrient compositions. For example, 1 carbohydrate choice is 15 g, which could be 1 slice of toast or $\frac{1}{3}$ cup of rice. In addition, because "choices" are based on grams, the standard unit on food labels, each goal also includes the target amount in grams. While grams may still present a challenge to individuals not accustomed to measuring their foods, it is the most common unit of measure and is the one typically used in diabetes education.

In addition, CDEs pointed out that some automatically generated recommendations might be inappropriate irrespective of their impact on BG. For example a goal to eat 100 g of fat in a single meal would not be appropriate for any individual regardless of its impact on BG levels. To mitigate this concern, we added a set of guardrails to filter out recommendations inconsistent with population-level nutrition guidelines.

The GlucoGoalie App

The computational engine described above generated personalized nutritional goals tailored to patterns in each individual's self-monitoring meals and BG levels. We used an mHealth app, GlucoGoalie, to present these goals to individuals, engage them in personalized goal setting and help them work towards achieving these goals with daily personalized meal-time decision support.

Users begin by choosing one or more nutritional goals from a list in the app (see Table 17.1 for a selection of goals). To compensate for the lack of self-monitoring data at the beginning of individuals' engagement with the app, all users begin by choosing from the same set of "generic" goals. These generic goals were developed by experts in nutrition and diabetes and include a set of generally healthy behaviors, such as "Choose whole fruits" and "Drink water with your meals" [43]. Twice per week, GlucoGoalie analyzes the data of each user with the aim of identifying new patterns and generating personalized nutritional goals. If new goals are available, GlucoGoalie sends a push notification, and users can view the new, personalized recommendations and choose any they wish to follow (Fig. 17.2d).

Once the goals are set, users can log their meals and enter their pre-meal BG. Two hours after the meal, GlucoGoalie sends a push notification reminder to enter a post-meal reading. To simplify the logging process, users log meals by taking a picture of the meal and typing a free text description (Fig. 17.2a). Macronutrient data are entered by a team of Registered Dietitians (RDs) who assessed each meal following a standard protocol based on the USDA nutrition database [44], but similar results could be attained via crowdsourcing [45].

To provide individuals with in-the-moment decision support and keep goals as a central part of individuals' self-management, GlucoGoalie prompts users to assess whether their meal fits with each of their chosen goals while logging with either "Yes" or "Not Really" (Fig. 17.2b). Users can view their current goals, remove or choose new goals, and review a summary of goal attainment in the My Goals section of the app (Fig. 17.2c).

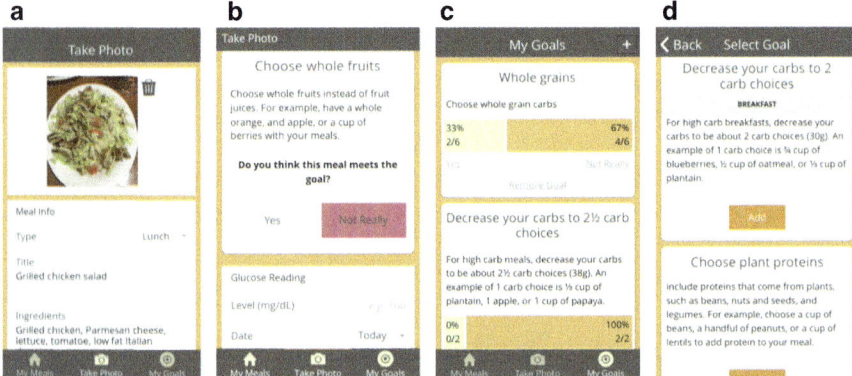

Fig. 17.2 The GlucoGoalie mobile application. (**a**) Logging a meal with a photo and free text description. (**b**) Users self-assess whether they met their chosen goals. (**c**) A summary of goal achievement. (**d**) Reviewing and choosing new personalized goals to work on after receiving a push notification

GlucoGoalie Evaluation

In order to evaluate feasibility of GlucoGoalie and its potential impact on individuals' self-management experience, we conducted two user studies. The first study was conducted in controlled lab settings and focused on whether goals generated by GlucoGoalie could be understood and acted on by individuals with T2D. The second study was conducted in naturalistic settings and focused on individuals' engagement and experience using the app. We describe these studies below.

Controlled Evaluation

Methods

Participants were recruited from two types of health centers in New York City: (1) a Federally Qualified Health Center (FQHC) in Brownsville Brooklyn, and (2) clinics affiliated with Columbia University Irving Medical Center. To be included, participants needed to be between 18- and 65-years-old, have a self-reported diagnosis of type 2 diabetes (T2D), and be proficient in English. After collecting consent, participants received a 10-min, in-person nutrition training introducing the concept of food "choices" and reviewing macronutrients. Participants then completed the following three tasks:

To assess *comprehension* of goals generated by GlucoGoalie, participants were presented with an example goal "for a friend with diabetes," and asked to choose which of two meals were a better fit with the goal. This task included two different components. First, individuals were presented with meals as images with a free text description with a nutrition label in the style of Facts Up Front [46]; this allowed us to test whether individuals could comprehend the goals even if they had little knowledge of nutrition and could not discern nutritional composition of a meal. This task was repeated twice. In the second portion of this task, we removed the food label; in this version, individuals needed to not only comprehend the goal, but to also have enough nutritional knowledge to compare each meal with a chosen goal. For both tasks, meal images were selected from a dataset collected in ongoing research with individuals from a similar population. For each assessment, we selected two meals that included similar ingredients but varied in macronutrient content; the incorrect answer was at least 1 macronutrient "choice" different from the correct answer, and the difficulty varied across scenarios. To account for higher variability in meal images, this task was repeated for eight goal/meal-pair combinations.

To assess whether goals were *actionable*, participants were asked to compose meals that aligned with selected nutritional goals using paper cutouts of different common foods, thus simulating an experience of choosing foods at a buffet. First, we asked participants to use the food cutouts to assemble a baseline meal for each type of meal (breakfast, lunch, and dinner) that was "closest to what you would normally eat." Participants then chose a nutritional goal that aligned with their general nutritional aspirations and were asked to compose additional meals with that goal in mind. Importantly, while participants were limited only to foods available in the buffet, they could vary the amount of each food by selecting multiple cutouts/portions. We used images from a web-based resource [47] and our ongoing research and sought to include common staples like bacon and eggs as well as culturally relevant foods like fried plantains.

The baseline meals were used to identify goals that would require participants to deviate from their typical macronutrient behavior by 1–1.5 macronutrient choices. For example, if a participant's baseline meal had 3.5 carb choices and 1 protein choice, they would receive two goals: one to decrease carbs to 2 choices and another to increase protein to 2 choices. Participants chose one of the two goals, and then assembled "breakfast," "lunch," and "dinner" for 3 days in a row, with the chosen goal in mind (nine total meals). Researchers tallied the chosen food items to calculate nutrient compositions. During the 1-on-1 activity, researchers made note of participant comments and feedback, for example, questions about missing or inappropriate food items.

Data Analysis

For the goal comprehension and goal/image matching tasks, we calculated binary accuracy as a percentage (#correct/[#correct + #incorrect]). For the "virtual buffet" experiment, we analyzed the data in two dimensions: direction and accuracy. First, we examined whether participants' meals were consistent with the *direction* of their chosen goal. For example, if the goal was to increase protein to 2 choices at lunch, we assessed whether subsequent lunches had more protein than baseline. A binomial test was used to determine whether performance was better than chance. Second, accuracy in meeting the goal target was measured with mean absolute error between participant choices and the goal target. For example, if the target was 2 choices, we assessed how close participant's meals were to the target, on average.

To synthesize participants impressions from their comments during the study, research met to debrief and aggregate notes in a series of meetings to summarize key themes.

Controlled Evaluation Results

We recruited and enrolled a total of 19 participants, including ten from a Federally Qualified Health Center, and nine from university-affiliated clinics. Four participants were excluded because of a data collection error for a total of 15 participants included in the analysis. As seen in Table 17.2, participants were predominantly female, and Black or Hispanic. Most were overweight or obese (body mass index ≥ 25).

Table 17.2 Participant demographics for both studies

Demographics	Study 1: controlled experiment	Study 2: deployment study
N enrolled (Incl. in Analysis)	19 (15)	10 (8)
Sex	80% Female	71% Female
Ethnicity	47% Hispanic	86% Hispanic
Race	17% White 42% Black 41% Other/Refused	43% White 29% Black 29% Other/Refused
Age	54 ± 9 years	55.7 ± 9.5 years
Body mass index (BMI)	37.4 ± 13.9	41.8 ± 14.4
Median household income	$20,000–$39,999	$40,000–$59,999
Median education level	Some College	Some College

For the goal comprehension task, when choosing which of the two nutrition labels met a given goal participants were correct 89% (SD = 21%) of the time. When choosing which of two meal images was a better match with a goal, participants chose the correct meal 49% (SD = 25%) of the time. When composing meals at the virtual buffet, meals were consistent with the direction of chosen goals 67% (68 of 102) of the time, significantly more than chance per a binomial test ($p < 0.001$). There was no difference in the percentage of meals consistent with the direction of chosen goals by meal type, macronutrient, or direction of goal. At the same time, there was a high degree of variability in precisely meeting the goal target. On average, meals selected by participants were <1 meal choice away from the target goal (mean = 0.83, SD = 0.56) which means that on average individuals were able to follow goal recommendations within the allowable margin of error.

Thematic analysis of individuals' comments during debriefing sessions identified two common themes. First, most participants felt that the virtual buffet included limited food options, which made it difficult for them to construct meals that resemble their dietary patterns. However, most participants were able to make choices that at least partially represented their daily diets. Second, most participants felt comfortable understanding and following the goals. However, some had challenges with some of the words used within nutritional goals. Specifically, use of the word "choice" as a measurement unit was confusing, with some participants interpreting "2 choice" as two different foods rich in a given macronutrient (e.g., rice and bread), rather than as its intended meaning as a measure of quantity (e.g., 30 g).

Study 2: Deployment Study

In the second study, we sought to better understand participants' experience engaging with setting and attaining personalized goals in the context of their daily lives. To this end, we conducted a 4-week deployment study of GlucoGoalie with individuals with T2D.

Deployment Study Methods

Participants and Procedure

For this deployment study, we recruited participants from Columbia University Irving Medical Center, using the same inclusion criteria as in the controlled experiment described above. In an initial visit, participants received a 1-h nutrition training; this training focused on relevant concepts, which were also identified as somewhat confusing in the previous study, like food "choices" and macronutrients. An investigator introduced participants to the GlucoGoalie application and helped them set an initial goal of their choice. After that participants were asked to use GlucoGoalie independently for 4 weeks. During this time, participants were asked to log their meals and BG levels, review and set new nutritional goals, including personalized goals if and when those become available, and review their progress towards meeting goals at their convenience. When new personalized goal recommendations became available, participants received push notifications and a text message from the study coordinator. After the 4-week period, participants returned for 1-h semi-structured interviews. To minimize barriers to participation, individuals without smartphone received an Android phone and could keep it after completing the study (participants who had their own smartphones received its monetary equivalent, $150). All participants received $20 for the initial visit and another $20 for the debrief interview.

Data Analysis

We used participants' usage logs to calculate descriptive usage statistics including the numbers of meals logged, goals selected, and goals used. Qualitative interviews were audio recorded, transcribed verbatim, and analyzed using inductive thematic analysis [48]. The investigators coded two transcripts (25%) collaboratively to create an initial codebook. Then the first two authors independently coded an additional two transcripts (25%), and met in person to discuss coding schemes and resolve all discrepancies through discussion. The remaining interviews were coded independently by EM with periodic discussion of emerging themes with the research team. Participant meal logs, usage, and goal attainment were considered throughout the coding process to contextualize user statements.

Deployment Study Results

Below, we briefly describe participants' demographics and their general experience managing diabetes and usage of the GlucoGoalie app, and then continue to describe the four main themes from the thematic analysis: (1) receiving goal suggestion informs self-discovery, (2) choosing goals highlights individual preferences, (3) following goals demonstrates the importance of feedback and context, and (4) challenges understanding and following goals in practice.

Participant Background and Demographics

A total of ten participants were enrolled in the deployment study. Two participants were lost to follow-up or withdrew for personal reasons, for a total of eight participants who completed the deployment study and were included in the analysis. There was some overlap between the controlled experiment and the deployment study, with two participants completing both studies. As shown in Table 17.2, the demographic breakdown was comparable across the two studies. While median income was higher in the deployment study, the distributions were similar, and the deployment study clinics were in an area with a higher cost of living (Manhattan vs. Brooklyn).

Diabetes Experiences

Participants had mixed and often poor experiences with self-management prior to enrolling in the study. Many reported poor eating habits and being indiscriminate about their meals:

> ... before that I eat whatever. Yeah, whatever. Dinner time, I eat whatever. P2

Along with challenges with nutrition, participants described challenges keeping their BG within target ranges:

> Sometimes [my blood sugar] goes very high or goes very low. P4

Some participants had tried prior bouts of focused self-management, with mixed success in the long run. Three participants had previously tracked their meals on paper, but none had any experience with self-monitoring apps.

Overall Impressions and Usage

Overall, participants reported that they enjoyed the experience of using GlucoGoalie, and found it fun, easy, and direct.

> It was fun. They laugh about me because every time I was going to eat — no, wait a minute. I can't start eating. I've got to take a picture of it... It was fun to play. P2

They also actively engaged with the main part of the app: setting and following goals.

> I try to follow the goals and instructions if I'm trying to improve my intake. That's what I'm trying to do most of the time. Because every day I try to follow a better diet and try to have more greens. P4

Usage statistics over the 4-week study are presented in Table 17.3. Participants showed high engagement with logging features: on average they recorded more than three meals per day, and all participants set at least one goal. Regarding personalized goals, 88% of participants (7 of 8) received personalized goals while in the study; one participant did not receive any personalized goals because their BG levels were well-controlled. Of those who received a goal recommendation, 71% (5 of 7) selected at least one of these goals in the app. However, 3 participants did not notice a push notification informing them of a new goal suggestion, and only selected one after a call from the study coordinator.

Below we describe the main themes in individuals' experiences that emerged from thematic analysis.

Theme 1: Receiving Goal Suggestion Informs Self-Discovery

One of the main aims of GlucoGoalie was to reduce the cognitive burden of self-tracking by relying on ML to automatically identify meaningful patterns in self-monitoring data and to use these patterns to generate concrete and actionable self-management goals. However, many participants of the study found the process of self-tracking to be insightful in and of itself. In particular, tracking meals in conjunction with BG levels often helped participants to notice dependencies between different foods in their meals and changes in their BG levels after meals that included these foods.

> *I did it for two days and I tested my sugar, oh, this is the rice… So, I stopped eating rice for two days, and then when I stopped eating rice, it got lower.* P6

In addition to these more common benefits of tracking, participants found that the goals they saw in the app prompted them to reflect on their choices and provided scaffolding for the self-discovery process. For example, when P2 saw the goal to "eat whole fruits instead of juice", it alerted them to the impact of juices on BG, which was confirmed by their observations:

Table 17.3 GlucoGoalie usage statistics over the 4-week study ($N = 8$)

Usage variable	Value
# meals logged	Median: 93.5 Range: 14–158
# BG readings logged	Median: 173 Range: 21–314
% received personalized goals	88% (7 of 8)
% used personalized goals	63% (5 of 8)
# unique personalized goals used during study period	Median: 3 goals Range: 0–8
Pre-meal BG (mean ± SD)	135.0 ± 36.7 mg/dL
Post-meal BG (mean ± SD)	156.1 ± 47.7 mg/dL

When I drink the juice, I see that sugar is what was high. And I learned that that was the problem.... Now, when I eat, I don't drink juice. P2

In many cases, the personalized goal recommendations provided additional opportunity to reflect on behaviors individuals already suspected as problematic.

And I know that, my carbs like I said, are usually high. I think that, my first, what I gravitate to first in any meal is the carb and that's what I want more of... So, I'm not like surprised that it recommends reducing the carbs and trying to replace it with something else. P3

In these situations, personalized goals were not only guiding individuals' future choices, but also helped them to critically reflect on their past behaviors and their self-management needs and pitfalls.

Theme 2: Choosing Goals Highlights Individual Preferences

All participants selected at least one goal while in the study; however, they varied widely not only in the number of goals they selected overall, but also in their reasons and motivations for choosing different goals. Some gravitated towards goals that appeared relatively easy to achieve and were not too different from their current behaviors. These participants viewed goals as a checkpoints or reminders to be more consistent.

I like that it was a goal that it was more feasible to me. So, it was just a good like a checkpoint for me not sort of a reminder but kind of like, oh it's going with what I'm doing. So, it's just reminding me. P8

In contrast, other participants took their participation in the research study as an opportunity to challenge themselves and chose goals that were farther from their current nutritional patterns.

Yes, I go to the notification and started looking at the new one. That's why, when I first took the other substitute of water for over sodas. I realized, well that's not really a goal because I've been doing that already. So, I need to change to something more difficult because I was done with the other one. P4

Another factor that played an important role in selection of goals was inclusion of foods that individuals liked among examples that accompanied each goal. For many participants, these examples were critical factors to deciding whether to try a goal or not, often more so than the goals themselves.

That one is okay, because I used to eat the oatmeal, one slice of toast, yeah that one is okay. P1

However, whilst for some participants seeing comfortable familiar foods and ingredients was an attraction, others wished for variety and novelty and saw these examples as an opportunity to break away from their existing routines. For example, P2 was looking for examples of vegetables they could eat other than broccoli:

I don't know, like, if I want to eat like broccoli, I will be tired. And I'm not going to eat it every day. P2

Theme 3: Following Goals Demonstrates the Importance of Feedback and Context

A persistent theme that ran through the interviews was the importance of context and its influence on individuals' willingness and ability to pursue different goals. Given its persistent nature, it was important for GlucoGoalie to fit with individuals' daily habits and routines and their daily lives. Many participants had established patterns they were reluctant to change, for example a favorite breakfast food; others struggled to establish such routines because of busy and unpredictable schedules. In either of these cases, participants expected GlucoGoalie to adjust to their routines or lack thereof and to have enough flexibility to accommodate different circumstances:

> *Since I'm a busy woman… it kind of just has to go back to like how my day is. So, I know that if I didn't meet it for one of my meals, I'll have to meet it for the next meal.* P8

Furthermore, daily patterns could change overtime, or during different seasons, presenting additional need for context-awareness and sensitivity.

> *I don't want to have a hearty breakfast compared to like in the winter.* P8

Finally, nutritional goals individuals set within this study were situated within a broader set of diabetes self-management activities. For example, many were mindful of the synergistic impact of diet and exercise on BG levels and wanted to be able to adjust their nutritional goals based on the planned exercise routines.

> *So, I know, if I have exercise, walking or an exercise routine after a meal that's going to be a little bit more high carbs. That has made an impact.* P5

In addition to the need to accommodate context, participants spoke of the importance of feedback on their progress. This included more specific feedback on attainment of selected nutritional goals:

> *Everybody would like to know how they're doing… Because if I'm eating less and it's not doing no good, what's the point of me doing it?* P2

Even more broadly, however, they wished to connect more specific nutritional goals in GlucoGoalie with their broader goals for diabetes self-management and healthy lives. Whilst nutritional goals were important, participants often viewed them as a step towards a broader goal, such as improvement in BG levels, or weight loss:

> *Definitely in terms of weight loss but like also my actual numbers in terms of my blood sugar.* P3

Theme 4: Challenges Understanding and Following Goals in Practice

Personalized nutritional goals within GlucoGoalie were formulated on the level of macronutrients, and only included specific foods as examples. This approach has several important advantages as it greatly reduces the number of features for ML and allows users flexibility in choosing different foods within the same macronutrient categories. However, in practice, many participants struggled to translate these somewhat abstract goals into specific meal choices.

> *The replacement, it was, you know was dropping, half a carb replacing, half carb. That was a little harder to figure out. So, it will require a little more thinking.* P5

This was particularly the case for participants who described themselves as lacking nutritional knowledge needed to identify macronutrients and estimate portion sizes. For these participants, goals formulated using macronutrients and "choices" as units presented an impassable barrier and were often dismissed. These participants often referred to using visual proportions of different types of foods on their plate to gauge how healthy their meals were:

> *I use my plate, but I try to go as they show me in the program, you see the plate then half it's a vegetable or fruit, this is a protein and that one is a carbohydrate.* P1

These challenges were further exacerbated by ambiguities in formulation of goals and lack of ability to clarify these ambiguities with follow-up questions. For example, P2 interpreted the word "choice" not as a unit of measure but as its more natural and common meaning, as a selection of several items one might choose from. Given that, this participant felt they accomplished their goal of including 2 "choices" of fat when they included two different fat-containing foods, rather than 10 g (2 choices) of any fat-containing foods.

> *Sometimes I put it together, the mozzarella on top of the egg which means I'm taking two fats.* P2

In general, static text alone was limited in its ability to convey the more abstract nutrition goals. During the interviews, participants asked many clarifying questions, for example which foods count as which macronutrients. Some participants suggested that visual aids for portion size estimation would be a welcome addition.

In contrast to the more abstract personalized goals, generic goals were simpler, focused on specific foods and food families that participants were familiar with, and were generally perceived as easy to implement without additional knowledge.

> *Those were right. Those were easy and I've been, I have been intentional to drink a bottle of water at every main meal and then have a bottle or two in between.* P5

Perceived Results

Despite these barriers, and as a result of following the goals they had chosen, many participants developed new habits, and internalized personalized goal suggestions to the point that they became integrated with their daily practice:

> *Even anything longer than two weeks will probably just make it into more of a habit for me. I'll probably eat two weeks to get comfortable with how much fat I'm taking, let's say the goal was on fat, so then after that it would just be more of a habit.* P8

At the end of the study, many participants described seeing changes not just in their behaviors, but also in their actual blood glucose levels.

I did notice because sometimes it was 200. When I see that it was 200, it was after I eat. Oh yeah. After I—but before, 250, 270—because I was eating a lot of food. Five or six in the night. P2

Discussion

In this research, we examined individuals' experiences with receiving, selecting, and following computationally generated nutritional goals for T2D. In designing GlucoGoalie, we took the approach of combining ML analysis of individuals' self-tracking data with an expert system to computationally generate recommendations for nutritional goals that are likely to lead to improvement in BG levels. Furthermore, we incorporated several interactive features for reviewing and selecting goals, for in-the-moment meal-time reflection, and for monitoring goal attainment overtime. We evaluated this approach in two studies that examined whether individuals can understand and follow nutritional goals generated by the expert system using ML inferences, and what experiences would result from receiving and following such goals in the context of individuals' daily lives.

In the first controlled study, we found that, to a large degree, participants could understand nutritional goals and correctly chose meals that met a goal 89% of the time when these meals were accompanied by corresponding nutritional labels. Furthermore, when asked to compose a meal that aligned with a particular nutritional goal, they created meals in the direction of the goal 67% of the time, and their meals were within 1 "choice" of their nutritional target. However, without a nutritional label, the participants' accuracy in choosing meals that align with goals dropped to 49%. This finding is consistent with prior research highlighting challenges in accurately assessing nutritional composition of meals [49]. This was supported by qualitative findings that indicated some confusion with nutrition terminology in goals, particularly in relation to macronutrients and "choices" as units of measure.

Similarly, the deployment study uncovered both successes and challenges for participants in understanding and acting on goal recommendations. The study showed that participants engaged with goals, generally found them easy to understand and follow and often found goals insightful and promoting reflection and learning. At the same time, participants sometimes struggled with integrating goals with the context of their daily lives, wished for more direct feedback on attainment of goals, and for more opportunities to disambiguate and negotiate goals and actions through a conversation. Below we discuss these themes and relate them to our design choices.

Cognitive Support: Balancing Reflection and Action

Supporting individuals' cognition is a long-standing goal and an active area of research in human-computer interaction and biomedical informatics. In the context of personal informatics, this often takes the form of promoting self-knowledge through collection of and reflection on self-tracking data, which, in turn, informs future action [9]. However, reflecting on data can be burdensome, and not everyone has the necessary time, mental energy, and literacy. In contrast, recommender systems provide more direct support for action, are easy to use and do not typically require effort or knowledge. However, there is a concern that focusing entirely on recommendations may inadvertently jeopardize learning and reduce the positive impact of reflection. These questions are particularly acute given the rapid rates of adoption of AI-powered systems in many domains and increasing body of research highlighting the dangers of over-reliance on AI [50] and the potential of cognitive disengagement from AI-powered decision support [51].

Our study suggested that it is possible to reach a middle ground between reflection and action, particularly in the context of AI-powered tools for health self-management. GlucoGoalie leveraged expert knowledge of nutrition to translate patterns identified with ML into concrete suggestions for nutritional goals, thus reducing the need for data examination and analysis. As a result, participants were able to make concrete changes to their diets, which often led to perceived improvements in BG levels. At the same time, because goals were based on participants' own dietary histories, they often inspired reflection as participants wondered which nutritional choices triggered specific goals. Participants compared goal suggestions to their own self-perceptions of their eating habits and used them as a mirror to re-examine their past choices.

These findings highlight new opportunities to provide synergistic support for both reflection and action. For example, future work could examine ways to more explicitly use data to support selection of specific goal recommendations, for example by incorporating visual summaries of pertinent trends [15, 52]. This additional information can serve as a form of explanation for the recommendations, and prior work has demonstrated the importance of explanations in facilitating nutritional learning [49]. A growing body of research in explainable ML may offer potential avenues to make recommendations in support of action and ground them with an explanation to support reflection [53]. Future work could further incorporate advances in explainable ML to personal informatics applications.

Aligning Goals with Eating Experiences and Personal Aspirations

GlucoGoalie used macronutrients as a foundation for identifying patterns and making recommendations for nutritional goals [38]. This approach greatly simplifies the task for machine learning: finding trends common to three main macronutrients that repeat in every meal is considerably easier than finding trends using concrete foods given a much larger set of food options with many occurring only infrequently. Furthermore, given the emphasis on macronutrients in diabetes education, this approach could further promote nutritional literacy and enable greater flexibility in making nutritional choices.

However, the study showed that macronutrients continue to present a barrier to many individuals who prefer to think of their meals in terms of specific foods they put on their plates. An alternative approach to recommendations could leverage this comfort and familiarity with foods and help to translate a macronutrient-level goal into a specific meal suggestion, in the style closer to the one used by contemporary nutritional RecSys. RecSys excel at making concrete suggestions based on personal preferences, learned from users' past behavior or characteristics [27], and can incorporate additional constraints like food allergies and other health-related considerations [35, 54]. Meal logs and macronutrient-centered goals from GlucoGoalie could be used as inputs to a preference-based RecSys to generate concrete suggestions that would help individuals connect their goals to what's on their plate.

Furthermore, when making these more concrete recommendations, future systems should take steps to integrate and incorporate individuals' context, both person-specific, such as context of previous meals and activities, and more general, such as time of year. Mobile phones and sensors can offer clues to the user's current state, and there is a rich body of research in context-aware computing within HCI and Ubiquitous Computing [55]. In health, location-based prompts have been used to help prevent relapse triggers [56], and step counts can inform adaptive fitness goals based on recent activity levels [57], but have not been widely used in nutrition [58]. Furthermore, future systems could aim to generate recommendations that align not only with individuals' immediate behavioral goals, such as nutritional goals, but also with their broader goals and aspirations in health and life. Niess and Woźniak observed the relationship between tracking goals and qualitative health goals in the context of individuals setting goals with fitness trackers [59]. Previous researchers have explored methods to elicit these values and motivations [60] and future work could explore how to connect them to more specific and quantitative goals that could be generated using ML and AI [59].

Interactivity, Negotiation, and Feedback

Integrating ML with an expert system enabled GlucoGoalie to generate personalized nutritional goals expressed in natural language. However, these goals were delivered as static text, which was not always easy to interpret, given its reference to nutritional abstractions (macronutrients and measurement "choices"). One approach to making nutrition goals more understandable is to incorporate illustrations. In health risk communication, illustrations and infographics have been used successfully to improve comprehension of complex information [61–63]. A similar visual approach has been applied to assist low literacy adults with portion size estimation [64], and could be used here to better convey numerical content in personalized goals.

Another approach is to transition from a static text as a goal delivery mechanism to a conversation. Such a conversation could enable individuals to ask follow-up questions, negotiate priorities, ask for explanations, and otherwise ensure that the resulting goals and suggestions are fully aligned with an individual's broader goals and priorities. Along these lines, conversational agents have been used to support interactive goal setting, health coaching, and motivational interviewing [65, 66]. Recent advances in generative AI and Large Language Models (LLM) made general-purpose conversational agents available to general public. These models are trained on vast amounts of text-based data amassed on the Internet, and are able to generate human-like responses to questions in a variety of domains and contexts. And while traditional conversational agents require complex dialog structures, for fully-scripted ones, or extensive training on specialized datasets, for those that incorporate ML, LLMs produce many of the same benefits with no additional training or effort on the part of the investigators. However, there remain many open questions as to the feasibility of using general-purpose LLMs in health contexts, mostly due to the tendency to incorporate widely inaccurate statements, not grounded in any facts or data. In GlucoGoalie, we used expert system to impose guardrails on inferences generated with ML. Similar efforts are needed to impose expert knowledge and common sense guardrails on LLMs to prevent them from generating erroneous and misleading statements. Machine learning approaches like mechanistic, controller, or reinforcement learning models are a potential vein for future exploration [67–69].

Limitations

As an initial step towards exploring actionable health recommendations, this work has a number of limitations. Both studies had small sample sizes, and while the sample was recruited from economically disadvantaged communities, it was not representative: participants were skewed female, and predominantly black or Latino. This cohort from a single United States metro area may not account for important cultural differences nationally or globally [70]. In addition, the deployment sstudy ran for 4-weeks, and usage patterns and engagement may change with extended use. Finally, while we report qualitative perceptions, we did not quantitatively examine changes in BG or other health outcomes because of the small sample and short timeframe [71].

Conclusion

While self-tracking data hold potential to inform action, deriving actionable insights is challenging and burdensome for individuals. In this work, we explored an approach that combines ML with an expert system to generate goals that are personalized based on an individual's health data. We found that support for action can also support, augment, and inform reflection. We connected our findings with both prior research and open questions in personal informatics, goal-setting, and health-based recommender systems, and argue that future interventions could incorporate more interactive, dialog-based components with conversational agents.

Acknowledgements This research was funded by the National Institute of Diabetes and Digestive and Kidney Diseases award number R56DK113189 and the National Library of Medicine award number T15LM007079. Thank you to the fellow students of Columbia's Department of Biomedical Informatics, who earned the undying gratitude of the corresponding author by arts-and-crafting food images for the virtual buffet.

References

1. National diabetes statistics report, 2020. CDC [Internet]. 2020 [cited 2021 Sep 8]. Available from: https://www.cdc.gov/diabetes/data/statistics-report/index.html
2. Bodenheimer T, Lorig K, Holman H, Grumbach K. Patient self-management of chronic disease in primary care. JAMA. 2002;288(19):2469.
3. American Diabetes Association. 4. Lifestyle management: standards of medical care in diabetes-2018. Diabetes Care. 2018;41(Suppl 1):S38–50.
4. Zeevi D, Korem T, Zmora N, et al. Personalized Nutrition by Prediction of Glycemic Responses. Cell. 2015;163(5):1079–95.
5. Matthan NR, Ausman LM, Meng H, Tighiouart H, Lichtenstein AH. Estimating the reliability of glycemic index values and potential sources of methodological and biological variability. Am J Clin Nutr. 2016;104(4):1004–13.
6. Centers for Disease Control and Prevention. Racial and ethnic approaches to community health. DNPAO [Internet]. 2018 [cited 2019 Jan 3]. Available from: https://www.cdc.gov/nccdphp/dnpao/state-local-programs/reach/
7. Hayward MD, Miles TP, Crimmins EM, Yang Y. The significance of socioeconomic status in explaining the racial gap in chronic health conditions. Am Sociol Rev. 2000;65(6):910.
8. Peek ME, Cargill A, Huang ES. Diabetes health disparities: a systematic review of health care interventions. Med Care Res Rev MCRR. 2007;64(5 Suppl):101S–56S.
9. Li I, Dey A, Forlizzi J. A stage-based model of personal informatics systems. Paper presented at: Proceedings of the SIGCHI Conference on Human Factors in Computing Systems (CHI

'10). New York: ACM; 2010 [cited 2017 Feb 21]. p. 557–66. Available from: http://doi.acm.org/10.1145/1753326.1753409
10. Epstein DA, Caldeira C, Figueiredo MC, et al. Mapping and taking stock of the personal informatics literature. Proc ACM Interact Mob Wearable Ubiquitous Technol. 2020;4(4):1–38.
11. Li I, Dey AK, Forlizzi J. Understanding my data, myself: supporting self-reflection with Ubicomp Technologies. Paper presented at: Proceedings of the 13th International Conference on Ubiquitous Computing (UbiComp '11). New York, NY, USA: ACM; 2011 [cited 2016 Dec 8]. p. 405–14. Available from: http://doi.acm.org/10.1145/2030112.2030166
12. Anderson I, Maitland J, Sherwood S, et al. Shakra: tracking and sharing daily activity levels with unaugmented mobile phones. Mob Netw Appl. 2007;12(2–3):185–99.
13. Consolvo S, McDonald DW, Toscos T, et al. Activity sensing in the wild: a field trial of Ubifit Garden. Paper presented at: Proceedings of the SIGCHI Conference on Human Factors in Computing Systems (CHI '08). New York: ACM; 2008 [cited 2014 Dec 10]. p. 1797–806. Available from: http://doi.acm.org/10.1145/1357054.1357335
14. Medynskiy Y, Mynatt E. Salud!: an open infrastructure for developing and deploying health self-management applications. Paper presented at: 2010 4th International Conference on Pervasive Computing Technologies for Healthcare. 2010. p. 1–8.
15. Epstein D, Cordeiro F, Bales E, Fogarty J, Munson S. Taming data complexity in lifelogs: exploring visual cuts of personal informatics data. Paper presented at: Proceedings of the 2014 Conference on Designing Interactive Systems (DIS '14). New York: ACM; 2014 [cited 2016 Dec 8]. p. 667–76. Available from: http://doi.acm.org/10.1145/2598510.2598558
16. Liang Z, Ploderer B, Liu W, et al. SleepExplorer: a visualization tool to make sense of correlations between personal sleep data and contextual factors. Pers Ubiquitous Comput. 2016;20(6):985–1000.
17. Mamykina L, Levine ME, Davidson PG, Smaldone AM, Elhadad N, Albers DJ. Data-driven health management: reasoning about personally generated data in diabetes with information technologies. J Am Med Inform Assoc. 2016;23(3):526–31.
18. Hollis V, Konrad A, Springer A, et al. What does all this data mean for my future mood? Actionable analytics and targeted reflection for emotional well-being. Hum-Comput Interact. 2017;32(5–6):208–67.
19. Clawson J, Pater JA, Miller AD, Mynatt ED, Mamykina L. No longer wearing: investigating the abandonment of personal health-tracking technologies on craigslist. Paper presented at: Proceedings of the 2015 ACM International Joint Conference on Pervasive and Ubiquitous Computing - UbiComp '15. New York: ACM; 2015. p. 647–58.
20. Lazar A, Koehler C, Tanenbaum J, Nguyen DH. Why we use and abandon smart devices. Paper presented at: Proceedings of the 2015 ACM International Joint Conference on Pervasive and Ubiquitous Computing - UbiComp '15. New York: ACM; 2015. p. 635–46.
21. Veinot TC, Mitchell H, Ancker JS. Good intentions are not enough: how informatics interventions can worsen inequality. J Am Med Inform Assoc. 2018;25(8):1080–8.
22. Veinot TC, Ancker JS, Cole-Lewis H, et al. Leveling up. Med Care. 2019;57:S108–14.
23. Gulshan V, Peng L, Coram M, et al. Development and validation of a deep learning algorithm for detection of diabetic retinopathy in retinal fundus photographs. JAMA. 2016;316(22):2402–10.
24. Rajkomar A, Oren E, Chen K, et al. Scalable and accurate deep learning with electronic health records. NPJ Digit Med. 2018;1(1):18.
25. Bentley F, Tollmar K, Stephenson P, et al. Health mashups: presenting statistical patterns between wellbeing data and context in natural language to promote behavior change. ACM Trans Comput-Hum Interact. 2013;20(5):1–27.
26. Desai PM, Mitchell EG, Hwang ML, Levine ME, Albers DJ, Mamykina L. Personal health oracle: explorations of personalized predictions in diabetes self-management. Paper presented at: CHI '19: Proceedings of the 2019 CHI Conference on Human Factors in Computing Systems. New York: ACM; 2019. p. 1–13.

27. Ricci F, Rokach L, Shapira B. Recommender systems: introduction and challenges. In: Recommender systems handbook. Boston, MA: Springer US; 2015. p. 1–34.
28. Swearingen K, Sinha R. Beyond algorithms: an HCI perspective on recommender systems. Paper presented at: ACM SIGIR 2001 Workshop on Recommender Systems. 2001. p. 1–11.
29. Harvey M, Ludwig B, Elsweiler D. You are what you eat: learning user tastes for rating prediction. In: Kurland O, Lewenstein M, Porat E, editors. String processing and information retrieval. Cham: Springer; 2013. p. 153–64. (Lecture Notes in Computer Science).
30. Lawo D, Böhm L, Stevens G. Veganaizer: AI-assisted ingredient substitution. Paper presented at: European CSCW, 2021. 2020.
31. Elsweiler D, Harvey M. Towards automatic meal plan recommendations for balanced nutrition. Paper presented at: Proceedings of the 9th ACM Conference on Recommender Systems. 2015. p. 313–6.
32. Karkar R, Zia J, Vilardaga R, et al. A framework for self-experimentation in personalized health. J Am Med Inform Assoc. 2016;23(3):440–8.
33. Zitar RA, Al-Jabali A. Towards neural network model for insulin/glucose in diabetics-II. ResearchGate. 2005;29(2):227–32.
34. Yang L, Hsieh CK, Yang H, et al. Yum-me: a personalized nutrient-based meal recommender system. ACM Trans Inf Syst. 2016;36(1):7.
35. Elsweiler D, Ludwig B, Said A, Schaefer H, Trattner C. Engendering health with recommender systems. Paper presented at: Proceedings of the 10th ACM Conference on Recommender Systems - RecSys '16. New York: ACM; 2016. p. 409–10.
36. Schäfer H. Personalized support for healthy nutrition decisions. Paper presented at: Proceedings of the 10th ACM Conference on Recommender Systems - RecSys '16. New York: ACM Press; 2016. p. 455–8.
37. Reading Turchioe M, Burgermaster M, Mitchell EG, Desai PM, Mamykina L. Adapting the stage-based model of personal informatics for low-resource communities in the context of type 2 diabetes. J Biomed Inform. 2020;110:103572.
38. Evert AB, Dennison M, Gardner CD, et al. Nutrition therapy for adults with diabetes or prediabetes: a consensus report. Diabetes Care. 2019;42(5):731–54.
39. Wheeler ML, Daly A, Evert A, et al. Choose your foods, food lists for diabetes. Chicago IL: Academy of Nutrition and Dietetics and American Diabetes Association; 2014.
40. Tabak EG, Trigila G. Explanation of variability and removal of confounding factors from data through optimal transport. Commun Pure Appl Math. 2018;71(1):163–99.
41. Aschner P. New IDF clinical practice recommendations for managing type 2 diabetes in primary care. Diabetes Res Clin Pract. 2017;132:169–70.
42. Mitchell EG, Tabak EG, Levine ME, Mamykina L, Albers DJ. Enabling personalized decision support with patient-generated data and attributable components. J Biomed Inform. 2021;113:103639.
43. Cole-Lewis HJ, Smaldone AM, Davidson PR, et al. Participatory approach to the development of a knowledge base for problem-solving in diabetes self-management. Int J Med Inf. 2016;85(1):96–103.
44. Kato S, Waki K, Nakamura S, et al. Validating the use of photos to measure dietary intake: the method used by DialBetics, a smartphone-based self-management system for diabetes patients. Diabetol Int. 2016;7(3):244–51.
45. Noronha J, Hysen E, Zhang H, Gajos KZ. Platemate: crowdsourcing nutritional analysis from food photographs. Paper presented at: Proceedings of the 24th Annual ACM Symposium on User Interface Software and Technology. New York: ACM; 2011. p. 1–12.
46. Facts Up Front [Internet]. [cited 2018 Sep 15]. Available from: http://www.factsupfront.org/
47. Nazario B. Portion size plate. Recommended serving sizes for portion control [Internet]. 2013 [cited 2018 Apr 15]. Available from: https://www.webmd.com/diet/healthtool-portion-size-plate
48. Braun V, Clarke V. Using thematic analysis in psychology. Qual Res Psychol. 2006;3(2):77–101.

49. Burgermaster M, Gajos KZ, Davidson P, Mamykina L. The role of explanations in casual observational learning about nutrition. Paper presented at: Proceedings of the 2017 CHI Conference on Human Factors in Computing Systems - CHI '17. New York: ACM; 2017. p. 4097–145.
50. Buçinca Z, Malaya MB, Gajos KZ. To trust or to think: cognitive forcing functions can reduce overreliance on AI in AI-assisted decision-making. Proc ACM Hum-Comput Interact. 2021;5(CSCW1):188:1–21.
51. Gajos KZ, Mamykina L. Do people engage cognitively with AI? Impact of AI assistance on incidental learning. Paper presented at: Proceedings of the ACM Conference on Intelligent User Interfaces. 2022.
52. Schroeder J, Karkar R, Fogarty J, Kientz JA, Munson SA, Kay M. A patient-centered proposal for bayesian analysis of self-experiments for health. J Healthc Inform Res. 2019;3(1):124–55.
53. Wang D, Yang Q, Abdul A, Lim BY. Designing theory-driven user-centric explainable AI. Paper presented at: Conference on Human Factors in Computing Systems - Proceedings. New York: ACM; 2019. p. 1–15.
54. Hsu P, Zhao J, Liao K, Liu T, Wang C. AllergyBot: a chatbot technology intervention for young adults with food allergies dining out. Paper presented at: Conference on Human Factors in Computing Systems - Proceedings. New York: ACM; 2017. p. 74–9.
55. Dey AK. Understanding and using context. Pers Ubiquitous Comput. 2001;5(1):4–7.
56. Chih MY, Patton T, McTavish FM, et al. Predictive modeling of addiction lapses in a mobile health application. J Subst Abuse Treat. 2014;46(1):29–35.
57. Korinek EV, Phatak SS, Martin CA, et al. Adaptive step goals and rewards: a longitudinal growth model of daily steps for a smartphone-based walking intervention. J Behav Med. 2018;41(1):74–86.
58. Rabbi M, Aung MH, Zhang M, Choudhury T. MyBehavior: automatic personalized health feedback from user behaviors and preferences using smartphones. Paper presented at: UbiComp 2015 - Proceedings of the 2015 ACM International Joint Conference on Pervasive and Ubiquitous Computing. New York: ACM; 2015. p. 707–18.
59. Niess J, Wozniak PW. Supporting meaningful personal fitness: the tracker goal evolution model. Paper presented at: Proceedings of the 2018 CHI Conference on Human Factors in Computing Systems - CHI '18. New York: ACM; 2018. p. 1–12.
60. Berry ABL, Lim C, Hartzler AL, et al. Eliciting values of patients with multiple chronic conditions: evaluation of a patient-centered framework. AMIA Annu Symp Proc. 2017;2017:430–9.
61. Arcia A, Suero-Tejeda N, Bales ME, et al. Sometimes more is more: Iterative participatory design of infographics for engagement of community members with varying levels of health literacy. J Am Med Inform Assoc. 2016;23(1):174–83.
62. Zikmund-Fisher BJ, Scherer AM, Witteman HO, et al. Graphics help patients distinguish between urgent and non-urgent deviations in laboratory test results. J Am Med Inform Assoc. 2016;24(3):ocw169.
63. Grossman L, Feiner S, Mitchell E, Masterson Creber R. Leveraging patient-reported outcomes using data visualization. Appl Clin Inform. 2018;09(03):565–75.
64. Chaudhry BM, Schaefbauer C, Jelen B, Siek KA, Connelly K. Evaluation of a food portion size estimation interface for a varying literacy population. Paper presented at: Proceedings of the 2016 CHI Conference on Human Factors in Computing Systems - CHI '16. New York: ACM; 2016. p. 5645–57.
65. Bickmore TW, Schulman D, Sidner CL. A reusable framework for health counseling dialogue systems based on a behavioral medicine ontology. J Biomed Inform. 2011;44(2):183–97.
66. Lee J, Hekler EB, Chiauzzi E, Towner A, Fitz-Randolph M. Helping users set rules for defining short-term activity goals. Paper presented at: Proceedings of the 2016 CHI Conference Extended Abstracts on Human Factors in Computing Systems - CHI EA '16. New York: ACM; 2016. p. 2178–84.
67. Albers DJ, Levine ME, Stuart A, Mamykina L, Gluckman B, Hripcsak G. Mechanistic machine learning: how data assimilation leverages physiologic knowledge using Bayesian

inference to forecast the future, infer the present, and phenotype. J Am Med Inform Assoc. 2018;25(10):1392–401.
68. Martín CA, Rivera DE, Hekler EB, et al. Development of a control-oriented model of social cognitive theory for optimized mHealth behavioral interventions. IEEE Trans Control Syst Technol. 2020;28(2):331–46.
69. Lei H, Tewari A, Murphy SA. An actor-critic contextual bandit algorithm for personalized mobile health interventions; 2017 Jun 27. https://doi.org/10.48550/arXiv.1706.09090.
70. Stowell E, Lyson MC, Saksono H, et al. Designing and evaluating mHealth interventions for vulnerable populations. Paper presented at: Proceedings of the 2018 CHI Conference on Human Factors in Computing Systems - CHI '18. New York: ACM; 2018. p. 1–17.
71. Klasnja P, Consolvo S, Pratt W. How to evaluate technologies for health behavior change in HCI research. Paper presented at: Conference on Human Factors in Computing Systems - Proceedings. 2011. p. 3063–72.

Part V
Future Directions

Chapter 18
Looking Forward: The Role of Human Computer Interaction and Cognition in Healthcare

Andre W. Kushniruk, David R. Kaufman, Thomas G. Kannampallil, and Vimla L. Patel

Introduction

A deeper understanding of Human-computer interaction (HCI) is critical to the success of efforts to advance healthcare using technology. Central to this, is a focus on understanding the cognitive basis of human interactions with systems, and the cognitive processes that underlie that interaction [1]. In this book the authors have reported on the current state of HCI with a focus on the cognitive underpinnings of HCI in healthcare.

The authors of the chapters in this book have described their work in a range of healthcare areas. This has included a focus on perspectives around the design and evaluation of emerging health technologies through an HCI lens focused on the users' cognitive processes and capabilities. Much of this work has been informed by theories and evaluation frameworks emerging from the study of cognitive science

---

A. W. Kushniruk (✉)
School of Health Information Science, University of Victoria, Victoria, BC, Canada
e-mail: andrek@uvic.ca

D. R. Kaufman
Health Informatics Program, School of Health Professions, SUNY Downstate Health Sciences University, Brooklyn, NY, USA

T. G. Kannampallil
Institute for Informatics, Data Science, and Biostatistics, Washington University School of Medicine, St Louis, MO, USA

V. L. Patel
Cognitive Studies in Medicine and Public Health, The New York Academy of Medicine, New York, NY, USA

Department of Biomedical Informatics, Columbia University, New York, NY, USA

and applied in a variety of healthcare contexts. This has also included a discussion of a wide range of HCI models and frameworks, including the consideration of socio-technical and distributed cognition perspectives and approaches.

The range of applications described in this book has also been varied. This has included the study of user interactions with a variety of clinical information systems, mobile devices, computer visualizations, dental systems, clinical decision support systems, patient-facing applications as well as artificial intelligence (AI) applications in healthcare. With the increasing use of health technologies by patients and the general population, the diversity of healthcare information technology users has grown exponentially. This has necessitated new ways of modeling, representing and thinking about user needs and capabilities, and underscores the importance of understanding the limits and cognitive capabilities of technology users [2].

Work in developing and refining new methods and approaches to analyzing HCI in healthcare have also been reported in this book. This includes work in evaluating health technologies in laboratory experimental settings, and the evaluation of technologies in actual healthcare work environments. This reflects a trend reflecting a move from the study of health technology in artificial settings to the analysis of the impact of technology within situated contexts and real-world healthcare settings.

Some of the current trends in this area, reported in this book, are related to the design, analyses and evaluation of AI systems in healthcare. As intelligent technologies and applications become more ubiquitous and impact more of our daily lives, an improved understanding of the interaction and interplay between human and machine will become increasingly critical. This also necessitates a deeper understanding of how technology affects key aspects of human reasoning, decision making and work activities.

Current State: Cognition and HCI in Healthcare

This book has focused on cognitive aspects of user interaction and user experience in healthcare. The chapters reflect a number of trends that have emerged and accelerated since the publication of the first edition of the book. This includes research in areas that mirror the organization of the book, including updated discussion of the following topics: theoretical foundations of HCI, user-centered approaches to clinical information system design and evaluation, as well as application of the methods discussed to a wider range of applications in healthcare. Throughout the book, it has been argued that a cognitive, human-centered perspective to understanding of the impact and role of technology on human processes will be central to understanding the role and integration of technology in healthcare [1, 2]. This will be needed in order to develop and deploy more effective healthcare systems that interact with users in more effective and efficient ways and has formed the basis of a number of chapters in this book.

Understanding the complex interaction among health professionals and technology will be essential to maximize the potential for technology to streamline healthcare processes. At the same time, such an understanding can inform our understanding of the interplay between human and machine in reducing medical errors. In order to reduce the potential inadvertent introduction of new errors emerging from the introduction of a new technology itself, developing an improved understanding of how such technology supports and interacts with human cognition is needed, as well as how it impacts human reasoning and decision-making processes [1]. These are areas that have begun to be explored and which are also the focus of a number of the chapters in this book.

There is an increasing recognition that a broad perspective on HCI is needed that focuses not only on the interaction of individual users of systems with individual systems or applications, but which also examines user interactions with technology in the healthcare context at multiple levels of abstraction. This includes understanding how the technology fits within complex clinical activities and cognition that is distributed amongst multiple people and technologies in healthcare. The application of models based on distributed cognition and an understanding of how technology can support human collaboration and communication has become an important area of focus and study. This has been reflected in a number of publications [3, 4]. Along these lines, advances in evaluation that focus on understanding use of systems in terms of evaluating impact of health technologies on work practices have also emerged [5–7]. For example, methods from computational ethnography have emerged to collect data from live user interactions [8]. Advances in user-centered design approaches for modelling users (in terms of their capabilities, limitations and contexts of use) are also reported on in this book [9].

The widespread use of mobile devices and applications by health professionals, patients and the general population has fueled the development of a wide range of mHealth devices and systems [10–12]. The need for mobile usability testing has emerged, particularly in the face of increased virtual care, and ubiquitous computing. This includes the use of a wide range of devices including computers, smart phones, smart watches and wearable devices and has also had a profound impact on the scope and reach of healthcare applications. Along these lines, an improved understanding of how to effectively design and deploy mobile health applications to match user needs and processing requirements is needed [10]. This will require an improved understanding of how to best integrate such technologies into work practices as well as daily living of patients and lay people. Remote usability testing approaches have become key methods for studying user interactions as much of healthcare moves to becoming virtual, including the remote use of telehealth applications [9, 13].

As reported in this book, there has been a movement away from the study of HCI exclusively in artificial laboratory settings towards the evaluation of human interaction within complex health technology in real-world settings [13, 14]. Although laboratory-based studies and approaches are reported on (and critiqued) in this book, there is also the need to understand HCI within the complexity of healthcare with an emphasis on understanding use of technology "in-situ". This represents a move towards understanding technology use within its cognitive as well as social-technical contexts. Both the cognitive as well as socio-technical aspects of use of technology are critical and form the focus of much of the current work in medical cognition in relation to system usability. This is reflected in a number of the chapters focusing on how socio-technical theory and models can be applied to enhance the usability and effectiveness of healthcare information technology [3, 4]. Approaches that have also attempted to integrate both cognitive perspectives with socio-technical perspectives have also emerged [14]. An improved understanding of how technology fits within the complex healthcare environment has become increasingly recognized as being essential in order to develop systems that effectively support human healthcare activities.

Advanced computer-based visualization tools are currently changing healthcare practice in many health related areas from radiology to the analysis of large patient data sets. Based on work in visual analytics, the study of analytical reasoning, which is facilitated by visual interfaces, has become another important area of current focus [15]. The increased use of advanced visualization and data analytic techniques are founded on methods for allowing human health professionals to comprehend the rapidly increasing amount of information data made available for the diagnosis and treatment of diseases. This trend will continue as the amount of health related data grows, well beyond human capability for processing and requiring an understanding of how technology can support human cognitive processing.

As reported in this book, there has been an increasing use of health technology designed for use by patients and lay people and there have been many advances in the field of consumer health informatics [11]. This trend has greatly expanded the range of user backgrounds, understanding and capabilities that need to be considered, when designing health information systems and technologies. This requires new ways of representing patient needs and requirements, and is an area needing an improved understanding of cognition and lay person reasoning about health and technology. This includes consideration of aspects of e-health literacy and cognitive capabilities, including understanding the cognitive processing limitations of technology users. This understanding will be needed in order to design technologies that better match patient and lay person information needs, capabilities and cognitive processing in order to effect positive behaviour change and disease self-management using technology.

Finally, the role of HCI in relation to an increasingly automated world, in particular involving AI applications, is another current area of focus of considerable research interest. This has been discussed in several chapters in this edition of the book [16, 17]. Designing systems that empower and augment human decision making and reasoning, rather than replacing human decision making and reasoning, has become the goal of researchers interested in cognitive aspects of HCI in healthcare and the integration of human factors research with technological advances. Technology-centered thinking will need to be replaced by human-centered approaches that focus on user experience design methods, including improved methods for user observation, and increased engagement with stakeholders [18]. In order to achieve this, an increased focus on the cognitive underpinnings of user interaction with intelligent systems will be required as a sound basis [19].

Future Directions

In the coming years, the above trends are expected to continue and accelerate. In addition, work will be needed to ensure emerging healthcare applications are safe and usable for human use in healthcare. A number of new trends in HCI are emerging related to data science and automated approaches to studying and predicting usability and user experience. It is expected that these trends will increasingly underscore the need for improved understanding of the impact systems have on human cognition. This includes understanding the impact of technology on human reasoning and decision making, and well as understanding how technology can be integrated into complex social environments and contexts.

Looking forward into the near future, these trends will be greatly accelerated as technology rapidly advances and brings an increasing range of applications, capabilities and new forms of interactions with humans in the healthcare space. These range from advances in existing healthcare applications themselves, to the increased use of intelligent systems. In addition, the need for developing scientific methods for automating the collection and analysis of large amounts of data obtained from usability studies will grow. At the same time, the need for conducting in-depth smaller scale cognitive studies to provide meaning to results from large-scale studies will also continue and will complement large scale studies.

Advances in Healthcare Applications

In the coming years as AI and intelligent applications proliferate in healthcare, understanding the integration of humans and information systems will become increasingly critical [18–21]. This will include an improved understanding of human-robot interaction and how intelligent applications can be designed to synergistically work with humans most effectively in domains such as healthcare. This will necessitate an improved understanding of the advantages and limitations of both human and machine intelligence. Striking the appropriate balance between the human and machine in complex areas including clinical reasoning and decision making will be critical. Achieving this balance will require an improved understanding of HCI in healthcare from a cognitive perspective. In particular, research will be needed examining aspects of HCI related to understanding how systems impact, alter and augment human reasoning and decision making in healthcare. This will become increasingly important in order to ensure that emerging applications are safe, effective and efficient in amplifying rather than replacing humans in critical healthcare processes and activities. Along these lines, HCI research into new modes of user interaction that are compatible with human work processes will be needed. Advances in evaluating the impact of design decisions on workflow in healthcare will need to be studied in order to design systems that clinicians find useful and usable.

Increased automation and changes to healthcare work involving greater use of AI will underlie the need to better understand impact of information systems on reasoning, decision making, and human work practices. Research will be needed into understanding how to effectively balance locus of control in human and machine interactions. Models and frameworks from distributed cognition and pervasive computing may prove to be useful for this [22]. Complex decisions made by clinicians in diagnosis and treatment planning can be augmented by technologies such as natural language processing applications (e.g. using generative AI), intelligent search engines designed to support clinical decision making, and increased application of robotics in healthcare. Popular tools such as ChatGPT and DALL-E show considerable potential for supporting information seeking, diagnosing and for automating reporting and documentation. However, the challenge will remain as to how those technologies can be appropriately integrated into human cognitive activities involved in clinical decision making and reasoning.

Safety Informatics in Healthcare and Cognitive Modelling

An increased focus on safety of healthcare technology will grow in importance as health information technology proliferates in healthcare [23–25]. This includes the emergence of a range of applications, increased sharing of patient data, a wider range of use and an increase in dependence on technology. The area of technology-induced error focuses on understanding human error that may result from use of technology in complex healthcare settings [23]. Such error may not be exclusively from programming bugs or errors, but rather emerge when complex technology is deployed in real-world settings, where even systems that have undergone traditional testing approaches still lead to (or induce) human users to make errors.

Poor usability has led to technology-induced error [24]. However, the relationship between usability and error has remained to be fully explored. Central to this will be understanding how technology fits with the end user's goals, motivation, skill, and context of use. This will necessitate a cognitive approach to understanding and mitigating such error. A greater emphasis on safety of healthcare systems will also emerge as AI systems proliferate. This will require the need for an HCI perspective that takes into account users' cognitive processes, applying methods from cognitive modelling. A promising direction here is in the development of a "safety net" approach to testing systems that involves applying methods such as usability inspection, usability testing, clinical simulations and near-live testing within an integrative and step-wise model for evaluating systems prior to widespread release [25].

Patient-Centered Design of Healthcare Systems

Perhaps one of the most important trends is the greater involvement of patients and the general population in their own healthcare [11]. Information technology has provided a powerful vehicle for effecting and supporting this change. With the advent of a wide range of health applications and patient-facing systems, such as patient portals, the role of patients in their own healthcare decision making has accelerated since the development of the first patient clinical information systems that allowed patients to access their own medical record data over the World Wide Web (WWW) [26]. This trend will require the development of new methods for modelling user understanding when designing systems targeted to patient populations. This argues for advances in participatory design approaches that put the patient at the centre of design and evaluation processes [27, 28]. Such work will necessarily have to take into account not only patient preferences, but also their cognitive capabilities, limitations, and ability to use information presented to them by information systems in a way that will effect positive health behaviours and support self-management of chronic diseases by patients. This trend will accelerate in the future as a greater proportion of the population interact with health information technology, both in conjunction with their healthcare providers as well as in standalone interaction with health applications and health promotion technologies [11].

HCI for Virtual and Home Healthcare

Virtual healthcare, involving the remote interaction among patients and healthcare providers using communication or information technology, has and continues to emerge as a major trend. This move promises to transform healthcare by making it more accessible, equitable and economic [29]. Wearable technologies and advances in mobile health applications are allowing for the continuous monitoring of vital signs, blood pressure, etc. and can now provide additional clinical information in a continuous data stream [28]. Such technologies will directly impact clinical as well as patient reasoning and decision making. However, the amount of data collected is becoming enormous. As a result, challenges remain in understanding what information is relevant and useful for human clinical decision making and how continuous data streams can be integrated in clinical practice [12]. Along these lines, advances in telehealth involving integration of remote monitoring in the home will allow the elderly and disabled to stay at home. The interaction between remote monitoring technologies and patients is another area that has remained to be fully explored from a cognitive perspective. This will require an improved understanding of lay reasoning and cognitive processing to match the impressive technology with actual human use and application.

Usability Data Quantification and Analytics

An important and rapidly emerging trend in HCI is related to the large amounts of data being collected on usability of health information systems. Such data lends itself to quantification of the user experience in terms of user preferences, error rates and user satisfaction with systems. Along these lines the use of automated test scripts for online usability trials will continue to expand [30]. Areas where advances will be made include research in big data analytics for usability data, predictive analytics (e.g. for predicting user acceptance of different interface designs) and automated data mining of large data sets obtained from online usability studies. A range of advanced statistical methods are being applied to support decision making around features and functions to be offered by systems to users (e.g. statistically comparing user reactions to different user interface designs) and this trend will continue. This includes statistically comparing outcomes such as completion rates, user satisfaction ratings, as well as frequency of errors and usability problems associated with different user interface designs [31–33].

Automated Collection and Analysis of Usability Testing Data

Automated collection and analysis of usability and usage data has transformed research and evaluation in clinical workflow, user experience and HCI. This includes methods from remote usability testing and analysis applied in rapid usability engineering (including video and audio data collected from user studies). This has also begun to include automated analysis of qualitative HCI data collected from usability studies and is part of a trend towards conducting larger scale usability studies [14]. Computational ethnography represents an important trend and is discussed in one of the chapters in this book [8]. This approach refers to a family of methods for the automated and unobtrusive collection of HCI data. Remote usability analysis, includes current work in the development of low-cost, portable and virtual approaches to collecting and analyzing usability data [9, 14]. Automating the normally time-consuming analysis of qualitative data from these studies is currently advancing. This trend is moving usability engineering from the usability lab and into real healthcare settings and will be required to determine patterns emerging from usability studies worldwide [31, 33].

Increased Multi-Modal User Interaction

The range of user interaction modes will increase in use in healthcare, including an increase in multi-modal applications, incorporating multiple ways of interacting with systems and technology [34]. This will include advances in areas such as visual computing, spatial computing, haptic interfaces, augmented reality, along with improved natural language understanding and speech capabilities of future healthcare systems and technologies. New and emerging interfaces and greater application of multi-modal applications will necessitate new approaches to designing and evaluating such applications. This will in turn require improved understanding of human capabilities, information needs and how multi-modal applications can be effectively incorporated into human cognitive processing and workflow.

Advances in HCI Study Designs

Advances in HCI study designs and methods will continue as the technology itself being evaluating rapidly evolves. There is a need for empirical approaches to inform system design in healthcare, as well as model-based approaches to analyzing HCI data and making predictions about impact of different design choices. In addition, there is the need for integration of both quantitative approaches on large-scale data with in-depth qualitative data from cognitive studies. Greater understanding will be required of how new technologies affect and impact healthcare processes at multiple levels, from the level of individual user cognition to impact at a broader societal level [32]. Hybrid methods that involve the consideration of the multiple levels of HCI will be required. For example, layered approaches to ensuring the usability and safety of healthcare technologies can involve the systematic application of multiple methods prior to deployment of new systems in live settings. This can involve application of usability inspection and usability testing approaches, to "near-live" testing of systems and technologies prior to implementation [35]. Improved software engineering approaches that integrate a range of user testing methods within agile system development cycles will also be needed. In addition, there is a trend towards development of repositories of usability data (e.g. publicly available results from regulatory testing of healthcare systems such as vendor based electronic health records). New methods will be needed to evaluate these large and growing data banks of usability related data. In addition, evidence-based guidelines and design principles specifically for healthcare applications will also be needed, and work along these lines involving mining of the human factors literature shows promise. These advances represent a trend towards developing evidence-based approaches to HCI in healthcare. Given the large investments involved in healthcare information systems there is a critical need to evaluate evidence related to organizational decisions around design and implementation. This can include consideration of measures of success or failure of information systems in relation to different approaches that can be taken for designing and implementing healthcare information systems. Ultimately this could form a more scientifically sound basis for making future decisions, thereby increasing the likelihood of successful system adoption when implementing systems, while minimizing the potential for lack of user adoption and implementation failure.

Advances in Knowledge Translation

Over the past several decades, a great many academic research studies have been conducted in the area of HCI in healthcare. This has included numerous reports about usability testing results, application of socio-technical design principles and descriptions of new evaluation methods. However, despite these efforts there are continued reports of unusable and potentially unsafe healthcare systems being deployed globally. An area that is needed will be improved translation of research findings and methods to actual improvements in the usability and effectiveness of health information systems. In particular this includes feedback into design and implementation of complex vendor-based systems such as electronic health records and clinical decision support systems. This will require greater sharing and application of research methods and approaches from the academic sector to the vendor and healthcare IT industry [32]. This in turn argues for improved approaches to knowledge translation. Along these lines, approaches that blend both academic and pragmatic objectives in evaluating and studying health information technology have been reported [36]. Such approaches are needed that blur the distinction between academic research and pragmatic application of HCI methods in practice. This can involve including cycles of pragmatic feedback directly in project planning (e.g. feedback around user issues when implementing new health information technology during agile development cycles) while at the same time collecting detailed HCI data that can be later analyzed for academic purposes and future publication [36]. This requires consideration of how to integrate academic objectives (and data collection) within the time and financial constraints of real-world projects and initiatives involving healthcare information technology.

Advances in HCI Education

Increased awareness and understanding of HCI theories, methods and approaches, such as those described in this book, will be needed to ensure the success of healthcare IT initiatives into the future. In considering trends in the area of education around HCI in healthcare, there is a need for training of health informatics students, professionals, researchers and practitioners. This will necessitate education and training for an increasingly wide range of skills and competencies to help adapt to the use of AI and intelligent systems in clinical settings [21]. An awareness of the critical importance of HCI in health informatics is needed as a basis for such advancements [32]. Along these lines, courses focused on HCI in healthcare are beginning to be incorporated in the curricula of undergraduate as well as graduate programs in health and biomedical informatics. This trend will likely continue into the future, with certifications in health informatics beginning to require a basic understanding of HCI and its relevance in healthcare. There is a clear need for training on aspects of HCI related to designing and evaluating systems and technologies to be both usable and useful to end users. In addition to covering topics related to developing technology for supporting communication, collaboration and decision making, additional coverage of topics around data analytics for collecting and analyzing large sets of data from user studies will also be needed. As a foundation for this, understanding of the importance of considering the impact of systems on basic human cognition will also be required. It has been shown that complex information systems that are designed and implemented without an understanding of end users' capabilities and processing are less likely to be adopted by the users they are designed for [37].

Although more human factors specialists are needed, many HCI practitioners in healthcare will continue to have academic backgrounds in health and biomedical informatics, the health sciences and other allied areas, and this trend will likely continue in the foreseeable future. The number of undergraduate and graduate programs in health informatics at leading institutions has increased and many universities and colleges now offer specific courses around topics including usability evaluation, human factors in healthcare and design and implementation of healthcare systems that are user-centered. A growing number of workshops and short training courses are also available in these areas. In addition to academic programs and training, there is a growing awareness that healthcare management (e.g. chief information officers and managers) need to be educated as to the critical importance of topic areas around HCI when procuring, implementing and managing large health related IT projects [32]. This will necessitate continuing education of those responsible for healthcare information technology procurement, design, and implementation. This will be required in order to increase the chance of technology and system adoption while maximizing the benefits from increased automation in healthcare.

Concluding Thoughts

The future success of efforts at improving and streamlining healthcare using technology will depend on the extent to which these systems and technologies fit with and augment healthcare processes and activities. Central to this tenet is the importance of HCI and the development of systems and user interfaces that are usable, effective and safe. To date, many systems have failed to be adopted due to a lack of adequate consideration of the end users of these technologies, including their cognitive processes and the socio-cultural environments of their use. Novel methods and approaches from a variety of domains, which are grounded in theoretical perspectives that can lead to a better understanding of HCI in healthcare, are desperately needed.

The need for understanding HCI from a cognitive perspective will only accelerate as technology becomes more sophisticated and integrated with all aspects of healthcare decision making in the clinical workplace [20]. In addition, the broader adoption and use of technology, by the general population will further spur work in HCI focused around elucidating the cognitive requirements of end users, including their capabilities and preferences. As a basis for this, considerations regarding human expertise, information processing, decision making and collaboration will become increasingly important. Current trends towards intelligent and ubiquitous computing in healthcare will only increase the importance of understanding how to successfully integrate advanced technology into human activities, processes and practice.

References

1. Patel VL, Kannampallil T, Kaufman D. A multi-disciplinary science of human computer interaction in biomedical informatics. In: Kushniruk A, Kaufman D, Kannampallil T, Patel VL, editors. Human computer interaction in healthcare – the role of cognition. 2nd ed. Springer; 2024.
2. Kaufman D, Kannampallil T, Patel V. Cognition and human computer interaction. In: Kushniruk A, Kannampallil T, Kaufman D, Patel VL, editors. Human computer interaction in healthcare – the role of cognition. 2nd ed. Springer; 2024.
3. Morrow D, Lopez KD. Theoretical foundations for health communication research and practice. In: Kushniruk A, Kaufman D, Kannampallil T, Patel VL, editors. Human computer interaction in healthcare – the role of cognition. 2nd ed. Springer; 2024.
4. Sittig D, Singh H. A new socio-technical model for studying health information technology in complex adaptive healthcare systems. In: Cognitive informatics for biomedicine: human computer interaction in healthcare; Springer; 2015.
5. Tang C, Xiao Y, Chen Y, Gorman P. Design for supporting healthcare teams. In: Kushniruk A, Kaufman D, Kannampallil T, Patel VL editors. Human computer interaction in healthcare – the role of cognition. 2nd ed. Springer; 2024.
6. Kalenderian E, Walji M. Applying HCI principles in designing usable systems for dentistry. In: Kushniruk A, Kaufman D, Kannampallil T, Patel VL, editors. Human computer interaction in healthcare – the role of cognition. 2nd ed. Springer; 2024.
7. Franklin A. The unintended consequences of the technology in clinical settings. In: Kushniruk A, Kaufman D, Kannampallil T, Patel VL, editors. Human computer interaction in healthcare – the role of cognition. 2nd ed. Springer; 2024.
8. Zheng K, Hanauer DA, Weibel N, Agha Z. Computational ethnography: automated and unobtrusive means for collecting data in situ for human–computer interaction evaluation studies. In: Kushniruk A, Kaufman D, Kannampallil T, Patel VL, editors. Human computer interaction in healthcare – the role of cognition. 2nd ed. Springer; 2024.
9. Kushniruk A, Monkman H, Borycki E, Kannry J. User-centered design and evaluation of clinical information systems: a usability engineering perspective. In: Kushniruk A, Kaufman D, Kannampallil T, Patel VL, editors. Human computer interaction in healthcare – the role of cognition. 2nd ed. Springer; 2024.
10. Turchioe M, Lai A, Siek K. Designing and deploying mobile health interventions. In: Kushniruk A, Kaufman D, Kannampallil T, Patel VL, editors. Human computer interaction in healthcare – the role of cognition. 2nd ed. Springer; 2024.
11. Jimison H, Pavel M, Parker A, Mainello K. The role of human computer interaction in consumer health applications: current state, challenges and future. In: Kushniruk A, Kaufman D, Kannampallil T, Patel VL, editors. Human computer interaction in healthcare – the role of cognition. 2nd ed. Springer; 2024.
12. Johnson T, Thimbleby H, Killoran P, Diaz-Garelli F. Human computer interaction in medical devices. In: Kushniruk A, Kaufman D, Kannampallil T, Patel VL, editors. Human computer interaction in healthcare – the role of cognition. 2nd ed. Springer; 2024.
13. Kannampallil T, Abraham J. Evaluation of health information technology: methods, frameworks and challenges. In: Kushniruk A, Kaufman D, Kannampallil T, Patel VL, editors. Human computer interaction in healthcare – the role of cognition. 2nd ed. Springer; 2024.
14. Kushniruk A, Borycki E. Analyzing video-based human-computer interaction in healthcare using a cognitive-socio-technical framework. In: Kushniruk A, Kaufman D, Kannampallil T, Patel VL, editors. Human computer interaction in healthcare – the role of cognition. 2nd ed. Springer; 2024.
15. Bhavnani S. Visual analytics: leveraging cognitive principles to accelerate biomedical discoveries. In: Kushniruk A, Kaufman D, Kannampallil T, Patel VL, editors. Human computer interaction in healthcare – the role of cognition. 2nd ed. Springer; 2024.
16. Hutch M, Luo Y. Applications and challenges on human computer interaction and AI interfaces for healthcare. In: Kushniruk A, Kaufman D, Kannampallil T, Patel VL, editors. Human computer interaction in healthcare – the role of cognition. 2nd ed. Springer; 2024.

17. Mamykina L. Human-centered AI to support everyday decisions in health. In: Kushniruk A, Kaufman D, Kannampallil T, Patel VL, editors. Human computer interaction in healthcare – the role of cognition. 2nd ed. Springer; 2024.
18. Shneiderman B. Human-centered AI. Oxford University Press; 2022.
19. Shortliffe EH, Sepùlveda MJ, Patel VL. Framework for the evaluation of clinical AI systems. In: Cohen TA, Patel VL, Shortliffe EH, editors. Intelligent systems in medicine and health: the role of AI. London: Springer; 2022.
20. Patel VL, Cohen TA. Clinical cognition and AI: from emulation to symbiosis. In: Cohen TA, Patel VL, Shortliffe EH, editors. Intelligent systems in medicine and health: the role of AI. London: Springer; 2022.
21. Patel VL, Dev P. Intelligent systems in learning and education. In: Cohen TA, Patel VL, Shortliffe EH, editors. Intelligent systems in medicine and health: the role of AI. London: Springer; 2022.
22. Hollan J, Hutchins E, Kirsh D. Distributed cognition: toward a new foundation for human-computer interaction research. ACM Trans Comput-Hum Interact (TOCHI). 2000;7(2):174–96.
23. Borycki EM, Kushniruk AW. Health technology, quality and safety in a learning health system. Healthc Manage Forum. 2023;36(2):79–85.
24. Kushniruk AW, Triola MM, Borycki EM, Stein B, Kannry JL. Technology induced error and usability: the relationship between usability problems and prescription errors when using a handheld application. Int J Med Inform. 2005;74(7–8):519–26.
25. Kushniruk A, Senathirajah Y, Borycki E. Towards a usability and error "safety net": a multi-phased multi-method approach to ensuring system usability and safety. Stud Health Technol Inform. 2017;245:763–7.
26. Cimino JJ, Patel VL, Kushniruk AW. The patient clinical information system (PatCIS): technical solutions for and experience with giving patients access to their electronic medical records. Int J Med Inform. 2002;68(1–3):113–27.
27. Simonsen J, Robertson T, editors. Routledge international handbook of participatory design. Routledge; 2012.
28. Househ M, Borycki EM, Kushniruk AW, Alofaysan S. mHealth: a passing fad or here to stay? In: Telemedicine and E-health services, policies, and applications: advancements and developments. IGI Global; 2012. p. 151–78.
29. Borycki EM, Kushniruk AW. Reinventing virtual care: bridging the healthcare system and citizen silos to create an integrated future. Healthc Manage Forum. 2022;35(3):135–9.
30. Albert B, Tullis T, Tedesco D. Beyond the usability lab: conducting large-scale online user experience studies. Morgan Kaufmann; 2009.
31. Fritz M, Berger PD. Improving the user experience through practical data analytics: gain meaningful insight and increase your bottom line. Morgan Kaufmann; 2015.
32. Kushniruk AW, Borycki EM. Human factors in healthcare IT: management considerations and trends. Healthc Manage Forum. 2023;36(2):72–8.
33. Fritz M, Berger PD. Improving the user experience through practical data analytics. Morgan Kaufmann; 2015.
34. Kortum P. HCI beyond the GUI: design for haptic, speech, olfactory, and other nontraditional interfaces. Elsevier; 2008.
35. Li AC, Kannry JL, Kushniruk A, et al. Integrating usability testing and think-aloud protocol analysis with "near-live" clinical simulations in evaluating clinical decision support. Int J Med Inform. 2012;81(11):761–72.
36. Mann DM, Chokshi SK, Kushniruk A. Bridging the gap between academic research and pragmatic needs in usability: a hybrid approach to usability evaluation of health care information systems. JMIR Hum Factors. 2018;5(4):e10721. https://doi.org/10.2196/10721.
37. Kujala S. User involvement: a review of the benefits and challenges. Behav Inform Technol. 2003;22(1):1–6.

Further Reading

Albert B, Tullis T, Tedesco D. Beyond the usability lab: conducting large-scale online user experience studies. Morgan Kaufmann; 2009.

Borycki EM, Kushniruk AW. Health technology, quality and safety in a learning health system. Healthc Manage Forum. 2023;36(2):79–85.

Cohen TA, Patel VL, Shortliffe EH, editors. Intelligent systems in medicine and health: the role of AI. London: Springer; 2023.

Fritz M, Berger PD. Improving the user experience through practical data analytics. Morgan Kaufmann; 2015.

Kushniruk A, Borycki E. The human factors of AI in healthcare: recurrent issues, future challenges and ways forward. In: Multiple perspectives on artificial intelligence in healthcare: opportunities and challenges. Cham: Springer; 2021. p. 3–12.

Shneiderman B. Human-centered AI. Oxford University Press; 2022.

Index

A
Agency for Healthcare Research and Quality (AHRQ), 113
Aggregated medical information tools and patient portals, 115
AIDS, 189, 190
AliveCor Kardia device, 306
AlphaFold protein structure database, 80
Ambient documentation technology in healthcare, 135
Ambulances, 327
Ambulatory patient care, 50
Ambulatory schedules, 51
American Reinvestment and Recovery Act (ARRA), 93
American Society for Testing and Materials (ASTM) International standard, 126, 137
Analytic evaluation techniques, 111
Analytical approaches, 95, 97–106
Anticipation, 377
Anti-vaxxer conspiracy theories, 187–189
Apache Cordova, 299
Apple Watch, 12
Apple's iOS, 299
Applied science, 3
Armed Forces Health Longitudinal Technology Application (AHLT) user interface, 104
Arthritis, 402
Artifact analysis, 124
Artificial intelligence (AI), 5, 12, 168, 300, 301, 320, 404, 408, 409
  types, 74
  in healthcare, 12
  health computing, 12
  recommendations or decisions, 12
Association for the Advancement of Medical Instrumentation (AAMI), 322
Asthma-Guidance and Prediction System (A-GPS), 77
Asynchronous communication technologies (closed loop communication), 54
Asynchronous voice communication, 45
Attributable component analysis (ACA), 420
Audit logs, 7, 126
Aviation, 37
AwareMedia, 275
AwarePhone, 275
Axure, 244

B
Back-stage activities, 280, 281
Bandwagon heuristic, 192
Bar code medication administration systems (BCMA), 267
Bayesian statistics, 70
BBraun Infusomat infusion pump, 336
Biclustering, 229, 230
Biological complexity in health care, 37
Biomedical informatics, 4, 103
  challenges related to HIT evaluation, 6–7
  and cognition, 7
  curriculum, 6
  research, 94
  research literature, 100
Black boxes, 72

Bluetooth technology, 296
Burnout, 269

C
Center for Medicare and Medicaid
    Services, 55
Chat app, 275
ChatGPT, 82, 83, 408
ChronoViz, 144, 145
Circos ideograms, 228
Classical cognitive or symbolic information
    processing theory, 4
Clinical care, 20
Clinical decision support (CDS)
    systems, 67, 76
Clinical informatics, 5
Clinical work processes and tasks, 105
Coding dictionary, 164
Cognition, 9, 444–446
Cognitive artifacts, 46
Cognitive burden of sense-making, 24
Cognitive complexity of health care, 49
Cognitive foundations of HCI, 4
Cognitive informatics (CI), 4, 5
Cognitive load, 49, 50
Cognitive models of risk communication, 41
Cognitive operating system, 24
Cognitive processes in communication, 41
Cognitive psychology, theories and empirical
    research, 4
Cognitive Reflection Test (CRT), 199
Cognitive resources, 46
Cognitive system, processing limitations, 19
Cognitive task analysis (CTA), 99, 100, 154
Cognitive theory, 13
    benefits, 11
    and HCI, healthcare, 7
        adaptation, 12
        descriptive, 12
        effectiveness, 12
        explanatory, 12
        generative, 13
        in health and biomedicine, 13
        interactive tasks, 12
        partial space, 13, 14
        predictive, 12
        prescriptive, 13
        usability, 12
        user experience, 12
    health information technology design and
        usage, 11
Cognitive walkthrough (CW), 102

Cognitive-socio-technical model, 160
Collaborative effort and communication
    success, 43
Collaborative filtering methods, 405
Common ground theory, 42
    in health care, 44, 45
Communication among clinicians, 37
Communication challenges, 38
Communication media, 44, 54
    and participant resource constraints, 54
Communication problems during handoffs, 54
Communication technologies, 52
Complex task-dependencies in clinical
    work, 122
Comprehension, 40
Computational ethnography, 7, 123
    coding schema, 137, 138
    cultural and social contexts, 124
    data sources, 137
    definition, 123–125
    distributed cognition perspective, 144
    EHR system, 143
    formal/informal interviews, 124
    in-depth drilldown analysis, 145
    limitations, 124, 139
    multiparty multimodal interactions, 144
    paging/phone logs tracked by
        telecommunication systems, 137
    patient–clinician–computer
        interactions, 147
    personal and professional experiences, 124
    sources, 125, 126, 128
    specific tracking devices, 125
    types, 136
    usability of technological systems, 147
Computational theory of mind, 14
Computer and information technology, 3
Computer logs, 125, 126
Computer supported cooperative work
    (CSCW), 4
Computerized physician order entry (CPOE),
    29, 99, 114, 374
Computerized provider order entry (CPOE)
    systems, 4
Computers on wheels (CoW), 380
Computer-supported cooperative work
    (CSCW), 122, 183
Computing power and memory, 63
Conceptual integration and inference
    processes, 40
Concurrent think aloud, 109
Consolidated Framework for Implementation
    Research (CFIR), 311

CONSORT-AI leveraged Delphi consensus, 84
Consumer health applications
  aging
    age-related declines, 400
    chronic conditions, 401, 402
    cognitive and sensory-motor skills, 401
    communication style, 400
    U.S. population, 400
    video-based communication, 401
  culture
    access issues and digital divide, 399
    communication styles, 398
    health disparities, 398, 399
    user interfaces, 397
    user testing, 397
  health literacy, 402–404
  human computer interaction
    artificial intelligence and machine learning, 408, 409
    distributed computing, 407, 408
    real-time remote usability testing, 404
    remote usability testing, 406, 407
    user designs, 404
    user interfaces, 404, 405
  interface design, 396, 397
  overview of, 394–396
Consumer health information tools, 115
Context dimension, 239
Contextual inquiry methods, 307
Continued influence effect (CIE), 198
Continuity and context-aware model, 107
Conversational agents, 435
Conversational partners, 42
Convolutional neural network (CNN), 75
Copy-paste function, 383, 384
COVID-19 pandemic, 192, 267, 274, 295, 387, 388
  fake news
    anti-vaxxer conspiracy theories, 187–189
    diabetes, 186, 187
    fabricated legitimacy, 186
    misinformation and disinformation, 184
    Pizzagate, 184
  human-computer interaction, 182, 183
  machine learning prediction model, 78
  misinformation, 181, 200–203
  social media, 182, 183
  social media platforms (*see* Social media platforms)
  social, cultural and cognitive factors
    anti-science and anti-vaccination, 196
    anxiety and irrational thinking, 198
    beliefs, 198
    CIE, 198
    CRT, 199
    ethnic minority communities, 196
    information literacy, 196
    IPC, 199
    lockdowns, business shutdowns, and mask mandates, 198
    MMR vaccine, 195
    racial resentment, 197
    safety and effectiveness, 196
    trust, 197
    worldview/mental model, 198
  xenophobia and AIDS, 189, 190
Cross-boundary working, 30
Culture
  access issues and digital divide, 399
  communication styles, 398
  health disparities, 398, 399
  user interfaces, 397
  user testing, 397

D

Data capture methods, 63
Data elements for EHR documentation, 137
Databases and interactive web-based applications, 79–81
Data-driven approach, 418
DCog theories, 32
D-dimer, 75
D-dimer levels, 75
Deep learning algorithm, 75, 76
Deep Motif Dashboard (DeMo), 81
Degree assortativity, 222
Dendrogram, 223
Dental Diagnostic System (DDS), 345, 346
Dentistry
  characteristics, 346, 347
  collaborative teams, 360–362
  DDS, 345, 346
  DxTMs, 365
  EHR, 345
    design challenge, 350–352
    development and refinement, 359
    ethnography, 353, 354
    findings, 354–358
    implementation of mockups, 359, 360
    semi-structured interviews, 354
    think-aloud user testing, 353
    treatment planning module, 351–353, 360
    usability, 350

Dentistry (cont.)
  use and usability, 350
  vendor and broad-based research team, 358
  inter-professional practice, 363–365
  secondary use of data, 362, 363
  standardized dental diagnostic terminology, 348, 349
  utilization and validity, 365
  workflow, 347, 348
Deployment
  data analysis, 426
  diabetes experiences, 427
  feedback and context, 430
  overall impressions and usage, 427, 428
  participants and demographics, 427
  participants and procedure, 426
  perceived results, 431
  in practice, 430, 431
  preferences, 429
  self-discovery, 428, 429
Designer's model, 17
Desirability, 375
Device-specific tasks, 328
Dietary intake monitoring application (DIMA), 307
Digital health coaching, 9
Digital traces, 123
Direct perception solicitation, 123
DISCERN instrument, 200
Discipline-specific terminologies and taxonomies, 52
Disinformation Dozen, 188
Distributed cognition (DCog) approach, 4, 27–29, 122
  individual cognition in context, 42, 43
  systems-level analysis, 47, 48
  theories, 46
Distributed Cognition of Teamwork (DiCoT), 30, 31
Distributed computing, 407, 408
Distributed health information systems, 4
Distributed resources model, 28, 29
Drilldown analysis, 145
DrugExplorer, 80

E
Early intelligent systems for health care, 67
Ecological Momentary Assessment (EMA), 406
E-health, 403
  literacy, 446

organization, 106–107
Electrical Impedance Tomography (EIT), 297
Electronic handoff tools, 54
Electronic health records (EHRs), 12, 21, 83, 93, 241, 242, 345
  benefits of, 271
  design approach
    development and refinement, 359
    ethnography, 353, 354
    findings, 354–358
    implementation of mockups, 359, 360
    semi-structured interviews, 354
    think-aloud user testing, 353
    treatment planning module, 351–353, 360
    vendor and broad-based research team, 358
  design challenge, 350–352
  documentation system, 113
  documentation tool, 271
  formal and informal work, 272, 273
  implementation, 63
  navigation behavior, 140–142
  relational coordination and social interaction, 272
  sequential patterns, 140, 142
  support collaboration, 272
  transition probabilities, 140
  usability, 350
  visible and invisible work, 273, 274
Electronic white boards, 46
Emergency Room (ER) using observational techniques, 95
Evaluation approaches
  brief categorization, 95
  classification, 96
Evidence-based medicine (EBM), 201
Expert inspection, 122
Expert system interpretation, 421
ExplodeLayout, 229, 230
Exploratory learning approach, 102
External cognition, 21–26
  framework, 26
Eye tracking, 130, 132, 133
EZCodes, 349

F
Facebook, 202
Face-to-face communication, 44, 270
Face-to-face handoffs, 54
Fact-checking pipelines, 202
Fake news

anti-vaxxer conspiracy theories, 187–189
  diabetes, 186, 187
  fabricated legitimacy, 186
  misinformation and disinformation, 184
  Pizzagate, 184
Fast Health Interoperability Resource (FHIR), 364
Federal Food, Drug, and Cosmetic Act (FFDCA), 322
Field studies, 122
Field/observational approaches, 111
Fitbit, 12
Fitts law, 14, 105
Focus groups, 108, 109
Formal usability testing, 106
Formative evaluation, 95
Friedman, Charles, 70
Front-stage-back-stage model, 280, 281
Fuzzy trace memory theory, 41

G

Gab, 192
General analytic evaluation approaches and usability testing, 95
General usability testing approaches, 106–110
Genomic and proteomic sequencing of biologic samples, 63
GlucoGoalie, 416
  controlled evaluation, 423–425
  deployment study
    data analysis, 426
    diabetes experiences, 427
    feedback and context, 430
    overall impressions and usage, 427, 428
    participants and demographics, 427
    participants and procedure, 426
    perceived results, 431
    in practice, 430, 431
    preferences, 429
    self-discovery, 428, 429
  expert system interpretation and guardrails, 421
  goal setting, 419, 420
  goals, 421, 422
  machine learning, 420, 421
  overview, 418, 419
Goals, Operators, Methods and Selection Rules (GOMS) analytical framework, 16, 103–105
Google's Android, 299
Graph-based methods, 222
Graphical user interfaces (GUIs), 18, 73

Group walkthroughs, 102
Grudin, Jonathan, 65
Guardrails, 421
Gulf of evaluation, 17

H

Health and treatment of illness, 50
Health care
  cognitive demands, biological complexity, 49, 50
  communication and communication technologies, 55
  domain, 37
Health communication, 38–48
Health disparities, 398, 399
Health information and communication technologies, 38
Health information dissemination, 77
Health information technology (HIT), 3, 25
  adoption and use, 93
  analytical evaluation studies, 114
  characterization of interactivity activities, 4
  clinical environments, 8, 94
  comprehensive evaluation studies, 94
  conducting evaluation studies, 114, 115
  coordination of care, 4
  design and development phases, 93
  evaluation methods, 94
  evaluation studies, 93
  generic usability and situated testing of systems, 94
  implementations on clinical workflow, 114
  in-situ and field-based, 94
  patient safety, 4
  preliminary considerations for evaluations, 114
  quality and safety, 93
  socio-technical system, 94
  systematic evaluation, 93
  tasks and decision-making, 114
  theoretical and methodological scaffold, 114
  theories and methods, 4
  unintended and unanticipated consequences, 93
Health literacy, 402–404
Health professionals, 266
Health technology, 13
Healthcare professionals, 267, 325
Healthcare providers, 269

Healthcare teams
  burnout, 269
  characteristics of, 264–267
  code team, 263
  continuous coverage, 268
  diversity of, 264, 265
  information media, 268
  locations, 267, 268
  loosely formed team
      collaboration, 277–279
  medical records, 268
  PICU, 279–281
  sociotechnical aspects
    COVID-19 pandemic, 274
    dynamic communication behaviors, 270, 271
    EHR, 271–274
  supporting coordination, 275, 276
  supporting distributed communication, 275
  supporting information access, 276, 277
  team effectiveness, 268
Health-focused apps, 298
HealthVault, 300
Heathfield, Heather, 69
Heuristic evaluations (HE), 100–102
  and walkthroughs, 100
Hick-Hyman law, 105
Hierarchical task analysis (HTA), 97–99, 353
HIMSS survey, 3
Home care environment, 328
Human augmented system, 75
Human cognitive operating system, 24
Human-computer interaction (HCI), 14, 247, 249, 250, 254
  and allied disciplines, 3
  analysis of usability testing data, 450
  artificial intelligence, 444
  and artificial intelligence (AI) interfaces, for health care (*see* Human computer interaction and artificial intelligence (HCI-AI))
  automated collection, 450
  for biomedical informatics (BMI) students, 6
  in biomedicine and healthcare, 5
  cognition, 444–446
  cognitive approaches, 7
  cognitive science, 4
  cognitive theories, 4
  consumer health
    applications, 6
      artificial intelligence and machine learning, 408, 409
      distributed computing, 407, 408
      real-time remote usability testing, 404
      remote usability testing, 406, 407
      user designs, 404
      user interfaces, 404, 405
  COVID-19 pandemic, 182, 183
  cultural backgrounds, 8
  dentistry (*see* Dentistry)
  design and evaluation, 3
  developments in technology and software, 4
  devices, 3, 330
  education, 452, 453
  environments, 327, 328
  evaluation methods, 7
  evaluation studies in healthcare, 121–122
  expert inspection, 122
  external representation, 7
  field of, 320, 321
  field studies, 122
  and global health informatics, 5
  in health care, 9, 11
  healthcare applications, 447, 448
  health-related content, 6
  human factors, 332–335
  human information processing, 7
  human reasoning and decision making, 447
  human-centered AI, 6
  knowledge translation, 451, 452
  laboratory style usability testing, 7
  low-cost rapid usability engineering methods, 7
  medical device, 321, 322
  medical device interface design and evaluation, 331, 332
  medical device users, 325, 326
  models and frameworks for evaluation, 5
  multi-modal user interaction, 450
  patient safety, 324, 325
    and clinical workflow, 5
    and HCI design considerations, 8
  patient-centered design, 448, 449
  perception solicitation through questionnaire surveys, interviews, or focus groups, 122
  productive use and acceptance of technology, 5
  regulatory history and human factors engineering requirements, 322–324
  requirements, 319
  safety informatics, 448
  SaMD, 320

socio-technical and distributed cognition
      perspectives, 443
  socio-technical approach, 4, 5
  study designs, 451
  tasks, 328–330
  theoretical and methodological basis, 6
  theories, 13
  transformation and development, 4
  usability data quantification and analytics,
      449, 450
  usability experiments, 122
  user interface, 336–338
  variability, 326
  video analysis, 158, 159
  virtual and home healthcare, 449
  visualization for data analysis and
      interpretation, 8
Human computer interaction and artificial
      intelligence (HCI-AI)
  activity trackers, 70
  AI explainability, 72
  applications, 63
  biological data, 79
  biomedical research, 64
  CDS sepsis prediction system, 83
  in clinical health care setting, 74
  classifications, 75
  clinical deterioration, 67
  clinical factors and trajectories, 78
  clinical health care setting, 69, 74
  clinical interventions and
      therapeutics, 76, 77
  clinical utility, 86
  continuous evaluation and
      monitoring, 86
  data collection, 77
  data collection and preparation, 86
  databases and interactive web-based
      applications, 79
  design and implementation, 70
  development and implementation, 81
  design approach for modeling the
      interactions, 66
  for diabetic glycemic control, 82
  diagnostic support, 74
  educational system, 66
  ethical and moral human values, 84
  health care providers, 82
  historical review, 64
  human decision making, 65, 66
  human input and cognition, 66
  human psychology and behavior, 66
  integration, 69
  intelligent clinical decision support
      systems, 64
  interactive web-based databases, 79
  interactive websites, 78
  linear-based models, 72
  literacy over proficiency, 82
  machine learning studies, 84
  mathematical functions, 70
  model explainability, 74
  model predictions, 78
  molecular pathways and genetic factors, 72
  neural network derived probabilities, 74
  passive smartwatch and mobile phone data
      collection, 79
  policies, guidelines, and regulations, 85
  predictive and prescriptive analytics, 82
  pre-specified probability, 68
  rule-based HCI system, 75
  scientific reproducibility, 84
  sepsis prediction, 82
  smartphones, 70
  surveillance efforts, 77
  system usability, 68
  system's data collection capabilities, 79
  technical considerations, 81
  timely policies and guidelines, 81
  training process, 71
  treatment strategies, 64
  usability and clinical utility, 68
  web application's development and
      implementation, 78
Human error, 323
Human factors (HF), 320, 322–324, 332–335
  and HCI, 5
  unintended consequences, 385, 386
Human factors engineering (HFE), 320
Human immunodeficiency virus (HIV), 189
Human information processor, 14, 249
Human intelligence, 66
Hybrid methods, 451
Hypertext Markup Language (HTML), 402

I

Identity Protective Cognition (IPC), 199
Inadequate communication between health
      care team members, 51
In-depth linguistic analysis of the
      verbalizations, 109
Individual differences in cognitive resources, 40
Individual interviews, 107
Infection control, 329
Informal social interactions, 272

Information analytics, 215–217
Information consumers, 214, 215
Information density, 281
Information processing approach, 15, 40, 45
Information retrieval, 12
Information systems and computer-mediated communication technologies, 124
Infusomat, 336
Inpatient environment, 327
Input-output model, 15, 379
Inspection-based evaluation, 100
Inspection-based/model-based approaches, 95
Instant data analysis (IDA), 256
Institute of Medicine (IOM) report, 93
Intelligent user interfaces (IUI), 4
Interactive approaches, 43
Interactive Sociotechnical Analysis (ISTA), 377–378
Interactive Team Cognition theory, 48
Interactive theories, 41, 45, 49
Interdisciplinary communication problems, 38
Interface design, 396, 397
Internet connectivity, 298
Internet-connected applications, 298
INTERNIST, 68
Interpersonal relationships, 272
Inter-professional practice, 363–365
Interviews, 106, 107
IV medication errors, 24

K
Kardex, 273
Keystroke level model (KLM), 16, 104
Kinect, 134, 135
Kinect Software Development Kit (SDK), 134
Knowledge translation, 451, 452

L
Laboratory-based evaluations, 114
Large-scale usability studies, 254–256
Large language model (LLM), 73, 82, 435
Limited English proficiency (LEP), 144
Linear-based models, 72
Log file, 168
Long-term observational studies, 114
Loosely formed team collaboration, 277–279
Loss-of-activation error, 139
Low-cost rapid usability testing
  in health informatics, 240, 241
  in practice, 243, 244
  rapid prototyping, 244–246
Lower-middle-income countries (LMIC), 293

M
Machine learning (ML), 9, 76, 408, 409, 416
Machine learning derived COVID-19 Pandemic Vulnerability Index, 78
Macroergonomic models, 385
Markov chain analysis, 140, 143
Massive expansions in technology, 63
Meaningful Use program, 300
Measles, mumps, and rubella (MMR) vaccine, 195
Media, communication within health care organizations, 38
Media-related constraints on communication, 45
Medical Emergency Decisions Assistance System (MEDAS), 69
MedWISE, 25
Mental model theory, 41
Mental models, 19–21
Mental representations in memory, 14
Mental simulation process, 20
Message comprehension and grounding, 46
Microcomputers, 16
Microsoft Kinect™, 135
Mobile and ubiquitous computing (UbiComp), 4
Mobile Application Rating Scale (MARS), 298
Mobile applications, 297–299
Mobile health (mHealth) interventions
  artificial intelligence, 300, 301
  definition, 291
  design, 306–308
  evolution of, 292, 293
  implementation, 309–311
  mobile applications, 297–299
  patient- and wellness-centric model, 291
  PHRs, 300
  smartphone, 293, 294
  tablets, 294, 295
  text messaging, 302, 303
  wearable systems, 295–297
Mobile technology, 330
Model-based evaluation approaches, 103
Model human processor (MHP), 15, 16
Modern eye-tracking technologies, 130
Morae, 130
Motion capture, 7, 132, 134
Multi-faceted data collection methods, 107
Multi-faceted model, 379
Multi-modal user interaction, 450

Multiple sclerosis (MS), 394, 395
Multiple usability experts, 102
MyChart, 300

N
Narrative interviewing, 107
NASA-TLX scales, 110
National Institute of Standards and Technology's (NIST) EHR usability evaluation protocol, 130
National Research Network for EHR Audit Log Data, 126–128
Nature of Science (NOS), 201
Needs assessment techniques, 396, 397
Network analysis
 edges, 217
 exploratory visual analysis, 218–222
 limitations, 228
 quantitative verification, 222–224
 strengths, 227
 sub-phenotypes and biological mechanisms, 225, 226
 theoretical, practical, and pedagogical hurdles, 228, 229
NightScout Project, 297
Non-observable perceptional measures, 122
Non-professional users, 326
Norman's theory of action, 15–18, 31

O
Office of the National Coordinator for Health Information Technology (ONC), 126
Off-the-shelf wearable sensing system, 296
Off-the-shelf wellness monitoring systems, 295
Online Health Information (OHI), 191
Open-ended questionnaires, 110
Open source tools, 81
Operators, 104
Organizational shell, 265
Outpatient clinics, 328

P
Paper-based records, 23
Parking lot compliance, 309
Participatory design, 361
Patient-assembled teams, 51
Patient care errors, 54
Patient care in acute settings, 54

Patient-centered care, 394
Patient-centered design, 448, 449
Patient-provider communication, 38
PatientsLikeMe, 214, 408
Pediatric intensive care unit (PICU), 279–281, 381
Perception solicitation methods, 122
Personal health coaching programs, 9
Personal health data, 306
Personal health records (PHRs), 300
Personal informatics, 415, 417, 418
Pervasive computing in healthcare, 5
Pluralistic walkthroughs, 102
Post-processing tasks, 134
Predictive modeling approaches, 103
Pre-hospital emergency settings, 327
Proactive artificial intelligence, 86
Professional/disciplinary teams, 266
Proof-of-concept testing, 311
Propagation of representational states, 29, 30
Psychiatric clinical narratives, 111

Q
Quantified self, 408

R
Radio-frequency identification (RFID) technology, 7, 136
Rapid diffusion of health information technologies, 52–54
Rapid Iterative Test and Evaluation (RITE) method, 256
Rapid prototyping, 244–246
Rapid Usability Evaluation (RUE) method, 256
Reach Effectiveness Adoption Implementation Maintenance (RE-AIM), 311
Real-Time Locating Systems (RTLS), 136
Recommender systems (RecSys), 416, 418
RecSys, 434
REDCap, 303
Remote usability analysis, 450
Remote usability evaluation studies, 114
Remote usability testing, 254–256, 406, 407
Representational effect, 22–24
ResearchKit, 299
Respiratory syncytial virus (RSV), 219
Retrospective think aloud, 109
Routine use of standardized diagnostic terminologies (DxTMs), 365
Rule-based systems, 70, 72, 78

S

Safety net, 448
Safety-critical devices, 327
Safety-critical settings, 331
Sample screen activity log, 131
Sample security audit log, 126–128
Scenario-based design, 114
Screen activities, 128–130
Security audit log, 126, 128
Selection rules, 104
Self-discovery process, 428, 429
Semantic Platform for Adverse Childhood Experiences Surveillance (SPACES) system, 78
Semi-structured interviews, 107, 354
SensoMotoric Instruments (SMI), 132
Sensor-based technologies, 134
Sequential pattern analysis, 138, 139
Shadowing and time and motion studies, 113
Shadowing techniques, 112
SHAP values, 76
Share responsibility, 266
Shared knowledge for communication, 46
Shared mental models (SMM), 20, 21, 50, 51
Shared situation model, 45
Sharing responsibility, 266
Simple rule-based systems, 75
Situation models, 40
Smartphone, 293, 294
Social and behavioral sciences, 3
Social and/or distributed nature of computing, 12
Social computing, 122
Social desirability bias, 123
Social media platforms, 187
    attention-driven design, 192
    bandwagon heuristic, 192
    computational capture and analytic methods, 192
    CSCW, 183
    democratization, 182, 183
    disinformation, 194, 195
    dissemination, 182
    fake news, 193
    Gab, 192
    live streaming services, 191
    misinformation, 182, 193, 194
    monthly users and modes of engagement, 191
    personalization algorithms, 193
    research, 183
    YouTube, 192
Social-organizational processes, 47
Social-psychological problems, 41

Sociotechnical system models, 382
Software as a Medical Device (SaMD), 320, 321
Software programming, 12
Software psychology, 3
Spatial transcriptomics, 79
Specialized teams in hospitals, 51
Speech Analysis, interpreter-mediated communication session, 145, 146
Speech production and comprehension on cognitive resources, 46
Speech recognition, 402
St. Jude Cloud Ecosystem, 80
Stimulus-response paradigm, 14
Structured interviews, 107
Summative evaluation, 95, 122
Surveys and questionnaires, 110, 111
Swarm's GUI, 75
Synchronous remote communication, 46
System development life cycle (SDLC), 239
Systematized Nomenclature for Dentistry (SNODENT), 348
System-based interactive communication theories, 48
System-based theories of communication interaction, 50
Systems Engineering Initiative for Patient Safety (SEIPS) model, 47, 386
Systems-based theories, 48

T

Table-mounted eye tracker in an outpatient exam room, 132
Tablets, 294, 295
Task analysis, 97–100
Task dimension, 239
Tasks and task transition probabilities, 142
Task, User, Representation, Function (TURF)), 114, 130
Team composition, 266, 267
Team effectiveness, 268
Team game, 12
Team performance
    COVID-19 pandemic, 274
    dynamic communication behaviors, 270, 271
    EHR
        benefits of, 271
        documentation tool, 271
        formal and informal work, 272, 273
        relational coordination and social interaction, 272
        support collaboration, 272

visible and invisible work, 273, 274
TeamSTEPPS, 51
Technology-based tools, 46
　use of, 47
Technology-centered thinking, 446
Technology-induced error, 448
Telecommunication systems, 123
Teleconferencing, 46
Telemedicine, 327, 387
Televaluation, 254
Temporal data mining, 138
Text editing, 12
Text messaging, 302, 303
Texting, 45
Text-to-speech technology, 402
Theories of external cognition, 24, 31
Theory-based technology design, 55
Theory of bimanual control, 14
Theory of intelligent spaces, 24–26
Think aloud evaluations, 109
Think aloud data, 155
Think aloud methods, 109, 310
Three-dimensional model, 238
Three rule-based system, 75
Time and motion studies, 112, 113
Time-consuming analysis, 450
Time-motion data in clinical workflow studies, 113
Tobii Technology, 132
Transition analyses, 138
Transition probabilities, 139
Trust, 197
Type 2 diabetes (T2D), 186, 307
　balancing reflection and action, 433
　diabetes self-management, 417
　eating experiences and personal aspirations, 434
　GlucoGoalie, 416
　　controlled evaluation, 423–425
　　deployment study, 426–431
　　expert system interpretation and guardrails, 421
　　goal setting, 419, 420
　　goals, 421, 422
　　machine learning, 420, 421
　　overview, 418, 419
　interactivity, negotiation, and feedback, 435
　limitations, 435, 436
　machine learning, 416
　personal informatics, 415, 417, 418
　personalization, 417
　recommender systems, 416
　RecSys, 418
　self-management, 415

U
Ubiquitous computing (UbiComp), 4
Unintended consequences (UCs)
　adherence, 382
　copy-paste function, 383, 384
　corrective actions, 386
　Covid pandemic, 374, 387, 388
　CoW, 380
　definition, 375–380
　distributed system community, 385
　doctor-patient interaction, 374
　documentation, 373, 386
　drug-drug or drug-allergy problems, 381
　emergency medicine, 381
　formative testing, 387
　healthcare quality and safety, 374
　human factors, 385, 386
　paper persistence, 384
　PICU, 381
　professional organizations, 387
　rapid adoption, 384
　SAFER guidelines, 387
　sensitivity, 381
　social and organizational structures, 386
　sociotechnical system models, 382
　summative testing, 387
　technology-induced errors, 380
　unbounded delays, 384, 385
　workarounds, 382, 383
Unsupervised learning method, 222
Usability data quantification, 449, 450
Usability engineering
　approaches, 236
　challenge, 235
　definition, 236
　development process, 236
　health information systems, 249, 250
　information needs and user cognitive requirements, 237–240
　low-cost rapid usability testing
　　in health informatics, 240, 241
　　in practice, 243, 244
　　rapid prototyping, 244–246
　multi-level usability analysis, 251, 252
　reasoning and decision making, 241, 242
　remote and large-scale usability studies, 254–256
　system design and evaluation
　　cost-effective approach, 248
　　development, 246
　　in-situ testing, 246, 248
　　limitations, 249
　　medication administration system, 247
　　post-task audio-recorded semi-structured interview, 248

Usability engineering (*cont.*)
    UCD, 248
        user-task-context approach, 247
        video analysis, 247, 248
    UCD, 236
    user-centered design, 252, 253
Usability experiments, randomized controlled design, 122
Usability inspection methods, 236, 245
Usability studies and market research, 130
Usability testing, 95, 106
    into field-based studies, 95
    methods, 95
Usefulness codes, 163–164, 169
User centered design (UCD), 235–238, 321
User dimension, 239
User experience (UE), 236, 321
User interface (UI), 122, 141, 336–338
User's mental model, 19
User's model, 18
User-centered design (UCD), 114, 252, 253, 361
    and evaluation of clinical Information systems, 8
    principles, 12
Users' mental models of system behavior, 17
User-Task-Context approach, 247

V

Verbal think aloud, 109, 110
Video analysis, 247
    annotation, 172
    audio portion, 152
    automated coding research, 173
    clinical guidelines, 174
    clinical workflow, 151
    coding system, 153
    cost effectiveness, 174
    human-computer interaction codes, 161–162, 164, 166
    identification, 153
    inductive approaches, 153
    reconciliation software, 174
    socio-technical level codes, 165–166, 169
    summarization, 172, 173
    system safety, 166, 170, 171
    think-aloud studies, 174
    transcription and log file creation, 172
    usability data analysis
        coding dictionary, 164
        coding schemes, 158, 160
        cognitive-socio-technical model, 160
        conceptual framework, 158
        human-computer interaction, 158, 159
        measuring time, 157
        mixed-method approach, 157
        phases, 158
        pragmatic, 156
        social, policy/organizational aspects, 160
        user experience, 157
        user interaction, 159, 160
        user interactions, 157
        visual evidence and feedback, 156
    usability data collection, 154–156
    usability testing, 152
    user interactions, 152
    video analysis tools, 173
    video coding, 167, 168
    workflow codes, 163–164, 168, 169
Virtual-reality technology, 14
Virtual Usability Laboratory (VuLab), 255
Visible and invisible work, 273, 274
Visual analytics
    classification, 212, 213
    definition, 210
    development, 209
    disciplines, 212
    goals, 214
    information analytics, 215–217
    information consumers, 214, 215
    interactivity, 211, 212
    mental model, 213
    network analysis
        biclustering, 229, 230
        edges, 217
        exploratory visual analysis, 218–222
        limitations, 228
        quantitative verification, 222–224
        strengths, 227
        sub-phenotypes and biological mechanisms, 225, 226
        theoretical, practical, and pedagogical hurdles, 228, 229
    parallel processing, 210
    road map pointing, 211
    systolic blood pressure, 210, 213
    working memory, 213
Voice Dialog Extensible Markup Language (VoiceXML), 402
Voice loops, 270
Voice recordings and clinical conversation transcripts, 135, 136

W

Walkthroughs, inspection-based approach, 102, 103
Wearable systems, 295–297
Wearable technologies, 449
Web-based social support tools, 115
WeChat, 191
WhatsApp, 191, 275
Workflow codes, 163–164, 168, 169
Working memory (WM), 15, 16
World Health Organization (WHO) COVID-19 guidelines, 78

X

Xenophobia, 189–191

Y

YouTube, 192

Z

Zoom®, 155

SPRINGER NATURE

GPSR Compliance

The European Union's (EU) General Product Safety Regulation (GPSR) is a set of rules that requires consumer products to be safe and our obligations to ensure this.

If you have any concerns about our products, you can contact us on ProductSafety@springernature.com

In case Publisher is established outside the EU, the EU authorized representative is:

Springer Nature Customer Service Center GmbH
Europaplatz 3
69115 Heidelberg, Germany